Major Incidents, Pandemics and Mental Health

Professor Richard Williams is Emeritus Professor of Mental Health Strategy at the University of South Wales. He was previously Presidential Lead on Disaster Management for the Royal College of Psychiatrists, Presidential Lead on COVID-19, Emergency Preparedness, and Mental Health, and Director of the Psychosocial and Mental Health Programme of the Faculty of Pre-Hospital Care of the Royal College of Surgeons of Edinburgh.

Ms Verity Kemp is an independent consultant specialising in emergency preparedness, resilience, and response, with prior senior management experience in the NHS and healthcare management working at all levels from hospital to central government.

Professor Sir Keith Porter is a former Consultant Trauma Surgeon and major trauma clinical lead for Queen Elizabeth Hospital Birmingham and the West Midlands Trauma Network. He was also civilian clinical lead for the interface between Queen Elizabeth Hospital Birmingham and the Royal Centre for Defence Medicine, Chairman of Trauma Care and co-founder of citizenAID, and Honorary Colonel of 202 Field Hospital.

Dr Tim Healing trained in clinical microbiology at the Royal London Hospital. He was on the staff of the Communicable Disease Surveillance Centre before working for 30 years in humanitarian aid with NGOs and the UN. He also ran the Conflict and Catastrophe Medicine Course at the Worshipful Society of Apothecaries of London.

Professor John Drury is a social psychologist and a Director of Research and Knowledge Exchange at the University of Sussex. His research on collective resilience informs the Civil Contingencies Secretariat's National Risk Assessments. During the COVID-19 pandemic he participated in the UK government's SAGE behavioural science subgroup SPI-B.

Major Incidents, Pandemics and Mental Health

The Psychosocial Aspects of Health Emergencies, Incidents, Disasters and Disease Outbreaks

Edited by

Richard Williams
University of South Wales

Verity Kemp
Independent Health Emergency Planning Consultant

Keith Porter
University of Birmingham

Tim Healing
Worshipful Society of Apothecaries of London

John Drury
University of Sussex

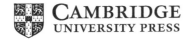
CAMBRIDGE
UNIVERSITY PRESS

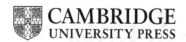

Shaftesbury Road, Cambridge CB2 8EA, United Kingdom

One Liberty Plaza, 20th Floor, New York, NY 10006, USA

477 Williamstown Road, Port Melbourne, VIC 3207, Australia

314–321, 3rd Floor, Plot 3, Splendor Forum, Jasola District Centre, New Delhi – 110025, India

103 Penang Road, #05-06/07, Visioncrest Commercial, Singapore 238467

Cambridge University Press is part of Cambridge University Press & Assessment, a department of the University of Cambridge.

We share the University's mission to contribute to society through the pursuit of education, learning and research at the highest international levels of excellence.

www.cambridge.org
Information on this title: www.cambridge.org/9781009011211

DOI: 10.1017/9781009019330

First published 2024

A catalogue record for this publication is available from the British Library.

A Cataloging-in-Publication data record for this book is available from the Library of Congress.

ISBN 978-1-009-01121-1 Paperback

Cambridge University Press & Assessment has no responsibility for the persistence or accuracy of URLs for external or third-party internet websites referred to in this publication and does not guarantee that any content on such websites is, or will remain, accurate or appropriate.

....

Every effort has been made in preparing this book to provide accurate and up-to-date information that is in accord with accepted standards and practice at the time of publication. Although case histories are drawn from actual cases, every effort has been made to disguise the identities of the individuals involved. Nevertheless, the authors, editors, and publishers can make no warranties that the information contained herein is totally free from error, not least because clinical standards are constantly changing through research and regulation. The authors, editors, and publishers therefore disclaim all liability for direct or consequential damages resulting from the use of material contained in this book. Readers are strongly advised to pay careful attention to information provided by the manufacturer of any drugs or equipment that they plan to use.

This book is dedicated to the memory of the late David Alan Alexander, DSc, PhD, MA(Hons), CPsychol, FRCPsych(Hon) FBPS, Honorary Fellow of the Royal Society of Medicine (1943–2020).

David was Emeritus Professor of Mental Health at Robert Gordon University in Aberdeen. He was Director of the Aberdeen Centre for Trauma Research, and he held a personal professorial chair at Aberdeen University.

David was elected an Honorary Fellow of the Royal College of Psychiatrists in 2002. He received the Scottish Governments' Humanitarian Medal in 2005 and the Aberdeen MedChi President's Medal in 2016. In 2017, the University of Abertay made him an Honorary Doctor of Science.

David's untimely death was not only a shock to the many people who knew him, but also a huge loss to the world of disaster mental healthcare. His pioneering wisdom and experience reached out to touch all of us. David was hugely respected as a person, a scientist, and a clinician, but especially as an inspirational, kind, and hugely supportive colleague. He was a pioneer in the field of distress and traumatic stress occasioned by major incidents, war, policing, and healthcare, and his innovative work received widespread plaudits. We hope he would think that his work continues in the pages of this book.

Contents

Section 1. The Nature and Impacts of Twenty-First-Century Healthcare Emergencies

Contents

Figures

Tables

Boxes

Contributors

Professor, the Lord Alderdice
Executive Chairman, The Changing Character of War Centre, Pembroke College, Oxford; Senior Research Fellow, Harris Manchester College, Oxford; Professor of Practice, Global Humanity for Peace Institute, University of Wales Trinity St David; Liberal Democrat Member of the House of Lords, UK

Dr Khalifah Alfadhli
Psychology Department, King Saud University, Saudi Arabia

Professor David E Alexander
Institute for Risk and Disaster Reduction, University College London, UK

Dr Kate Allsopp
Research Fellow, Complex Trauma and Resilience Research Unit, Manchester Academic Health Science Centre, Greater Manchester Mental Health NHS Foundation Trust, and Division of Psychology and Mental Health, School of Health Sciences, University of Manchester, UK

Dr Nick Ambler
Consultant Clinical Psychologist, Intensive Care Unit, Southmead Hospital, North Bristol NHS Trust, UK

Professor Richard Amlôt
Behavioural Science and Insights Unit, UK Health Security Agency, UK

Dr Golnar Aref-Adib
Consultant Psychiatrist in General Adult Psychiatry, Camden and Islington NHS Foundation Trust, London, UK

Dr Dominic Aubrey-Jones
General Adult Psychiatry, South Westminster Community Mental Health Hub, Central and North West London NHS Foundation Trust, UK

Professor Alan Barrett
Greater Manchester Resilience Hub, Pennine Care NHS Foundation Trust and School of Health and Society, University of Salford, UK

Dr Claire Bayntun
Independent Consultant in Global Public Health, UK

Mr Emir Battaloglu
Consultant in Trauma and Orthopaedic Surgery, Queen Elizabeth Hospital Birmingham, University Hospitals Birmingham NHS Foundation Trust, UK

Professor Jonathan I Bisson
Clinical Professor in Psychiatry, Division of Psychological Medicine and Clinical Neurosciences, Cardiff University School of Medicine, UK

Professor Chris R Brewin
Emeritus Professor of Clinical Psychology, Research Department of Clinical, Educational and Health Psychology, University College London, UK

Dr Samantha K Brooks
Senior Research Associate, Department of Psychological Medicine, Institute of Psychiatry, Psychology and Neuroscience, King's College London, UK

Dr Jennifer Burgess
Research Fellow and General Adult Psychiatry Specialist Registrar, Translational and Clinical Research Institute, Faculty of Medical Sciences, Newcastle University, and Cumbria, Northumberland, Tyne and Wear NHS Foundation Trust, UK

Dr Penelope Campling
Medical psychotherapist now working independently, and retired psychiatrist and former Clinical Director at Leicester Partnership NHS Trust, UK

Dr Holly Carter
Behavioural Science and Insights Unit, UK Health Security Agency, UK

Professor Prathiba Chitsabesan
Pennine Care NHS Foundation Trust and Visiting Professor, University College London and Manchester Metropolitan University, UK

Dr Chris Cocking
Principal Lecturer in Psychology, School of Humanities and Social Sciences, University of Brighton, UK

Dr Anna Conolly
Research Fellow, School of Health Sciences, University of Surrey, UK

Mr Lewis Doyle
Doctoral Researcher, University of Sussex, UK

Professor John Drury
Professor of Social Psychology, School of Psychology, University of Sussex, UK

Dr Michael Duffy
Consultant Cognitive Psychotherapist & Senior Lecturer, School of Social Sciences, Education and Social Work, Queen's University, Belfast, UK

Mr Neil Dufty
Principal Consultant for Water Technology Pty Ltd, Australia

Dr Matthew J Easterbrook
Reader in Social Psychology, University of Sussex, UK

Professor Daisy Fancourt
Associate Professor of Psychobiology and Epidemiology, University College London, UK

Dr Maria Fernandes-Jesus
Lecturer in Psychology, School of Psychology, University of Sussex, UK

Professor Paul French
Clinical Researcher, Research and Innovation Department, Pennine Care NHS Foundation Trust, Manchester, UK

Group Captain Andrew D Green CBE KHP
Defence Consultant Adviser in Communicable Diseases, Royal Centre for Defence Medicine, UK

Professor Neil Greenberg
Professor of Defence Mental Health, King's College London, UK

Dr Talya Greene
Associate Professor, Research Department of Clinical, Educational and Health Psychology, University College London, UK

Dr Vladislav H Grozev
Post-Doctoral Research Associate, Sheffield University Management School, UK

Dr Tim Healing
Worshipful Society of Apothecaries of London, UK

Professor Rowena Hill
Department of Psychology, Nottingham Trent University, UK

Professor Stevan E Hobfoll
STAR: Stress, Anxiety, and Resilience Consultants, Sandy, Utah, USA

Ms Christine Howard
Trauma Impact Prevention and Wellbeing Trainer Derbyshire Constabulary, UK

Dr Sharon Irvine
Consultant in Medicine and Infection, Dumfries and Galloway Royal Infirmary, NHS Dumfries and Galloway, UK

Dr Brian Jacobs
Consultant Emeritus, South London and Maudsley NHS Foundation Trust, UK

Dr Adrian James
President of the Royal College of Psychiatrists, UK

Dr Trevor K James
Assistant Professor (Social Psychology), Psychology Department, Durham University, UK

Professor Krzysztof Kaniasty
Professor of Social Psychology, Department of Psychology, Indiana University of Pennsylvania, USA, and Institute of Psychology, Polish Academy of Sciences, Warsaw, Poland

Dr Raphael Kelvin

National Clinical Lead MindEd Programme, NHS England, Technology Enhanced Learning; Workforce, Education and Training Directorate. Consultant Child and Adolescent Psychiatrist, UK

Ms Verity Kemp

Independent Health Emergency Planning Consultant, UK

Mr Thomas König

Consultant General, Vascular and Trauma Surgeon, Royal London Hospital Trauma Service, Barts Health NHS Trust and Defence Medical Services, UK

Dr Alison Lacey

Research Fellow, University of Sussex, UK

Miss Justine Lee

Major Trauma Service, Queen Elizabeth Hospital, Birmingham, UK

Dr Claire Leppold

Research Fellow, Centre for Health Equity, School of Population and Global Health, University of Melbourne, Australia

Dr Kathryn J Lester

Senior Lecturer in Psychology, University of Sussex, UK

Professor David Lockey

Gibson Professor, and Immediate Past Chair of the Faculty of Pre-Hospital Care, Royal College of Surgeons of Edinburgh, UK

Professor Jill Maben OBE

Professor of Health Services Research and Nursing, School of Health Sciences, University of Surrey, UK

Ms Morwenna Maddock

Intensive Care Department, North Bristol NHS Trust, UK

Mr Guanlan Mao

Trainee Clinical Psychologist, Medical Sciences Division, Oxford Institute of Clinical Psychology Training and Research, University of Oxford, UK

Professor Sir Jonathan Montgomery

Faculty of Laws, University College London; Chair of Oxford University Hospitals NHS Foundation Trust, UK

Dr Sarah Moslehi

Division of Psychiatry, University College London, UK

Dr Yvon Motreff

Santé publique France, Non-Communicable Diseases and Trauma Division, Saint-Maurice, France

Professor Orla Muldoon

Department of Psychology, University of Limerick, Ireland

Dr Ciaran Mulholland

Clinical Senior Lecturer, School of Medicine, Dentistry and Biomedical Sciences, Queen's University, Belfast, UK

Dr Esther Murray

Reader in Health Psychology, Faculty of Medicine and Dentistry, Queen Mary University of London, UK

Dr Evangelos Ntontis

Lecturer in Social Psychology, School of Psychology and Counselling, The Open University, UK

Dr Janet Obeney-Williams

Consultant Psychiatrist, Camden and Islington NHS Foundation Trust, UK

Dr Elise Paul

Institute for Global Health, University College London, UK

Professor Betty Pfefferbaum

George Lynn Cross Research Professor Emeritus. Department of Psychiatry and Behavioral Sciences, College of Medicine, University of Oklahoma Health Sciences Center, Oklahoma, USA

Dr Philippe Pirard

Santé publique France, Non-Communicable Diseases and Trauma Division, Saint-Maurice, France

Professor Sir Keith Porter CStJ

Emeritus Professor of Clinical Traumatology, University Hospitals Birmingham NHS Foundation Trust, UK

Dr Clare Rayner

Member of Society of Occupational Medicine Long COVID Taskforce; Specialist Occupational Physician (retired) and former Honorary Lecturer, Centre for Occupational and Environmental Health, University of Manchester, UK

Professor Julian Redhead
Consultant, Emergency Medicine, Medical Director, Imperial College Healthcare NHS Trust, UK

Dr Lennart Reifels
Centre for Mental Health, Melbourne School of Population and Global Health, University of Melbourne, Australia

Dr Tom Renninson
Consultant in Anaesthetics, Gloucester Royal Hospitals NHS Foundation Trust; Consultant in Prehospital Emergency Medicine, Emergency Medical Retrieval and Transfer Service Wales (EMRTS Cymru), UK

PC Sarah Robbins
Citizens in Policing Support & Development Officer. Derbyshire Constabulary, UK

Professor James Ryan OBE OStJ
Emeritus Professor, St George's, University of London; formerly Professor of Military Surgery, Royal College of Defence Medicine, UK

Dr Stefan Schilling
Lecturer in Social and Organisational Psychology, Department of Psychology, Faculty of Health and Life Sciences, University of Exeter, UK

Dr Louise E Smith
Research Fellow. Department of Psychological Medicine, Institute of Psychiatry, Psychology and Neuroscience, King's College London, UK

Dr John Stancombe
Consultant Clinical Psychologist (retired) formerly of Pennine Care NHS Foundation Trust, Manchester, UK

Dr Suzy Stokes
Consultant in Pre-Hospital and Emergency Medicine, Oxford University Hospitals NHS Foundation Trust and Thames Valley Air Ambulance, UK

Mr Gary Strong
College of Paramedics and Department of Clinical Education, University of Plymouth, UK

Dr Charles Symons
Behavioural Science and Insights Unit, UK Health Security Agency, UK

Dr Selin Tekin
Assistant Professor, Psychology Department, Karabük University, Turkey

Dr Anne Templeton
Senior Lecturer in Social Psychology, Department of Psychology, University of Edinburgh, UK

Mr Mark Thomas
Chair, National Fire Chiefs Council Mental Health Board. Area Manager and Head of Prevention, Merseyside Fire and Rescue Service, UK

Dr Derek K Tracy
Chief Medical Officer, West London NHS Trust, UK; Honorary Senior Lecturer, King's College London, Imperial College London, and University College London, UK

Ms Beata Urbańska
Doctoral Student, Institute of Psychology, Polish Academy of Sciences, Warsaw, and SWPS University, Warsaw, Poland

Miss Toni Wallace
Registered General Nurse, Anaesthetic Associate, and Expert by Experience of Trauma, Anaesthetic Department, Dorset County Hospital, Dorchester, UK

Dr Sonya Wallbank
Senior Leadership and Organisational Development Consultant, The King's Fund, UK

Dr Rebecca K Webster
Department of Psychology, University of Sheffield, UK

Dr Dale Weston
Behavioural Science and Insights Unit, UK Health Security Agency, UK

Professor Richard Williams OBE TD
Emeritus Professor of Mental Health Strategy, Welsh Institute for Health and Social Care, University of South Wales, UK; Presidential Lead for Disaster Management (2008–2014 and 2017–2020) and Presidential Lead for COVID-19, Emergency Preparedness, and Mental Health (2020–2023), Royal College of Psychiatrists, UK

Dr Andrew Wood
Consultant in Anaesthesia and Pre-Hospital Emergency Medicine, Royal London Hospital, Barts Health NHS Trust and London's Air Ambulance, UK

Ms Lisa Woodland
Department of Psychological Medicine, Institute of Psychiatry, Psychology and Neuroscience, King's College London, UK

Dr Liam Wright
Centre for Longitudinal Studies, Social Research Institute, University College London, UK

Professor Hanna Zagefka
Department of Psychology, Royal Holloway University of London, UK

Dr Meng Logan Zhang
Teacher of Psychology, and formerly School of Psychology and Neuroscience, St Andrews University, UK

Foreword by Dr Adrian James

The timing of this book could not be more apt. The last few years have alerted the world to the significant mental health impacts of emergencies, incidents, disasters, and disease outbreaks.

I was President of the Royal College of Psychiatrists during the first global pandemic in 100 years. This, despite its significant challenges, allowed me to see first-hand the way that the mental health needs of populations around the world became increasingly central to the healthcare response.

The world faced a truly unprecedented situation and, as mental health professionals, many of us had an understandable desire to assist our colleagues working on the frontline as they contributed to the national effort to save lives. We all had to understand quickly how to support each other in a considerate, timely, and – above all – evidence-based way.

We also now know that the impacts of the pandemic were not equal. Those especially vulnerable to developing severe illness and dying from COVID-19 were people from Black, Asian and ethnic-minority backgrounds, people living in deprived areas, and people with physical health conditions. These groups were more likely to experience some impact on their mental health as a result. Similarly, I know from colleagues working in child and adolescent psychiatry that the pandemic has had a devastating impact on the mental health of many young people, and we are still trying to understand the true extent of this. Ultimately, as we emerge from the acute phase of the pandemic, comprehending how to address the fallout will be central to helping us to prepare for future disease outbreaks.

The pandemic experience has led me to believe that we have a duty, now more than ever, to understand the psychosocial aspects of these kinds of events. Emergencies and disasters are not going away.

The climate and ecological emergency, which is leaving vast populations exposed to extreme weather, is also a mental health emergency. Populations are already experiencing the health effects of more severe storms, floods, wildfires, and droughts.

Furthermore, the conflict in Ukraine and the devastating earthquakes in Turkey and Syria are displacing millions of people, leaving them vulnerable. These are just a few examples, but mental health professionals must grapple with the impacts of events of this kind with some urgency. We must be prepared to address the growing numbers of people who are experiencing mental ill health as a result.

Fortunately, we are quickly amassing evidence to guide us, as demonstrated not least by the fantastic chapters in this book. Professor Richard Williams OBE, the lead editor of this title, has been crucial in developing my own understanding in his role as Presidential Lead for Disasters at the Royal College of Psychiatrists. The pages of this book are filled with expert perspectives from people who have genuine experience. They eloquently set out the nature and impacts of present-day healthcare emergencies, clinical perspectives on them, and the role of the public in emergencies. They have equally eloquently captured the differing population needs and, importantly, the value of understanding when to act.

I welcome this book, which is a true testament to the authors' dedication to helping some of the most vulnerable people around the world.

Dr Adrian James
President, Royal College of Psychiatrists
April 2023

Foreword by Professor David Lockey

Although, in most countries, major incidents of one kind or another occur regularly, it takes a long time for people who work in the emergency services to accrue meaningful experience based on their own practice. We have a duty to learn from tragic events to try to constantly improve our performance, and this can best be achieved by learning from the pooled experience of others. This book provides an opportunity to do just this.

I am one of many who have responded to multiple major incidents over a long career, and who have observed at close quarters the changes in how we approach and manage them. The management of incidents has become increasingly structured and better organised. Each emergency service has governance arrangements and accountability for its actions, and must work seamlessly with other services.

Despite this, inquests and inquiries often reveal opportunities for improvement, and sometimes expose errors. Press and social media interest is intense, and the public demand to know what happened and who might be to blame. Dissection of events retrospectively can sometimes be brutal, and can be almost as stressful for survivors, families, and emergency responders as were the events themselves. Sadly, when we look at conclusions and recommendations, we often recognise them because they are repeated from previous incidents, which occurred years or decades before. Often the drive and resource to implement meaningful change fades as the next incident takes centre stage.

The ability to provide an effective response includes preparation, infrastructure, training, and predetermined plans. These actions require time, effort, and tenacity, and are achieved well away from the adrenaline of actual incidents. Despite the challenges, it is vital to get this work done if the major incidents of the future are to be dealt with by resilient and effective emergency medical services.

This book is an impressive achievement. Using carefully selected topics, it comprehensively explores the effect of major incidents not only on survivors and responders, but also on their families and the wider community. It considers a diverse range of incident types, from localised incidents to global pandemics. Much of the material is also directly relevant to 'significant' and multi-casualty incidents. Despite their smaller scale, these more common scenarios can be just as disturbing, because they can generate equal distress but without the support and attention generated by major incidents.

The book consists of short multi-author chapters on a fascinating range of topics, and illustrative case studies that focus on real experiences and incident types. The core material is covered in detail, and there are also valuable expert views on issues which are rarely addressed elsewhere. The authors are subject specialists drawn from many disciplines, and in presenting their topics they reference much of the up-to-date existing research on the subject. The material covered is not specific to one readership group. It is as relevant to the professional community who arrive on scene as it is to those who manage the complex aftermath of incidents.

This book provides the essential material to help to embed mental health considerations into every aspect of major incident management and provide support for all who are affected by tragic events. The editors and authors should take pride in having delivered this work, which combines comprehensive coverage and clear presentation on a really challenging subject – how to support the diverse groups of people affected by major incidents.

Professor David Lockey
Gibson Professor and Immediate Past Chair, Faculty of Pre-Hospital Care, Royal College of Surgeons of Edinburgh
April 2023

Emergencies, Incidents, Disasters, Disease Outbreaks, and Mental Health

The Scope of This Book

Richard Williams

This Book

This book is about some of the psychosocial aspects of emergencies, incidents, disasters, and disease outbreaks.

My clinical and academic engagement with the mental health consequences of, and responding to emergencies and disasters began when the *Herald of Free Enterprise* capsized in Zeebrugge Harbour on 6 March 1987, causing the deaths of 193 passengers and crew. Many more people survived; some were injured, and the impacts on the mental health of the survivors became a major long-term issue. I learned a huge amount from patients who were referred to me. This incident occurred relatively soon after the American Psychiatric Association had first included post-traumatic stress disorder (PTSD) in its *Diagnostic and Statistical Manual of Mental Disorders (DSM)* in 1980. There have been huge developments in science and practice relating to the mental health aspects of disasters in the 37 years that have elapsed since the Zeebrugge ferry tragedy.

Subsequently, I have had the privilege of being interested in, researching, working directly on, and advising governments and the responsible authorities about their management of a range of incidents and disease outbreaks. This privilege stems from the enormous generosity of people directly affected by what might loosely be termed emergencies and disasters. At the worst moments of their lives, often while they were worried about the survival and whereabouts of close family members, they have allowed me into their lives. Thus I have come to see how people behave in extreme situations, and the truth is very often substantially different from the perceptions of the public, the media, and films. Therefore one motivation for writing this book is the need to provide a balanced account.

I have also met and worked with a great many talented and dedicated people from around the world, whose role is to reduce the impacts of disastrous events on the people who are affected by them. I have worked extensively in the UK and with all four governments there, in the USA, and in Australia and New Zealand.

I have worked through three pandemics. The first was in the 1980s, when I was engaged in advising young people and education authorities on how to cope with the rapid spread of HIV/AIDS. Colleagues and I published a journal paper describing how young people reacted adversely to the stark messages in the UK government's public campaign. This drew me into involvement in creating better educational material that was explicit but also helpful and acceptable to young people. The next few years were quite an experience. Like so many disastrous events, HIV/AIDS raised a number of challenging ethical issues about the nature and content of the advice that people requested, and which might be offered to them. The pop song 'Street Life', which was used to promote the content of the package for young people with which I became associated and which was created in South West England, is still being played! And HIV/AIDS is still a pandemic, despite the huge scientific advances in finding effective treatments for it.

Next was the flu pandemic of 2009–2010, when I was directly involved in developing policy and practice that was intended to protect people in the UK. There were huge and persistent anxieties about the potential impacts of the pandemic on the public, healthcare, and other services, and on the people who deliver them. I very rapidly learned a lot about the relevant public health principles. Again there were great challenges to public ethics. I was involved in working on a fascinating committee that reported to the Cabinet Office and the Department of Health, and which was charged with creating a framework for ethical decision making. That pandemic resolved reasonably rapidly, whereas the next one, in which I am involved now – the pandemic caused by the SARS-CoV-2 virus – has not. What stands out for me about the COVID-19 pandemic is the substantial way in which people's socioeconomic circumstances have affected both the risks that they face and the impacts on their psychosocial and mental health.

In all of these circumstances, kindness has come to the fore as an important component of responding, as has the power of families and communities to shape how people cope under duress. Early in the present pandemic, much research focused on the evident primary stressors imposed by dealing with the health effects of the virus, but many other stressors, which we term secondary stressors, are now recognised as major influences on outcomes. If readers wish to see further validation of the social determinants of mental health, they need look no further. This leaves me to speculate about the potential for long-term effects on the mental health of populations that may not be visible for some years yet.

Between the last two pandemics was the Ebola outbreak in West Africa. Again I learned a lot about communities and the impacts on those volunteers who went to Freetown of working in conditions that demanded such rigour in donning, doffing, and working in personal protective equipment. The lasting impacts on the volunteers were substantial. Once more we saw the huge relevance of colleagues, communities, and culture to that event.

I have spent substantial amounts of time since the Manchester Arena bombing in May 2017 working as a member of a group that is researching the mental health impacts on the people involved. Most recently, I have contributed a small amount of indirect input to the work of healthcare practitioners in Ukraine. In scientific terms, this is a very large-scale complex emergency as well as a war. It has caused death, loss, misery, and suffering for so many people, but has also reached out to engage so much of the world. In the midst of the enormity of what is happening, the capacity of people for good is also evident. Again, similar issues emerge from these events despite the fact that they have different origins. The horrific effects of the earthquakes in Turkey and Syria were occurring as our editing this book was drawing to a close. These two most recent large-scale emergencies emphasise the signal importance of the socioeconomic conditions in which people live to virtually all emergencies and incidents.

All of my experiences have left me thinking that there are core principles which, arguably, apply across the many varying types of untoward events with

which this volume is concerned. That is why the editors have drawn together the contributions in this book.

Signposting the Sections in This Book

As a consequence of these thoughts, and before the SARS-CoV-2 pandemic began, colleagues and I agreed that we should endeavour to distil what we have learned over the years. We wanted to take a broad approach to searching for common principles, and to add in information and evidence from the pandemic to set alongside our wider experiences with regard to terrorism, conflict, flooding, and earthquakes.

Therefore we commissioned expert authors from a range of disciplines to contribute their learning and wisdom. Much of that material is based on research. High-quality studies are hard to put in hand rapidly and with authority during emergencies and disasters, but many of our contributors have applied considerable ingenuity in doing so. The diversity of topics in this book provides evidence of how broadly the world of disaster healthcare has burgeoned in the last 50 years.

We start, in Section 1, by laying a foundation for all the other sections by including four introductory chapters, followed by eight chapters that deal with a range of powerful generic topics that are raised by many emergencies. Early on, we realised that it was important to agree on definitions of common terms, which experience shows may often be used loosely. Therefore this book includes a glossary of recurring terms. We struggled with a summary term to describe the contents of the book, but settled on *emergencies, incidents, terrorist events, disasters, disease outbreaks and conflicts (EITDDC)*. Part of Chapter 49 covers these terms in more detail. Importantly, Chapter 4 introduces the human element of common emergencies in the UK. The first short account is provided by a woman who was involved in a serious car crash, and the second is by a person who was previously a trainee in pre-hospital emergency medicine. What is very clear from both accounts is that human contact is hugely important to sufferers, their relatives, rescuers, staff of Blue Light services, and healthcare practitioners alike in dealing with extraordinary events.

Section 2 covers two very important sources of impacts – often unpredicted – on the mental health of people who are involved in emergencies and disease outbreaks. Thus in this section we review the massive developments in our capabilities for responding to the needs of people injured in emergencies, and the vital importance of realising that civilian and military healthcare practices are linked. We also offer three chapters on the impacts of disease outbreaks. Although not directly about mental health, each of these six chapters is clearly linked to the ways in which people respond to, adapt to, and face the risks of possible mental disorders that arise from being involved directly and indirectly in events that are beyond the majority of everyday experiences.

Section 3 embraces directly the huge contributions made by the social sciences to our understanding of the vital connections of EITDDC with people's social circumstances and relationships. These chapters illustrate the importance of including people's social relationships when designing and delivering responses for them. We learn about the importance to outcomes of the legitimacy with which the public views the emergency services and, in Chapter 22 in particular, of the importance of so-called bystanders to the effectiveness of responses mounted by societies to all untoward events. This might be a hard lesson for our Blue Light services, but we have learned that it is vital that they accommodate the willingness of some members of the public to be involved if our emergency responses are to be maximally effective.

Sections 4 and 5 cover the responses required by the public, and the importance of caring for and supporting the staff of services who respond to EITDDC. The chapters in each of these sections demonstrate the importance of social support that was established by the authors of Chapter 5 and explained in detail in Section 3. They contain a wealth of well-researched material and accounts of actions taken in recent EITDDCs presented as case studies.

In Section 6 the book returns to the importance of effective effective managers and caring leaders in designing and delivering emergency services that are capable of reducing the profiles of mental health consequences. Thus the book establishes the vital legitimacy of including mental health considerations in all plans and through emergency preparedness and responses. Chapter 52, on public ethics, shows how important it is for governments to behave ethically in EITDDC. COVID-19 has been accompanied by a challenging mix of public populism, and social media posts, which have given vast numbers of people a voice, and a distrust of experts that was emerging before the pandemic began. Chapter 52 paints a picture of the challenges and of the need to find a public approach to ethics that can incorporate many viewpoints.

Finally, the editors draw together the major conclusions of the book in Chapter 56 in Section 7 in a future-orientated endeavour to highlight what we see as the core issues in dealing with the mental health aspects of all EITDDC.

At this point I should like to take this opportunity to thank sincerely all of the authors, and especially my colleagues – Verity Kemp, Keith Porter, John Drury, and Tim Healing – for all their wisdom and for the industry that they have brought to this book.

Chapter

2

How the World Views Trauma and Trauma Care

Julian Redhead

Trauma remains the leading cause of death worldwide in the first four decades of life. Estimates for 2014 suggest that there were around 14,000–16,000 trauma-related deaths per day, with road traffic collisions being the most common cause. The burden is especially high in low- and middle-income countries, where over 90% of injury-related deaths occur. However, this figure hides a much wider and deeper burden of trauma on communities. For every person who dies, many more are left with physical and mental sequelae of trauma. Disability-adjusted life years (DALYs) take this into account by combining the number of life years lost from a premature death with the number of years lived with disabilities due to non-fatal injuries, with one DALY being one lost year of healthy living. Such data for 1998 indicated that 16% of the world's burden of disease was attributable to trauma, and predictions for 2020 suggested that this figure would rise. In 1999 it was acknowledged that around 60 million DALYs were lost due to trauma in India and China combined.

These data can drive the perception that trauma is a disease of young people, with much of the focus of training and trauma management being on this age group. However, there is growing evidence of the challenge of elderly patients who are involved in trauma. Increasing life expectancy across the world means that that trauma in older people is likely to become a growing concern. In many countries there is an expanding population of older patients, who are enjoying better health and mobility than in previous generations at their age. However, greater independence, health improvements, and improved longevity also result in an increase in the potential for injuries. This, combined with increasing use of medications that may affect trauma outcome, such as anticoagulants, lowers physiological reserve and can impair people's ability to recover, also affecting outcomes and hence ongoing healthcare and social needs in this important group.

The numbers of road traffic collisions are increasing in low- and middle-income countries, with costs estimated to be up to 3% of gross domestic product (GDP). However, the wider effects on households are now being recognised, with studies suggesting that road traffic injuries result in significant personal and household economic hardship; more than a third of patients report having to sell assets in order to meet their basic needs.

Yet the perception of trauma is that emergencies occur as a result of accidents or random events. Consequently, they have not had the public health focus that they deserve. This attitude is changing as we are recognising that accidents are preventable, and that early systematic management of trauma can improve both survival and the incidence of disability. Legislation has led to significant reductions in injuries – for example, through using helmets, child restraints, and seatbelts, efforts to limit alcohol use in risky situations, and attempts by the water leisure industry to reduce the number of drownings. Seatbelt legislation has consistently led to reductions in morbidity and mortality of 25–65%. However, many countries have not introduced such measures. Wider prevention campaigns have also led to reductions in trauma – for example, alcohol reduction campaigns have led to a decrease in violent injuries. More focused campaigns, such as those on using social media, and on childhood injuries, have all had positive results.

In order to improve trauma outcomes, it is important to have data to support and refute improvements. In the UK, the development of the Trauma Audit and Research Network (TARN) has allowed systematic recording of outcomes for trauma patients across healthcare systems. This database enables comparisons of the actual and expected outcomes for an injury that take into account age, gender, physiological response, and the nature of the injury. In turn, this knowledge enables researchers to compare outcomes for different interventions and between different hospitals and systems. Many countries have struggled to set up similar databases, often due to the perception of initial costs involved rather than the overall improvements in economic burden due to improvements in care.

Coordinated systems of care have consistently demonstrated improvements in patients' outcomes. Studies have indicated that where coordination of this nature does not exist, a 20% higher inpatient mortality may be found. In 2009 the first National Clinical Director for Trauma Care was appointed in England, with trauma networks in London following in 2012. By 2013, an independent report had concluded that 20% more patients were surviving severe trauma since the introduction of formal trauma centres and networks. Since 2019 the World Health Organization (WHO) has identified the lack of universal health coverage, which is affecting provision of timely care for injured patients, as an important area of focus. It recognises that barriers to accessing healthcare lead to increased mortality and morbidity for patients across all emergency conditions, including injuries. An emergency care system must deliver care from the scene of an accident, through transport to a hospital, care within that hospital, with timely access to theatre and intensive care services, to discharge and rehabilitation within the community. There is a perception that high-quality emergency trauma care is too expensive for low- and middle-income countries, but the WHO has identified a number of relatively low-cost interventions to improve emergency care, such as formal triage processes, checklists, and education about life-saving and life-changing interventions, improvements to Morbidity and Mortality (M&M) meetings, and preventable death panels. There are worldwide examples of the cost benefits of organised care – for example, in Malawi, where establishing a dedicated emergency unit with formal triage in one hospital halved patient mortality, at a cost of US$ 1.95 per patient.

Standards of care within hospital emergency departments and operating theatres also have an impact on outcomes. Development of Advanced Trauma Life Support (ATLS) courses has led to a standard approach to caring for trauma patients. Development of damage control surgery, whole body imaging, interventional radiological techniques, blood product ratios, and the use of the WHO Trauma Care Checklist have all led to improvements in outcomes. Uptake of these standards has varied between countries, and the need to develop international support and education for all healthcare systems is an important issue for the future if we are to influence international outcomes and reduce the global burden of injuries.

Increasingly we are recognising that trauma outcomes depend not only on the initial management of patients, but also on their ongoing rehabilitation. This is particularly evident in the management of brain injuries, with significant improvement occurring within 2 years of injury, but continuing improvement occurring over 5–10 years. It is important to note that the majority of injuries occur in young patients, with consequences for their psychological and social development, resultant social isolation, and a significant impact on their families and sometimes also their communities. There is also a high incidence of psychiatric disorders associated with brain injury, with substance abuse and depression being more common in people with head injuries. However, the psychiatric and socioeconomic consequences of trauma are not limited to head injuries. Follow-up of patients with thoracic trauma has found that the mental health impacts are under-recognised and affect a large number of these patients, and that there is wide variation in the time taken for them to return to work. Follow-up of patients who have experienced trauma is important, and often requires input from a number of specialties, both hospital and community based. The trauma systems that the WHO has identified as being necessary for better care should also include these wider aspects of patient care.

The psychosocial impacts on patients of being in intensive care are well recognised, and a large number of studies have emphasised the importance of identifying these aspects early in these patients' care. The importance of providing strong social support for every patient should not be underestimated, and the impacts on family members must also be recognised.

Patient Reported Outcome Measures (PROMs) related to certain specialties, such as orthopaedics, have increasingly influenced how patients are managed. These outcome measures are vital as they reflect what is important to patients, and not necessarily the procedural outcome. In some forms they represent the psychosocial and socioeconomic impacts of injuries, and the options that should be considered in caring for patients.

This is not the only area in which a more multi-disciplinary approach to trauma care is required. End-of-life decisions and defining the goals of care may require input from a wide variety of specialists, including palliative care and elder care specialists. Discussions with patients and their families can be challenging, especially in emergencies.

As I have already mentioned, it is important to keep in mind the impact of trauma on patients' family members and carers. The recent COVID-19 pandemic has highlighted the importance of ensuring support for healthcare staff. However, this has often been under-recognised in clinical teams involved in caring for patients who have suffered trauma.

Chapter

3

How the World Views the Mental Health Implications of Traumatic Events, Major Incidents, and Serious Contagious Diseases

John Alderdice

I grew up in a divided community where people had conflicting views on many issues, because of their differing religious, political, social, and cultural backgrounds. As I trained in psychiatry, I learned how biological, psychological, and sociological perspectives competed for allegiance in the profession. Later the diversity of views within our scientific communities was brought home to me when I was invited by the World Federation of Scientists to help them with a major division that had opened up as they tried to apply their expertise in the aftermath of the 9/11 terrorist attacks. Western scientists wanted to assist in the fight against Al Qaeda, whereas those from Eastern countries insisted that we must understand why the attacks were taking place. These conflicting perspectives among scientists showed how, even within the rational scientific community, we develop different narratives to explain and explore traumatic events and major incidents.

We see similar divergence with the COVID-19 pandemic caused by the SARS-CoV-2 coronavirus. Epidemiologists give a response based on their developing understanding of the community transmission of the virus. Clinicians focus on treating the disease resulting from the over-reaction of the immune system that occurs in a minority of individual patients, and which may lead to serious illness and death. The impact on the healthcare system as a whole is the concern for people on lengthening waiting lists, and government officials are constantly balancing these pressures and the economic and societal consequences. More profound divergences are seen between those who accept the need for social distancing, mask wearing, and the vaccination rollout, and those 'anti-vaxxers' who, for personal, political, religious, historical, or cultural reasons, do not accept this narrative. Even within our communities, at this time in history, facing a global pandemic, there is no one view.

Four years ago my wife and I moved from the city of Belfast, where we had lived and worked during the Troubles, to a quiet village in rural Oxfordshire. We wanted to be closer to my activities in Westminster and Oxford, and to our children and grandchildren living in England and Scotland. We thought that we had planned for most eventualities, but we did not expect the pandemic. We were fortunate. Spending the lockdown in an Oxfordshire village is not a hardship. We were not locked in, suffering the ravages of the pandemic in crowded city housing. Nor were we suffering directly from the increasing geopolitical instability, the risk of terrorist attacks, or other such traumatic incidents. However, this was not always the case in our rural idyll.

The early pre-Norman settlement grew up away from the nearby Roman road for safety reasons, since that was the route taken by the Viking marauders. Even so, during the English Civil War there was a military skirmish because of the proximity of the settlement to the Royalist centre of Oxford, and the Anglican rector in the village was replaced by a religious non-conformist until the restoration of Charles II. Walking the local bridle paths, we noticed that some historic villages no longer exist because almost all of their inhabitants died during the plague years. I tell this story because – from the parables of Jesus to the case histories of Sigmund Freud and the broadcasts of current affairs – it is not through theory that we learn most easily, remember best, and construe our lives, but through the medium of 'human interest' stories. We view traumatic events, including violence, pandemics, and their mental health implications, through the stories we tell ourselves and the reactions of our communities moulded by history, place, and culture.

The Astronomer Royal, Lord (Martin) Rees, has pointed out that when the Black Death swept across Europe in the fourteenth century, communities continued to function even if they lost half of their population, because the survivors had a fatalistic attitude to the massive death toll [1]. 'In contrast,' he says, 'the feeling of entitlement is so strong in today's wealthier countries that there would be a breakdown in the social order as soon as hospitals overflowed, key workers stayed at home, and health services were overwhelmed. This would occur when those infected were still a fraction of 1 percent'. One might imagine that with a scientific education, the ready availability of expert medical professionals, the prospect of protection through vaccination, and measures such as social distancing, disinfection, approved personal protective equipment, and an effective healthcare system, people would be less anxious and more resilient. Paradoxically, however, we have seen the fear that has gripped responsible governments with the appearance of each new variant of COVID. Despite the relief of financial hardship for many people through furloughing schemes for those who could not work remotely, and the ease of online social communication, there are still daily reports of 'serious mental health consequences' across wealthy countries, instead of a sense of confidence that the pandemic will be contained, and that life can continue. There are many reasons for this twenty-first-century response, and Rees identifies one of them. When we live with a narrative that focuses on 'me' as an individual, living only in the here and now, and expecting that all ought to be well for me, any deviation from that 'entitlement to wellbeing' is experienced as more frightening and unfair than if I expect to live with uncertainty, and am sustained by a mixture of religious belief and fatalism.

Such 'paradoxical' responses can be found in other contexts, too. When people are told that everyone can achieve anything they want, this does not bring reassurance and confidence about life. Instead, it results in anxiety and unhappiness as people discover that life is not like that for them, and they either blame themselves or 'the system'. The philosopher Onora O'Neill pointed to another apparently paradoxical outcome in her 2002 Reith Lectures, showing that current approaches to openness and accountability have reduced rather than increased public trust – the opposite of what had been expected [2]. Dominic Johnson has recently shown how cognitive biases that were assumed to lead inevitably to catastrophic defeats in war may instead result in remarkable successes [3]. These and other findings are raising questions about whether what are regarded as 'rational' views of how to address societal problems are not as successful as we might expect.

A further problem of expectation, specifically with regard to mental wellbeing, has been created by widening the meaning of 'mental health problem'. In the past, disturbed mental functioning was regarded as being caused by moral weakness or the influence of evil spirits. More recently, mental illnesses, which might have physical, psychological, or social contributors, have been viewed through a medical lens that sees definable categories of mental illness whose diagnoses have pathological and therapeutic implications. Such an approach regarded low spirits and anxiety as symptoms of mental illness only when they were experienced in an inappropriate context or to an excessive degree. In bereavement, disappointments in love, miserable life circumstances, and unhappy relationships, low spirits are a normal reaction. Anxiety is also an appropriate response to a threatening situation, such as receiving worrying news about one's health, uncertainty about employment, or environments where security is an issue. Symptoms such as low spirits or anxiety may be an indication of mental illness if they arise without external disturbances, but otherwise they are appropriate responses to challenging life circumstances. Today such symptoms are regarded by many people as 'mental health problems', and there are many referrals to mental health services of people whose complaints are a reaction to the vicissitudes of normal life, rather than a sign of abnormal mental functioning. In a time of pandemic, when the vast majority of people are experiencing challenging life circumstances, the majority of the population might be regarded as suffering from mental health problems. Is this an appropriate use of scarce professional resources? Does it mislead people into thinking that they are suffering from a disorder when they may simply be showing a normal reaction to an abnormal circumstance?

Focusing on adverse reactions to trauma, major incidents, and disease outbreaks also diverts us from studying the resilience of individual people and communities. After major terrorist incidents, most people do *not* suffer from post-traumatic stress disorder (PTSD) or other adverse mental health consequences, and a greater focus on how and why some people are more resilient than others might be as productive as trying to understand why a minority break down or do not recover [4]. Studying why some countries are stable and suffer less conflict, rather than why some break down into violence, has been the focus of the Institute for Economics and Peace. Its founder, Steve Killelea, recently described how he arrived at this approach, and the benefits that arise from it [5]. His approach has resulted in the identification of eight pillars of 'Positive Peace', rather than a list of reasons why things break down into conflict. These pillars – well-functioning government, equitable distribution of resources, a sound business environment, low levels of corruption, free flow of information, acceptance of the rights of others, high levels of human capital, and good relations with neighbours – were identified through the analysis of many data sets, are followed up globally each year, and are applied using a systems approach to understanding communal relations.

Another reason for the wide range of worldviews is the dramatic pace of change in technology. One example is a consequence of the insatiable appetite of the 24/7 news cycle and pervasive social media. Both of these excite emotional responses rather than merely providing information that can be rationally processed, and the uncertainty and anxiety that they stimulate are now being exacerbated by hostile politically motivated actors using synthetic bots driven by artificial intelligence to deepen splits and foment social and political instability. This new element of 'hybrid warfare' is producing a global conflict in cyberspace. Although most people are unaware of it, there are significant impacts on mental and physical healthcare as well as on industry, politics, and security. One example of this was the WannaCry ransomware attack on 12 May 2017.

Although this was a relatively unsophisticated attack, it had a major impact on National Health Service hospitals in England and Scotland, and up to 70,000 devices – including computers, MRI scanners, blood-storage refrigerators, and theatre equipment – may have been affected. On 12 May 2017, some NHS services had to turn away non-critical emergencies, and ambulances were diverted. In 2016, thousands of computers in 42 separate NHS trusts in England had already been reported to be still running the Windows XP operating system, although support for the latter had ended 3 years previously and Microsoft was no longer providing security updates or technical support. The system should have been replaced before the attack, but in 2018, a year after the WannaCry attack, a report by British Members of Parliament concluded that all 200 NHS hospitals or other organisations checked in the wake of the attack still failed cybersecurity checks. This failure to address necessary protections before and after a major attack in a major developed country with a uniquely networked and government-funded healthcare system shows that the threat we face may not just be external, or solely a consequence of financial pressures. It may also be a form of denial seen in the absence of a serious public debate about these new threats, which are increasing at an exponential rate and are a form of psychological warfare that is having significant impacts on our mental wellbeing.

In his interview study after the 2001 Al Qaeda attacks in New York, Charles Strozier described 'zones of sadness' in which the distance from the scene of death affected people's experience. *Survivors* who saw people die in real time were not just those who escaped from the buildings, but those who saw people die by jumping from the buildings [6]. *Witnesses* experienced the destruction, but remained just far enough away not to actually see people die. *Participants* felt the danger, but all they saw was a lot of smoke. *Onlookers* watched the attacks on television, distanced from the actuality of the scenes of death. These four cohorts – survivors, witnesses, participants, and onlookers – were defined by both physical and psychological distance. Recently, Strozier has also applied this perspective to the pandemic, showing how the four similar groups can be identified in that context, too. Apart from the differences between the people in the four groups, the one-off attack that they experienced is very different from situations where people live in a community traumatised by ongoing wars or constant terrorist campaigns. Victims such as these suffer repeated and sometime regular traumatic experiences. Mental disturbance in response to trauma is affected not only by psychological distance but also by whether people have one-off or repeated experiences.

This chapter has outlined why there can be no single worldview of the mental health implications of traumatic events, major incidents, and serious contagious diseases. It also implies that although our perspectives have evolved from previous views, we shall continue to change those perspectives. With the further passage of time and changes in culture and technology, current views will become substantially modified. We can only wonder how future generations will assess our views, how they will understand what we now refer to as 'mental health', and whether the separation that we observe between physical and mental health will survive.

References

1. Rees M. *On the Future: Prospects for Humanity*. Princeton University Press, 2018.

2. O'Neill O. *A Question of Trust: The BBC Reith Lectures 2002*. Cambridge University Press, 2002.

3. Johnson DDP. *Strategic Instincts: The Adaptive Advantages of Cognitive Biases in International Politics*. Princeton University Press, 2020.

4. Bonanno GA, Galea S, Bucciarelli A, Vlahov D. Psychological resilience after disaster: New York City in the aftermath of the September 11th terrorist attack. *Psychol Sci* 2006; **17**: 181–6.

5. Killelea S. *Peace in the Age of Chaos: The Best Solution for A Sustainable Future*. Hardie Grant Books, 2020.

6. Strozier CB. *Until the Fires Stopped Burning: 9/11 and New York City in the Words and Experiences of Survivors and Witnesses*. Columbia University Press, 2011.

Chapter

4

Two Personal Perspectives on Trauma and Recovery

Toni Wallace and Tom Renninson

11 August 2018

Toni Wallace

I've always been a massive music fan, and I love seeing live bands. About 15 years ago, I was able to use my role as a registered nurse and an anaesthesia associate to work as a volunteer medic at huge events such as the Glastonbury Festival, Reading Festival, and other big live music events. I loved it, combining the two things I am passionate about. The trade-off for attending these festivals was to also volunteer at less glitzy events and so, on Saturday 11 August 2018, I set off at 04:30 from my home in Dorset for the Bristol Balloon Festival, where I was providing medical cover.

I had been driving for about 20 minutes when I saw the first car of my journey – pinpoint headlights on a long remote country road which bears the national speed limit. Seconds later, there was a horrendous explosion, a huge roaring, a smash, and enormous impact. It was black and incredibly noisy, and all I could do was cough because of the thick smoke, which I now know was caused by the airbags deploying. I was completely disoriented and had no idea what had happened. I was conscious throughout.

I realised quickly that I had been in a big accident, but I didn't know why. I felt really calm and thought 'At least I'm not dead'. Weirdly, I then said out loud, 'AM I dead?', because I had never felt this way before – I truly wondered whether this was what it was like to be dead. Then the pain in my pelvis started and I realised I definitely wasn't!

I heard a man groaning very close by, and saw a car alongside mine, facing the same way. The passenger door was missing and I could not see the man, but I could hear gurgling agonal sounds. My instinct, and training, was to help to support his airway, but I was trapped in my car both by his car and by the intrusion of my dashboard. A few minutes later he stopped

groaning, and I suspected he was dead. His phone kept ringing and I was yelling for him to answer it. I also thought it was weird his phone was ringing at that exact time … strange the things you think of!

I was alone in the middle of nowhere, my phone was gone, and I was in the most indescribable agony. I suddenly had the idea that I would die here from internal injuries, having done well to survive the impact. Eventually, after I think about 20 minutes, a car appeared, and a man got out but would not come to the scene. I was begging for help, but he stayed well back and called the emergency services. Weirdly, all I wanted was for him to come over and tell me it was going to be OK – a bit of human contact I suppose. I heard from the police since that he was too concerned to approach, as the scene was such a mess.

Because of the rural location, the emergency services took a long while to come, but in the meantime a doorman from one of the clubs came across the scene on his way home from work. I shall never forget his manner. I thought he was a police officer. He was so calm and reassuring, and stayed with me. He turned off my engine (I hadn't realised it was still running) and told me he would help me. I was pleading for him to get me out of the car, and remember him saying 'You know I can't do that'. I was glad he didn't when I found out the severity of my injuries. The fact that he was there, however, was such a reassurance to me, and I shall never forget his kindness that morning.

Eventually the emergency services arrived and assessed the scene. It was very unpleasant being on the other side. I suspected I had broken my pelvis and my spine, and I could not feel my legs, which were trapped under the pedals; the pain was horrific, but I had an overwhelming desire to get out of the car. Everyone had their role and was dedicated to it, but all I wanted was for someone to hold my hand and tell me what was going to happen and that it would all be alright. I understand that there aren't a lot of spare folk at these things, but I'm definitely a strong advocate for a 'designated hand-holder'!

Something that really sticks in my mind is that somebody assessed the scene and took control. Hearing the words out loud, 'one male deceased and one female with life-threatening injuries', is very scary. Even though I am medically trained and knew the other driver was dead, it was an awful thing to hear out loud. I was convinced I would die before they got me out of the car.

It has been 5 years now since the accident, and I do think about it fairly often. I have had superb counselling support, but it is odd how a sudden seemingly small event, like the smell of burning or the crump of a car's impact, can take me right back. This is not necessarily a bad thing – I know I am very lucky to have survived and done so well, but I do wish it hadn't happened, as it has definitely changed my life.

I am not a 'touchy-feely' person, but that morning I needed someone who was there just for me, telling me what was going to happen, holding my hand, and telling me it was going to be OK. I have never felt so alone in my life – frightened out of my life and in agony. I consider myself to be quite brave and stoic, but until something that you never think will happen to you happens, you have no idea how you will respond. To me, human kindness throughout my whole journey from my accident until now is the thing I searched for, and meant so much when I got it – even to a 'toughie' like me!

A Personal View of the Reality of Training in Pre-Hospital Emergency Medicine

Tom Renninson

Many common mental health themes are described in different medical training programmes and also across many different professions within healthcare. The last decade has seen the development of the new subspecialty of *pre-hospital emergency medicine (PHEM)*, which has been identified as frequently delivering trainees to stressful work environments. This was recognised by the Faculty of Pre-Hospital Care, which collaborated to produce a report with recommendations to improve the wellbeing of pre-hospital practitioners. This included organisational and personal strategies to prevent serious mental health outcomes by intervening early and supporting the mental health of all staff. Every trainee's experience is different, and there are very different delivery models and case mixes between services. Here I shall relate my personal experience of PHEM's impact on me, and how I ultimately continue to thrive in this environment.

I started training in PHEM in 2020 as a senior anaesthetic trainee. I had spent 10 years training in anaesthetics and intensive care, much of this in a Major Trauma Centre. I was unable to get a PHEM training post locally, so I transferred to an Air Ambulance Service with bases 50 to 200 miles from home to spend 12 months training full-time. Like many others undertaking subspecialty training at this stage of their life, I was a home owner and had three young children in school; my wife was working full-time as a doctor. The training year placed a significant burden on my family, who tried to maintain normality despite my frequent absences. This added considerably to the stress at work.

I had some understanding of the challenges of PHEM prior to starting the training. I understood that the case mix would mainly consist of severely ill and injured patients, and I was well trained and familiar with in-hospital management of this patient group. However, like many new trainees, I had not been able to achieve really regular pre-hospital clinical exposure in advance of taking up my post. I knew there would be challenges in transferring the care that I delivered in hospital on a daily basis out of hospital, but I underestimated how much impact the other stresses of commuting, fatigue, and guilt about working away from home would have on me.

In my year in PHEM, I attended approximately 200 incidents – about 50% major trauma and 50% medical emergencies, including cardiac arrests. Aside from the heart attacks and road traffic incidents I attended two multi-patient major incidents, 26 critically ill or injured children (9 of whom were in cardiac arrest), 37 patients who required an anaesthetic at the scene, and 15 patients who needed a blood transfusion to stabilise them prior to transfer. I attended gunshot wounds and stabbings, I resuscitated children in front of their parents, and I saw burns, industrial injuries, strangulation, and drowning in adults, children, and newborns. Despite our considerable capacity and best work, many of these patients died prior to, during, or soon after our call to resuscitate and stabilise them.

In time I would learn about primary and secondary stressors, which gave me the terminology to describe, be honest about, and mitigate stressors. I found that this improved my overall performance, and it has been vital to my longevity in this specialist field. The unit I worked in had multiple mechanisms in place to support staff after particularly stressful events, and had considered and attempted to mitigate secondary stressors. They had stocked kitchens and bedrooms on the bases, mitigated the impact of commuting by adapting shift patterns to suit each person, and allowed for commuting by providing overnight accommodation before shifts. This was also one of the UK services that have invested in a dispatch system, which includes a clinician from the service who is separate from the duty crew. This is very helpful in a number of ways – for example, by deflecting further inputs into the active team during a mission, and by protecting the team after challenging and traumatic cases.

I was faced with three significant mental wellbeing challenges that I had not anticipated before I started. First, I had for the last 10 years relied on debriefing with my wife as the 'backbone' of my coping mechanisms. Debriefing these types of difficult cases and shifts with someone outside risks affecting their own mental health, by association. This forced me to adapt and establish new coping strategies while still encountering new and frequent situations that required processing. Second, treating patients in their own environments made it much more difficult to avoid emotional engagement in the cases. Emotion obviously has strengths and weaknesses, but it can make objective decision making very challenging. For me, it made moving on from a case harder than I had found with similar patients in the 'sterilised' environment of a hospital. Third, hospital colleagues and the general public showed enormous variation in the level of respect and value that they placed on the very challenging work I was performing. At worst, the public think you have superpowers, and are surprised, disappointed, and angry when you don't know the answer or can't make things better. Hospital staff are often casually scornful or belittling about the specialty, and are sceptical — sometimes even hostile – about the care you have been trying so hard to deliver.

It is very difficult to summarise all the challenges experienced and support received during a year of shifts, but one particular episode which took me weeks to process gives a good example of how this specialty brings multiple primary and secondary stressors together to create circumstances that can induce trauma. The particular challenge of pre-hospital care is that these cases and shifts, although exceptional, are not uncommon, and so it is entirely possible to do two shifts like this 'on the bounce'.

It was a night shift, and I started without adequate sleep because I had spent the previous hours picking up my children from school and clubs, and getting them fed and changed before exchanging childcare responsibilities with my wife and commuting the hour to work. I was new to working solo with a critical care practitioner, having recently completed the sign-off required to work under remote supervision. No sooner had we arrived on base than the klaxon sounded and we headed straight out. A toddler in cardiac arrest – my fourth really sick child in as many weeks. When we arrived, we found the child upstairs and in cardiac arrest, and we started our treatments; I noticed that the child had the same changing mat as my youngest had had when she was their age. After the initial treatments, I left my colleagues to run the arrest while I went downstairs to speak to the family. During the conversation it became clear that I might be attending a case of non-accidental injury. I kept up my facade of calmness, called in the police, and coaxed the details from the family, listening to a detailed timeline to aid our decision making. I then went back upstairs and joined my colleague who was working on the child. As we were considering whether we should stop resuscitation, we felt a pulse. We rapidly moved the child into the back of the ambulance and set off to the children's hospital, working hard all the way, but we all knew the outlook was grim. In the emergency department the atmosphere was very intense, with many police officers and other people. Emotions were running high all round with such a young patient. We wrote down all the details we could, as we knew that we would be relying on that detail for reference over the coming days and months for statements, interviews with the police, and possibly even court appearances. As soon as we were done, we were back to base and restocking our trashed kit. While we were working we talked through the sequence of events and our actions, looking for things that went well and things that could have gone better. Both of us have young children, and we were disturbed by the case and the surrounding detail. By the time we had finished it was late evening. We finally got to eat something (the first meal since lunch), and then we were out again. We were sent out to a couple of small jobs – one we got to, and the other did not require our input.

Then we were tasked again in the early hours. A young adult had been ejected from a car and was critically injured. We went by helicopter, arriving 30 minutes after the call to find a teenager who had been thrown down the road during a high-speed collision with a tree. The passenger side of the car was completely destroyed. It was no exaggeration to say that the teenager had broken everything – they were the most broken patient who still had a pulse whom I have seen before or since. They were deeply unconscious, not breathing, with a weak central pulse, and just moments from bleeding to death. The driver – who had walked away from the crash – was in the background, full of alcohol and drugs, and swearing and spitting at the emergency services. We scrambled a resuscitation using everyone on the scene to help with an anaesthetic, central venous access, surgical procedures to decompress the patient's chest, binding and splinting bones, and giving all the blood and blood products we carried with us as rapidly as possible. While still doing this, we loaded into the ambulance and bounced around in the back as we raced to the Major Trauma Centre. We got the patient into the resuscitation department alive but still critically unstable, and handed them over to the expectant hospital team. Again we started on the paperwork. Now we were 12 hours into shift, tired and coming down off the adrenaline of the last hour, and the department was swarming with staff working to resuscitate this young sick patient. Then the emergency department consultant marched out of the computerised tomography (CT) suite and started to loudly criticise an aspect of my management in front of the whole department. Deep down I knew what they were saying was incorrect, but in that moment I couldn't think of a response, and my mind was so full that all I could do was apologise. Head down, I started questioning what I did. Did I cause the patient harm? Other members of the team reassured me that what I did was right, but I left feeling angry, with a deep sense of unfairness, and only now were all of the sensible and smart responses I could have given going round in my head.

I finished this shift late, having had a hot debrief with the critical care practitioner (CCP) and the oncoming crew, and set off on the hour's drive home with thoughts circling in my head about the last interaction and the memory of talking to a parent. These thoughts took weeks to fade, and inevitably took a toll on me during that time. I derived benefit from a number of texts, used as a follow-up tool, sent from managers and senior staff who checked in during subsequent shifts with the offer to talk. I spoke to some of them, both informally and formally, in a structured cold debrief. I confirmed that my management had been sound, and the follow-up team gave updates about the patient's continued forward progress. I was supported in raising an incident report for the interaction with the emergency department consultant. I found the promise that more support and time would be available very reassuring, which I believe helped me not to need them. Over the year, I found that my coping strategies held up, but the experience I have described here did force me to inspect and understand my stressors and adapt my coping strategies to a degree that I hadn't expected.

PHEM will continue to challenge trainees, who often have to leave their usual working, domestic, and family lives to travel far from home to new teams and places of work, with limited first-hand experience. They all need to be supported in this transition by systems that educate them and actively look for and mitigate the primary and secondary stressors which they will face from day one. The effective support in pre-hospital organisations may well be applicable to other organisations whose staff face similar challenges.

Chapter

5

How Emergencies, Incidents, Disasters, and Disease Outbreaks Affect People and Healthcare Practitioners

John Stancombe, Suzy Stokes, Andrew Wood, and Richard Williams

Introduction

There are common challenges and demands that we all face when involved in major events. They are likely to include direct stress from the experience of pain, injury, threat to life, frightening treatment, and exposure to other people's suffering with severe illness and injury, death, bereavement, and loss. They may also include indirect stress associated with social, employment, educational, and community disruption, and people's socioeconomic circumstances. Regardless of the nature of the event, these experiences and circumstances have the potential to affect us, and we are highly likely to experience some level of distress. The term distress describes emotional, social, spiritual, or physical pain or suffering that may cause us to feel sad, afraid, depressed, anxious, or lonely, and these experiences challenge our tolerance and adaptation. This chapter first outlines some of the features of distress, and then provides a commentary on the experiences of staff of healthcare services.

The Impacts on People Affected by Emergencies, Major Incidents, Disasters, Conflict, and Communicable Diseases

General Principles That Emerge from Science

Distress can range from mild to severe, with short-lived or long-lasting impacts on psychological and social wellbeing. People's immediate reactions to events and direct stressors are of most importance for short-term distress. However, exposure to secondary stressors – that is, circumstances, events, or policies that are indirectly related to or a consequence of emergencies, or which are present before the event, and stressors that emerge in the aftermath – influence the long-term course of distress and functional impairment [1].

Psychosocial factors, in terms of people's personal and collective attributes and resources, play a crucial part in determining the various ways in which they react to adversity. People's responses also vary according to the particular range or types of stressors pertaining to each situation or event, and the way in which or the extent to which people are involved or exposed. Moreover, how people subjectively appraise their experience is pivotal in shaping how they are affected, as are the social support systems available to them. Factors such as relationships with friends and family members, how they share their traumatic experiences, how other people validate their concerns, and the social support that they receive may mitigate their distress and stress responses [2]. The psychosocial and behavioural consequences of disasters result from interactions between all of these factors. Therefore there is no such thing as a universal response, although we can discern patterns.

A Description of the Short-, Medium-, and Long-Term Impacts

The Common Reactions and Trajectories

Although there is considerable individual and population variability, there are consistent findings of identifiable patterns or trajectories of stress responses, across a range of indicators and diverse contexts [3,4], that fall into four main groups (see Table 5.1).

This suggests that these trajectories are phenotypic stress responses, in which recovery is the most common response to even the most severe stress or adversity.

The Spectrum of Experiences That People Describe as Distress

There is a broad spectrum of ways in which people react emotionally, cognitively, socially, behaviourally, and physically after events. The usual initial response is a range of experiences of distress (see Table 5.2).

Table 5.1 Trajectories of stress responses after major incidents (© Williams R, 2015, updated 2020, all rights reserved.)

1. **Common responses**
   Depending on the nature of events, most people (c. 50–60%) cope reasonably well. They may suffer distress, usually mild to moderate, that decreases in severity if they receive support that they perceive as adequate

2. **Slower recovery**
   Some people (c. 10–30%) experience distress of moderate severity initially and then recover over time. The duration and severity of their distress are likely to be increased by secondary stressors

3. **Deteriorating responses/prolonged stress***
   Some people (c. 10%) experience distress of moderate severity initially, and these stress levels may deteriorate and later become prolonged or associated with significant dysfunction

4. **High stress responses***
   Some people (c. 10%) may experience high levels of stress after events (at above a level that is consistent with a psychiatric diagnosis). The symptoms, signs, and dysfunction of about 50% of these people may be prolonged, whereas the remainder improve

* People who follow deteriorating or high stress trajectories tend to have had greater exposure to events, greater exposure to secondary stressors after the events, and they may experience persisting adversity.

Table 5.2 Common experiences of people affected by emergencies, major incidents, and disasters (Adapted from Alexander DA, 2005 [5], and reproduced with permission of *BJPsych Advances*.)

Emotional reactions	Cognitive reactions
Fear and anxiety	Impaired concentration
Fear of recurrence	Impaired memory
Anhedonia	Confusion or disorientation
Helplessness or hopelessness	Intrusive thoughts
Shock and numbness	Dissociation or denial
Anger	Reduced confidence or self-esteem
Guilt and shame	Hypervigilance
Social reactions	**Physical reactions**
Regression	Insomnia
Withdrawal	Reduced appetite
Irritability	Reduced energy
Interpersonal conflict	Hyperarousal
Avoidance	Headaches
	Somatic complaints

This represents a highly variable and heterogeneous set of experiences and emotions that can disrupt everyday life and prevent people from functioning. People are likely to report a mix of these experiences that can change over time.

To date, the research has been dominated by biomedical models with minimal focus on the majority of people with mild and moderate distress and their lived experiences in the short and long term [5]. There is growing evidence that qualitative research methods can provide a more nuanced and deeper understanding of people's subjective experiences of distress, and its impact on their interpersonal relationships, leisure, work, and health and wellbeing [6–8]. The Social Influences on Recovery Enquiry (SIRE) is a recent exemplar [9].

SIRE explored the experiences and opinions of people who used the Manchester Resilience Hub, which was established in the wake of the Manchester Arena bombing to provide a central point for psychosocial care, mental health advice, and a programme to identify people who might require specialist mental health services. One arm of the study involved qualitative interviews with survivors of the event who registered with the Hub and completed its mental health triage measures 3 months after the event and at regular intervals up to 3 years. The interviews were split across three subgroups of people who showed personal responses typical of three broad patterns of severity – mild, moderate, and severe distress. These interviews produced rich and detailed accounts of survivors' experiences of distress over time and its impact on their everyday everyday lives. We believe that the key findings from this and other qualitative studies have implications for our understanding of distress and the responses to it.

Distress During and After Incidents Is Ubiquitous But Not Necessarily a Function of Psychopathology, Including Mental Illness

The literature on people's reactions to disasters has traditionally drawn on the contents of measures designed to identify psychopathology, as evidenced by re-experiencing the event and hyperarousal. The survivors of the Manchester Arena bombing reported a much wider range of experiences. The intensity and duration of distress differentiated the three distress subgroups. The common experiences that distressed people reported include feeling upset, fears, anxiety, fear of recurrence of the event, excessive vigilance at social gatherings and in public places, avoiding uncomfortable feelings, and social withdrawal.

The interviewees reported re-experiencing the event uncommonly, and anger, moral distress, survivor guilt, and shock were rare. Thus the experiences listed in Table 5.2 are shown in two fonts (the common or milder experiences in roman font and the more severe ones in italics). Distress was extremely common and was enduring in many cases, even for people who were only mildly affected. However, the majority of the interviewees did not have high levels of mental health symptoms in the initial months after the event. Therefore they did not reach the threshold for early intervention. Yet they represent a large group of people whose suffering warranted validation, and many of them required access to appropriate psychosocial care.

Distress May Be Intense and May Persist Over Long Periods of Time

Previous work on the impact of major events indicates that the intensity of initial distress is strongly associated with enduring and debilitating distress [10], and some longitudinal studies suggest that distress reaches a peak in the year following the event and then slowly improves with recovery, ranging from several months to 2 years. However, there is accumulating evidence that distress of longer duration and greater suffering are experienced by some people [11,12]. After the Manchester Arena bombing, some of the people who experienced mild distress, and many of those with moderate distress, were still experiencing a certain degree of distress and impaired functioning more than 2 years after the event. This suggests that the existing literature might underestimate the number of people who take a long time to recover.

Intriguingly, in the SIRE study, there were some reactions, which have drawn less attention in previous research, that appear to be distinctive to certain subgroups of distressed people. For example, physical reactions – such as sleep difficulties, loss of appetite, somatic complaints, and physical inability to perform everyday functions – were more likely to be reported by people with higher levels of initial distress and more enduring functional impairment. This association has also been reported elsewhere, after the terrorist attacks in Paris in 2015 and in Norway in 2011 [13,14]. Similar findings have also been reported in studies of disasters due to so-called hazards [10]. In addition, the Manchester study showed that shame and guilt were common emotions in the acute phase, and that they were more often associated with longer duration of distress. These findings suggest that certain types of early distress might serve as markers of the risk of enduring distress, and possibly of developing mental health disorders.

A Worrying Feature Is Social Iisolation of Some People Who Are Distressed

SIRE identified the worrying tendency of some people to isolate themselves in the short and longer term, and their intrinsic reluctance to seek help. Social withdrawal, which was not associated with reminders of the event or fear of recurrence, was common early on, when it tended to be short-lived. However, some people who were moderately or severely distressed reported early social withdrawal that became more enduring. In some of these cases, social withdrawal was linked to long-term changes in lifestyle, friendships, and membership of social groups. Similar findings have been reported elsewhere in other contexts [6,8]. This points to the importance of tracking over time the severity of people's experiences and their behaviour.

Negative Self-Appraisal Can Intensify Distress

People who normally cope well with the mundane stresses of life often feel overwhelmed in the face of emergencies, and emotional regulation can become difficult. This natural response can be construed as weakness or inadequacy, which can intensify their experience of distress. Many SIRE interviewees were surprised by the intensity and duration of their distress and the impact that it had on their everyday lives. As they struggled to make sense of their distress, they tended to make self-evaluations of their reactions and coping that were predominantly negative, and this compounded their suffering. The scientific evidence shows that it is the subjective experiences of adverse events that shape the psychosocial outcome, rather than the objective markers of the severity of stress, worry, fear, disease, injury, or life threat [15]. How people make sense of their experiences is pivotal in shaping their emotional and behavioural responses, including their distress levels, suffering, and coping actions.

The Impact of Secondary Stressors on Distress

Secondary stressors (see Chapter 9) can compound and maintain distress after major events [16]. The findings from SIRE elucidate the common and potent stressors that affected the interviewees' coping and recovery. They show that inappropriate responses by survivors' friends and families, in the form of social invalidation of their distress, acted as an important secondary stressor. Wider social contexts – for example, the actions of employers, news and social media coverage, and the public responses of support – also acted as secondary stressors, as did inappropriate forms of psychosocial care and mental healthcare.

The Implications for Intervention

The emerging evidence that distress is extremely common, and can be debilitating even for people who are only mildly affected, has implications for service planning and delivery. First, it emphasises that it is important to recognise distress because the number of people affected is much greater than the number who screen positive for a possible mental health disorder. While not wanting to pathologise natural reactions, the distress and suffering of people who do not present with symptoms that are indicative of mental health disorders must not be ignored. Second, it challenges the orthodox view that major events have only minimal impact and very short-term effects for the majority of people, and hence this group does not warrant intervention. Major events may leave a lasting legacy for some people. Given the epidemiology of how many people in populations have experienced an emergency or major incident, the burden of psychosocial consequences is likely to be substantial for the general population and needs to be addressed by public health and social initiatives. Fostering personal and collective psychosocial resilience for all has the potential to buffer the ill effects of untoward events, and to decrease the risk of negative mental health outcomes.

Distress can be intense and may persist over long periods of time. The implication is that planning and

systems of surveillance should take into account these longer trajectories, not only for groups of people who suffer mental disorders but also for those whose distress does not come to the attention of services. In addition, it is important to recognise the breadth of possible long-term psychosocial consequences that are not best described as mental disorders for people who are exposed to emergencies and major incidents.

Certain experiences of distress – for example, somatic reactions – might serve as early markers of more severe and enduring difficulties, and including them in enhanced psychosocial screening and targeted psychosocial interventions may mitigate the risk of distress becoming chronic. Furthermore, more research drawing on ethnographic description of the wider range of experiences of distress, which is not limited by the search for symptoms and identifying pathology, could provide a more comprehensive understanding of people's common experiences of distress and enlighten the approach to intervention.

Social connectedness is a key predictor of well-being and recovery. Therefore the patterns of social withdrawal that are common in some distressed people have implications for assessment, surveillance, and intervention if people's access to the potentially positive effects of social support is limited. This points to the importance of tracking over time the severity of people's experiences and their behaviour, in order to reduce the risks of them withdrawing from social contacts.

Social support is often considered protective and central to coping and recovery. The findings from the Manchester Arena study suggest that a more nuanced and multidimensional understanding of social support is needed, which recognises that inappropriate types of informal social support, and of psychosocial care and mental healthcare, are not only unhelpful but may also function as secondary stressors, potentiate distress, and affect coping and recovery. Importantly, this research showed that secondary stressors were consequential and socially mediated, and therefore preventable with timely and appropriate psychosocial care and intervention.

Practical Aspects of Implementing the Principles

The fact that distress in the aftermath of emergencies is ubiquitous but not necessarily a function of psychopathology draws attention to unresolved matters in our use of language. One of these is the way in which the term distress is used. We recommend use of the term in relation to people who, during and after emergencies, have a range of experiences that are anticipated, and which are usually much broader than symptoms of common mental disorders. Viewing distress as composed of symptoms of undiagnosed disorders is less helpful. People have their own preferences and understandings with regard to making sense of their experiences, and there is often a large gap between how people understand and express their distress and suffering, and what professional practitioners and researchers 'count' as symptoms associated with abnormality and disorders in response to major events [12]. This suggests that the view of distress that is often used in mental healthcare and portrayed in public-facing information leaflets and digital resources may unintentionally reduce the likelihood that people's needs will be recognised. Therefore it may be necessary to modify the lists of common features of distress that are often included in these materials.

The ways in which we understand distress have real practical implications for the ways in which we respond to it. Assessments of distress that engage with the meaning and detail in a person's life are more likely to aid our understanding of the personal, social, and contextual factors that might mitigate or exacerbate their distress, in a way that 'screen and treat' algorithms designed to identify mental health disorders do not. Over-reliance on or inappropriate use of triage processes based on these algorithms is likely to underestimate distress and its impact on people's psychosocial functioning and potential demand for services. Hence some people are less likely to receive support when they might need it, or more likely to receive premature and inappropriate offers of biomedical intervention when they are not needed.

SIRE found that people who are distressed seek early and open access to authoritative sources of information and emotional support. This finding emphasises the importance of planning, care pathways, and outreach for all those people who are affected by major events. It argues for coordinating outreach and offering the expertise of professional practitioners employed at Mental Health Hubs by specialist mental health services. It also emphasises the importance of ease of early access to professional validation of people's distress, and access to psychosocial care if their distress persists.

The Impacts on People Affected by Emergencies, Incidents, and Disease Outbreaks

Next we hear directly three perspectives on the impacts of the same event, given by three members of a helicopter emergency medicine service (HEMS) team who work together within the subspecialty of pre-hospital emergency medicine (PHEM). All names have been changed.

The Consultant's Perspective

Today was challenging. As always, I have a lot on at work. Working in HEMS effectively means that I have two jobs, with all the meetings, projects, and extras that go with that, but my day of HEMS is always one of the highlights of my week. I often get to be really hands on, delivering care for my patients and training my colleagues.

It was my first time working with Sam, the new PHEM trainee, and I was planning to go over some of the basics with him, including procedures and policies, as I know he has a lot to get through before his official sign-off. Of course, you never really know how your HEMS day is going to go, and on this day we were particularly busy bouncing from job to job, which meant that all my well-intended plans for the day had to be put aside. It also meant that when this particular call came in during the late afternoon, we had not yet finished all of our routine equipment checks, I still had a pile of cases to review for governance from the previous few days, and we had not even had a chance to sit down to have our lunch!

When you receive a call-out, there's always a slight sense of foreboding, knowing that someone out there has been injured and needs your help. There are so many unknowns ahead, from being stood down en route because the case is not as serious as was first thought, to the unpredictable conditions on-scene, through to potentially arriving in the midst of a developing major incident. We had been told that two young children had been injured in a road traffic collision. Cases involving children always seem to heighten the emotions. I know that for patients to have their best chance of survival, I will need to apply my judgement, decision making, and skills with rapidity and without error or hesitation.

When we arrived on-scene there was a lot going on. A speeding car had hit a mother and her two children as they were crossing a quiet residential road, and the driver had not stopped. The mother was not hurt, but her 4-year-old and 2-year-old children had been badly injured. It was good to have Alex on the team that day. She is an experienced HEMS paramedic with whom I have developed a close working relationship over the years, and I know that she can be relied upon to deliver calm and meticulous care in the most difficult situations.

One of the challenges of being a consultant can be achieving the right balance between delivering optimum clinical care for your patients, and, at the same time, ensuring the best training experience possible for more junior members of the team, so that they are ready to handle the most difficult cases independently in the future. During this case, my trainee was having difficulty managing the airway and providing oxygen to one of the patients, and I knew that I had to step in to help immediately. I tried to do so in a way that did not undermine him, but knew that this would probably have knocked his confidence. Ultimately, though, I have a burden of responsibility to make sure that the patients get the treatment they need, when they need it.

Dealing with the emotional side of cases like this is really difficult. I am aware that Alex did a lot of the communication with both of the parents during the journey to hospital, while I was treating one of the children in the back of the ambulance. I know that Alex has two young children about the same age as our patients, and I wish I could have done more to support her with those conversations, which can be the most difficult part of the job. I tried to check in with her when we got back to base, and she said she was fine, but she was quieter than usual. I understand how important it is not to pressure people to talk about things if they are not ready to do so, and I know she has a close support network both at work and at home should she need to talk about how the case had made her feel.

We had a 'hot debrief' of some of the technical aspects of the case at the end of our shift, but I was mindful that we were already late off after a busy day. The trainee had a considerable amount of paperwork to complete for his training portfolio, and I knew that the case would be discussed again at our local governance meeting and also at the hospital's governance meetings. The trainee appeared to be receptive to my feedback, and we identified the skills that he needs to develop to enable him to handle difficult cases like this independently. I know how it can feel to have

your work scrutinised, especially when you think you could have performed better, and I am mindful of the need to prepare trainees for the extra level of scrutiny and visibility that working in pre-hospital care entails.

After a HEMS shift I try to switch off during my commute home, listen to a podcast, and try to create a buffer to separate my day at work from my evening at home. It can be hard to do this after days like today. I heard details of our case on the news this evening; the police had arrested someone whom they suspected had been under the influence of alcohol. I know that this will be one of those days that I think about a lot and which stays with me, probably for the rest of my career.

The PHEM Trainee's Perspective

Today was challenging. My day always starts very early. I chose to live near to the hospital where I do the other part of my job, and I accepted that it would be a long commute to the HEMS base. I had to move into a rental property hundreds of miles away from my family home, leaving my partner and children behind. However, this was my dream job that had been offered to me, and I could not pass up the opportunity to take it. Living so far away from home is quite isolating, I know very few people around here, and I try to work shifts close together so that I can get back to my family on my days off.

I have only been working in pre-hospital care for a few months, and there is still a novelty factor to it. As every case is so different, even though we practise and simulate all eventualities, this can never cover everything. Today came as a real shock, and I am not sure any amount of training can properly prepare anyone for what we see. We had lots of paperwork planned for today as I am working towards my sign-off, but I was glad to get out on the road. We did not fly to the scene – in fact we most often go by road, particularly to residential areas – so we had time to chat in the car on the way and to divide up tasks for when we arrived. Time seemed to stand still for a few seconds when we reached the scene, and there was so much noise and apparent chaos that I could not focus. I could hear someone screaming, whom I realised was the mother of the injured children. Then the consultant took charge and allocated me a task to focus on. He led confidently and showed a situational awareness I hope to emulate one day, but nevertheless I could see that he was shaken as well. I did my best to manage the airway of one of the patients, but my hands and brain did not seem to be connected. The harder I tried, the less effective I became, and the consultant had to step in and take over. Part of me felt embarrassed, but mostly I was just relieved. What if I had been on my own? I wonder if maybe I am not cut out for this, after all. The expectations are high, and I often feel that I fall short.

All of the other emergency services swung into action, and I could see the police taking statements. The driver had clearly fled the scene, and I felt immense, nauseating, almost distracting anger at this. I know moral distress is common, and I often wonder whether experienced clinicians eventually develop an ability to block this out.

Once we had dropped the patients off at the paediatric emergency department, conversation on the drive home was muted. I felt as if I had suddenly hit a wall of tiredness, but the day was not over. We managed a 'hot debrief', and I was relieved that the consultant and paramedic recognised how junior I am and helped me to identify some learning needs. Working in a small team has its benefits, and the camaraderie is certainly one of them.

I have a mountain of paperwork to finish for this shift and for several days earlier in the week. Although training in two specialties has its rewards – such as more career choices and a variety of practice environments – it also doubles the paperwork and exams, at huge financial and emotional cost. I feel as if I have been in training for ever, and look forward to the day when I do not have to be constantly assessed. However, I also recognise that governance and continuing professional development are an essential part of any clinician's practice, and nowhere more so than in the pre-hospital world, where certain emergencies are fortunately rare.

After I had spoken to my partner on the way home, I shed a few tears. It is hard to talk to someone who does not work in the medical field. How can I expect them to understand? I felt that I should have done better, I felt anger towards the driver, and I felt immense sadness for the parents. But I have to come back tomorrow for another shift, this time at night, when we see more stabbings and alcohol-related problems. I have never been good at sleeping during the day, and shift work really messes up my body clock. My parents ask me why I could not have chosen a specialty that works office hours! That is easy to answer – it is because I love my job. But today was a challenge, and I know that this will be one of those days that I think about a lot and which stays with me, probably for the rest of my career.

The HEMS Paramedic's Perspective

Today was challenging. Even though I have been a paramedic for over 20 years, and still enjoy my job, sometimes things get to me. Today I am working with one of the senior doctors and a new trainee. I like seeing the trainees come and go – you can watch them learn and grow as pre-hospital professionals and help to support them. Some days we operate independently as a small medical team, whereas other days we are working with different emergency services with dozens of other staff. Of course, pre-hospital teams are so much more than just the medical staff. Our pilots fly us to the scene, our control room staff and dispatchers make sure we get as much information as possible, and our blood delivery service drivers make sure we are stocked up with blood products that might save someone's life.

I try to fit in some physical exercise before work, though it is particularly unappealing on cold dark winter mornings. It is important to be physically fit in order to be able to lift equipment and patients without causing personal injury. Proportionally, women are under-represented in PHEM, but the only barriers I have come across are people's perceptions! I also feel that exercise helps to keep my mind balanced. It was certainly an important part of my return to work a few years ago after I had been experiencing burnout. It is not uncommon for pre-hospital staff to experience compassion fatigue, irritability, self-doubt, and feelings of defeat or isolation, and it is even more common for this not to be recognised at the time. It is often only with hindsight that such feelings are easy to spot. Now I am back on form I have spoken to colleagues and helped them to develop coping mechanisms when they experience similar feelings.

This afternoon's job was a hard one. I know the geography of the area like the back of my hand, so I drove us there quickly. I felt that I helped to keep the team together, and I supported the family meanwhile. The medical treatment and transport are what the public tend to see, but there is a lot that goes on both at the scene and afterwards with regards to family support, liaison with the police for reports, and debriefing. I could tell that both doctors were upset and angry about what had happened. It's hard not to sympathise with the family. I have children myself, and I often think 'What if it had been them?'

Later on, we heard that both children had died. I could not find a way of expressing my emotions in words, and I think I was pretty quiet for the rest of the shift. Was there anything we could have done differently? Did I say the right thing to those parents? Have they caught the driver? This will be a case for the coroner and maybe even for the criminal courts.

When I got home from work I snuck into my sleeping children's bedrooms, and I hugged them tight. We never know what each day holds. I am proud of what I do, but am reminded daily of the fragility of life. I know that this will be one of those days that I think about a lot and which stays with me, probably for the rest of my career.

References

1. Cerdá M, Bordelois PM, Galea S, Norris F, Tracy M, Koenen KC. The course of posttraumatic stress symptoms and functional impairment following a disaster: what is the lasting influence of acute vs. ongoing traumatic events and stressors? *Soc Psychiatry Psychiatr Epidemiol* 2013; **48**: 385–95.

2. Woodhouse S, Brown R, Ayers S. A social model of posttraumatic stress disorder: interpersonal trauma, attachment, group identification, disclosure, social acknowledgement, and negative cognitions. *J Theor Soc Psychol* 2018; **2**: 35–48.

3. Bonanno GA, Brewin CR, Kaniasty K, Greca AM. Weighing the costs of disaster: consequences, risks, and resilience in individuals, families, and communities. *Psychol Sci Public Interest* 2010; **11**: 1–49.

4. Galatzer-Levy IR, Huang SH, Bonanno GA. Trajectories of resilience and dysfunction following potential trauma: a review and statistical evaluation. *Clin Psychol Rev* 2018; **1**; 41–55.

5. Alexander DA. Early mental health interventions after disasters. *Adv Psychiatr Treat* 2005; **11**: 12–18.

6. Mennecier D, Hendrick S, De Mol J, Denis J. Experience of victims of Brussels' terrorists attacks: an interpretative phenomenological analysis. *Traumatology* 2020; https://doi.org/10.1037/trm0000249

7. Massazza A, Brewin CR, Joffe H. Feelings, thoughts, and behaviors during disaster. *Qual Health Res* 2021; **31**: 323–37.

8. Freh FM, Dallos R, Chung MC. An exploration of PTSD and coping strategies: response to the experience of being in a bomb attack in Iraq. *Traumatology* 2013; **19**: 87–94.

9. Stancombe J, Williams R, Drury J, Collins H, Lagan L, Barrett A, et al. People's experiences of distress and psychosocial care following a terrorist attack: interviews with survivors of the Manchester Arena bombing in 2017. *BJPsych Open* 2022; **8**: e41.

10. Garfin DR, Thompson RR, Holman EA. Acute stress and subsequent health outcomes: a systematic review. *J Psychosom Res* 2018; **112**: 107–13.

11. Thoresen S, Birkeland MS, Arnberg FK, Wentzel-Larsen T, Blix I. Long-term mental health and social support in victims of disaster: comparison with a general population sample. *BJPsych Open* 2019; **5**: e2.

12. Arnberg FK, Hultman CM, Michel PO, Lundin, T. Fifteen years after a ferry disaster: clinical interviews and survivors' self-assessment of their experience. *Eur J Psychotraumatol* 2013; **4**: 20650.

13. Vandentorren S, Pirard P, Sanna A, Aubert L, Motreff Y, Dantchev N, et al. Healthcare provision and the psychological, somatic and social impact on people involved in the terror attacks in January 2015 in Paris: cohort study. *Br J Psychiatry* 2018; **212**: 207–14.

14. Stensland SØ, Thoresen S, Jensen T, Wentzel-Larsen T, Dyb G. Early pain and other somatic symptoms predict posttraumatic stress reactions in survivors of terrorist attacks: the Longitudinal Utøya Cohort Study. *J Trauma Stress* 2020; **33**: 1060–70.

15. Ehlers A, Clark DM. A cognitive model of posttraumatic stress disorder. *Behav Res Ther* 2000; **38**: 319–45.

16. Williams R, Ntontis E, Alfadhli K, Drury J, Amlôt R. A social model of secondary stressors in relation to disasters, major incidents and conflict: implications for practice. *Int J Disaster Risk Reduct* 2021; **63**: 102436.

The Impact of Emergencies, Terrorism, and Disease on Children and Their Families

Prathiba Chitsabesan, Brian Jacobs, and Raphael Kelvin

Introduction

Emergencies, terrorism, and disease have impacts on children's and families' mental wellbeing, lives, and routines. Psychosocial reactions are influenced by the nature and extent of their exposure, by vulnerabilities and strengths, and particularly by family and social support. Almost all adverse childhood experiences are likely to amplify the effects of pandemics and disasters. Social support, connectedness, and social scaffolding help to mitigate adversity, and promote wellbeing and recovery. This chapter highlights the evidence base and some implications for policy and practice.

Mental Health and Wider Impacts on Children and Young People

Childhood traumas are defined as events that include death or threatened death, serious injury or accident, or sexual violence [1]. After traumatic events, most children show transient responses – for example, they may become tearful, anxious, or withdrawn. They may struggle to sleep, complain about headaches or stomach aches, or become irritable as they struggle to cope with their emotions. These are anticipated psychosocial responses that usually subside within a few weeks or months in most children. However, sometimes they persist and may impair children's or young people's functioning.

A range of surveys conducted in England during the COVID-19 pandemic found that children commonly worried about the possibility that family members might die from the virus, about their own education, and about the future [2]. Most young people also reported increased loneliness; this increased with their age. Young people linked this loneliness to feeling anxious and to lower life satisfaction [3]. Children and young people who were lonely were also 5.8–40 times more likely to reach the clinical cut-off score on rating scales for depression, and were 1.63–5.49 times more likely to report feeling anxious [3].

A literature review of the mental health consequences for children and young people who were exposed to disasters and major incidents also found significant increases in such consequences overall [4]. Data from meta-analyses of symptoms of post-traumatic stress disorder (PTSD) suggest that 15.9% of children and young people aged 2–18 years who were exposed to severe stressors met the clinical threshold for PTSD [5], and the prevalence of depression was in the range of 7.5–44.8% [6].

Unfortunately, many studies lack comparison data gathered before the disaster or incident under consideration, and rely on convenience samples based on screening programmes rather than random or controlled samples. In England, a national survey was conducted in 2017 and followed up in 2020 during the COVID-19 pandemic. This research, which used the Strengths and Difficulties Questionnaire (SDQ), a screening measure that is widely employed in children's mental health services, showed that one in six children (16.0%) aged 5–16 years in England was identified as having a probable mental disorder in 2020. This is an increase from one in nine children (10.8%) in 2017 [7].

Approaches to responding to the needs of children, young people, and their families during the COVID-19 pandemic are examined in more detail by Betty Pfefferbaum in Chapter 30.

Poor mental health among children and young people usually peaks within 1 year after a disaster or incident, and then often, but not always, declines [8,9]. A large group of young people appears to be unaffected, but some of them develop mental health difficulties later; some have problems that endure for years [9]. These different patterns are associated with many personal factors as well as with secondary stressors (see Chapter 5 and 9), such as the economic impact on the family, or stressors that arise from the trauma and its effects on the family through, for example, divorce or domestic violence [10,11].

Social and Economic Factors That Place Children and Families at Higher Risk: Secondary Stressors

It is important to identify whether emergencies are sudden, brief, and transient, or whether they are repeated events that result in sustained stress or circumstances that alter people's lifestyles, or continuing events that persist over a long period (see Chapter 30). Different patterns vary in their social and financial impacts.

The law of unintended consequences is centrally important. Secondary stressors (see Chapters 5 and 9) can be created as accidental side effects of well-intentioned and otherwise sensible policies. It is often the case that these secondary stressors affect the mental health of many more children and young people than do the direct effects of a disaster. They also include the impacts of social isolation, disturbance to daily routine, exposure to domestic violence, family illness, effects of home schooling or shielding, parental anxiety, and financial pressures. Disruptions to the support linked to going to school or college, which provides education, social interactions, stability, and routine, can lead to some children and young people feeling isolated. This has been linked with worse wellbeing and mental health for some children who have pre-existing needs [2].

The Ebola epidemic in 2014–2016 had a pronounced socioeconomic impact in the countries affected by it. There was substantial loss of investment, as well as reduced agricultural production and cross-border trade, due to restrictions. There was also a significant impact on the workforce, reflecting breakdown of important aspects of society.

Unemployment is a particular risk factor for young adults, with an association between unemployment and poor mental health outcomes having been identified in 16- to 30-year-olds [12].

In summary, both direct and indirect effects of emergencies, incidents, and disease outbreaks have an impact on the mental health of children and young people.

Factors That Affect the Risk of Mental Health Problems

Few studies have established whether the nature of the incident influences the mental health consequences for young people. Rates of post-traumatic symptoms (PTS) appear to be comparable across disasters due to human activity and natural hazards [8], which suggests that the type of disaster does not influence outcomes as much as the factors involved in each person's experience (for further information, see Chapter 30).

There are many factors that affect the risk of children and adults developing more serious problems, such as mental health disorders. A number of studies have reported a dose–response relationship between the amount and intensity of traumatic exposure and the risk of developing PTSD and other psychological problems [13]. It is not just being nearby, but also the 'severity' of the experience that matters – for example, injury, witnessing death, or experiencing the destruction of one's home [8,14].

Trickey et al. found in their meta-analysis that perceived life threat during trauma was reported as a risk factor for PTSD, together with negative appraisals and emotions [15]. They concluded that the relationship between pre-trauma life events and PTSD is significant but modest by comparison with certain peri-trauma and post-trauma factors. A study of young people directly affected by the Omagh Bomb also found that exposure alone is not a precise predictor of risk, but rather it is the aspects of trauma to which young people are exposed (seeing someone they think is dying), what they are thinking during the event (thinking they themselves are going to die), and the cognitive mechanisms employed thereafter, particularly if the young person develops negative beliefs about him- or herself or ruminates [16]. A review of post-trauma factors for children and adolescents also identified social support as important, and poor family functioning was a stronger risk factor for PTSD than was poor parental mental health [15].

Children and young people of all ages can be affected by disasters. However, the impact may be greater for those who are older young people through loss of opportunities, including job insecurity, increased by the societal crisis.

The importance of gender is uncertain; some studies have found that girls have poorer mental health outcomes. The association between female gender and PTSD in children and adolescents increases with age [15], which may be partly explained by the tendency for rumination to be more common in girls.

The ways in which ethnic background influences mental health outcomes in children and young people remain relatively little understood. Most studies do not have sufficient power to analyse subgroup differences in ethnicity, while others have found no significant differences during disasters [7]. There is as much difference within ethnic groups as between them, which suggests that responses are heterogeneous and personal.

Children who have pre-existing mental health or neurodevelopmental needs may be at greater risk of poor mental health outcomes. For example, a prospective study of Hong Kong students during the SARS epidemic found that a pre-existing tendency to experience anxiety may predict higher levels of anxiety during a pandemic [17]. Young people with a disorder on the autism spectrum seemed to have heightened anxiety and more mental health difficulties during COVID lockdown compared with their neurotypical peers [18].

Social factors – for example, being the child of key workers – may also have a negative effect on mental health. A survey of 13- to 24-year-olds in England found higher reporting of COVID-related trauma and PTSD symptoms, somatic symptoms, and depression among children of key workers [19]. Most varieties of adverse experiences in childhood increase or intensify during pandemics and following disasters due to natural hazards or human activity. Table 6.1 lists the risk factors for poor mental health outcomes.

Relative poverty or being a young carer may have an impact due to loss of routine, sleep, or support networks [2]. Children with caring responsibilities may need to look after siblings who are not in school,

Table 6.1 Risk factors for poor mental health outcomes

- Degree of injury sustained
- Witnessing death (seeing someone one thinks is dying)
- Perceived life threat (thinking one is going to die)
- Experiencing the destruction of one's home
- Negative cognitions about oneself or anxious ruminations after the event
- Gender (female)
- Age (older adolescents and young adults)
- Pre-existing mental health or neurodevelopmental needs
- Parental mental health needs
- Poor family functioning
- Limited access to social support
- Children of keyworkers
- Young carers
- Children living in poverty/social deprivation

may lose contact with local services, and may have difficulty with home learning, and have unremitting responsibilities.

A study of mental health outcomes for parents and children in the USA who were affected by recent epidemics and pandemics, including SARS and H1N1 events, found that 85.7% of parents who reached cut-off scores on scales for PTSD had children who also reached clinical cut-off scores for PTSD. Among parents who did not meet the criteria for PTSD, only 14.3% had children with PTSD symptoms – that is, there is a sixfold increase in the risk of developing childhood PTSD if a parent has the disorder [10].

In England, a national survey conducted during the COVID-19 pandemic [7] found that the proportion of children with a probable mental disorder increased to 30.2% (from 23.2% in 2017) for children with a parent who showed distress, compared with 9.3% (from 8.5% in 2017) for children whose parents showed no distress. This represents a 2.7- to 3.2-fold increase in risk. However, these associations are complex and cannot explain causality.

Childhood Development and the Neurobiological Impact of Trauma

We are beginning to obtain clues about the biological paths that underlie some of these observations. They include an interplay of genetic inheritance with environmental experiences. Early relationships are pivotal for people's development. The way in which parents interact with their children relates to their own attachment relationships, capacity for reflective functioning, and current experiences, including having mental health problems.

Adverse experiences in early life have profound effects on developing brains. Repeated early-life stress alters the corticotropin-releasing factor system, leading to increased sensitivity to stress. Subsequent exposure to traumatising events, including emergencies, terrorism, or disease outbreaks, may reactivate memories of stress and loss. This can have lifelong impacts on physical and mental health.

Psychosocial problems may also have neurobiological consequences for the offspring of exposed people. The epigenome can be viewed as the interface between the genome and the environment. It can shape gene function and phenotypic expression in response to the environment. Studies on children of survivors of the Holocaust and prisoner-of-war camps during the Second World War have questioned whether trauma-induced epigenetic modifications can be passed from traumatised people to subsequent generations of offspring. A review of the emerging literature found accumulating evidence of an enduring effect of trauma exposure being passed to offspring transgenerationally via the epigenetic inheritance mechanism of DNA methylation alterations, which have the capacity to change the expression of genes [20]. However, further research is required, including longitudinal studies.

Exposing Health Inequity and Inequality: Their Relationship to Pandemics and Disease Clustering

In the 1990s, Merrill Singer and his colleagues realised that diseases, social context, and related factors interact synergistically to multiply the impact on the health of individual people and whole populations – an approach they called syndemics [21]. That approach examines the patterns and pathways through which these factors interact biologically and socially both for individual people and within populations. It also examines the ways in which social inequity contributes to disease clustering as well as to enhanced vulnerability.

Healthcare services are not used equally by everyone. Income, ethnicity, employment status, and education affect whether people access healthcare. This is an important driver of healthcare inequity. It drives poorer outcomes during times of crisis for some sections of society, demonstrating the notion of syndemics. Wider governmental and societal responses can amplify this disparity quite accidentally, as in the impacts of pandemic lockdowns on education and on vulnerable families' finances. Critically, these factors combine in complex ways to put some people at much greater risk [22]. In addition, measures taken to control the spread of a pandemic or of other disasters, such as fire or flood, may have unequal socioeconomic impacts, which are likely to deepen health inequities in the long term. Some of the social and educational aspects of epidemics and pandemics are covered in Chapter 31.

Children from the poorest 20% of households are four times more likely to have serious mental health difficulties by the age of 11 years than those from the wealthiest 20% [23]. Poverty is associated with poor mental health. This effect is compounded by the economic impact of critical events [23]. Increased family financial strain during a pandemic is strongly associated with poor mental health of the children [7]. This impact is likely to last for several years.

Another inequality is concern about the digital divide. Some young people, including those living in poverty or those with a disability, may be less likely to have good access to or even engage with digital support from schools or healthcare services following emergencies or pandemics. This contributes to further inequity.

There are limitations to approaches that identify and address personal risk factors without recognising the complex non-linear interrelationships between them. In contrast to the situation with infectious diseases research, systems modelling has yet to pervade mental health research [24]. Potentially it can help us to understand complex causal pathways to and from psychosocial distress, mental ill health, suicidal behaviour, and utilisation of healthcare services. Better understanding would allow development of more sophisticated tools for rapid deployment in response to national and regional threats to mental health after incidents, disasters, and pandemics. Infrastructure to support collection of data from across different systems, including health, education, and social services, is essential for developing and refining models that recognise the importance of the socioeconomic determinants of mental health.

Resilience and Protective Factors

Psychosocial resilience is built on relationships – it is systemic and social. It is dynamic with time and circumstance, and affects people's ability to respond to stress. It includes people's own psychosocial resources, as well as offers of and acceptance of support from families, friends, and other important adults, such as teachers. This social scaffolding has substantial effects on how people can mitigate adversity, promote well-being, and recover during and after emergencies and pandemics [25,26]. It can offer access to wider community support networks. Our capacity and capability for learning from experience and personal growth in all of its forms are critical throughout life (for more information, see Section 3 of this book).

We know that people's social connectedness and access to social support have substantial effects in building their resilience and promoting their well-being and recovery after emergencies and pandemics. In a systematic review of survivors of the Wenchuan

Table 6.2 Key principles to support children and families affected by emergencies, incidents, and disease outbreaks

- Create a coordinated strategic approach delivered and working across government, systems, and agencies to support children and their families
- Focus on the pivotal importance of relationships for parents, family, education, and peer environments for children's wellbeing and mental health
- Consider the wellbeing and mental health of parents, carers, and education staff, and their ability to support and nurture children and young people
- Recognise the importance of public health initiatives to build resilient empowered communities that can address health inequalities and inequities
- Recognise the importance of prevention and early intervention to support resilient responses and limit the risk of escalation of mental health needs and poorer outcomes
- Create stepped/graduated support facilities which acknowledge that children and young people are likely to have a range of different experiences, needs, and symptoms
- Provide clear and consistent communication to all key stakeholders, including young people, parents, and professionals, in relation to the expected course and outcome of people's psychosocial responses and effective strategies for responding to their needs
- Ensure that support is coordinated with pathways to access a range of multi-agency services as needed, in which there is joint work involving all professionals and the voluntary sector
- Monitor children and young people in a low-level manner, but include clear escalation processes/pathways and access to specialist mental healthcare
- Identify active support for vulnerable groups of children and young people, including those who have pre-existing mental health and neurodevelopmental needs
- Plan for fluctuation of impacts over time depending on other factors, including secondary stressors
- Recognise the importance of interventions that are based on best evidence as well as positive relationships
- Aim to do no further harm, and recognise that providing inappropriate support may do harm

Earthquake, it was noted that support from teachers and social support were positive factors for children's mental health [11]. Lack of social support is associated with an increased risk of developing depression [6] and PTSD [15].

Other factors associated with positive mental health for children after emergencies and pandemics include:

- positive coping behaviour
- strong family relationships
- being able to make change happen, and having a sense of owning what one does (agency)
- the emotional tools to self-regulate and manage stress
- peer and community engagement
- enjoying and engaging in education
- using support
- physical activities.

Conclusion: Implications for Policy and Practice

The information presented in this chapter has emphasised the importance in emergencies, incidents, and disease outbreaks of coordinated system-wide strategic responses that are delivered across government, systems, and agencies to support children and their families (see Table 6.2).

The mental health of caregivers is pivotal to the mental health and wellbeing of children and families, and should be a prime focus of intervention [27]. Interventions provided early on after an incident that validate people's experiences (see Chapter 5), early access to empathic reassurance, and explanation of children's and young people's anticipated responses should be universally available, because social scaffolds buttressed by parents, teachers, and other key adults facilitate recovery. Non-specialist support (psychosocial care) of this kind provided by relatives and friends but supported by other adults trained in the principles of psychological first aid is not the same as professionally delivered mental healthcare. The two have different intentions but share some key principles [28].

Schools and colleges also have important roles in prevention by supporting resilient responses and maintaining the wellbeing of children and young people and staff alike.

The majority of children and young people who experience distress are likely to improve over time, especially if they are not exposed to secondary stressors. Screening after large-scale events can help to identify at-risk children [29]. Children and young people who experience mental health disorders should have access to evidence-based interventions and treatment [30] (for further information, see Chapter 30).

References

1. American Psychiatric Association (APA). *Diagnostic and Statistical Manual of Mental Disorders* 5th ed. APA, 2013.

2. Public Health England. *Impact on Mental Health. Chapter 7: Children and Young People.* Public Health England, 2020 (www.gov .uk/government/publications/ covid-19-mental-health-and-wellbeing-surveillance-report/7-children-and-young-people).

3. Loades ME, Chatburn E, Higson-Sweeney N, Reynolds S, Shafran R, Brigden A, et al. Rapid systematic review: the impact of social isolation and loneliness on the mental health of children and adolescents in the context of COVID-19. *J Am Acad Child Adolesc Psychiatry* 2020; **59**: 1218–39.

4. Thomas-Meyer M, Allan S, Tyrrell C, Bealey C, Cross M, Gathercole C, et al. *A Rapid Review of Mental Health Impacts of Infectious Disease Epidemics and Major Incidents on Children and Young People: Prevalence, Risk Factors and Interventions; Summary and Key Points.* Public Health England, 2020.

5. Alisic E, Zalta AK, Van Wesel F, Larsen SE, Hafstad GS, Hassanpour K, et al. Rates of post-traumatic stress disorder in trauma-exposed children and adolescents: meta-analysis. *Br J Psychiatry* 2014; **204**: 335–40.

6. Tang B, Liu X, Liu Y, Xue C, Zhang L. A meta-analysis of risk factors for depression in adults and children after natural disasters. *BMC Public Health* 2014; **14**: 623.

7. NHS Digital. Mental Health of Children and Young People in England, 2020; Wave 1 follow up to the 2017 survey, 2020 (https:// digital.nhs.uk/data-and-information/publications/ statistical/mental-health-of-children-and-young-people-in-england/2020-wave-1-follow-up [cited 4 Jan 2021])

8. Furr JM, Comer JS, Edmunds JS, Kendall PC. Disasters and youth: a meta-analytic examination of posttraumatic stress. *J Consult Clin Psychol* 2010; **78**: 765–80.

9. Wang C, Chan CL, Rainbow TH. Prevalence and trajectory of psychopathology among child and adolescent survivors of disasters: a systematic review of epidemiological studies across 1987–2011. *Soc Psychiatry Psychiatr Epidemiol* 2013; **48**: 1697–720.

10. Sprang G, Silman M. Posttraumatic stress disorder in parents and youth after health-related disasters. *Disaster Med Public Health Prep* 2013; **7**: 105–10.

11. Hong C, Efferth T. Systematic review on post-traumatic stress disorder among survivors of the Wenchuan earthquake. *Trauma Violence Abuse* 2016; **17**: 542–61.

12. Bartelink VHM, Ya KZ, Guldbrandsson K, Bremberg S. Unemployment among young people and mental health: a systematic review. *Scand J Public Health* 2020; **48**: 544–58.

13. Slone M, Mann S. Effects of war, terrorism and armed conflict on young children: a systematic review. *Child Psychiatry Hum Dev* 2016; **47**: 950–65.

14. Gordon-Hollingsworth AT, Yao N, Huijing C, Mingyi Q, Sen C. Understanding the impact of natural disasters on psychological outcomes in youth from Mainland China: a meta-analysis of risk and protective factors for post-traumatic stress disorder symptoms. *J Child Adolesc Trauma* 2018; **11**: 205–26.

15. Trickey D, Siddaway AP, Meiser-Stedman R, Serpell L, Field AP. A meta-analysis of risk factors for post-traumatic stress disorder in children and adolescents. *Clin Psychol Rev* 2012; **32**: 122–38.

16. Duffy M, McDermott M, Percy A, Ehlers A, Clark D, Fitzgerald M, et al. The effects of the Omagh bomb on adolescent mental health: a school-based study. *BMC Psychiatry* 2015; **15**: 18.

17. Cheng C, Cheung MWL. Psychological responses to outbreak of severe acute respiratory syndrome: a prospective, multiple time-point study. *J Pers* 2005; **73**: 261–85.

18. Pearcey S, Shum A, Waite P, Creswell C. *COVID-19: Supporting Parents, Adolescents and Children during Epidemics. Supplementary Report 03: Differences in Pandemic Anxiety, Parent/Carer Stressors and Reported Needs Between Parent/ Carers of Children with and without ASD; Change Over Time in Mental Health for Children with ASD.* Westminster Foundation, 2020 (https://cospaceoxford.org/ wp-content/uploads/2020/04/Co-SPACE-supp-report-03_06-09-21 .pdf).

19. Levita L, Gibson Miller J, Hartman TK, Murphy J, Shevlin M, McBride O, et al. *Report 2: Impact of Covid-19 on Young People Aged 13–24 in the UK – Preliminary Findings.* Center for

Open Science, 2020 (https://psyarxiv.com/s32j8/)

20. Youssef NA, Lockwood L, Su S, Hao G, Rutten B. The effects of trauma, with or without PTSD, on the transgenerational DNA methylation alterations in human offsprings. *Brain Sci* 2018; **8**: 83.

21. Singer M, Bulled N, Ostrach B, Mendenhall E. Syndemics and the biosocial conception of health. *Lancet* 2017; **389**: 941–50.

22. Marmot M, Allen J, Boyce T, Goldblatt P, Morrison J. *Health Equity in England: The Marmot Review 10 Years On*. Institute of Health Equity, 2020.

23. Morrison GL, Joshi H, Parsonage M, Schoon I. *Children of the New Century*. Centre for Mental Health and University College London, 2015.

24. Cassidy R, Singh NS, Schiratti PR, Semwanga A, Binyaruka P, Sachingonu N, et al. Mathematical modelling for health systems research: a systematic review of system dynamics and agent-based models. *BMC Health Serv Res* 2019; **19**: 845.

25. Williams R, Drury J. The nature of psychosocial resilience and its significance for managing mass emergencies, disasters and terrorism. In *Rebuilding Sustainable Communities for Children and Their Families After Disasters: A Global Survey* (ed. A Awotona): 57–75. Cambridge Scholars Publishing, 2010.

26. Haslam C, Haslam A, Cruwys T. Social scaffolding: supporting the development of positive social identities and agency. In *Social Scaffolding; Applying the Lessons of Contemporary Social Science to Health and Healthcare* (eds R Williams, V Kemp, SA Haslam, C Haslam, S Bhui, S Bailey): 244–56. Cambridge University Press, 2019.

27. Rousseau C, Uzma J, Kamaldeep B, Boudjarane M. Consequences of 9/11 and the war on terror on children's and young adults' mental health: a systematic review of the past 10 years. *Clin Child Psychol Psychiatry* 2015; **20**: 173–93.

28. Williams R, Kemp VJ, Alexander DA. The psychosocial and mental health of people who are affected by conflict, catastrophes, terrorism, adversity and displacement. In *Conflict and Catastrophe Medicine: A Practical Guide* (eds J Ryan, BA Hopperus, C Beadling, A Mozumder, DM Nott): 805–49. Springer, 2014.

29. French P, Barrett A, Allsopp K, Williams R, Brewin C, Hind D, et al. Psychological screening of adults and young people following the Manchester Arena incident. *BJPsych Open* 2019; **5**: e85.

30. Danese A, Smith P, Chitsabesan P, Dubicka B. Child and adolescent mental health amidst emergencies and disasters. *Br J Psychiatry* 2020; **216**: 159–62.

Chapter

7

The Impacts of Urbanising the World's Population on Emergencies, Incidents, Disasters, and Disease Outbreaks

Tim Healing

Introduction

Over half of the world population of 7.6 billion now lives in urban areas, and UN-Habitat estimates that the world urban population will increase to 6.7 billion by 2050 (68% of the world's population), with 90% of the expected growth occurring in low- and middle-income countries in Asia and Africa, driven by expanding economies [1]. At present about one-third of urban dwellers live in informal settlements, many of which have little in the way of services or infrastructure, and at least 1 billion live in slums. The global rural population is expected to decline from 3.4 billion to 3.1 billion by 2050 [2]. This chapter reviews the impacts that increasing urbanisation has on the ability of people to respond to emergencies.

The World Bank has noted that expansion of urban areas is expected to add 1.2 million square kilometres of new urban built-up area to the world by 2050, putting pressure on agricultural and recreational land and on natural resources [3]. It also reports that cities already account for two-thirds of global energy consumption and more than 70% of greenhouse gas emissions. By 2030 the world is likely to have 43 megacities (cities with more than 10 million inhabitants), mostly in developing regions. At present there are 33 megacities, with about one in twelve people living in them, but about half of the world's urban dwellers live in smaller cities, with fewer than 500,000 inhabitants, and a number of these smaller cities in Africa and Asia are among the fastest-growing urban areas [2].

The increase in urbanisation is likely to influence all aspects of human activity – economic, social, and environmental. Many of the low- and low-middle-income countries where so much of this development is likely to occur are those least able to support it. Urban development in these countries is likely to produce large amounts of inadequate housing, the cities will lack proper infrastructures, and healthcare provision is likely to be inadequate or lacking. Stagnant economies, corruption, poor governance, and a lack of planning skills

are likely to produce environments in which poverty will abound. These trends can already be seen with slums and informal settlements proliferating, especially in developing countries.

Until quite recently, much of the focus of humanitarian activity was on rural environments. More people lived and worked there, and many of them were among the poorest members of the populations of low-income countries, with least resilience to disasters. Many major disasters (e.g., famines) occur in rural environments, and refugee camps are often located there. Now the emphasis is moving towards urban areas. However, urban and rural areas cannot be considered separately. Disruption of food production in rural areas in turn disrupts supplies of food to urban centres, and disruption of goods and services in urban areas has impacts on farmers and rural populations.

Box 7.1 Some definitions with examples

The terms city and town are used to refer to large urban areas, although the nomenclature often depends on local usage. In the UK, a city is frequently a town with a cathedral, and may be quite small. Either term may refer to the urban area (the area of continuous urban development) or the metropolitan area (largely an economic definition comprising a densely populated urban core with its less populated, economically connected, surrounding territories, sharing industry, infrastructure, and housing, parts of which may be quite rural).

Tokyo, for example, is the most populous metropolitan area in the world, with a population of over 37 million. It has an urban area of 3,925 square kilometres, but the metropolitan area as a whole covers 14,034 square kilometres.

Many cities are very densely populated, particularly in less well-developed parts of the world. For example, Manila has 1.8 million people living in an area of 42.9 square kilometres, which corresponds to a population density of around 41,500 per square kilometre, compared with 6,160 per square kilometre in Tokyo.

The Nature of Urban Areas

Sphere is a project initiated by humanitarian non-governmental organisations (NGOs) and the International Red Cross and Red Crescent Movement. It is designed to improve the quality of their actions during disaster response, and to be held accountable for them. The *Sphere Handbook* is an internationally recognised set of common principles and universal minimum standards for humanitarian response. It notes that urban areas typically differ from other contexts in terms of density, with a higher density of people, houses, infrastructure, laws, and cultures in a relatively small area, and with social, ethnic, political, linguistic, religious, and economically diverse groups living in close proximity to each other [4]. The social dynamics of urban environments tend to be more fluid and changeable than those of rural areas, with high mobility and rapidly shifting power relationships. Urban environments tend to impose more market pressures on populations, and low-income groups struggle to find jobs, affordable accommodation, and health services.

Urban areas are inherently fragile. Many cities in lower- and middle-income nations are desperately overcrowded, and their populations are faced with challenges that include poor building construction, poor access, poor or absent waste disposal and drainage, limited access to water (which is also likely to be contaminated), irregular supplies of food, unsafe and unreliable power supplies, inadequate emergency services, and crime and violence. Healthcare is often poor or absent, and this lack is associated with an increased risk of communicable diseases [5].

Climate change has the potential to increase risks to urban inhabitants, especially poor urban people, by damaging and degrading systems and infrastructure and by increasing the risk of disease [2]. Cities in low-lying areas and close to the sea are particularly at risk from storm surges and rising sea levels, and almost 500 million urban residents live in coastal areas. In the 136 largest coastal cities, 100 million people are exposed to coastal floods [6]. About 90% of urban expansion in developing countries – much of it informal and in unplanned settlements – is in or near hazard-prone areas [6].

Supply Chains and Infrastructure

The populations of cities are wholly dependent on functioning supply chains. Few urban dwellers can maintain stores of food for more than a few days, and many live wholly from day to day due to poverty, lack of storage capacity, or both. Much of the world's supply of food and goods is provided on a 'just-in-time' basis, and interruptions of this system can rapidly lead to shortages.

Provision of power, food, and clean water, as well as disposal of solid and liquid waste, requires a complex infrastructure that has to be maintained. The populations of cities need healthcare facilities, emergency services, educational and recreational facilities, and public transport. Urban areas require competent local government and sufficient finance to ensure that all of these services are provided in an equitable fashion and function effectively.

Urban Poverty

As the population of the world and of urban areas has increased, there has been a concomitant increase in the numbers of people who live in urban poverty, mostly in low- and middle-income nations. UN-Habitat reports that about 1 billion urban dwellers still live in poor-quality overcrowded housing, in slums or informal settlements with a lack of basic infrastructure and services [1].

Urban dwellers in high-income nations have at least some capacity to cope with adverse events, due to a whole network of institutions, infrastructure, insurance, services, and regulations. Often people who are living in low- and middle-income nations lack such protection. In nations (mainly high-income ones) that have undertaken measures such as earthquake-proofing buildings, earthquakes that affect urban areas are less likely to cause large losses of life and damage to property. For example, on 12 January 2010 the island of Haiti experienced an earthquake that registered at 7.0 on the Richter scale. On 27 February 2010 an earthquake of magnitude 8.8 struck Chile, releasing about 500 times as much energy as the Haiti earthquake. Although both countries were devastated, the destruction was far worse in Haiti, where an estimated 230,000 people were killed, compared with a death toll of 525 in Chile. The difference appears to have been largely due to the far more stringent building codes in Chile compared with those in Haiti [7].

Although economic losses due to a disaster, such as an earthquake, may be large in high-income nations, they can generally be absorbed by society. By contrast, similar disasters in cities in low- and middle-income nations not only cause major loss of life, but also poverty. Lack of financial resilience, and the absence of a safety net mean that even quite small economic losses can be catastrophic.

Informal Settlements and Slums

People who live in informal settlements usually lack any official documentation of ownership of their land and home. Settlements of this nature lack infrastructure, such as piped water, sewers, drains, and paved roads, and most have little or no public provision for healthcare or emergency services.

About 1 billion urban dwellers live in slums [8]. In operational terms, UN-Habitat defines a slum household as lacking one or more of the following indicators: a durable housing structure; access to clean water; access to improved sanitation; sufficient living space; secure tenure.

Urban dwellers who live in informal settlements and slums, including those in wealthier cities, frequently inhabit poorly built dwellings. Yet the importance of a dwelling, however badly built, cannot be overestimated. It provides a home for a family, a focus for social life, and a measure of privacy and safety. It is also a place of work for many families, and a means by which they can access income and services. Its location in relation to income-earning opportunities and services is often more important than its size, quality, or legality, which is why so many informal settlements are located on marginal lands, such as flood plains, river banks, and steep slopes. These are often the only sites within a city close to centres of employment that low-income groups can occupy. Loss of this housing exacerbates poverty, and usually there is little or no compensation when homes in these areas are damaged or destroyed. Few of these householders have insurance. Rehousing may mean relocation and loss of local contacts, familiar social structures, and easy access to earning opportunities [5].

Disasters in Urban Settings

Urban poverty and disaster risk are often closely linked [9]. The nature of urban areas, especially overcrowded cities in poorer countries, can magnify the effects of many of these risks. Urban dwellers, particularly those who are economically disadvantaged, are frequently compelled to live in high-risk areas. They are also limited in their capacity to reduce risk, due to inadequate income, the need to live close to work and

earning opportunities, high land prices, limited political influence, and corruption. Equally, urban authorities often lack the knowledge, financial capacity, and, sometimes, willingness to reduce risks and vulnerabilities.

Frequently, poorly constructed buildings collapse, and they are vulnerable in earthquake zones. Often buildings such as these are crowded, and collapses frequently lead to disproportionate numbers of injuries and deaths. One of the worst such events was the collapse of the eight-storey factory building in Savar, on the outskirts of Dhaka, in April 2013, due to structural failure. The death toll was 1,134, and approximately 2,500 people were injured. Poor access, combined with inadequate emergency services, means that disasters such as this, and others such as fires, may be difficult to deal with effectively in this type of environment.

Disaster Resilience

Cities can be made more resilient to disasters, but this requires many different and interwoven activities [10]. Organisation and coordination are needed if disaster risks are to be understood and reduced. The participation of citizen groups and civil society is essential, and local alliances must be built. All government departments must understand their roles in disaster risk reduction and preparedness, and should budget for disaster risk reduction. However, many urban authorities lack the knowledge, financial capacity, or willingness to reduce the risks and vulnerabilities facing their constituents, especially the most deprived people. Corruption frequently prevents progress towards support for those people most at risk.

There must be incentives for all sectors of society to invest in risk reduction. Education programmes are of great value in building resilience, by ensuring adequate emergency preparedness and effective disaster responses. These programmes need to be developed in conjunction with local communities, and if those communities are to accept the programmes, they must have ownership of key aspects of developing and performing them. Local people need to be trained to share advice on risk reduction with the members of their communities. They should be advised to work with the planners to assess the impact of this advice on the risk reduction behaviour of those communities and to modify the advice in the light of feedback from their communities. However, these steps must be accompanied by the development of centres in which training and support can be provided, stocks of necessary materials can be established, and work can be undertaken. Funds must be made available to pay for these facilities, materials, and worker's salaries, so that the completed training can be put to use without delay.

Exciting developments in appropriate technologies and novel solutions to problems are showing that major improvements in resilience, lifestyle, and health can be achieved at low cost.

The COVID-19 Pandemic

Close-packed cities with poor infrastructure are fertile grounds for the uncontrolled spread of communicable diseases, and a lack of good healthcare can worsen the situation. Crowded urban areas are particularly vulnerable to outbreaks of readily transmissible diseases, especially those which, like COVID-19, are spread by the respiratory route [11,12]. In July 2020 the UN published a document entitled 'Policy Brief: COVID-19 in an Urban World' [8], which pointed out that, at the time of publication, urban areas had become the epicentre of the pandemic, with 90% of all reported COVID-19 cases. The brief also noted that 'the size of their populations and their high level of global and local interconnectivity make them particularly vulnerable to the spread of the virus'. The report went on to note that 'In many cities every facet of urban life has been affected, including access, equity, finance, safety, joblessness, public services, infrastructure and transport, all of which are disproportionately affecting the most vulnerable people in society'.

Many countries have reported that the sharpest increases in numbers of COVID-19 cases occurred in urban areas, and that rates of infection were much higher in those areas. In the UK, the Department for Environment, Food & Rural Affairs (DEFRA) reported that by 6 March 2021 there had been a total of 4,350 cases per 100,000 people living in rural areas, compared with 7,217 per 100,000 people living in urban areas (excluding London, where numbers were even higher) [13]. In the USA, Rajib Paul and his colleagues examined the data on urban and rural spread of the infection over a 3-week period in April 2020, and found that the mean prevalence of COVID-19 increased from 3.6 to 43.6 per 100,000 people in the rural counties that they studied, whereas it increased from 10.1 to 107.6 per 100,000 in the urban counties [14]. However, this urban

link is not invariable, and higher rates in rural areas have been reported [15]. The balance between rural and urban areas can be affected by applying controls and mitigation activities in each type of area [16]. Ethnic minorities may also be at greater risk, affecting rates in cities where there are substantial numbers of ethnic-minority residents [14,17].

The pandemic has radically affected cities, and has induced major changes in urban life [18]. Measures in response to COVID-19 that involved lockdowns in urban areas have had economic impacts far beyond the boundaries of those areas. In April 2020, the World Bank [3] noted that:

> COVID-19 is a massive challenge for cities on the frontline, rich and poor alike. The measures taken to control the spread of the virus are having massive implications on cities due to their economic structure, their preparedness for such a crisis – especially the state of their public health and service delivery systems – and the extent to which their population's health and livelihoods are vulnerable, all of which are a function of the effectiveness of their urban governance systems.

COVID-19 and Informal Settlements

People who live in inadequate housing or slums are especially vulnerable to diseases, such as COVID-19, that are transmitted by the respiratory route, and which spread rapidly in overcrowded and closely situated dwellings. The lack of basic amenities such as clean water, functional waste and sewage disposal, and effective healthcare worsens the situation. Basic sanitary measures such as handwashing, ventilation, disinfection of surfaces, physical distancing, isolation for people who are infected, and quarantine for those who are exposed, all of which are essential elements of COVID-19 prevention, are often impossible to implement due to overcrowding and lack of money. In addition, the health of slum dwellers is often poorer than that of people living in wealthier areas, due to malnutrition, contaminated food and water, and poor sanitation. Furthermore, socioeconomically disadvantaged people frequently have a higher than average incidence of conditions such as cardiovascular diseases, lung damage, diabetes, and high blood pressure [19], all of which have been shown to result in more severe COVID-19 infections [20,21].

A UN Human Rights Special Procedures COVID-19 Guidance Note entitled 'Protecting Residents of Informal Settlements' notes that 'Housing has become the frontline defence against the coronavirus. Home has rarely been more of a life-or-death situation' [22]. In order to prevent the spread of COVID-19, nations across the world asked people to stay at home, and in some cases legislated to insist that they do so. This assumes that one's home provides protection against contracting and spreading the virus. However, this is not always the case. It has been pointed out that many of the actions needed to reduce person-to-person transmission of COVID, including personal distancing and observance of lockdowns, are virtually impossible for the majority of urban poor people, whose dwellings are crowded and poorly ventilated, and who need to leave their homes every day to earn an income if they are to eat [23].

The UN document 'Policy Brief: COVID-19 in an Urban World' pointed out that COVID-19 has highlighted the critical role played by local governments as frontline responders in crisis response, recovery, and rebuilding [8]. However, the ability of authorities and external agencies to respond to the needs of the inhabitants of informal settlements is often complicated by limited or absent healthcare services, lack of finance, and shortages of healthcare staff. Their ability to act may be further limited by a lack of data on the health needs and problems that are already faced by people living in these settlements [24,25], and by a serious shortage of information about the number of inhabitants of informal settlements, as there is substantial variation in estimates of the number of people who live in these settlements [26]. Adequate support by national governments is also vital.

The Future

UN-Habitat states that its 2016 World Cities Report 'unequivocally demonstrates that the current urbanization model is unsustainable in many respects. It conveys a clear message that the pattern of urbanization needs to change in order to better respond to the challenges of our time' [1]. The UN Policy Brief of July 2020 states that 'Avoiding a return to the pre-pandemic status quo and instead transforming cities globally for future resilience, inclusion, green and economic sustainability has never been more urgent' [8]. The COVID-19 pandemic does provide an opportunity to take this agenda forward. A great deal of material has been published about the planning needed for recovery after the COVID-19 outbreak, and studies have focused on the urban dynamics of the outbreak because cities are centres of economic activity, are densely populated, and frequently have high levels of COVID infections [27,28].

An essential part of the development of cities in the future must include planning for future pandemics as a priority [6]. In June 2020, in a joint piece, the UN-Habitat Executive Director and the UN Special Representative for Disaster Risk Reduction expressed their view that COVID-19 demonstrates an urgent need for cities to prepare for pandemics. They noted that COVID-19, like most epidemics, is largely an urban problem, and that local strategies for disaster risk reduction must include pandemic preparedness as a priority. This needs to be part of the process of better recovery and building resilience to future disease outbreaks [29].

References

1. UN-Habitat. *World Cities Report 2016. Urbanization and Development: Emerging Futures.* UN-Habitat, 2016.

2. UN Department of Economic and Social Affairs (UN DESA). *World Urbanisation Prospects: The 2018 Revision.* UN DESA, 2019 (www.un.org/development/desa/publications/2018-revision-of-world-urbanization-prospects.html).

3. World Bank. *Urban Development.* World Bank, 2020 (www.worldbank.org/en/topic/urbandevelopment/overview).

4. Sphere Association. *The Sphere Handbook: Humanitarian Charter and Minimum Standards in Humanitarian Response* 4th ed. Sphere Association, 2018.

5. International Federation of Red Cross and Red Crescent Societies (IFRC). *World Disasters Report 2010: Focus on Urban Risk.* IFRC, 2021.

6. World Bank. *Urban and Disaster Risk Management Responses to COVID-19.* World Bank, 2020 (bdocs.worldbank.org/en/575581589235414090/World-Bank-Urban-DRM-COVID-19-Responses.pdf).

7. Lovett RA. Why Chile fared better than Haiti. *Nature* 2010. Available from: https://doi.org/10.1038/news.2010.100.

8. UN. *Policy Brief: COVID-19 in an Urban World.* UN, 2020 (https://unsdg.un.org/resources/policy-brief-covid-19-urban-world).

9. International Institute for Environment and Development (IIED). *Understanding the Nature and Scale of Urban Risk in Low- and Middle-Income Countries and its Implications for Humanitarian Preparedness, Planning and Response.* IIED, 2012 (assets.publishing.service.gov.uk/media/

57a08a6940f0b652dd0006fe/
UrbanRisk_andResponse-
IIEDforDFID-211012.pdf).

10. Watson GB. Designing resilient
cities and neighbourhoods.
In *Urban Disaster Resilience* (eds
D Sanderson, JS Kayden, J Leis):
39–52. Routledge, 2016.

11. Alirol E, Getaz L, Stoll B,
Chappuis F, Loutan L.
Urbanisation and infectious
diseases in a globalised world.
Lancet Infect Dis 2011; **11**: 131–41.

12. Norwegian Institute of Public
Health (NIPH). *Urbanization and
Preparedness for Outbreaks with
High-Impact Respiratory
Pathogens*. NIPH, 2020 (apps.who
.int/gpmb/assets/thematic_
papers_2020/tp_2020_4.pdf).

13. Department for Environment,
Food & Rural Affairs (DEFRA).
*Official Statistics. Rural Economic
Bulletin for England (updated
1 April 2021)*. Defra, 2021.

14. Paul R, Arif AA, Adeyemi O,
Ghosh S, Han D. Progression of
COVID-19 from urban to rural
areas in the United States: a
spatiotemporal analysis of
prevalence rates. *J Rural Health*
2020; **36**: 591–601.

15. Centers for Disease Control and
Prevention (CDC). COVID-19
stats: COVID-19 incidence, by
urban-rural classification –
United States, January 22–
October 31, 2020. *MMWR Morb
Mortal Wkly Rep* 2020; **69**: 1753.

16. Huang Q, Jackson S, Derakhshan
S, Lee L, Pham E, Jackson A, et al.

Urban–rural differences in
COVID-19 exposures and
outcomes in the South: a
preliminary analysis of South
Carolina. *PLoS One* 2021; **16**:
e0246548.

17. Iyanda AE., Boakye KA., Lu Y,
Oppong JR. Racial/ethnic
heterogeneity and rural-urban
disparity of COVID-19 case
fatality ratio in the USA: a
negative binomial and GIS-based
analysis. *J Racial Ethn Health
Disparities* 2022; **9**: 708–21.

18. Acuto M, Larcom S, Keil R,
Ghojeh M, Lindsay T,
Camponeschi C, et al. Seeing
COVID-19 through an urban lens.
Nat Sustain 2020; **3**: 977–8.

19. Howard G, Safford MM, Moy CS,
Howard VJ, Kleindorfer DO,
Unverzagt FW, et al. Racial
differences in the incidence of
cardiovascular risk factors in older
black and white adults. *J Am
Geriatr Soc* 2017; **65**: 83–90.

20. Friesen J, Pelz PF. COVID-19 and
slums: a pandemic highlights gaps
in knowledge about urban
poverty. *JMIR Public Health
Surveill* 2020; **6**: e19578.

21. Jordan RE, Adab P, Cheng KK.
Covid-19: risk factors for severe
disease and death. *BMJ* 2020; **368**:
m1198.

22. Farha L. *COVID-19 Guidance
Note: Protecting Residents of
Informal Settlements*. UN Human
Rights Special Procedures, 2020
(www.ohchr.org/Documents/
Issues/Housing/SR_housing_

COVID-19_Guidance_
informaettlements.pdf).

23. Du J, King R, Chanchani R.
*Tackling Inequality in Cities is
Essential for Fighting COVID-19*.
World Resources Institute, 2020
(www.wri.org/insights/tackling-
inequality-cities-essential-
fighting-covid-19).

24. Ezeh A, Oyebode O, Satterthwaite
D, Chen Y-F, Ndugwa R, Sartori J,
et al. The history, geography, and
sociology of slums and the health
problems of people who live in
slums. *Lancet* 2017; **389**: 547–58.

25. Wilkinson A. Local response in
health emergencies: key
considerations for COVID-19 in
informal urban settlements.
Environ Urban 2020; **32**: 503–22.

26. Kuffer M, Pfeffer K, Sliuzas R.
Slums from space—15 years of
slum mapping using remote
sensing. *Remote Sensing* 2016; **8**:
455.

27. Sharifi A, Khavarian-Garmsir AR.
The COVID-19 pandemic:
impacts on cities and major
lessons for urban planning,
design, and management. *Sci
Total Environ* 2020; **749**: 142391.

28. Teller J. Urban density and Covid-
19: towards an adaptive approach.
Build Cities 2021; **2**: 150–65.

29. UN-Habitat. *OPINION: COVID-
19 Demonstrates Urgent Need for
Cities to Prepare for Pandemics*.
UN-Habitat, 2020 (unhabitat.org/
opinion-covid-19-demonstrates-
urgent-need-for-cities-to-prepare-
for-pandemics).

Chapter

8

Myths About Disasters

David E Alexander

Introduction: Disaster Mythology

It is both a truism and a fact that disasters are much misunderstood phenomena. Whether their origins lie in natural events or in technological problems, disasters tend to be complex events, and their impacts range from abrupt to insidious. Human nature compels many people to underestimate or ignore disaster risk. Despite more than a century of research, only since the 1960s has there been a concerted worldwide effort to understand disasters and deal seriously with their risks and consequences. This is true despite the early work of authors such as the psychologist Irving L. Janis, who in 1954 lamented the scarcity of data and studies capable of turning disasterology itself from a myth into a reality [1, p. 14]. Much still remains to be addressed, including the need to improve communication of what we know about disasters, in order to induce people to do more to mitigate and prepare for them. Meanwhile, misunderstandings abound.

The *Oxford English Dictionary (OED)* defines myth as 'a widespread but untrue or erroneous story or belief; a widely held misconception; a misrepresentation of the truth'. Despite its Greek and Latin origins, the term did not become widely used in English as a description of contemporary events until the nineteenth century. At that point, as forms of mass communication began to proliferate, more and more opportunities to perpetuate incorrect ideas began to present themselves.

In this context, myths are dismissible statements which are widely believed, and easily communicated and adopted, but unlikely to be true. Misconceptions are incorrect framings of circumstances, often as a result of prejudice, ignorance, or failure to verify prior beliefs against reality. Finally, misassumptions are incorrect beliefs that are held without adequate attempts to measure them against real conditions. All of these forms of belief postulate the existence of a mismatch between a measurable verifiable form of reality and what people perceive to be true. *Caveat lector* ('let the reader beware'), as most myths about disaster are statistical, not absolute. This means that there are exceptions which confirm the rule, or perhaps even bring it into question. Benigno Aguirre saw some of the 'myths' as hypotheses rather than facts [2].

Among disaster scholars, attitudes to the myths are quite variable. Some professionals, such as Norris Johnson [3] and Jeffrey Arnold [4], seem to have taken it for granted that disasters will be misunderstood. Others, such as Aguirre [2], have questioned such assumptions. If one follows the latter school of thought, then one might be dealing with a 'myth about myths'. However, the consensus that disasters are frequently misunderstood is strong and enduring. Aguirre contested the use of the term 'myths', and noted that entire cultures are founded on myths as systems that help to explain events and beliefs [2]. However, that involves a different use of the term 'myth' to the one employed here. In this respect, this chapter uses the term 'myths' as a shorthand expression for phenomena that are misunderstood.

The most forthright statement about disaster myths was put forward in 1999–2000 by Dr Claude de Ville de Goyet, then Director of the Emergency Preparedness and Disaster Relief Coordination Programme of the World Health Organization (WHO) regional office for the Americas – the Pan American Health Organization (PAHO) [5]. In order to prepare the ground for better disaster management, de Ville de Goyet wrote a polemic about how these events are misunderstood. He sent it to a variety of academic journals and leading newspapers, and it was published in several of the former [5] but in none of the latter.

What Is Misunderstood?

There are many misconceptions about disasters and major incidents. One is that they are exceptional events. Their frequency around the world belies this. Another misconception is that they are unpredictable events. Even among people who study disasters, they are often portrayed as black swans, using the analogy coined by Nassim Nicholas Taleb in 2007 [6]. Taleb was referring to completely unexpected developments in the field of economics, the perceptual impact of which he likened to the first arrival of European travellers in Australia. They believed that all swans were white, and were suddenly confronted by black examples. However, in disasters there is little that has not happened before, and the concept of black swans is generally misleading. Perhaps it is an excuse for not properly thinking through the roots and antecedents of events. Although magnitude–frequency relationships are usually incomplete for natural hazards, both events of natural origin and those with technological causes have a history that can be reconstructed and scrutinised. For example, when two jet aircraft were deliberately crashed into the World Trade Center on 11 September 2001, it was not the first time that an aircraft had collided with a tall building in Manhattan; that was in 1945 when an aircraft accidentally crashed into the Empire State Building.

A significant proportion of misconceptions about disasters concern their impacts on human health. One of the most strongly held ideas is that dead bodies, if they are not rapidly buried, create a health hazard. Careful investigation by epidemiologists has revealed no significant connection between outbreaks of disease and failure to bury dead bodies, except in relation to certain specific diseases [7]. Although this misconception is enduring, there have been occasions when it has been successfully counteracted. For example, during the aftermath of the Haiti earthquake in 2010, thousands of unburied dead bodies accumulated in courtyards and at roadsides. A concerted information campaign by the International Federation of the Red Cross and the WHO reduced the amount of misreporting of this myth in international news media [8]. More than 20 years previously, work by the US Centres for Disease Control and Prevention had conclusively shown that less than 1% of disasters are associated with epidemics [9]. When they are, this tends to be the result of a rise in endemic diseases, which may in any case be a regular seasonal phenomenon. Although it is perfectly possible for disruption of life and healthcare caused by disaster to cause a rise in the incidence of diseases, in any major disaster this is likely to be counteracted by

an increase in medical assistance. Enhanced disease surveillance may increase the diagnosis rate [10] but not necessarily the true incidence rate.

I have identified 72 common misconceptions about disasters in an attempt to catalogue the myths [11]. They cover a considerable range of phenomena. We have considered misconceptions about the incidence and health-related effects of disasters, but special consideration needs to be given to two particular phenomena – panic and looting. That people commonly panic during disasters is perhaps the most widespread and enduring misassumption of all [12]. It deserves close examination in the light of both the research on and the experience of panic. Looting is rather different, as it is common enough to call into question its status as a myth [13]. It also deserves close examination.

The supposed prevalence of both panic and looting has much to do with a popular model of disasters that is most easily visualised, and perhaps depicted at its most extreme, in Hollywood disaster movies [14]. It is counterbalanced by the scholarship of social scientists working in post-disaster communities. The contrast between these two viewpoints is discussed later in this chapter.

Panic

The term 'panic' appears to have been received into English from middle French (*panique et terreurs*) in the sixteenth century. In ancient mythology, it referred to the ability of the rustic god Pan to inspire terror, even in armies of Titans, with his echoing shout. The *OED* defines it as 'a feeling of sudden terror' and 'wild or unreasoning'. The occurrence of panic in disasters, or even the fear that panic will happen, is perhaps the most enduring myth or misassumption of all. My research suggests that the assumption that there will be panic in disasters cuts across social groupings, professions, and walks of life, and is quite rigidly adhered to [12].

As with other negative phenomena that are uncommon in disaster, panic is not entirely absent. I have found myself prey to it on several occasions in disasters. However, it is also probably the most difficult phenomenon to define and analyse, in part because it is elusive. Nevertheless, there has been a large amount of work on panic by both sociologists and psychologists [15]. In a previous study [16] I noted a striking difference between the sociological and psychological views of panic. The former tends to regard it, predictably, as a social phenomenon, or perhaps an 'asocial' one [17], whereas the latter sees it as an innate tendency in certain people, representing a form of loss of control [18].

Most of the research on panic in the context of disasters has been sociological. It is difficult to summarise, as some sociologists have regarded panic as practically a non-phenomenon [3], whereas others see it as more common [e.g., 19]. If one can have the temerity to try to explain panic, it involves a spontaneous withdrawal of perceptual contact between people who perceive an immediate, probably life-threatening hazard and an instinctive need to protect themselves from it. This ushers in the idea of fight or flight, with a heavy emphasis on the latter [20].

There are several problems with the definition and identification of panic. One is that most studies have taken place after the event, and have therefore had to reconstruct circumstances from the testimonies of witnesses who have been through a harrowing experience, which may be distorted when viewed in retrospect [17]. Another problem is that panic is frequently connected with flight, and is regarded as an arational response. Indeed, flight may lead people into danger rather than out of it. However, not all flight is unconsidered or ill-considered. Once panic has been rationalised, it ceases to exist.

In many instances, panic is more of a metaphor than a fact. Imposition of authoritarian measures or withholding information because 'people may panic' is usually a misjudged move, based more upon prejudice than upon fact. Looking down on a chaotic scene in the aftermath of a sudden-impact disaster, it could well be a mistake to assume that what one is witnessing is panic. Apparent chaos may mask a complex series of rational actions that have nothing to do with the phenomenon. Finally, there is ample evidence that people do not usually panic in situations of grave danger. For example, when bombs were exploded on underground trains in London on 7 July 2005, and it was feared that the trains would catch fire while people were trapped in the tunnel, incidences of panic were severely limited or absent, despite the presence of dead bodies and people with horrendous injuries. Women tended to be more level-headed than men, which might be because they are less likely to assume a 'fight or flight' mentality [21]. Despite these observations, Mirko Draca and his colleagues published a paper about the bombings entitled 'Panic on the streets of London'

[22]. Aside from the title, it contained no references at all to panic during the incident.

In a previous analysis [16], I concluded that panic may be rare, but it is liable to be culturally conditioned and a function of persistent instability in a particular environment that makes people susceptible to heightened anxiety. Panic itself tends to be a transient phenomenon and a reaction to extreme situations, whether these are real or perceived. Observation of participants suggested to me that panic is contagious [16,17]. In addition to the practical assessment of panic, the phenomenon has two other observable features. One is that identifying panic where it does not exist owes much to the 'Hollywood model' of disaster [23]. The other is that panic is most commonly used as a metaphor for an ungovernable situation, but not necessarily an irrational or arational one. In my opinion, this represents a misuse of the term.

Looting

In the mismatch between the Hollywood model of disaster as the breakdown of society and the 'therapeutic community' model of disaster as a trigger for community solidarity, none of the so-called disaster myths, except panic, is more contentious than looting. This is the (usually violent) theft of property under circumstances that normal policing functions have failed to control [24]. It is mainly associated with riots, and less commonly with disasters. Nevertheless, there are plenty of reports of looting having occurred in the immediate aftermath of disasters [25].

In the aftermath of Hurricane Katrina on 29 August 2005, two photographic images were widely circulated, showing people up to their chests in floodwater. One photograph showed two white people who had 'found' a source of food and drink. The other showed a black person who had 'looted' a grocery store. There was little difference between the circumstances depicted in the two photographs (see https://digitalresource.center/content/what-fairness-how-do-i-find-it). On examining the discrepancy between reports of looting and its actual occurrence in Hurricane Katrina, Lauren Barsky and her colleagues noted that 'there is no clear definition of what separates looting from appropriating behaviour, particularly in the minds of responders' [26, p. 5].

In riots, looting tends to occur when property norms are abandoned, perhaps spontaneously [25].

In both riots and disasters, the propensity for looting to take place clearly depends on pre-existing conditions. Despite Allen Barton's 'therapeutic community', which is discussed later in this chapter, one cannot expect that criminal activity will cease because there is a disaster. Indeed, criminals and people with delinquent tendencies may see the disruption caused by a disaster's impact as an opportunity to intensify illicit activities. There is no doubt that community solidarity keeps looting at bay, but it cannot entirely prevent it. On the other hand, after a disaster has struck, reports of looting are often wildly exaggerated. In the case of the earthquake sequence that struck central Italy in early 1997, newspapers reported an out-of-control epidemic of looting, which on closer analysis turned out to be a grossly exaggerated report of one person robbing an electrical goods shop. In a thorough social analysis, Gabriele Prati and his colleagues found only two relatively minor cases of theft relating to this 3-month emergency [27]. The conclusion on looting and disasters is that it does occur, but in relatively few disasters, and usually in response to prior conditions that make it relatively predictable [24]. Whether antisocial and criminal behaviour occurs is a measure – indeed a barometer – of the strength of pre-existing tensions in society [28]. Nothing exemplifies this better than looting.

The Hollywood Model of Disaster, and Its Antidote

Film studios in California have made countless movies in which disaster is the theme. Most of them include the standard ingredients – a hero and heroine battling against impossible odds to achieve something right and laudable, misguided efforts to control the situation by lesser characters, antisocial behaviour, technology as the saviour of society, and so on. The films strive to achieve an entertaining story based on a spectacular threat, a stereotyped and none too precise view of human suffering, and the eventual triumph of reason, love, and fairness [29].

What emerges is a picture of disaster that portrays it as unpredictable, capricious, uncontrollable, and a dark force. A common thread that runs through these films is the breakdown of society. Even when natural disasters, such as earthquakes, storms, and volcanic eruptions, can be regarded as morally neutral impacts, the result abruptly uncovers the naked savage that lurks within us, and the competitive struggle for survival. Human social organisation is deemed to be fragile, and a major disruption may cause it to collapse altogether. There is a smidgen of truth in this [30]. If violence erupts, it must be met with corrective violence – if naked competition takes over, one must outcompete one's neighbour. Many people will become casualties because they are essentially helpless in the face of the breakdown of the support function of society. In this 'accelerated Darwinism', the survival of the fittest becomes the norm, and where there is any reference to charity, it is at the beck and call of an emergent leader [29].

About 700 disasters occur each year, perhaps two-thirds of them being generated by natural hazards and one-third by anthropogenic phenomena. The reality of these events is a world apart from the Hollywood portrayal. Early sociological research was based on observation of the effects of strenuous efforts to bring relief and social solidarity [31]. Eventually a model emerged in which the early stages of disasters were distinguished by what Barton termed the 'therapeutic community' – a situation in which there was a heightened consensus about what is good and right, and a stronger than usual desire to help one's neighbour [32]. Students of the therapeutic community argued that, during disasters, people do not shoot their fellow citizens, turn to aggression and violence, or shy away from charitable acts. Law and order do not break down, social norms and institutions do not disappear, and crime does not become rampant.

Like all efforts to debunk the myths of disasters, there are exceptions, although they tend to prove the rule rather than undermine it. The extent to which a pre-existing society or community is riven by conflict, dissent, repression, violence, or dysfunctionality does have a bearing on how it performs in a disaster. Nevertheless, at scales that range from the local to the international, cooperation tends to be greater than conflict. Indeed, disasters have been shown to play a role in peaceful diplomacy, perhaps thanks to reciprocal aid supplied by belligerent states. Thus was born the theory, if not the field, of disaster diplomacy, which is in direct opposition to the 'Hollywood model'.

Conclusion: Myth or Reality?

It is difficult to assess or measure the extent to which the myths of disaster are genuinely believed. One reason for this is that the myths are broad generalisations. If they have validity it is statistical, not absolute, and exceptions to the rule must be anticipated. As Barton noted, disasters foster community [32], but many others have argued that it is not always a therapeutic phenomenon, as it may be dysfunctional or riven by conflict. Disasters do not necessarily foster crime, but criminal enterprises are likely to see them as an opportunity [33]. On the other hand, the spontaneous development of disaster subcultures and emergent groups illustrates how people are willing to help each other in adversity rather than compete for scarce resources [34].

One substantial factor that allows disaster myths to survive is that people often have inaccurate perceptions of risk [35, p. 14]. This was particularly evident during the phases of COVID-19 infection in relation to behaviour that spread the disease [36]. Another lesson of COVID-19 is that good communication between the authorities and the public is an essential means of creating the collective endeavour to bring a disease under control. 'Good' means that communication must be clear, consistent, copious, and authoritative [37].

We live in times of accelerating change, in which people's concerns and preoccupations vary with the debate on what is considered important. Since the turn of the millennium, increasing emphasis has been placed on the concept of resilience [38]. Useful as this concept is, it risks generating its own misconceptions. One of these is that resilience can be achieved by tackling a particular hazard or reducing a particular vulnerability. In reality, specific resilience (e.g., against floods) can only exist in the context of general resilience to life's hazards and pitfalls, including homelessness, loss of employment, poverty, and susceptibility to illness. There is sometimes a tendency to see resilience as a panacea – a phenomenon with almost magical properties. It is nothing of the sort, but it does focus attention on the need to adapt to disasters. Thus resilience is not a myth, but it remains an elusive phenomenon.

As we look into the future, one major concern is the role of new means of communication in propagating a distorted view of disaster. In 2014, I published a review of social media in disasters and disaster risk reduction [39]. The new media began to be used for crisis management and response around 2008–2009. Although there were drawbacks, the consensus at the time was that social media were benign and constituted a valuable aid to safety and security. Subsequently the 'dark side' of social media has become much more prominent [40]. The full effects of this on mitigating, responding to, and recovering from disasters cannot yet be assessed. However, the ability of social media to distort facts, replace them with false information, alter images and films, and propagate harmful viewpoints raises a red flag.

In conclusion, many of the so-called myths of disaster have proved to be remarkably enduring. It appears that, as society is transformed by technology, these misassumptions are likely to persist, nurtured by new forms of communication. There is thus a pressing need to replace the 'myths' with better, more rational communication and education. This is an imperative. As we all know, in any disaster there are lives at stake.

References

1. Janis IL. Problems of theory in the analysis of stress behaviour. *J Soc Issues* 1954; **10**: 12–25.

2. Aguirre BE The myth of disaster myths. In *Oxford Encyclopaedia of Politics* (ed. WR Thompson): 1–20. Oxford University Press, 2020.

3. Johnson NR. Panic and the breakdown of social order: popular myth, social theory, empirical evidence. *Sociol Focus* 1987; **20**: 171–83.

4. Arnold JL. Disaster myths and Hurricane Katrina 2005: can public officials and the media learn to provide responsible crisis communications during disasters? *Prehosp Disaster Med* 2006; **21**: 1–3.

5. De Ville De Goyet C. Stop propagating disaster myths. *Prehosp Disaster Med* 1999; **14**: 213–14.

6. Taleb NN. *The Black Swan: The Impact of the Highly Improbable*. Penguin, 2007.

7. Morgan O, De Ville de Goyet C. Dispelling disaster myths about dead bodies and disease: the role of scientific evidence and the media. *Rev Panam Salud Pública* 2005; **18**: 33–6.

8. Alexander DE. News reporting of the January 12, 2010, Haiti earthquake: the role of common misconceptions. *J Emerg Manag* 2010; **8**: 15–27.

9. Gregg MB, ed. *The Public Health Consequences of Disasters*. US Centers for Disease Control and Prevention, 1989.

10. Babaie J, Ardalan A, Vatandoost H, Goya MM, Akbarisari A. Performance assessment of communicable disease surveillance in disasters: a systematic review. *PLoS Curr* 2015; **7**: 1–14.

11. Alexander DE. *Common Misconceptions about Disaster*. Disaster Planning and Emergency Management, 2019 (http://emergency-planning.blogspot.com/2019/03/).

12. Alexander DE. Misconception as a barrier to teaching about disasters. *Prehosp Disaster Med* 2007; **22**: 95–103.

13. Dynes RR, Quarantelli EL. What looting in civil disturbances really means. *Trans-Action* 1968; **5**: 9–14.

14. Mitchell JT, Thomas DSK, Hill AA, Cutter SL. Catastrophe in reel life versus real life: perpetuating disaster myth through Hollywood films. *Int J Mass Emerg Disasters* 2000; **18**: 383–402.

15. Tester K. *Panic*. Routledge, 2013.

16. Alexander DE. Panic during earthquakes and its urban and cultural contexts. *Built Environ* 1995; **21**: 171–82.

17. Quarantelli EL. The sociology of panic. In *International Encyclopedia of the Social and Behavioural Sciences* (eds N Smelser, PB Baltes): 11020–30. Pergamon Press, 2001.

18. Rachman S, Maser JD, eds. *Panic: Psychological Perspectives*. L. Erlbaum Associates, 1988.

19. Clarke L, Chess C. Elites and panic: more to fear than fear itself. *Soc Forces* 2008; **87**: 993–1014.

20. Grosshandler W, Bryner N, Madrzykowski D, Kuntz K. *Report of the Technical Investigation of the Station Nightclub Fire, Volume 1*. Report no. NIST NCSTAR 2. US National Institute of Standards and Technology, 2005.

21. Rose G. Who cares for which dead and how? British newspaper reporting of the bombings in London, July 2005. *Geoforum* 2009; **40**: 46–54.

22. Draca M, Machin S, Witt R. Panic on the streets of London: police, crime, and the July 2005 terror attacks. *Am Econ Rev* 2011; **101**: 2157–81.

23. Haney JJ, Havice C, Mitchell JT. Science or fiction: the persistence of disaster myths in Hollywood films. *Int J Mass Emerg Disasters* 2019; **37**: 286–305.

24. Alexander DE. Looting. In *Encyclopedia of Crisis Management* (eds KB Penuel, M Statler, R Hagen): 575–8. Sage, 2013.

25. Quarantelli EL, Dynes RR. Property norms and looting: their patterns in community crisis. *Phylon* 1970; **31**: 168–82.

26. Barsky L, Trainor J, Torres M. *Disaster Realities in the Aftermath of Katrina: Revisiting the Looting Myth*. Quick Response Report 184. Natural Hazards Center, University of Colorado at Boulder, 2006.

27. Prati G, Catufi V, Pietrantoni L. Emotional and behavioural reactions to tremors of the Umbria–Marche earthquake. *Disasters* 2012; **36**: 439–51.

28. Brown BL. Disaster myth or reality: developing a criminology of disaster. In *Disasters, Hazards and Law. Sociology of Crime, Law and Deviance, Volume 17* (ed. M Deflem): 3–17. Emerald Group Publishing, 2012.

29. Keane S. *Disaster Movies: The Cinema of Catastrophe* 2nd ed. Wallflower Press, 2006.

30. Butzer KW. Collapse, environment, and society. *Proc Natl Acad Sci USA* 2012; **109**: 3632–9.

31. Prince S. *Catastrophe and Social Change: Based Upon a Sociological Study of the Halifax Disaster*. Colombia University Press, 1920.

32. Barton AH. *Communities in Disaster: A Sociological Analysis of Collective Stress Situations*. Doubleday, 1970.

33. Aguirre BE, Lane D. Fraud in disaster: rethinking the phases. *Int J Disaster Risk Reduct* 2019; **39**: 101232.

34. Granot H. Disaster subcultures. *Disaster Prev Manag* 1996; **5**: 36–40.

35. Breakwell GM. *The Psychology of Risk* 2nd ed. Cambridge University Press, 2014.

36. Thiagarajan K. Why is India having a Covid-19 surge? *BMJ* 2021; **373**: n1124.

37. Finset A, Bosworth H, Butow P, Gulbrandsen P, Hulsman RL, Pieterse AH, et al. Effective health communication: a key factor in fighting the Covid-19 pandemic. *Patient Educ Couns* 2020; **103**: 873–6.

38. Adger WN. Social and ecological resilience: are they related? *Prog Hum Geogr* 2000; **24**: 347–64.

39. Alexander DE. Social media in disaster risk reduction and crisis management. *Sci Eng Ethics* 2014; **20**: 717–33.

40. Baccarella CV, Wagner TF, Kietzmann JH, McCarthy IP. Social media? It's serious! Understanding the dark side of social media. *Eur Manag J* 2018; **36**: 431–8.

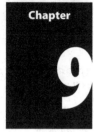

Chapter

9

Primary and Secondary Stressors
The Ways in Which Emergencies, Incidents, Disasters, Disease Outbreaks, and Conflicts Are Stressful

Richard Williams, Evangelos Ntontis, John Drury, Khalifah Alfadhli, and Richard Amlôt

Introduction

This chapter is a commentary on the origins of the adverse psychosocial experiences that people may develop after their exposure to a range of aversive, and disastrous events of long or short duration. As this book portrays, these events include emergencies, major incidents, outbreaks of high consequence infectious diseases (HCIDs) such as HIV/AIDS, severe acute respiratory syndrome (SARS), Middle East respiratory syndrome (MERS), and Ebola, terrorist attacks, and conflicts. In this chapter we use the phrase 'emergencies, major incidents, and outbreaks' to encompass all disastrous adverse events and circumstances.

Our experience of the COVID-19 pandemic has been that its psychosocial consequences have been broadly similar in nature to those that have emerged from single-incident events, such as the Manchester Arena bombing in 2017. However, these events are very different in terms of causes, consequences, duration, and geographical spread. Although this worldwide viral outbreak, which has wiped trillions of dollars off world economies, is very different in character to a range of terrorist events, they do share a number of problems, including that of agreeing definitions. In this chapter, we address the matter of how we conceptualise stress and the stressors that affect us in the face of all nature of disasters.

Our approach to stress is summarised from a paper by Richard Williams and his colleagues [1]:

> Stress is a term that is used widely and often
> inconsistently. Sometimes it refers to a stimulus (more
> appropriately described as a stressor) and sometimes to
> people's responses [2]. In respect of major incidents and
> emergencies, stress describes a collection of common
> human psychological, physical, and behavioural
> responses. It can be positive, when it motivates people,
> but is a problem when the level of stress people

experience is overwhelming and unpleasant. Then, the experiences are described as distress [3]. Stressors are events, circumstances, attitudes, and responses that stimulate people to experience a stress response, or which cause states of strain or tension because they are excessive [4].

There has been a temptation to think that all of the impacts of disasters and major incidents are directly referrable to the event that has occurred or is occurring. However, brief experience shows that this is too simple an analysis. For example, the spread of research published in 2020 and early in the evolution of the pandemic relating to the impacts of COVID-19 demonstrates that there was a temptation to focus on the SARS-CoV-2 virus alone as the cause of stress [5]. Research published since 2021 covers a wider range of influences, and clearly shows that the social conditions in which people live, relate, and work have implications for the impact of the virus on them. The factors considered in research published in 2022 were wider still. Neither the risk of contracting the disease nor its impacts are distributed equally across populations. These observations are far from novel. In a book about disasters published in 2014, Richard Williams and Neil Greenberg warned that 'leaders should be cautious about ascribing the stress that staff experience as, necessarily, resulting from . . . what they have witnessed, and the work they have done or not done' [6, p. 404].

In fact, there are many influences on how people respond, and on the psychosocial, behavioural, and psychiatric effects of emergencies and incidents of all kinds, which go well beyond considering the direct effects of noxious events alone. The term primary stressor was coined to describe the impacts of events, and many authors have written about secondary stressors as a collective descriptor for the other risk factors that affect the ways in which people respond to events. For example, it is clear that many secondary stressors describe people's socioeconomic circumstances, whereas others describe the impacts of policies and practices that have adverse effects in the changed circumstances created by emergencies, incidents, and disease outbreaks.

Given the growing interest, which began around 15 years ago, in better defining different types of stressor, and the importance of these distinctions to the ways in which government policy was developing in England at that time, work was put in hand to conduct a systematic review of the literature on secondary stressors. This resulted in a clearer definition of and a typology for secondary stressors [7]. However, it is evident that the concept has been used in different ways by a large number of researchers, and has been widely misunderstood. This led the authors of this chapter to review the subsequent literature and conduct a substantial review of the topic in order to develop a new definition that is more theoretically grounded and more practical, but also more consistent. It is intended to provoke discussion. We published the paper on that review and our proposed new definition during 2021 [1]. Our engagement in research on the Manchester Arena bombing and in advising the responsible authorities on managing the COVID-19 pandemic, as well as other adverse events and circumstances, has driven that work and provided opportunities to test our thinking. Recently one of us (RW) was involved in publishing a narrative paper on the impacts of COVID-19 on staff of the four National Health Services (NHS) in the UK [8]. In that paper the authors also explore the nature of secondary stressors in the pandemic. Socioeconomic disadvantage looms very large, much as has been portrayed in Chapter 7 of this book.

A very potent illustration of the impacts of both primary and secondary stressors comes from our mixed methods research involving people who registered with the Resilience Hub that was set up after the Manchester Arena bombing in May 2017. The aims of the Hub were to support, assess the needs of, and provide responses for people from across the UK who were directly or indirectly affected by that terrorist incident. Aspects of the Social Influences on Recovery Enquiry (SIRE) into the experiences of people who used the Hub are reported in several chapters in this book. In Chapter 5 we describe what we learned about the nature of the distress that was experienced by people who attended the Arena event, and which lasted longer than anticipated for a substantial number of people. Often distress arising from these kinds of events is described as lasting for brief periods of time, but our participants continued to be distressed to at least a mild degree for more than 2 years. Most important of all, they described – in semi-structured interviews and in answer to questions in a quantitative survey 3½ years after the event – a rich array of secondary stressors that had clearly shaped their experiences. These matters are reported in more detail in Chapters 27 and 28.

In this chapter we offer definitions of primary and secondary stressors, we provide a clear rationale for their importance, and we emphasise that the term secondary stressor certainly does not mean that these stressors have less impact than do primary stressors. We offer a worked example that is drawn from our assessments of academic papers published in 2020 and 2021 on which some of our advice to NHS England was based. Those papers reported research on the needs of and care required by staff of health and social care services. Finally, we explore the implications of primary and secondary stressors for responding to people's needs before, during, and after emergencies, incidents, and disease outbreaks.

Definitions of Primary and Secondary Stressors

Primary stressors are factors that are 'inherent in particular major incidents, disasters and emergencies and arising directly from those events' [3, p. 20]. They are therefore stressors that arise from the traumatic event. Examples include physical injury, damage to property, exposure to gruesome scenes and life-threatening danger, bereavement, and loss of homes, possessions, and amenities. Although some of these occurrences may be preventable by greater preparedness [9], we argue that they are inherent in the sense of being directly attributable to the action of the emergency, incident, or outbreak, which can include, for example, floods, fires, earthquakes, terrorist attacks, and pandemics.

We understand secondary stressors as processes that cause distress in relation to emergencies, incidents, and outbreaks, but which do not inherently have their origin in the events [1]. Instead they have two types of origin. First, they may be events, policies, practices, and social, organisational, and financial arrangements that have their origins in society and people's personal life circumstances before the extreme event occurs. Second, they can arise from society's responses to the emergency, incident, or outbreak. In each case, they can become sources of substantial stress in addition to, but separately from, the primary stressors.

Examples of secondary stressors that arise from prior events or arrangements include some of the rules by which insurance companies have operated to compensate property owners. For the people of Hull whose homes and businesses were flooded in June 2007, the damaging effects of these rules on how they tried to deal with the primary stressors – in this case, damage to property – caused great distress for people who had been flooded. In other words, prior to the floods the insurance procedures had few impacts, but after the floods they came to have a new and negative significance [10].

Examples of secondary stressors that arise from aspects of society's responses to an extreme event include the response of the local authority to the Grenfell Tower fire in June 2017. The authority failed to provide sufficient emergency housing locally, which resulted in some people becoming separated from their support networks [11].

Why Primary and Secondary Stressors are Important

The distinction between primary and secondary stressors, and a proper understanding of the distinctive features of secondary stressors, are important for a number of reasons.

First, the distinction helps us to properly understand and analyse the sources and dynamics of distress in relation to emergencies, major incidents, and outbreaks. Typically these events generate multiple sources of distress. Identifying the sources of distress is important both to validate the experiences of those people who are distressed, and to respond properly and effectively. Understanding the role of secondary stressors can serve to legitimise a focus – in addition to the direct impact of emergencies, major incidents, and outbreaks – on other sources of stress that may be just as or even more distressing than the effects of primary stressors, or that might significantly compound the effect of primary stressors. An example is the recent finding that having a mental disorder may pose a greater risk of death when people contract COVID-19, due to the impacts of cognitive changes, depressed mood, hallucinations and/or delusions, and

behaviour problems [12]. Thus secondary stressors may serve to increase the risks that are posed by primary stressors.

Second, a proper understanding of secondary stressors draws attention to the role of events, policies, practices, and social, organisational, and financial arrangements that have their origins in society and people's personal life circumstances before the extreme event occurs. It can thus serve to restore the balance between health promotion, prevention, and care for distressed people, and meeting the needs of people who receive a diagnosis, including their treatment and recovery.

Third, crucially in distinguishing between stressors that are inherent in the disaster and those that are contingent upon prior events or the emergency responses, the concept of secondary stressors highlights the fact that sources of distress are tractable. Prior life circumstances and societal responses to the disaster could have been different – society could have been organised differently so that these stressors did not exist, or at least caused less distress. The examples in this chapter show very clearly that many secondary stressors are a function of particular political and policy decisions or choices, rather than being inevitable, and these political and policy decisions or choices could have been different.

A Worked Example

We present a worked example from the context of the COVID-19 pandemic to illustrate our points regarding the nature of secondary stressors. In the first quarter of 2021, two of the authors of this chapter (RW and EN) were asked by NHS England to review a collection of published outputs on the experiences and effects of COVID-19 on healthcare staff, and to assess the robustness, reliability, and potential utility of the findings for policy and practice. We reviewed 148 papers.

A clear pattern emerged whereby the impact of the pandemic on healthcare staff seemed to be driven by structural and systemic problems and ineffective policies (i.e., secondary stressors) rather than by the virus itself (i.e., the cause of primary stressors, such as exposure to death and suffering).

Saied Ali and his colleagues showed that a large proportion of healthcare workers in acute hospital settings experienced symptoms of depression, anxiety, post-traumatic stress disorder, and stress [13].

Crucially, they noted that common responses from healthcare workers regarding how their working conditions during the pandemic could be improved included involvement in decision making, adequate and timely communication, the need for staggered rosters and rest areas, increased staffing levels to allow for leave entitlement, and the availability of childcare facilities [13].

A study on redeployed doctors conducted by Ryan Faderani and his colleagues showed that many participants felt unsupported by hospital managers and by their clinical and educational supervisors, and did not have confidence in the personal protective equipment (PPE)-related advice issued by the public health authorities; more than half of the sample did not feel safe while wearing PPE [14]. Crucially, some redeployed doctors felt that they were working in areas and facing incidents that were beyond their level of training and competence.

Imrana Siddiqui and her colleagues examined the causes of anxiety and the wellbeing support needs of healthcare workers in the UK [15]. Qualitative data from their questionnaire survey showed that participants experienced distress not only due to fears of the virus itself, but also because of their inability to work remotely where possible, and their concerns about the effects of reduced support networks and service provision. Among other topics, support requested by healthcare professionals included workplace-based support (e.g., information, visibility of managers, supervision), clearer signposting, peer support and safe spaces, staff helplines, wellbeing activities and relaxation sessions, bereavement support, effective leadership, and appropriate communication.

The papers in a thematic series in the journal *BJPsych Open* illustrate the impact of different research methods on the findings. Some papers focus on the use of questionnaires that are intended to identify mental health disorders, whereas others identify what we call secondary stressors as important factors that have an impact on risk. In this context, Norha Vera San Juan and her colleagues used qualitative methods to interview 33 frontline healthcare workers in the UK, in order to examine the applicability in practice of 14 sets of wellbeing guidelines that provided recommendations for supporting frontline staff during the current and future pandemics [16]. San Juan and her colleagues found that many of the guidelines emphasised the importance of staff receiving psychological support and avoiding mental health disorders and psychosocial problems, whereas the healthcare workers placed greater emphasis on structural conditions at work, responsibilities outside the hospitals, and the support of the community in dealing with what we take to be secondary stressors. These matters are raised in the paper by Esther Murray and her colleagues [8].

Mathew Nyashanu and his colleagues analysed interviews with workers in care homes in the UK [17,18]. The results showed that apart from fears of contracting the virus themselves or passing it on to family members (i.e., a primary stressor), participants also experienced a lack of recognition, felt that their contributions to the healthcare system were undervalued, and were worried about unsafe hospital discharges of untested patients, staff shortages, perceived disparities between the NHS and the private healthcare sector, and not receiving test results in a timely manner. Participants also felt unprepared, experienced shortages of PPE supplies, faced challenges in maintaining protection measures, and found it hard to keep track of constantly evolving PPE guidance.

Overall, the studies that we have highlighted here provide examples of the kinds of primary and secondary stressors that staff mentioned in relation to COVID-19. They show that healthcare and care workers experienced distress and identified potential mechanisms through which adverse psychosocial experiences emerge. It is worth emphasising that most adverse experiences were associated with structural problems (e.g., perceived lack of preparedness, ineffective leadership, poor communication, inequality) as well as exposure to the virus.

The Implications of Primary and Secondary Stressors for Responding to People's Needs Before, During, and After Emergencies, Incidents, and Outbreaks

The concept of secondary stressors has implications for the public, professional responders, and policymakers with regard to responding to emergencies and pandemics. In the case of the public, we illustrate the point with examples from the COVID-19 pandemic. Here non-pharmaceutical interventions, such as self-isolation, quarantine, and requirements for people to stay at home, entailed a degree of self-sacrifice and privation for many members of the public. However, they were more difficult and caused more distress for some people than for others. This variation in experiences of distress was a function of structures and policies that existed prior to the pandemic, as well as features of the response.

Thus Daisy Fancourt and Alexandra Bradbury's survey of 70,000 people found that their experiences of the pandemic were dependent on their life situations before it began [19]. Ethnic minorities, people who were more deprived, and young people struggled much more with distress and other problems than did the white adult majority, those who were better off, and older people. Some of these differential outcomes can be explained by primary stressors, such as the increased incidence of disease among some groups. However, in addition the UK's policies of austerity that pre-dated the pandemic created health inequalities, including a reduction in mental health services, which made it difficult for some groups to obtain formal assessment and care during the pandemic when their needs were acute [20]. Furthermore, these groups had only limited resources to help with mitigations, such as the option of working from home, home entertainments, and large gardens.

The difficulties and distress caused by people's responses to the pandemic also varied according to social group. For example, an international comparison of policies and practices regarding self-isolation found considerable variation in how much financial support people were given to stay at home if they were infected, and how much (if any) practical support was organised by the authorities [21]. The inadequate response in relation to poorer groups in some countries meant that people in these groups had less protection and experienced more worry. By contrast, comprehensive 'find, test, trace, isolate, support' (FTTIS) programmes would be more likely to properly reflect people's needs and would provide:

> type[s] of support ... tailored to the particular circumstances of different sections of the community: the homeless, multi-generational households, crowded households, single-parents, gig economy workers etc. A bold and imaginative support system, involving all sections of society – government, mutual aid community groups, and the private sector, is key to the success of FTTIS [22].

In relation to responders, some mitigations of the effects of secondary stressors might occur without the benefit of the conceptual framework outlined here.

However, our examples of changes to the working practices of healthcare workers in the COVID-19 pandemic demonstrates that the framework adds value and assists with positive change in two ways – first, through the recognition that it affords to the causes of some forms of distress, and second, through the priority that it suggests should be given to these causes. Without foregrounding the social and tractable nature of secondary stressors, it can be easy to discount all sources of distress in major incidents and emergencies as inevitable, intractable, or inherent.

In terms of policy, this is not the first time it has been argued that emergency preparedness, response, and recovery (EPRR) programmes require strategic investment to address inequalities and other factors (e.g., [23]). However, the concept of secondary stressors as explained here helps to demonstrate connections between mental health outcomes and social policies and practices that can inform spending, and to identify political priorities in terms of allocation of resources and development of resilient emergency response organisations.

In relation to societal responses to a major incident, our example of secondary stressors in the case of flooding points to how policy could be different. Here factors that can mitigate the impact of secondary stressors relate to integrating otherwise fragmented post-disaster support services [24], simplifying insurance procedures, and reducing waiting times for support [10].

Conclusions

The impact of both primary and secondary stressors on how members of the public and staff who respond are able to cope with emergencies, major incidents, outbreaks of diseases, and conflicts is striking.

Early on in the COVID-19 pandemic, there was a temptation to focus on the SARS-CoV-2 virus and people's fears about coping with it and reducing the risks of people becoming ill or dying. This was necessarily the case at that stage, but this focus rapidly moved to consider broader matters. A good example is provided by the work of Fancourt and her colleagues as described in this chapter with regard to social inequalities, stress, and coping with the changed circumstances required to contain the virus [19,25]. In addition, reports from clinicians have drawn attention to the importance of the conditions under which staff of the healthcare services work –

conditions which have existed for many years – to their experience of delivering clinical services during the pandemic. Our research on the Manchester Arena bombing has yielded similar observations.

Therefore we see an empirically based approach to understanding the sources of stress and broad patterns of stressors as important across all emergencies, major incidents, disease outbreaks, and conflicts.

References

1. Williams R, Ntontis E, Alfadhli K, Drury J, Amlôt R. A social model of secondary stressors in relation to disasters, major incidents and conflict: implications for practice. *Int J Disaster Risk Reduct* 2021; 63. Available from: https://doi.org/10.1016/j.ijdrr.2021.102436.

2. NATO/EAPC. *Psychosocial Care for People Affected by Disasters and Major Incidents: A Model for Designing, Delivering and Managing Psychosocial Services for People Involved in Major Incidents, Conflict, Disasters and Terrorism.* NATO, 2009.

3. Department of Health. *NHS Emergency Planning Guidance: Planning for the Psychosocial and Mental Health Care of People Affected by Major Incidents and Disasters: Interim National Strategic Guidance.* Department of Health, 2009.

4. Stokols D. A congruence analysis of human stress. *Issues Ment Health Nurs* 1985; 7: 35–64.

5. Williams R, Kaufman KR. Narrative review of the COVID-19, healthcare and healthcarers thematic series. *BJPsych Open* 2022; 8: 1–10.

6. Williams R, Greenberg N. Psychosocial and mental health care for the deployed staff of rescue, professional first response and aid agencies, NGOs and military organisations. In *Conflict and Catastrophe Medicine* (eds J Ryan, A Hopperus Buma, C Beadling, A Mozumder, DM Nott): 395–432. Springer, 2014.

7. Lock S, Rubin GJ, Murray V, Rogers MB, Amlôt R, Williams R. Secondary stressors and extreme events and disasters: a systematic review of primary research from 2010–2011. *PLoS Curr* 2012; 4. Available from: https://doi.org/10.1371/currents.dis.a9b76fed1b2?dd5c5bfcfc13c87a2f24f.

8. Murray E, Kaufman KR, Williams R. Let us do better: learning lessons for recovery of healthcare professionals during and after COVID-19. *BJPsych Open* 2021; 7: e151.

9. Maini R, Clarke L, Blanchard K, Murray V. The Sendai framework for disaster risk reduction and its indicators — where does health fit in? *Int J Disaster Risk Sci* 2017; 8: 150–5.

10. Tempest EL, Carter B, Beck CR, Rubin GJ. Secondary stressors are associated with probable psychological morbidity after flooding: a cross-sectional analysis. *Eur J Public Health* 2017; 27: 1042–7.

11. Tekin, S. A social psychological perspective on post-disaster justice campaigns. *PhD thesis* University of Sussex, 2022.

12. Boland B, Gale T. Mental and behavioural disorders and COVID-19-associated death in older people. *BJPsych Open* 2020; 6: e101.

13. Ali S, Maguire S, Marks E, Doyle M, Sheehy C. Psychological impact of the COVID-19 pandemic on healthcare workers at acute hospital settings in the South-East of Ireland: an observational cohort multicentre study. *BMJ Open* 2020; 10: e042930.

14. Faderani R, Monks M, Peprah D, Colori A, Allen L, Amphlett A, et al. Improving wellbeing among UK doctors redeployed during the COVID-19 pandemic. *Future Healthc J* 2020; 7: e71–6.

15. Siddiqui I, Aurelio M, Gupta A, Blythe J, Khanji MY. COVID-19: causes of anxiety and wellbeing support needs of healthcare professionals in the UK: a cross-sectional survey. *Clin Med* 2021; 21: 66–72.

16. San Juan NV, Aceituno D, Djellouli N, Sumray K, Regenold N, Syversen A, et al. Mental health and well-being of healthcare workers during the COVID-19 pandemic in the UK: contrasting guidelines with experiences in practice. *BJPsych Open* 2021; 7: e15.

17. Nyashanu M, Pfende F, Ekpenyong MS. Triggers of mental health problems among frontline healthcare workers during the COVID-19 pandemic in private care homes and domiciliary care agencies: lived experiences of care workers in the Midlands region, UK. *Health Soc Care Community* 2022; 30: e370–76.

18. Nyashanu M, Pfende F, Ekpenyong MS. Exploring the challenges faced by frontline workers in health and social care amid the COVID-19 pandemic: experiences of frontline workers in the English Midlands region, UK. *J Interprof Care* 2020; 34: 655–61.

19. Fancourt D, Bradbury A. We asked 70,000 people how coronavirus affected them – what they told us revealed a lot about inequality in the UK. The Conversation, 2021 (https://theconversation.com/we-asked-70-000-people-how-coronavirus-affected-them-what-they-told-us-revealed-a-lot-about-inequality-in-the-uk-143718).

20. Marmot M, Allen J, Goldblatt P, Herd E, Morrisson J. *Build Back*

Fairer: The COVID-19 Marmot Review. Health Foundation, 2020 (www.health.org.uk/publications/build-back-fairer-the-covid-19-marmot-review).

21. Patel J, Fernandes G, Sridhar D. How can we improve self-isolation and quarantine for COVID-19? *BMJ* 2021; 372: n625.

22. Independent SAGE. *Final Report on Find, Test, Trace, Isolate and Support System*. Independent SAGE, 2020

(www.independentsage.org/final_fttis_june2020/).

23. Savitt A, Montano S. Will someone please ask Biden & Trump about emergency management policy? *Disasterology*, 18 September 2020. (www.disaster-ology.com/blog/2020/9/18/will-someone-please-ask-biden-amp-trump-about-emergency-management-policy).

24. Medd W, Walker G, Mort M, Watson N. *Flood Vulnerability*

and Urban Resilience: A Real-Time Study of Local Recovery Following the Floods of June 2007 in Hull. Environment Agency, 2010.

25. Fancourt D, Bhui K, Chatterjee H, Crawford P, Crossick G, DeNora T, et al. Social, cultural and community engagement and mental health: cross-disciplinary, co-produced research agenda. *BJPsych Open* 2020; 7: e3.

Chapter

10

The Differing Challenges Posed by Big Bang, Rising Tide, and Longer-Term Incidents Affecting Local and Dispersed Populations

Chris R Brewin, Kate Allsopp, Talya Greene, and Richard Williams

Understanding Each Incident

The People Who Are Affected

In each incident, the first task in planning a response is to anticipate who has been, or may have been, affected. It may be helpful to think of a diagram with concentric circles, as depicted in Figure 10.1. The circles represent the spreading effect of the incident, but severe consequences may be present in each of them.

In the centre are the people who have been directly affected by the incident. Typically they are likely to have been physically present at the site of a major incident, such as a terrorist attack, earthquake, or other event, and may have been injured or have feared for their lives.

The second circle consists of people who were not directly in danger themselves, but witnessed the event or its aftermath, and may have been in continuing danger from, for example, infrastructure collapse, contamination, secondary devices, and secondary incidents. These people include bystanders, volunteers, and members of the emergency services and aid organisations such as the Red Cross. Initially, survivors and bystanders may be localised or dispersed, or, if they are initially localised, they may become dispersed later – for example, visitors returning home, and relocated or displaced survivors.

The third circle is formed of the many groups that are exposed to aspects of the event and its aftermath by virtue of their work, such as medical and social care staff, porters, cleaners, receptionists, mortuary attendants, and coroner's office staff.

The fourth circle consists of the families and close friends of people who died in the incident and of those who survived. Severe effects are frequently to be expected. For example, children are likely to be deeply affected by incidents in which their parents were involved.

The fifth circle consists of local communities and their leaders, including religious leaders, teachers, and council workers and administrators, whose tasks include responding to the short- and long-term needs of people who are affected.

Finally, large-scale events may have impacts on the attitudes, behaviour, and psychosocial wellbeing of the general population, even if those people have no direct connection to the locality, and live and work a long distance away from it.

Types of Incidents

Incidents fall into three broad categories: 'big bang' isolated events in which the immediate threat to people is time-limited; 'rising tide' incidents in which the levels of threat to people's lives or livelihoods grow and encompass more people as time goes on; and longer-term incidents, in which either threat to

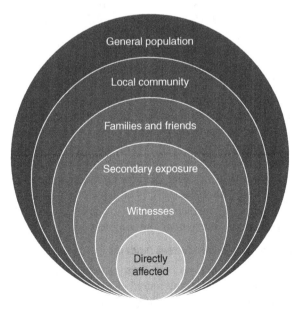

Figure 10.1 Circles of exposure to a traumatic incident.

General population

Local community

Families and friends

Secondary exposure

Witnesses

Directly affected

life or the consequent effects on people's livelihoods – including, for example, loss of employment or housing, and relocation – are long-lasting. The nature of each incident (e.g., terrorist attack, earthquake, hurricane, fire, pandemic) does not by itself determine the category, which is a product of both the nature of a particular incident and the specific contextual circumstances. Moreover, some incidents have the characteristics of more than one category, and there are also mixed categories.

Big Bang Incidents

Examples of big bang incidents include many terrorist events, such as the bombings in London in 2005 and in the Manchester Arena in 2017. Although the London bombings involved five separate explosions across the city, they nevertheless represented time-limited incidents. Many examples of big bang incidents are explosions, but other instances include the Tokyo subway sarin attack in 1995, shootings such as the Sousse attack in 2015, the shootings and bombings in Paris in 2015 (see Chapter 35 in this book), and vehicle ramming incidents, such as those in Nice and Berlin in 2016, and in Stockholm and London in 2017.

Despite the short-term nature of the incidents themselves, the secondary impacts on the people affected may be devastating for a significant number, including loss of life, bereavement, life-changing injuries, effects on mental health, and socioeconomic consequences. These incidents may also be accompanied by raised anxiety and perceived threat in the general population. For example, fear of future terrorist attacks has been identified both in London [1] and in the USA [2]. This perceived threat can also lead to altered behaviour, such as spending more time with loved ones, and avoiding public transport and plane travel [3].

Terrorist attacks may also contribute to a 'conservative shift' in which the general public's political views may become more right-wing in response to recent terrorist incidents. Studies have demonstrated a shift in the political views both of people who are directly exposed to terrorist incidents [4] and of the wider population. The impacts on the wider population after 9/11 in New York and the London bombings in 2005 included people developing more conservative views on issues such as increased military spending [5], and increased prejudice towards Muslims and immigrants [6].

Rising Tide Incidents

Often incidents are described as exemplifying a 'rising tide' pattern, when it is possible to forecast their occurrence in sufficient time to issue warnings to the populations who are likely to be involved. Another hallmark of rising tide events is that their impacts develop and persist over time. However, that criterion is more challenging to employ, and it could also be applied to many big bang events as we get to know more about them. The most common rising tide incident is flooding.

Flooding is now the most frequent calamity to strike populations across the world, and its frequency is continuing to increase as it is linked to global warming and climate change. 'The presence of water in areas that are usually dry' is the World Health Organization (WHO) definition of a flood. The water increases in volume often rapidly, and causes huge damage to infrastructure, including homes, workplaces, roads, railways, and communications [7]. Worldwide, the numbers of people affected by flooding are huge.

Although a significant number of people die in floods, most commonly by drowning, the risk of dying is low compared with other types of disaster. There are risks of electrocution, and people may suffer cardiac arrest as a result of this and because of the unaccustomed physical effort involved in protecting loved ones and their property. It is wise to assume that all flood water is contaminated, as deaths and serious illness can occur as a result of the contaminants. The toll on people's mental health is very significant [8], especially in areas that are subject to recurrent floods.

Recovery of homes, workplaces, communications, and communities may take a long time, during which people may become impoverished, which increases the risk that they will develop long-term psychosocial needs and experience distress over long periods. These circumstances raise the risk of mental ill health. Often people are displaced from their homes, with the attendant risks of dislocation from their families and friends and from the services on which they depend. The impacts of displacement on people's mental health can be substantial and long-lasting.

Longer-Term and Recurrent Incidents

Longer-term incidents are those in which either the threat to life or the consequent effects of the incident on people's livelihood are long-lasting. In some cases, the incidents themselves are prolonged or repeated, and thus there is an extended period of threat to people. These incidents include the Fukushima nuclear disaster in Japan in 2011 (caused by an earthquake and a tsunami), the earthquakes in Central Italy in 2016–2017, the rocket attacks on Israel which started in 2001 and have continued intermittently ever since, and the Northern Ireland 'Troubles'. Earthquakes, for instance, may be followed by a long-lasting pattern of aftershocks in addition to the infrastructure damage, leading to a sense of threat that may persist long into the future. A good example of the latter is the earthquake sequence in Canterbury, New Zealand, in 2010–2011; the process of recovery of the city's infrastructure is still taking place in Christchurch more than 10 years later. Other examples include the series of forest fires in Australia and California in 2020, which were related to climate and weather, and raged over a considerable number of months.

In other cases, even though the original event is relatively short-lived, the after-effects can continue to have psychosocial or material impacts for months or even years through, for example, loss of employment or housing, or relocation. Examples include the Grenfell Tower fire in the UK in 2017, the Beirut Port explosion in 2020, and Hurricane Katrina in the USA in 2005. In these incidents, many people were bereaved, lost their homes and possessions, and were displaced. Incidents that involve displacement and community dispersal cause loss of access to local and familiar support structures, such as schools, health services, and religious communities [9,10]. The people affected may be unable to get to their workplaces, either because they were destroyed or because the people no longer live near to them. It can take many years before communities are rebuilt, and this inhibits a sense of recovery from these incidents.

The Novichok poisonings in Salisbury in 2018 provide another example of a hybrid pattern of multiple incidents. The nature of the ill health and the method of delivery of the noxious agent to the people who were directly affected tempts us to categorise this as a big bang incident, because the casualties occurred as a result of a single attack, or as a rising tide incident, because the effects on the people involved took time to develop and originated on two distinct occasions. However, this incident really represents a compound category because, if nerve agents are not carefully and securely disposed of, they can lie dormant for a long time until they accidentally come into unintended contact with people who are then affected by them.

There is no clear endpoint for all types of longer-term incidents. People in the affected population may feel 'on edge', waiting for the next disaster or event. Populations of people who continue to live in an affected area may develop a sense that nowhere is safe, including their own homes and communities [11].

Cross-Cutting Dimensions

The Scale of the Incident

Determining the scale of each incident is complicated [9,12]. Incidents may be single or repeated, can be brief or of prolonged duration, may occur at single or multiple locations (including potentially across several different countries simultaneously, as happened with the Tsunami on Boxing Day 2004), and can cascade into a chain of additional incidents (as occurred in the wake of the Fukushima nuclear disaster). The extent of death, injury, and disruption, and of destruction of property, infrastructure, and livelihoods, can vary by many orders of magnitude.

It is often difficult to determine who has and who has not been 'exposed' to incidents [13]. Although it is reasonably straightforward to identify people who were at the epicentre of the event, those who were not present are likely to be affected, too, because they may suffer personal or material loss at personal or community levels. The ripple effects of these losses can encompass whole communities.

All of these aspects have an impact on the type of response that should be mobilised, the resources needed to mount that response, and the degree of regional, national, and international coordination that is required.

Dispersion of People Who Are Affected

Some events involve settled local communities (e.g., the Grenfell Tower fire in 2017, the shootings in Dunblane in 1996), or temporary communities formed by people having been present at a particular place and time (e.g., the Manchester Arena bombing in 2017, the attacks in Sousse in 2015). The population affected may disperse after the incident. It has been reported that 80% of the people affected by the Manchester Arena bombing who registered with a dedicated mental health support service, the Greater Manchester Resilience Hub, lived outside the Manchester region [14].

Membership of a temporary community may provide the opportunity in principle to directly identify those affected. Other events involve people who were there by chance, and who may be travellers or foreign tourists (e.g., the London terrorist attacks in 2017). Subsequently some of them may form a virtual community because of their involvement, but this activity is unlikely to be comprehensive.

Many disasters, such as major earthquakes and hurricanes, may be followed by the planned or unplanned relocation of large sections of communities. Socioeconomic factors may also affect people's dispersal – for example, those who did not evacuate during Hurricane Katrina in 2005 were more likely to be of lower socioeconomic status, and to have lacked the transportation or resources that would have enabled evacuation [15,16]. Uprooting communities can pose a threat to pre-existing social and support networks and community resilience, which might otherwise have helped to mitigate the negative impacts of disaster [17–19]. Relocating communities in ways that maintain pre-existing social ties may help [20], but may also have a negative impact on subsequent integration with new communities [21]. Damage to housing may continue to have negative implications for mental health and wellbeing many years after incidents [22]. We have a lot to learn about handling the need for people to be displaced to protect them in the face of major incidents, so that they do not lose contact with relatives, friends, and services on which they rely.

Still other events affect a population of varying size and dispersion that may change over time. Examples include chemical, biological, radiological, and nuclear incidents, and pandemics.

Types and Chronology of Presentation

As is depicted in Chapter 5, distress of varying durations is very common during and after major incidents of all kinds. Around 50% of the affected population and their relatives may recover fairly quickly, but 15–30% develop distress that persists. Although most people in this group are unlikely to have a mental disorder, they suffer restriction of their lives and have continuing needs for psychosocial care. Thus even though no overall increase in mental health disorders is usually observed among the general population who have not been directly affected, the secondary stressors (see Chapter 9) may interact with the primary stressors to place people at risk of developing mental disorders. This applies especially

to around 15% of people whose stress levels are very high or whose stress increases with the passing of time.

For example, the Three Mile Island disaster in 1979 was associated with increased reports of anxiety and physical health complaints among the people who were not directly exposed to radiation. The major mental health outcomes among directly affected, previously healthy people are likely to involve increases in anxiety, depression, post-traumatic reactions, and substance abuse. They may be combined with specific physical effects from, for example, smoke inhalation, deafening blasts, exposure to toxins, and post-viral syndromes. Different symptom trajectories are well established, with delayed onsets accounting for a substantial proportion, especially among members of the emergency services. People who have had mental health conditions previously, or who are already in vulnerable situations, are at additional risk of recurrence, exacerbations of previous symptoms, or developing new symptoms and disorders.

Involving the Public

There may be high levels of public involvement, and the degree of public interest depends on the timescale, societal implications, symbolic significance of traumatic events, and associated media coverage. In the past, we have said that signs of stress may increase temporarily after terrorist attacks, and there may be changes in behaviour even among those people who have no direct connection with the events [23]. However, it is now becoming clearer that the signs of stress may not be temporary but extend into the medium and longer term for a substantial proportion of those affected [24,25]. Public attitudes such as identifying with one's community or country may increase temporarily [26].

There is a clear need for an evidence-based but pragmatic communications strategy. This is because high levels of media exposure in the aftermath of attacks are associated with an increased frequency of symptoms of mental health disorders. There has been great interest in whether people can develop post-traumatic stress disorder (PTSD) after events even though their exposure is limited to media images and reports. Although PTSD symptoms related to attacks are often described in remote populations, they probably occur in people who already have mental health problems. There is little evidence for an overall increase in mental disorders in remote populations after such events [26]. However, a vicious circle may develop in which media exposure and associated PTSD symptoms predict, in turn, greater exposure to subsequent traumatic events [27]. Children in particular are vulnerable to the presentation of horrific images in the media, and these concerns should form part of any communications strategy. Even less is known about the impact of social media use in the context of major incidents, especially given that graphic and shocking images and videos may be shared among users without any filtering of the content. This may be particularly problematic among young people who are very frequent users of social media.

The content and the extent to which messaging aimed at the general public is required varies greatly. Messages should include statements that are designed to address the public mood following terrorist attacks (e.g., after the Oslo attacks in 2011), to advise on aspects of everyday life such as use of public transport (e.g., after the London bombings in 2005), to prepare people for the possibility of contamination (e.g., after the Salisbury poisonings in 2018), or to institute protective measures (e.g., after an earthquake or during a pandemic). More generally, messages that are designed to inform the public about stress responses and the resources available to help them to deal with distress will almost certainly be required, and should be prepared in advance. Advice about preparing and transmitting public messages was formulated for the H1N1 flu pandemic of 2009–2010, and has been revised subsequently [28].

Planning Responses

We recommend that, where appropriate, planners should consider each type of incident and the degree of dispersal of the people involved under each of the following headings.

Identifying Affected People

In principle, identifying affected people may be easier for localised events, through records of residence (e.g., the Grenfell Tower fire in 2017), attendance at events (e.g., the shootings on Utøya Island, Norway in 2011), or purchase of tickets for events (e.g., the Manchester Arena bombing in 2017).

The laws and regulations for sharing data need to be clear and enforceable across multiple private and public bodies if identification of those involved is to be effective. In the UK, mental health responses have consistently been impeded by the reluctance of organisations to share customer, patient, or employee contact details, despite their duties under the Civil Contingencies Act and data protection provisions that are designed to enable this [29].

Engagement with communities of survivors and relatives is often needed, because people may be hesitant about referring themselves to support services [30]. When large numbers of people are affected, consideration needs to be given to which of them are likely to be most vulnerable, and outreach approaches used to actively address barriers to care. This is particularly important when the incident is likely to exacerbate existing health inequalities, such as those related to ethnicity, gender, or socioeconomic status [31–33].

Recording Details of People Who Are Involved

An effective mental health response requires a central database of people who have been involved and who can be followed up and provided with advice, interventions, and treatment if required. Relevant information is likely to come from multiple sources, such as municipal authorities, customer or police witness lists, hospital attenders, the emergency services, and third-sector providers. Ideally, details of bystanders and volunteers should be taken during the incident. If data are not collected rapidly, people may be impossible to trace, particularly in the case of incidents that occur on the streets or in transport networks. However, a register can increase its coverage by permitting members of the public to identify themselves through, for example, a dedicated website.

Consideration needs to be given to how this disparate information can be brought together, integrated into a common register, handled securely, and made available for approved purposes. Relying on local organisations such as hospital or mental health providers, which happen to be involved, is unlikely to be effective, as they will have to develop the relevant expertise de novo. By contrast, public health bodies such as the UK Health Security Agency, or the Centers for Disease Control and Prevention in the USA, are well placed to do this. Some initial efforts have been made in this direction [34–37], but protocols are limited and not widely available or employed. Surveys in the UK suggest that centralised registers are likely to be acceptable to the great majority of the public [38].

Planning a Hierarchy of Interventions

In order to mitigate the impact of the incident, a suite of interventions is required for prevention and treatment. These range from public messaging to care for people who are distressed (including face-to-face contacts; see Chapter 5), psychoeducation and online support, access to mental health screening, formal assessments, and evidence-based treatments. Psychosocial support that spans multiple levels of intervention by being made available to individuals, through people's workplaces, and via community groups should be accessible to those who wish to use these services.

Psychosocial support can involve a wide variety of content and modes of delivery, including financial and housing advice, counselling, family intervention, and parenting advice, as well as additional support around anniversaries, criminal trials of perpetrators, and other significant times [39,40]. Training managers, providing peer support, and building team-based cohesion within organisations should be available to professional groups. There may be existing support structures in communities – for example, through schools and faith-based groups – and these can play valuable roles in secondary prevention and in adapting materials to the specific beliefs and needs of community members.

Active outreach may be necessary, as people may not know how to access support, or may not even know that it exists or that they could benefit from it. Mental health screening has been successfully used to direct affected people towards support and interventions following major incidents such as the Manchester Arena bombing in 2017 and the London 7/7 terrorist attacks in 2005 [24,25,29,30].

Formal assessments and evidence-based treatments are likely to be needed by a significant minority. Therefore planners should be prepared for a surge in the number of people seeking personal or group-based assessments and treatments. This may require redeployment of mental health professionals for a period of time, which is likely to have knock-on effects on routine mental health services.

Most critical of all is ensuring that interventions are coordinated between the various services, agencies, and organisations, in order to avoid duplication and provide support for those people who need it as effectively and efficiently as possible [10,29].

Organising and Resourcing Responses

Plans must be in place in advance of major incidents to clarify which are the responsible public bodies, who within them has responsibility for emergency preparedness, what procedures are to be followed, and how the additional requirements are to be financed.

For example, in the UK, integration of local authorities, the NHS, fire and rescue services, the police, and other statutory agencies, as well as non-statutory agencies such as the Red Cross and other voluntary bodies, is crucial. Coordination of planning, service design, and service delivery is the responsibility of the Local Resilience Forums. Discharging the tasks probably requires standing groups to be established involving advisers who have experience of the mental health aspects of major incidents. It is important to avoid the loss of knowledge and of relationships between key people that occurs all too often as a result of staff turnover, promotion, and changes in organisational structure.

Summary

General Principles That Emerge from the Science

The mental health response to an incident should be based on its estimated scale, how it is likely to unfold, the variety of groups that are potentially affected, and the type and chronology of stress reactions and mental health disorders that can be anticipated. These responses should be well integrated into every aspect of the response plan [40,41].

A Description of the Short-, Medium-, and Long-Term Impacts

Many people are likely to be distressed in the short term, and a smaller number will experience distress in the medium or longer terms. A minority of people who are directly affected are likely to show acute stress reactions in the days immediately following the incident. The other main short-term impact involves an increase in anxiety and avoidant behaviours, which in most cases are likely to resolve provided that there is no continuing source of threat, secondary stressors are reduced to a minimum, and the support of people's families or friends is available throughout this period [24,25]. However, the findings from research involving people affected by the Manchester Arena bombing estimate that perhaps 30% of affected people may develop more persistent distress [24,25]. Reactions of this nature may occur in many other major incidents, and can include people who were not directly affected. With time, more people who have persistent problems are likely to be identified, and some of them may require formal assessment and other interventions. Indeed, the later people come forward, the more likely they are to need formal intervention from specialised mental health services.

The Implications for Intervention

Knowledge about the principles and types of intervention required is constantly advancing. The main issue in major incidents is the timely mobilisation of an effective response. The key objectives are as follows:

- anticipation and mapping of all the groups that are likely to be affected
- involving key stakeholders and community leaders
- identifying the relevant affected people and determining how to contact them
- collecting and holding these details in a secure database with safeguards on data usage

- tailoring an appropriate suite of assessments, interventions, and treatments
- funding any addition to existing services that may be necessary to deliver what is required.

Practical Aspects of Implementing the Principles

There are considerable organisational problems in mobilising and delivering psychosocial support and formal interventions to the people who need them. These problems can only be effectively dealt with before incidents occur. This means that the right structures and processes must already be in place. At the very minimum, we suggest that these should include the following:

- a national major incident mental health response group that is permanently staffed
- the integration of mental health into emergency planning scenarios and exercises
- agreed funding mechanisms
- robust data-sharing agreements with public and private organisations
- a nominated body with a protocol for gathering and responsibility for information about affected people.

References

1. Fenn L, Brunton-Smith I. The effects of terrorist incidents on public worry of future attacks, views of the police and social cohesion. *Br J Criminol* 2021; **61**: 497–518.

2. Huddy L, Feldman S, Taber C, Lahav G. Threat, anxiety, and support of antiterrorism policies. *Am J Pol Sci* 2005; **49**: 593–608.

3. Huddy L, Feldman S, Capelos T, Provost C. The consequences of terrorism: disentangling the effects of personal and national threat. *Polit Psychol* 2002; **23**: 485–509.

4. Bonanno GA, Jost JT. Conservative shift among high-exposure survivors of the September 11th terrorist attacks. *Basic Appl Soc Psych* 2006; **28**: 311–23.

5. Nail PR, McGregor I. Conservative shift among liberals and conservatives following 9/11/01. *Soc Justice Res* 2009; **22**: 231–40.

6. Van de Vyver J, Houston DM, Abrams D, Vasiljevic M. Boosting belligerence: how the July 7, 2005, London bombings affected liberals' moral foundations and prejudice. *Psychol Sci* 2016; **27**: 169–77.

7. World Health Organization (WHO). *Floods in the WHO European Region: Health Effects and Their Prevention*. WHO and Public Health England, 2013.

8. Stanke C, Murray V, Amlôt R, Nurse J, Williams R. The effects of flooding on mental health: outcomes and recommendations from a review of the literature. *PLoS Curr* 2012; **4**: e4f9f1fa9c3cae.

9. Davidson JRT, McFarlane AC. The extent and impact of mental health problems after disaster. *J Clin Psychiatry* 2006; **67**: 9–14.

10. Norris FH, Friedman MJ, Watson PJ, Byrne CM, Diaz E, Kaniasty K. 60,000 disaster victims speak: Part I. An empirical review of the empirical literature, 1981–2001. *Psychiatry* 2002; **65**: 207–39.

11. Besser A, Neria Y. When home isn't a safe haven: insecure attachment orientations, perceived social support, and PTSD symptoms among Israeli evacuees under missile threat. *Psychol Trauma* 2012; **4**: 34–46.

12. Alexander D. A magnitude scale for cascading disasters. *Int J Disaster Risk Reduct* 2018; **30**: 180–85.

13. Norris FH. Disasters in urban context. *J Urban Health* 2002; **79**: 308–14.

14. French P, Barrett A, Allsopp K, Williams R, Brewin CR, Hind D, et al. Psychological screening of adults and young people following the Manchester Arena incident. *BJPsych Open* 2019; **5**: e85.

15. Stephens NM, Hamedani MG, Markus HR, Bergsieker HB, Eloul L. Why did they "choose" to stay? Perspectives of Hurricane Katrina observers and survivors. *Psychol Sci* 2009; **20**: 878–86.

16. Thiede BC, Brown DL. Hurricane Katrina: who stayed and why? *Popul Res Policy Rev* 2013; **32**: 803–24.

17. Bryant RA, Gallagher HC, Gibbs L, Pattison P, MacDougall C, Harms L, et al. Mental health and social networks after disaster. *Am J Psychiatry* 2017; **174**: 277–85.

18. Kaniasty K, de Terte I, Guilaran J, Bennett S. A scoping review of post-disaster social support investigations conducted after disasters that struck the Australia and Oceania continent. *Disasters* 2020; **44**: 336–66.

19. Masson T, Bamberg S, Stricker M, Heidenreich A. 'We can help ourselves': does community resilience buffer against the negative impact of flooding on mental health? *Nat Hazards Earth Syst Sci* 2019; **19**: 2371–84.

20. Koyama S, Aida J, Kawachi I, Kondo N, Subramanian SV, Ito K, et al. Social support improves mental health among the victims relocated to temporary housing following the Great East Japan earthquake and tsunami. *Tohoku J Exp Med* 2014; **234**: 241–7.

21. Fu T-H, Lin W-I, Shieh J-C. The impact of post-disaster relocation on community solidarity: the case of post-disaster reconstruction after Typhoon Morakot in Taiwan. *World Acad Sci Eng Technol* 2013; **7**: 1964–7.

22. Oishi S, Kimura R, Hayashi H, Tatsuki S, Tamura K, Ishii K, et al. Psychological adaptation to the Great Hanshin-Awaji Earthquake of 1995: 16 years later victims still report lower levels of subjective well-being. *J Res Pers* 2015; **55**: 84–90.

23. Rubin GJ, Brewin CR, Greenberg N, Simpson J, Wessely S. Psychological and behavioural reactions to the bombings in London on 7 July 2005: cross sectional survey of a representative sample of Londoners. *BMJ* 2005; **331**: 606–11.

24. Stancombe J, Williams R, Drury J, Collins H, Lagan L, Barrett A, et al. People's experiences of distress and psychosocial care following a terrorist attack: interviews with survivors of the Manchester Arena bombing in 2017. *BJPsych Open* 2022; **8**: e41.

25. Drury J, Stancombe J, Williams R, Collins H, Lagan L, Barrett A, et al. Survivors' experiences of informal social support in coping and recovering after the 2017 Manchester Arena bombing. *BJPsych Open* 2022; **8**: e124.

26. Bonanno GA, Brewin CR, Kaniasty K, La Greca AM. Weighing the costs of disaster: consequences, risks, and resilience in individuals, families, and communities. *Psychol Sci Public Interest* 2010; **11**: 1–49.

27. Silver RC, Holman EA, Garfin DR. Coping with cascading collective traumas in the United States. *Nat Hum Behav* 2021; **5**: 4–6.

28. Bish A, Michie S, Yardley L. *Principles of Effective Communication: Scientific Evidence Base Review.* Department of Health, 2021 (https://assets.publishing.service .gov.uk/government/uploads/ system/uploads/attachment_data/ file/215678/dh_125431.pdf).

29. Allsopp K, Brewin CR, Barrett A, Williams R, Hind D, Chitsabesan P, et al. Responding to mental health needs after terror attacks. *BMJ* 2019; **366**: 14828.

30. Brewin CR, Fuchkan N, Huntley Z, Robertson M, Thompson M, Scragg P, et al. Outreach and screening following the 2005 London bombings: usage and outcomes. *Psychol Med* 2010; **40**: 2049–57.

31. Nahar N, Blomstedt Y, Wu B, Kandarina I, Trisnantoro L, Kinsman J. Increasing the provision of mental health care for vulnerable, disaster-affected people in Bangladesh. *BMC Public Health* 2014; **14**: 708.

32. Keys C, Nanayakkara G, Onyejekwe C, Sah RK, Wright T. Health inequalities and ethnic vulnerabilities during COVID-19 in the UK: a reflection on the PHE reports. *Fem Leg Stud* 2021; **29**: 107–18.

33. Masozera M, Bailey M, Kerchner C. Distribution of impacts of natural disasters across income groups: a case study of New Orleans. *Ecol Econ* 2007; **63**: 299–306.

34. Behbod B, Leonardi G, Motreff Y, Beck CR, Yzermans J, Lebret E, et al. An international comparison of the instigation and design of health registers in the epidemiological response to major environmental health incidents. *J Public Health Manag Pract* 2017; **23**: 20–28.

35. Catchpole MA, Morgan O. Physical health of members of the public who experienced terrorist bombings in London on 07 July 2005. *Prehosp Disaster Med* 2010; **25**: 139–44.

36. Close RM, Maguire H, Etherington G, Brewin CR, Fong K, Saliba V, et al. Preparedness for a major incident: creation of an

epidemiology protocol for a health protection register in England. *Environ Int* 2014; **72**: 75–82.

37. Motreff Y, Pirard P, Lagree C, Roudier C, Empereur-Bissonnet P. Voluntary health registry of French nationals after the Great East Japan earthquake, tsunami, and Fukushima Daiichi nuclear power plant accident: methods, results, implications, and feedback. *Prehosp Disaster Med* 2016; **31**: 326–9.

38. Rubin GJ, Webster R, Rubin AN, Amlôt R, Grey N, Greenberg N. Public attitudes in England towards the sharing of personal data following a mass casualty incident: a cross-sectional study. *BMJ Open* 2018; **8**: e022852.

39. North CS, Pfefferbaum B. Mental health response to community disasters: a systematic review. *JAMA* 2013; **310**: 507–18.

40. Williams R, Bisson JI, Kemp V. Health care planning for community disaster care. In *Textbook of Disaster Psychiatry* 2nd ed. (eds RJ Ursano, CS Fullerton, L Weisaeth, B Raphael): 244–60. Cambridge University Press, 2017.

41. NHS England and NHS Improvement. *Responding to the Needs of People Affected by Incidents and Emergencies: Guidance for Planning, Delivering and Evaluating Psychosocial and Mental Healthcare*. NHS England and NHS Improvement, 2021.

Mental Health in the Context of Multiple Exposures to Disasters

Claire Leppold and Lennart Reifels

Introduction

We are now living in a time characterised by a multiplicity of incidents and disasters. The potential for disasters to overlap, cascade, and compound each other has been seen in a new light in recent years as disasters have occurred on top of the COVID-19 pandemic. The year 2020 saw a new record in terms of the most active Atlantic hurricane season to date, with 30 named storms, of which 14 became hurricanes and 7 became major hurricanes, occurring at the same time as the first wave of the pandemic [1]. Although disasters have historically been perceived as rare events, and often researched with a focus on single events, there is growing evidence that people and places are experiencing multiple disasters [2]. Climate change has been predicted to increase the frequency and severity of extreme weather events [3], and the number of people who experience multiple disaster exposures across their lifetime is likely to rise. Consequently, the field of disaster studies, and mental health research in disaster contexts, must continue to grow and develop to enable us to understand and address the complexity of multiple disaster exposures.

This chapter draws on our recent review of the public health impacts of multiple disaster exposures [2], and it unpacks findings on mental health. We present key review findings on cumulative exposures, re-activation of post-traumatic stress disorder (PTSD), and links between mental and physical health. Overall, we argue that multiple disaster exposures have some different implications for mental health compared with exposure to a single disaster, and should be prioritised as an emerging public health issue, given the projected increase in disasters due to climate change. Viewing disasters as single rare events is no longer accurate in the field of public health.

Multiple Disaster Exposure Contexts and Constellations

Certain multiple disaster scenarios have been well studied, generating valuable bodies of evidence for particular disaster contexts and constellations. For instance, the disaster that occurred in Fukushima, Japan, in March 2011 comprised an earthquake, tsunami, and nuclear disaster, and is sometimes referred to as a 'triple disaster'. Another well-studied location identified in this review was the Gulf Coast of the USA, where Hurricane Katrina occurred in 2005, followed by Hurricane Rita, also in 2005, and the BP oil spill in 2010, in addition to Hurricane Gustav in 2008, Hurricane Ike in 2008, and Hurricane Isaac in 2012, among others [2]. The events that occurred in Fukushima in 2011 are an example of a cascading disaster (an earthquake leading to a tsunami, which subsequently led to a nuclear accident at the Fukushima Daiichi nuclear power plant), whereas the Gulf Coast illustrates a case of recurring disasters of the same type (hurricanes), in addition to an unrelated oil spill in the same place.

There are also new disaster scenarios occurring all the time. During the first 3 weeks of 2021 alone, the Indonesian National Board for Disaster Management reported 185 disasters resulting from natural hazards [4]. In early 2022, the Hunga Tonga volcanic eruption led to a tsunami, and relief efforts were complicated by a COVID-19 outbreak. The floods in Eastern Australia in 2022 included some of the worst flooding disasters in Australian history, while many of the regions affected were still in the process of recovering from the devastating impacts of the Black Summer bushfires of 2019–2020. The total number of locations affected by multiple disaster trajectories is growing every month, and the full extent of these effects is still not understood. This scoping review was therefore conducted to document the public health implications of multiple disaster exposures, and it reflects the state of the literature as of August 2021.

For the purpose of our review of published science we used the UN Office for Disaster Risk Reduction (UNDRR) definition of disaster as a 'serious disruption of the functioning of a community or a society at any scale due to hazardous events interacting with conditions of exposure, vulnerability and capacity, leading to one or more of the following: human, material, economic and environmental losses and impacts' [5]. We took an inclusive view of disasters of different origins or causes, and included all types of disasters that fit the UNDRR definition, such as those resulting from natural hazards, technological disasters, war, and terrorism. Inclusion criteria were that 'articles focus on individuals or communities exposed to multiple disasters, and include discussion of the health, wellbeing, or social effects of these disasters; post-disaster activities; or economic, cultural, legal, or political effects that could influence health or wellbeing' [2]. After screening, 150 articles were included in our review, of which 53 articles focused on mental health. Full details of the inclusion criteria and screening process can be found in the paper [2].

Key Mental Health Findings

The subsections under this heading cover some key areas of mental health findings identified in our review, and highlight recommendations for practice and future research.

Cumulative Effects

One mental health finding of this review was evidence for cumulative effects. This review identified a group of studies, which found that exposure to two or more disasters was associated with a higher likelihood of adverse mental health outcomes compared with exposure to a single disaster. This cumulative effect was documented for outcomes including suicide, depression, probable generalised anxiety disorder, and PTSD, examined by studies across a range of different disaster settings [2]. For example, in Australia a nationally representative survey found that people who had been exposed to multiple disasters during their lifetime had a statistically significantly higher risk of suicide attempts compared with those who had been exposed to a single disaster [6]. Studies focusing on cumulative effects included those that examined exposure to multiple disasters of the

same type (e.g., multiple 'natural' disasters, compared with one such disaster) [6], as well as those which looked at exposure to multiple disasters of different types (e.g., exposure to Hurricane Katrina and the BP oil spill, compared with exposure to only one of these disasters) [7,8].

Although some scholars and practitioners have speculated that exposure to one disaster could potentially have positive effects, such as desensitising, inoculating, or better 'preparing' people for future disasters, and thereby reducing the likelihood of subsequent negative effects on mental health, our review could not find clear evidence to support this idea. On the contrary, Emily Harville and her colleagues studied the impacts of Hurricane Katrina in 2005 and Hurricane Gustav in 2008, and documented the cumulative risk to mental health associated with exposure to both hurricanes [9]. Importantly, this study found that even when people reported feeling a positive benefit of becoming more mentally prepared for disasters after Hurricane Katrina, this was not associated with protective effects on their mental health during Hurricane Gustav.

Some aspects of cumulative effects are still not well understood. One study identified in the review found differences in cumulative effects depending on the participant's age at the time of exposure, such that high levels of previous exposure to disaster were associated with an increased risk of developing PTSD symptoms after exposure to a subsequent disaster for younger adults, but not for older adults [10]. Other authors have pointed out that cumulative exposure may depend on the severity of exposures, and that it may be event- and experience-specific – for example, potentially relating to the types of exposure and secondary stressors, rather than just the crude number of exposures [11]. There is still a need for further research to consolidate and refine our understanding of these processes. However, the evidence to date clearly suggests that experiences of disasters can 'stack' on top of each other, and thus cumulatively increase risk.

Interactive Effects

The review also identified growing evidence for interactive effects, whereby two different disaster exposures can simultaneously have a joint effect that is greater and more complex than the sum of the exposures. This trend was clearly highlighted by evidence for the 're-activation' of PTSD from one disaster to the next, particularly from studies of populations in and around New York City which had been exposed both to the 9/11 terrorism attacks in 2001 and to Hurricane Sandy in 2012. Multiple sources found that people's exposure to Hurricane Sandy was associated with a recurrence of symptoms of PTSD that were originally related to their exposure to 9/11, even if the symptoms had resolved before the hurricane [12–14]. The evidence from New York is especially notable, given that 9/11 and Hurricane Sandy occurred 11 years apart and were completely different types of disaster. This highlights the need for potential interactive effects of disasters on mental health to be considered over a long timescale.

Our review also identified some evidence about the interactive link between mental and physical health across multiple disasters. For example, on the Gulf Coast of the USA, one study of Hurricane Katrina and the BP oil spill found that Katrina-related losses were associated with distress following the oil spill, which was subsequently associated with physical symptoms. The researchers outlined a pathway by which mental health effects translated into physical health risks in this context when multiple exposures occurred over a period of years [15]. The link between mental and physical health has also been studied in settings in which multiple disaster exposures occurred in quick succession. In Japan, for example, one study after the 'triple' disaster in March 2011 found that PTSD and insomnia were associated with an increased risk of bone fractures in older adults [16]. These studies represent a growing area of research. The links between multiple exposures to disasters, mental health, and physical health deserve greater research attention to enable us to better understand their causal pathways and wider implications for wellbeing and quality of life.

Overall, the evidence identified in our review suggests that multiple disaster exposures can have impacts on mental health that exceed the effects seen after single disasters. The literature identified at the time of the review does not necessarily suggest that multiple exposures are linked to the emergence of new types of mental health conditions. Rather, the complexity of cumulative and interactive effects appears to indicate the potential for the progression of mental health conditions to be accelerated or re-activated. Thus these cumulative and interactive effects have an impact on the overall scale of anticipated mental health outcomes in settings involving multiple exposures, compared with those involving single exposures.

Recommendations for Practice

It is notable that, at the time of this review, most guidelines and frameworks on disaster mental healthcare for people and communities have been based on the premise of a single disaster occurring. This is also true for broader psychosocial support interventions. As Joshua Miller and Gianluca Pescaroli note, 'Despite the strengthening of psychological guidelines in the last decade, the implications of cascading disasters have not yet been adequately considered in the psycho-social literature and in practice' [17, p. 167]. We suggest that the evidence for cumulative and interactive effects documented here should draw renewed attention to the need to actively support the resilience of communities in disaster-prone areas, and to ensure that relevant supports are put in place for populations that are exposed to multiple disasters.

The articles that have been cited in this chapter made various recommendations for practice. Some studies recommend that clinicians screen for past exposure to disasters, that counselling protocols take into account people's histories of symptoms of PTSD associated with previous disasters, and that post-disaster mental health interventions include screening for previous disaster exposure in order to identify groups of people who may be at high risk of adverse outcomes in subsequent exposures [2]. More widely, Yuval Palgi and colleagues have underscored the importance of considering the historical nature of trauma in an area, and therefore taking into account previous traumatic events in communities when interpreting the effects of current disasters [18]. We fully support these recommendations. Further research will also aid our understanding of the full extent of the potential impacts of overlapping, cascading, or compound disasters, so that we can continue to develop an understanding of what constitutes best practice in these circumstances.

Directions for Further Research

Research on mental health in settings of multiple disaster exposures is continuing to develop, and there is still more to be done. This review identifies a particular need for more nuanced research to examine different effects by timing and type of disaster exposure – for example, any differences in effects between disaster exposures that occur in rapid succession and multiple exposures that are spread over a long time period [2]. Furthermore, it is worth remembering that conducting research on the outcomes of multiple exposures to disasters involves being aware of methodological and theoretical questions (e.g., how to define what 'exposure' to a disaster means) that are also present in single-disaster settings [19], but which may be amplified in settings where multiple disasters occur. We also need to consider the wider context in which multiple disaster exposures are happening, including the structural inequalities that can influence which population groups are likely to be exposed to disasters [20], and personal experiences of other traumatic life events which may also accumulate with multiple disaster exposures to create an interactive risk profile. More broadly, there remains a need for research on practice and interventions. There is a significant knowledge gap with regard to which interventions and support models are effective in averting mental health risks in multi-disaster scenarios, and we suggest that this should also be a priority area for further research.

Conclusion

This chapter presents a brief summary of the findings about mental health from a scoping review of the public health impacts of multiple exposures to disasters, with a focus on cumulative and interactive effects. It makes the case that multiple disaster exposures have some different implications to single exposures to a disaster, and should be treated as a priority emerging public health issue, given the projected increases in the frequency and severity of disasters due to climate change.

This review was conducted at a time when there was rapidly growing attention to this area, and we hope that this body of research continues to expand. We emphasise the continuing need for researchers and policymakers to work creatively to improve strategies for disaster risk reduction, and for public health preparedness, response, and recovery to better account for the realities arising from scenarios of multiple disasters.

References

1. Shultz JM, Berg RC, Kossin JP, Burkle Jr F, Maggioni A, Pinilla Escobar VA, et al. Convergence of climate-driven hurricanes and COVID-19: the impact of 2020 hurricanes Eta and Iota on Nicaragua. *J Clim Chang Health* 2021; **3**: 100019.

2. Leppold C, Gibbs L, Block K, Reifels L, Quinn P. Public health implications of multiple disaster exposures. *Lancet Public Health* 2022; **7**: e274–86.

3. Intergovernmental Panel on Climate Change (IPCC). *AR6 Climate Change 2021: The Physical Science Basis. Summary for Policymakers.* IPCC, 2021 (www.ipcc.ch/report/ar6/wg1/).

4. Renaldi E. Indonesia's latest natural disasters are a 'wake-up call', environmentalists say. *ABC News*, 21 January 2021 (www.abc .net.au/news/2021-01-22/ indonesia-hit-by-series-of-disasters-in-the-first-weeks-of-2021/13075930).

5. United Nations Office for Disaster Risk Reduction (UNDRR). *Sendai Framework Terminology on Disaster Risk Reduction: Disaster.* UNDRR, undated (www.undrr .org/terminology/disaster).

6. Reifels L, Spittal MJ, Dückers MLA, Mills K, Pirkis J. Suicidality risk and (repeat) disaster exposure: findings from a nationally representative population survey. *Psychiatry* 2018; **81**: 158–72.

7. Harville EW, Shankar A, Schetter CD, Lichtveld M. Cumulative effects of the Gulf oil spill and other disasters on mental health among reproductive-aged women: the Gulf Resilience on Women's Health Study. *Psychol Trauma* 2018; **10**: 533–41.

8. Lowe SR, McGrath JA, Young MN, Kwok RK, Engel LS, Galea S et al. Cumulative disaster exposure and mental and physical health symptoms among a large sample of Gulf Coast residents. *J Trauma Stress* 2019; **32**: 196–205.

9. Harville EW, Xiong X, Smith BW, Pridjian G, Elkind-Hirsch K, Buekens P. Combined effects of Hurricane Katrina and Hurricane Gustav on the mental health of mothers of small children. *J Psychiatr Ment Health Nurs* 2011; **18**: 288–96.

10. Shrira A, Palgi Y, Yaira H-R, Goodwin R, Menachem B-E. Previous exposure to the World Trade Center terrorist attack and posttraumatic symptoms among older adults following Hurricane Sandy. *Psychiatry* 2014; **77**: 374–85.

11. Garfin DR, Silver RC, Ugalde FJ, Linn H, Inostroza M. Exposure to rapid succession disasters: a study of residents at the epicenter of the Chilean Bío Bío earthquake. *J Abnorm Psychol* 2014; **123**: 545–56.

12. Gargano LM, Li JH, Millien L, Alper H, Brackbill RM. Exposure to multiple disasters: the long-term effect of Hurricane Sandy (October 29, 2012) on NYC survivors of the September 11,

2001 World Trade Center attack. *Psychiatry Res* 2019; **273**: 719–24.

13. Li J, Alper HE, Gargano LM, Maslow CB, Brackbill RM. Re-experiencing 9/11-related PTSD symptoms following exposure to Hurricane Sandy. *Int J Emerg Ment Health* 2018; **20**. Available from: https://doi.org/10.4172/1522-4821.1000404.

14. Bromet EJ, Clouston S, Gonzalez A, Kotov R, Guerrera KM, Luft BJ. Hurricane Sandy exposure and the mental health of World Trade Center responders. *J Trauma Stress* 2017; **30**: 107–14.

15. Osofsky HJ, Hansel TC, Osofsky JD, Speier A. Factors contributing to mental and physical health care in a disaster-prone environment. *Behav Med* 2015; **41**: 131–7.

16. Hayashi F, Ohira T, Nakano H, Nagao M, Okazaki K, Harigane M, et al. Association between post-traumatic stress disorder symptoms and bone fractures after the Great East Japan Earthquake in older adults: a prospective cohort study from the Fukushima Health Management Survey. *BMC Geriatr* 2021; **21**: 18.

17. Miller JL, Pescaroli G. Psychosocial capacity building in response to cascading disasters: a culturally informed approach. *Int J Disaster Risk Reduct* 2018; **30**: 164–71.

18. Palgi Y, Shrira A, Hamama-Raz Y, Palgi S, Goodwin R, Ben-Ezra M. Not so close but still extremely loud: recollection of the World Trade Center terror attack and previous hurricanes moderates the association between exposure to Hurricane Sandy and posttraumatic stress symptoms. *Compr Psychiatry* 2014; **55**: 807–12.

19. Perry RW. Disasters, definitions and theory construction. In *What is a Disaster? New Answers to Old Questions* (eds RW Perry, EL Quarantelli): 311–24. Xlibris, 2005.

20. Reid M. Disasters and social inequalities. *Sociol Compass* 2013; **7**: 984–97.

Chapter 12

The Common Ground in the Mental Health Impacts of Emergencies, Incidents, Disasters, Disease Outbreaks, and Conflict, and a Framework for Responding to People's Needs

Richard Williams, John Stancombe, and James Ryan

Introduction

This chapter introduces several themes that recur throughout this book. It also reflects on a selection of topics that are the focus of chapters in this section. Our intention is to encourage readers to think about these themes, but not to provide comprehensive accounts this early in the book. One key matter concerns the common areas and differences in people's responses and needs before, during, and after emergencies, incidents, terrorist events, disasters, disease outbreaks and conflicts (EITDDC). First, we summarise the themes and look at people's responses in more detail. Later, we consider the interventions that people require to cope with the immediate impacts of events. Finally, we identify a strategic approach for communities.

The Common Ground

Typologies of Emergencies, Incidents, and Disasters

A common consideration in many accounts concerns typologies of disasters; they are often divided into natural and human-made disasters. In reality the distinction is much less clear-cut than these two categories suggest. We can detect the hands of humans in all disasters. Although it is possible to separate the hazards into those that stem from so-called natural events and those in which humans are directly involved, the frequency of natural hazards (e.g., floods, high winds) is plainly affected by human policies, plans, and activities, as the contemporary grave concerns about climate change demonstrate most strongly. This is as true for the COVID-19 pandemic as it is for recent terrorist incidents. Put another way, we may erect typologies of hazards, but humans influence the mediation, moderation, and mitigation of most disasters, and they may

be – deliberately, unwittingly, or otherwise – perpetrators of some incidents. Therefore we do not adopt a rigid typology in this book, but encourage readers to familiarise themselves with the core elements of how humans cope with untoward events and the problems that they may experience.

We think that a broad approach to understanding how people react is feasible, and that this is a good basis for planning and for setting responses in hand at the beginning of all emergencies. Once a broad plan for responding to people's needs has been engaged, more detailed consideration of the nature of what happened, how it did so, and with what effects becomes appropriate. Thus we based our work on this thesis when we researched the 7/7 London bombings of 2005, advised about and researched the Manchester Arena bombing of 2017, and advised the responsible authorities during the COVID-19 pandemic.

We think that, just as there are important differences in how different types of emergency affect people, there are also great similarities in how humans respond and in the mental health consequences. We refer readers back to Chapter 3 to see that it is not only the events but also their philosophical and societal contexts that impinge on the meaning of events, as well as people's personal or shared values, which may differ from or be similar to each other. These considerations raise fundamental issues – to which we return at intervals throughout this book – about the nature of society, and about public and personal expectations that may have as much to do with the similarities and differences of the impacts as do the events themselves.

Pragmatically, we identified three broad patterns of incident in Chapter 10:

1. big bang
2. rising tide
3. longer-term incidents.

However, we identify from the content of that chapter and the mixed categories of incident summarised there that there are also five more complicated sorts of incident that have an impact on healthcare services:

1. continuing incidents, such as the rapid onset of recurring incidents that evoke huge demands on responders, with major long-term consequences (e.g., the Australian bush fires of 2019–2020)
2. clouds on the horizon – protracted build ups to war and catastrophic incidents overseas
3. headline news – media-driven public alarm and health scares
4. internal incidents – internal workings of organisations affected by incidents (e.g., power outages, flooding)
5. deliberate or accidental releases of chemical, biological, radiological, or nuclear materials.

Typically, many agencies are involved in responding to incidents. In the UK, for example, they include:

- central government – for example, through COBR (COBRA)
- the police
- fire and rescue services
- the NHS, including ambulance services
- the Maritime and Coastguard Agency (MCA)
- the Royal National Lifeboat Institution (RNLI)
- local authorities
- the intelligence, security, and communication services
- voluntary agencies
- the public
- the military (for certain defined circumstances and tasks).

Therefore, coordinating planning, decision-making, and responding becomes a major challenge to safe and effective care. Reports on emergencies and major incidents often find that:

- there is a breakdown of communication between affected sites and between the scene, hospitals, and other healthcare services
- healthcare staff may receive good training, but it is often orientated to past events and not focused on possible future incidents
- there is a temptation for authorities to make assumptions about their capacities and capabilities that may not be borne out in practice.

The Impacts of Emergencies, Incidents, and Disasters on the People Directly Affected

We learned in Chapter 3 that there are four cohorts of people affected by emergencies – survivors, witnesses, participants, and onlookers – and that they are defined by both physical and psychological distance from the scene of the event. In this book we consider these four categories (described by Charles Strozier as 'zones of sadness)'. This chapter and many others focus on survivors, and we also refer readers to Section 3, where several other cohorts are considered in more detail.

Figures 12.1 and 12.2 are from the UN Office for Disaster Risk Reduction (UNDRR) [1]. They compare the impacts of a variety of types of disaster using the numbers of deaths and the numbers of people affected as indices. They emphasise just how many people are affected each year by disasters. We do not examine each of the types of events in this book – research has shown that different types of emergency have very broadly similar effects, although each hazard has its own unique features and therefore a varying range of impacts on humans of differing prominence. For example, different risks and horrors emerge from a tsunami compared with a seasonal flood in a temperate zone, or with being engulfed in a mudslide, which is arguably one of the worst experiences imaginable.

Chapter 8 offers a summary of the myths that surround disasters of all kinds, the most significant of which is that people panic in the immediate aftermath. Another misconception is that disasters are rare. This is not so. In fact they are so common that many people experience a number of incidents in the course of their lives. Chapter 11 refers to the growing evidence that people and places are experiencing multiple disasters. In that chapter, Claire Leppold and Lennart Reifels identify the cumulative and interacting effects on people who are exposed to disastrous incidents that occur in close proximity or many years apart. They also highlight the interactions between physical ill health and the mental health impacts of multiple exposure to disasters. Julian Redhead emphasises the mental health dimensions of major physical trauma in Chapter 2.

Yet the structural aspects of emergencies, incidents, communicable disease outbreaks, and warfare are very different. Furthermore, all pandemics, near pandemics, epidemics, and public health emergencies

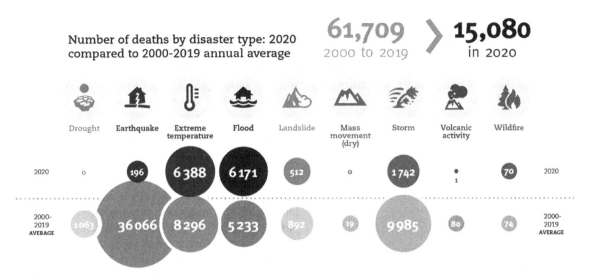

Figure 12.1 Deaths related to disasters. Reproduced from UNDRR [1].

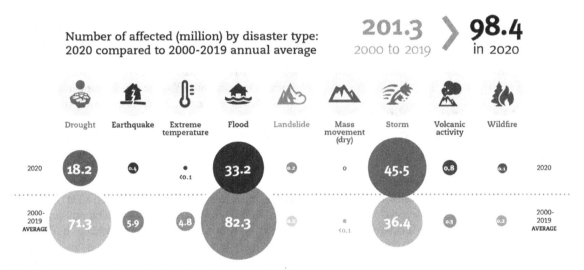

Figure 12.2 Numbers of people affected by disasters. Reproduced from UNDRR [1].

of international concern (PHEICs) are not the same. Nevertheless, we assert that there are basic public health principles in common about how we should respond to incidents and disasters of differing origins that take place in different parts of the world. Compare, for example, the H1N1 flu pandemic of 2009–2010 with the COVID-19 pandemic of 2019 onwards, and the WHO declaration of monkeypox as a PHEIC in July 2022.

The common ground of terrorist events, conflict and warfare may appear to be that they are deliberate acts of mass violence. However, all emergencies are violent to some degree, and the common nature of

many emergencies is arguably the intensity of the events and the intensity of their impacts on humans.

Two of us (JR and RW) have spoken at training events and have extracted lessons from a succession of urban terrorist incidents. They raise very similar questions about what are likely to be the better responses of the rescue and specialist health services, and about endeavours to protect responders and patients against the impacts on their mental health. In our talks, we progress from the impacts of 7/7 (multi-site coordinated transport bombings) in London in 2005, through the Bataclan shooting attack in 2015 in Paris (associated with atrocities at other sites in the city), to the Manchester Arena bombing in 2017 (a single incident, but one in which a high proportion of those involved were children and parents). There are lessons to be drawn from each of these incidents. Later in this chapter we return to comparing societal responses and how they have moved on over the last 20 years.

Despite these variations, we recognise that there are common broad patterns of serious physical injury, which include:

- penetrating injuries
- blunt injuries
- thermal injuries
- blast effects
- acute lung injury and/or other lung lesions
- cardiac risks
- traumatic amputation
- deafness.

There can be no doubt that the creation of generic major trauma centres in the UK has had huge effects on survival in the face of these kinds of injury, and in reducing persisting disability resulting from the kinds of event described in Chapter 2.

The Effects of Emergencies, Incidents, Disasters, and Disease Outbreaks on People's Mental Health

Having scoped in outline the nature of incidents, we offer an overview of the mental health impacts. It is based on recent research into the psychosocial and mental health impacts of terrorist incidents as well as the COVID-19 pandemic.

As the COVID-19 pandemic began, a number of people forecast that there would be a tsunami of mental ill health associated with morbidity and mortality directly due to SARS-CoV-2, and indirectly due to the socioeconomic stress and stringent social restrictions. Similar concerns were voiced about the health, wellbeing, and mental ill health of the health-care workforce [2]. Early studies were mainly based on single uncontrolled cross-sectional quantitative surveys of convenience samples using self-completed screening questionnaires for mental illness, which can yield higher rates of disorders than are later supported by clinical interviews. Hence many surveys reported high rates of probable mental ill health among both populations and health carers [3]. How should we interpret these claims? Do the high numbers reflect true levels of mental health disorders, do they reflect the adjustments being made by people faced with real challenges, or do they reflect short-term or more persisting distress? Also, is it possible that people who are suffering substantially are more inclined to come forward in convenience sampling? These are corollaries of questions raised by John Alderdice in Chapter 3.

Studies are now emerging that have used more exacting sampling and longitudinal methodologies. They show lower rises in the levels of disorder compared with the surveys based on convenience sampling. This challenges not only the survey methods but also the accuracy of the population normative data with which survey scores are usually compared.

There are other questions, too. For example, how does this circumstance compare with those in other types of emergency or disaster? Researchers with experience of major incidents, for instance, did not expect a tsunami of mental disorders early on, but predicted that the effects would emerge more gradually. They also anticipated that the severity of the impacts and compliance with restrictions to liberty would vary inversely with socioeconomic affluence [4]. A number of experts who advised nationally, as well as the locally responsible authorities, based their early advice with regard to the so-called '100-year event' of COVID-19 on their experience with other types of major incident. They were not sure whether that experience would hold up in the face of the very different and much longer-term series of events that this pandemic has raised. Yet we were impressed by how accurate this general advice was in predicting what should be offered initially during the pandemic. Thus, based on research on other emergencies, major incidents, conflict, and outbreaks of high consequence infectious diseases (HCIDs), we think that there may be more immediate impacts on people's wellbeing early on, but that the effects on the mental health of the public and professionals may be delayed, develop insidiously, and be protracted [5].

Trajectories of Psychosocial and Mental Health Impacts

We draw attention here to the trajectories over time of people's responses to all types of emergencies, incidents, and outbreaks. These public health trajectories apply to populations of people and are based on surveying people affected by a range of types of disaster. A number of authors offer graphs that show how

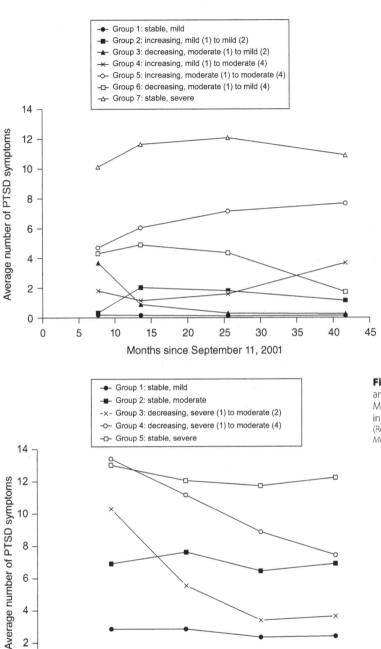

Figure 12.3 Trajectories of PTSD symptoms among residents of the New York City metropolitan area (n = 1,267) after the September 11, 2001 attacks [6]. Numbers in parentheses refer to the wave of assessment. (Reproduced with permission from *Social Science & Medicine*.)

Figure 12.4 Trajectories of PTSD symptoms among residents of Villahermosa and Teziutlan in Mexico (n = 561) after the 1999 flood [6]. Numbers in parentheses refer to the wave of assessment. (Reproduced with permission from *Social Science & Medicine*.)

the impacts of disastrous events vary with time. Often they are based on reported rates of symptoms of common mental disorders, especially post-traumatic stress disorder (PTSD). Examples are offered by Fran Norris and her colleagues [6].

Mobilisation and Deterioration of Support

Another matter to which we drew attention early on in this book concerns the impact of social support on how people respond to unwelcome events. Krzysztof

Kaniasty and Fran Norris have shown that there is usually an outpouring of altruistic responses that incorporate emotional and social support, sharing resources, innovative responses, and reductions in pre-existing tensions between groups of people very early on after major incidents [7]. These effects last for some time, and the levels of practical and emotional support in communities increase substantially. Thereafter, altruistic responses falter and the support falls away. We looked at this in relation to flooding in York and found a similar pattern [8].

This pattern is visible after many emergencies, incidents, and disasters, but our question in the first 4 months of 2020 was whether it would occur in response to the COVID-19 pandemic. Esther Murray and her colleagues believe that this is exactly what occurred during the initial months of the pandemic [9]. However, we believe that, although the COVID-19 pandemic has shown a wave pattern of waxing and waning case numbers as the SARS-CoV-2 virus has mutated, the mobilisation and deterioration phases of human response have been much more linear. The support mobilisation phase was very evident at the beginning of the pandemic, but it was followed by rapid decline, and that high level of support – for example, for healthcare staff – has not recurred.

The Psychosocial and Mental Health Impacts of Major Incidents on Survivors

Research has established that there is a broad spectrum of ways in which people who are directly or indirectly involved in emergencies, disasters, and disease outbreaks react emotionally, cognitively, socially, behaviourally, and physically [10,11]. An international review published in 2019 concluded that we understand little about the course of psychosocial distress after major incidents [12], but more recent research – for example, on the Manchester Arena bombing – has made a useful contribution to the literature, although there is still much further to go [13–15].

The Nature of Distress

One interesting challenge highlighted by the research involving people affected by the Manchester Arena bombing and by that on the COVID-19 pandemic, for example, is how we define and understand 'distress'. In our research we have used all three of the current approaches. This demonstrates the importance of agreeing definitions of terminology (see Chapter 27), and for that reason this book includes a Glossary.

John Alderdice provides a good example in Chapter 3 when he asks what constitutes a 'mental health problem'. The nature of distress is another example.

There have been three broad approaches to defining distress [15]. 'First, some of the literature refers to distress being comprised of sub-threshold symptoms of anxiety, depression, or post-traumatic stress disorder' [16]. 'The second common use of the term ... in relation to emergencies [is] to depict people who have a range of experiences that are anticipated, and usually much broader than symptoms of common mental disorders. Some accounts organise these potential experiences into emotional, cognitive, social, and physical domains' [17]. 'The ... third approach to defining distress [is based] on ... the experiences of people who say that they have been or are subjectively distressed. This is the way in which the term is applied in practice'.

Understanding People's Feelings, Behaviour, and Needs Before, During, and After Terrorism and War

Understanding how people feel and behave and their psychosocial and mental health needs before, during, and after emergencies is crucial to planning and delivering responses. Research on the psychosocial and mental health impacts of terrorist attacks has been predominantly quantitative, and has tended to focus on identifying specific psychopathology, usually PTSD or depression, within large cohorts of survivors. These studies privilege the prevalence of signs and symptoms while neglecting survivors' personal lived experiences, in terms of their experiences of distress over time and the impact of incidents on people's lives at the time and in the long term. However, recent studies have demonstrated that qualitative approaches can provide valuable insights into people's lived experience of psychosocial distress and its course [13,14]. We therefore recommend mixed methods approaches to studying the impacts of emergencies, incidents, disasters, and outbreaks of communicable diseases on humans.

Terrorist incidents are associated with multifaceted psychological and social reactions [18], with each type of event having its own stressors and potential for different mental health effects and psychosocial consequences [19]. Moreover, the burden of psychological and social consequences is substantial among large groups of people, even in those who are less exposed, such as witnesses, participants, and onlookers. The emotional wellbeing, physical health, social relationships, work, education, and quality of life of survivors may be affected for months or even years [20–23]. This pattern of early, medium- and long-term responses is identifiable in major incidents, such as 9/11 [24]. Serious effects on the physical and mental health of responders to 9/11 increased after the event and remain at substantial levels.

More than 40 years later, one of us (RW) read *Glimpses of the Falklands War*, a book of retrospective memories of people directly involved in the Falklands War of 1982, in which another of us (JR) served. He was a military surgeon, and later Professor of Military Surgery, who worked on East Falkland during that war [25]. Again, patterning of mental health responses and needs over time is visible in his and others' accounts. It consists of immediate calmness and not panic (see Chapter 8), early distress, which is almost ubiquitous, and which may persist and is accompanied by outpourings of altruistic concern and brave actions to care for and support injured colleagues, followed by personal mental retreat and reflection that lasts for much longer. The following extract describes part of JR's experience when the ship he was on was bombed from the air, severely damaged, and set ablaze, causing large numbers of soldiers and sailors to be killed or severely burned. He himself was not physically injured, and observed that:

> After the hit . . . I ended up on the floor. . . . We were in total darkness and all exits were buckled. A remarkable quietness ensued, and people just sat still and in silence. After a seemingly lengthy period, we heard the . . . voice of a young officer. He found a trapdoor leading outside. The officer . . . was cool and collected. He ushered us all to safety, only leaving when we were all safe   [25, p. 316].

It is clear how important the demeanour and leadership of such an inexperienced young man was to uninjured survivors. We read similar things in the accounts in Chapters 4 and 5. Time and again we learn similar lessons from accounts of severe events, such as the Manchester Arena bombing, demonstrating that people want authoritative acceptance and non-judgmental validation of their feelings early on. The non-intrusive support and care described by JR and offered naturally and spontaneously by such a junior officer represent exactly the kind of emotional, social, and practical support that is craved by people embroiled in most emergencies, and this links powerfully to the narrative account of Toni in Chapter 4. Thereafter, the majority of people may recover quickly

from their distress. However, a sizeable minority of unfortunate people may continue to be distressed and to retain memories that can persist for long periods of time in ways that risk becoming a way of life. At these times, people crave contacts with those who were also involved. Perhaps contributing to the book about the Falklands provided this kind of continuing care and support for some of the authors 40 years after the event. People's medium-term responses are likely to slowly diminish, or they may affect their social relationships and working lives; a minority of people in this group may have symptoms that are pathognomonic of mental ill health, for which specialist treatments are needed. We look at these paths in this book. For many of the people who were involved in the Falklands War, the impacts were clearly long-lasting, as is shown by the lucid and selfless contributions that so many people have made to *Glimpses of the Falklands War*.

Chapter 9 describes how the psychosocial effects of extreme events can be influenced by a complex combination of primary and secondary stressors. However, a lack of conceptual clarity about the nature of secondary stressors has hindered efforts to recognise and mitigate their effects through effective timely psychosocial interventions [26]. Moreover, systematic reviews have highlighted limitations of current research, including a lack of medium- to long-term follow-up and difficulties with separating the effects of primary and secondary stressors [12,27]. Again these matters came to the fore during the early waves of the COVID-19 pandemic. In response, a new social model of secondary stressors was proposed in 2021 [26]. That ushered in a more precise, practical, and heuristic definition of secondary stressors, and a growing awareness of their potential to exacerbate and prolong people's experience of distress after major events, and possibly contribute to longer-term social and relationship problems or the development of mental health disorders. Conversely, we hope that timely action to reduce the impacts of secondary stressors will reduce people's distress and suffering. The COVID-19 pandemic has clearly demonstrated the importance of tackling the risks that are most costly to the health and wellbeing of humans.

Using Psychosocial Care and Mental Healthcare After Emergencies and Major Incidents

Most studies of people after terrorist incidents examine the psychosocial impacts on them. However, the literature on using psychosocial care and mental healthcare after mass traumatic events is scarce. With a few notable exceptions [28–30], there has been a lack of studies that reflect survivors' voices. Consequently, relatively little is known about survivors' perceptions of, and experiences with, psychosocial care and mental healthcare response services. This is a key gap in the literature; we have little evidence on the effectiveness of psychosocial care and how models of stepped care and service delivery after major incidents work in practice. It is essential to learn more about consumers' experiences after incidents with outreach, psychosocial care, and mental healthcare services in order to identify the aspects of care that may be most important for meeting survivors' needs and strengthening preparedness for future incidents.

Our research on the Manchester Arena bombing draws attention to distress during and after incidents being ubiquitous among our participants. The numbers of people affected are much greater than the numbers who screen positive for a possible mental disorder. This means that screening scores cannot be used as a proxy for potential demand on services; there are likely to be people who are distressed, but do not report high levels of mental health symptoms, who are likely to wish to use services.

Current evidence suggests that people who develop distress in the wake of terrorist attacks may be reluctant to seek help, although the psychosocial factors underlying this apparent restraint are not clear [31]. It is possible that unidentified barriers prevent people from seeking or accepting care.

The findings from our interviews with people who attended the Manchester Arena event substantiate the importance of people's social connectedness and social support. As time passed after the event, people sought support initially from family members, subsequently from work or education colleagues, and then from other people who had attended the event. However, many people also reported that they wanted help with their distress but did not know how to get support, and they resorted to internet searches to help them to find services. Indeed, some felt that the delays in accessing psychosocial care were not favourable to their coping and recovery. By contrast, some interviewees said that the knowledge that services were available and accessible, if needed, helped to mitigate their distress.

General practitioners and primary care services were seen as an important source of care by people who were distressed, although they often reported receiving an unhelpful response. Many participants in the research described encountering limited knowledge of the psychosocial effects of major incidents and appropriate support services, and inappropriate offers of care.

Many interviewees reported that it was unhelpful to repeatedly encounter barriers when attempting to access mental healthcare. The barriers came in a variety of forms (e.g., being turned away due to not meeting services' threshold criteria for care, and the delays caused by long waiting lists). Some people thought that the stress of encountering these barriers compounded their experience of distress.

Unmet healthcare needs are associated with higher levels of psychological distress, post-traumatic stress, somatic symptoms, and less social support [30]. Our interviews with survivors of the Manchester Arena bombing have advanced our understanding of the relationship between unmet care needs and distress. Many interviewees' commentaries indicated their reluctance to approach support services if they felt that their distress was in some way invalid, or that support services were prioritising others. They reported that receiving validation of their suffering and their entitlement to care, particularly from someone whom they perceived to have special expertise, was a crucial component of the psychosocial care that they received [13]. However, people also report that being told their experiences are 'normal' can be invalidating. With good intentions, it is likely that service providers who used that term were trying to convey 'it's okay not to be okay'. However, the message that came across to many of our interviewees was that their distress was only minor, and it was part of normal experience. Thus the problem with 'normalising' reactions to major events is that it can minimise people's experience of distress and delegitimise their need for care [13].

Developments in Psychosocial Care and Mental Healthcare Since 7/7

More than 4,000 people were involved in some way in the effects of the London bombings on 7 July 2005, but there was no pre-planned mental health service available and there had been no prior financial planning. However, the government in England enabled an NHS Trauma Response Programme to be established in September 2005; it was centrally funded and ran until September 2007. This was the first service of its kind, and 596 adults returned at least one screening questionnaire to it. Realising the need for better planning, in 2005 the Department of Health in England established an expert advisory committee, which set out to improve planning in a way that integrated specialties, including mental health, from 2006. That work on integrating mental healthcare resulted in a report for England that was published in 2009, and in the same year, it also led to NATO publishing guidance on psychosocial care and mental healthcare after disasters [32,33]. However, implementation of the core elements of the guidance was slow.

Initially there was no psychosocial and mental health component in the major incident plan in place in Manchester on 22 May 2017. However, the advanced state of inter-agency partnership enabled effective and speedy 'hot planning' for services that were funded at risk. The local agencies recognised the mental health risks and the need to act, and were keen to accept external advice. This resulted in the Manchester Resilience Hub being put in place rapidly. This style of response has led the way in creating psychosocial and mental health services during the pandemic. Chapter 36 looks at that Hub in more detail as a case study. Despite the actions taken, children and young people affected by the attack had to wait 8 months for mental health support, and these delays have been replicated during the COVID-19 pandemic.

Nevertheless, we recognise that between 2005 and 2017 there had been continuing positive advances in:

- recognising the psychosocial and mental health impacts of disasters and terrorism both on the people involved (directly and indirectly) and on responders
- people's attitudes to psychosocial care – the notions of 'man up' and 'mollycoddling' are still extant but are rapidly being replaced with less fear-inducing injunctions.

However, the developments have been a long time coming and remain partial as this book is published [34]. Involvement of psychosocial care and mental healthcare in emergency planning is incomplete in the UK. Undoubtedly the pandemic has pushed matters forward, but long-term funding of a standing core of services is still not certain. Readers may wish to look again at Chapter 10 in this regard.

Epidemics and Pandemics

The Impacts of Serious Communicable Illnesses on Populations

As this chapter has opined, at the outset of the pandemic, advisers to governments and bodies responsible for mounting public responses based their advice on many types of incident or hazard. They were not clear whether that advice would hold true during the pandemic. Yet they had a certain amount of research to fall back on in relation to Ebola, severe acute respiratory syndrome (SARS), and several other highly infectious diseases. The profile of impacts of each pathogen was variable. However, the passage of time has shown that advice based on our accumulated knowledge from a rich variety of hazards was helpful. Thus we focus this part of our summary chapter on the research that has been done on the COVID-19 pandemic and other outbreaks.

Using Psychosocial Care and Mental Healthcare During and After Outbreaks of Communicable Diseases

The literature indicates that, during epidemics and pandemics, there is an initial increase in distress and mental health concerns, the majority of which do not require or reach primary or mental healthcare services [35]. Furthermore, a recent longitudinal study of the mental health of the UK population showed that, although mental wellbeing declined at the onset of the COVID-19 pandemic, most adults (89%) remained resilient or returned to pre-pandemic levels within a few months [36]. However, people suffering from pre-existing mental or physical ill health and/or financial difficulties were more likely to experience a sustained decline in their mental health over time during lockdown and after their infection with COVID-19. Unfortunately, the measures imposed to prevent the spread of disease, such as home confinement, social isolation, and the closure of schools and community infrastructure, disrupted people's access to natural sources of psychosocial care – that is, their families, friends, peers, and work and education settings. This may explain why, during the SARS epidemic [37] and COVID-19 pandemic [38], people utilised frontline telephone services to access psychosocial care. Initially they sought information about the disease, driven by uncertainty about how long it will last, the long-term impacts on health and society, and how to protect themselves and others. They then sought emotional support for their experiences of distress. Only a minority of these people request services. Instead they want to tell their stories of hardship and suffering, and their 'greatest need is to be listened to' by someone who can validate their distress. Moreover, it seems that this need is maintained across time during outbreaks [39].

Primary care practitioners, who provide patient-centred longitudinal care, are well placed to offer psychosocial care and mental healthcare during pandemics. However, there is evidence of public reluctance to use primary care services, which is associated with anxiety about contagion and stigma, not feeling worthy of support, and beliefs that help is not available or that services are already overburdened. In combination, these factors prevent people from accessing mental health and psychosocial support services and make it more difficult for service providers to effectively access affected people, families, and communities. Consequently, there are delays in people seeking help, reduced referrals to specialist mental health services, and fewer face-to-face consultations, due to missed appointments [40]. Thus, during outbreaks, there is a delay before mental health services see an increase in the numbers of new or relapsing cases. Given this, and the delayed morbidity associated with secondary stressors resulting from socioeconomic hardship and disparities during and after pandemics, we hypothesise that the mental health burden of the effects of outbreaks of communicable disease is likely to remain long after pandemics subside.

During pandemics, the opportunities to monitor needs and deliver care can be seriously affected by measures imposed to prevent the spread of disease [41]. There was a marked shift from face-to-face to remote consulting (tele-health) for primary care and mental healthcare providers during the COVID-19 pandemic. However, not everyone has internet access. Thus the effects of basic inequalities in access to care can be worsened by pandemics [42]. Also, although there is good evidence that tele-health has been well-received by the majority of service users during the COVID-19 pandemic, it has not been a positive experience for all. Qualitative research on lived experience is providing growing evidence that remote support is not a panacea [42]. Some people find the lack of physical presence problematic, and, most importantly, many of them feel less supported and less able to share emotional concerns [43,44].

Children, Young People, and Families and Emergencies of All Natures

Chapter 6 in this section introduces readers to the impacts of emergencies, incidents, disease outbreaks, and conflict on children and their families. This theme is developed in Chapter 30 in Section 4 of this book.

In the face of emergencies, children and young people experience distress of varying intensity and duration; the large majority of these experiences are not pathological or symptomatic of mental health disorders. In this respect, their responses are similar to those of adults. However, it is important to use a developmental lens when viewing the impact on children and young people of different ages and developmental capabilities, and in a variety of contexts that may contribute to a range of scenarios in which they are vulnerable. Nevertheless, there is growing evidence for commonalities in the pre-, peri-, and post-event risk factors and the recovery trajectories of children, young people, and adults [45]. The pre-existing and post-event psychosocial functioning and socioeconomic status of families play a pivotal role in influencing how they cope with and recover from their distress, as is shown in Chapters 5 and 6. Hence the best way in which we can promote the mental health of children and young people and mitigate the adverse effects of emergencies is to attend to the emotional and physical health of their caregivers and of the key adults in children's lives, and the quality of their family relationships, because these are all pivotal in facilitating social connectedness and access to social support.

Intervening to Aid People's Recovery

Principles and Models of Psychosocial Care and Mental Healthcare

Although the majority of people cope well in the face of disaster, a substantial proportion experience some, usually temporary, psychosocial impairment, and a smaller proportion are likely to develop mental disorders. Hence most people do not require access to services that deliver specialist mental healthcare. However, distress after emergencies is very common, with adverse psychosocial consequences and functional impairment for many people who may never meet the criteria for a mental health disorder [3,10]. The majority of people in this group are likely to benefit from lower-level – but nonetheless important – psychosocial interventions provided by their families, friends, colleagues, or statutory and non-statutory organisations. There is some evidence that people who are distressed may not proceed to develop disorders if they are offered sufficient support in a timely manner. In this context, Richard Williams and Verity Kemp have created what they call the integrated psychosocial approach [46]. This involves:

- distinguishing between people who are distressed and those who require biomedical interventions
- basing distinctions between the two sorts of conditions on trajectories of people's stress levels and dysfunction
- providing assistance for the greater number of distressed people through lower-intensity psychosocial care.

Therefore people affected by major incidents are likely to need a broad-based suite of evidence-informed support services, ranging from timely and appropriate psychosocial care through to specialist mental healthcare [46,47]. Although there is evidence for the effectiveness of specialist therapeutic interventions for disorders, and the evidence relating to the positive effects of social support is growing, there has been less research on the optimal provision of psychosocial care for the large proportion of people who develop mental health needs but do not meet threshold criteria for disorders [47–49].

This book uses the term psychosocial care to describe public mental health interventions and to differentiate them from the mental healthcare that is provided by primary healthcare or specialist mental health services. In its broadest definition, psychosocial care is a form of psychologically informed social care in which people set out to bolster the recovery environments of those affected by incidents, and provide social support. We are influenced by Kaniasty's work, and define social support as interactions that provide people with actual assistance, embedded in a web of relationships that they perceive to be caring and readily available in times of need, and which ensure that affected people are able to sustain their social connectedness [7,33,47]. The components of social support defined in this way can be emotional, informational, or operational.

Theoretical frameworks and the empirical literature suggest that the mental health needs of people affected by major incidents and disasters are met by a combination of public mental health and clinical components [10,50]. Several sources, based on evidence-informed principles, describe strategic frameworks for planning, designing, and delivering psychosocial and mental health services for survivors [33,50]. There is consensus for offering a strategic stepped model of care. For example, the guidance documents cited here advocate early and active responses that are available to all, and which consist of the following: increasing access to social support and promoting social connectedness and community support rather than psychological therapies; the practical resources necessary to assist people to cope reasonably well, and the expectation of recovery and ease of transition back to normality as soon as possible; and more targeted responses aimed at people with needs that require more extensive help.

However, many of the guidelines have not been implemented in practice [51]. Despite the widespread and long-lasting psychosocial and mental health effects of incidents, the protocols to deal with them are less well established, as they have attracted relatively little academic research [52,53].

A Framework for Responding: Comprehensive Responses to People's Needs After Major Incidents, Epidemics, and Pandemics

The Services Required

Our conclusions from research on the responses required after the Manchester Arena bombing support our earlier advice derived from other incidents. We conclude that it is very important for all of the agencies to come together well before any incident to agree a comprehensive plan with the intention of:

- sustaining the wellbeing of everyone affected (the Wellbeing Agenda)
- identifying and responding to the social and psychological needs for intervention and support of people who are distressed but who do not reach the thresholds for specialist mental health assessment and treatment (the Psychosocial Agenda)
- identifying, assessing, and meeting the needs for treatment of everyone who is identified as

potentially having a mental health disorder (the Mental Health Agenda).

This approach is espoused by recent guidance from NHS England [54], and we have applied it during the pandemic. It has several implications. First, it is important to be aware of the potential duration of the impacts of incidents on people who are affected, their relatives and friends, and the staff of services that intervene. Although a minority of people require mental health services, there is a much larger group of people who become distressed and who do not require specialist mental healthcare but do require psychosocial care. Provision for this group of people may not be adequate after many incidents.

Second, the researchers observe that there is a substantial agenda for all services to develop aware-ness of people's needs after incidents, and another agenda for training and developing practitioners.

Third, the matter of definitions and understand-ing is important. For example, wellbeing is a concept that is easily misunderstood. Some accounts use this term as a synonym for the whole spectrum of psycho-social care and mental healthcare that people require after incidents and during and after disease outbreaks. However, greater precision is required to enable effective planning, preparation, and rehearsal.

Fourth, people who struggle and are distressed during and after incidents may not only be affected by what has happened, but also by their background circumstances, as Chapter 9 well illustrates. Our research on people affected by the Manchester Arena bombing confirms these conclusions about the importance of psychosocial care, but also elevates its importance by finding that many people who were affected continued to have psychosocial needs 3 years later. Contrary to earlier doctrine, we found that a sizeable minority of people did not improve as rapidly as previously thought.

Fifth, some people require ease of access to mental healthcare for skilled assessments of their needs and circumstances, and for access to the evidence-based therapeutic services that they require.

A Framework for Cross-Agency Service Design, Development, and Delivery

In summary, the researchers recommend that plan-ners and practitioners recognise the importance of three broad agendas for services after incidents.

- The Wellbeing Agenda assists people to thrive at home, in work, or at school. Wellbeing is about feeling good and functioning well, and is influenced by each person's experience of life.
- The Psychosocial Agenda supports people who are struggling. Psychosocial care describes interventions for people who are distressed or struggling, or who have symptoms of mental health problems that do not meet the criteria for a diagnosis, whether or not they also experience social or work dysfunction.
- The Mental Health Agenda enables people whose needs appear to go beyond struggling to access mental healthcare for timely assessment and, if necessary, treatment, recovery, and support with returning to work or school.

This approach is summarised in Figure 12.5.

We shall return to the framework depicted in Figure 12.5 in Chapters 27 and 28.

Conclusion: A Summary of the Common Ground

Every emergency, incident, disaster, and disease out-break is different, and the differences do not turn solely on types of events. There are many matters of philosophy, value, and meaning in addition to the impacts of people's circumstances prior to untoward events occurring that are important in our coming to an understanding of how best to approach meeting people's needs. Yet there are also many commonal-ities with respect to people's social, psychological, and mental health needs across all disastrous events.

One of the most important recommendations to emerge thus far from the COVID-19 pandemic is that of the critical importance of preparedness. The ability of agencies to hit the ground running as incidents occur makes a vital difference to outcomes. This calls for substantial planning, preparation, and rehearsal. All plans require adjustment in the light of experi-ence, but communities that start their responses from a well-understood and agreed cross-agency plan that has been rehearsed are in a much stronger position than those that respond ad hoc. This general axiom applies to psychosocial care and mental healthcare, which must be fully integrated into the policies of communities and nations.

The second powerful learning point about responding effectively raises the importance of the

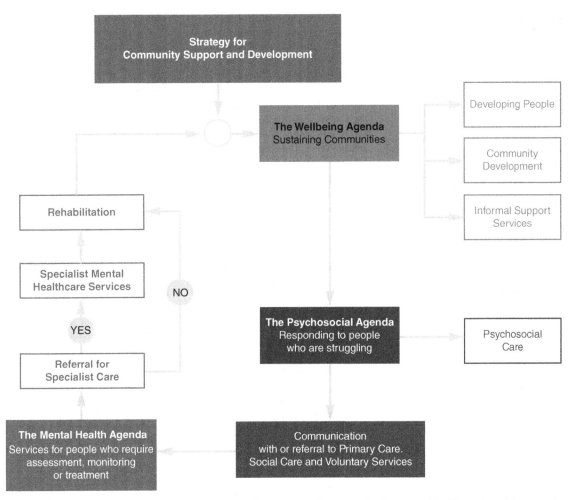

Figure 12.5 A strategic approach to meeting the needs of communities for support for their mental health, psychosocial care, and mental healthcare. (© R Williams, V Kemp. All rights reserved.)

wide range of stressors that have impacts both on people and on their needs and outcomes, in addition to the primary stressors that emerge from what has happened and/or is happening. Adversity and socioeconomic disadvantage result in further disadvantage in the wake of emergencies, incidents, and disease outbreaks. Deciding how to respond to these circumstances is another key aspect of preparation and planning.

A third learning point that should be emphasised relates to the huge impacts of displacement. This may be on a relatively small scale (e.g., when people are moved elsewhere from flooded homes, or are admitted to hospital) or on much larger scales (e.g., when populations of people move into accommodation that

is initially intended to be temporary, or flee their country to become refugees or asylum seekers). Often people in all of these circumstances are dislocated from the services on which they ordinarily rely, lose contact with relatives and friends, and are as socioeconomically disadvantaged by incomplete or inadequate responses to the events as they are by the actual events.

This chapter finishes by identifying the wellbeing, psychosocial, and mental health agendas of care that are required by survivors of EITDDC and also often by their relatives. It presents a strategic approach to meeting people's mental health needs, a subject to which we shall return in Sections 4 and 5 of this book.

References

1. UN Office for Disaster Risk Reduction (UNDRR). *The Human Cost of Disasters: An Overview of the Last 20 Years (2000-2019).* UNDRR, 2020.

2. Lamb D, Greenberg N, Stevelink S, Wessely S. Mixed signals about the health of the NHS workforce. *Lancet Psychiatry* 2020; 7: 1009–11.

3. Williams R, Kaufman KR. Narrative review of the COVID-19, healthcare and healthcarers thematic series. *BJPsych Open* 2022; 8: e34.

4. Fancourt D, Bradbury A. We asked 70,000 people how coronavirus affected them – what they told us revealed a lot about inequality in the UK. The Conversation, 2021 (https://theconversation.com/we-asked-70-000-people-how-coronavirus-affected-them-what-they-told-us-revealed-a-lot-about-inequality-in-the-uk-143718).

5. Jordan HT, Osahan S, Li J, Stein CR, Friedman SM, Brackbill RM, et al. Persistent mental and physical health impact of exposure to the September 11, World Trade Center terrorist attacks. *Environ Health* 2019; 18: 12.

6. Norris FH, Tracy M, Galea S. Looking for resilience: understanding the longitudinal trajectories of responses to stress. *Soc Sci Med* 2009; 68: 2190–98.

7. Kaniasty K, Norris FH. Distinctions that matter: received social support, perceived social support and social embeddedness after disasters. In *Mental Health and Disasters* (eds Y Neria, S Galea, FH Norris): 175–200. Cambridge University Press, 2009.

8. Ntontis E, Drury J, Amlôt R, Williams R, Rubin GJ. Endurance or decline of emergent groups following a flood disaster: implications for community resilience. *Int J Disaster Risk Reduct* 2020; 45: 101493.

9. Murray E, Kaufman KR, Williams R. Let us do better: learning lessons for recovery of healthcare professionals during and after COVID-19. *BJPsych Open* 2021; 7: e151.

10. Williams R, Bisson J, Kemp V. *OP94: Principles for Responding to People's Psychosocial and Mental Health Needs after Disasters.* Royal College of Psychiatrists, 2014.

11. Forbes D, O'Donnell M, Bryant RA. Psychosocial recovery following community disasters: an international collaboration. *Aust N Z J Psychiatry* 2017; 51: 660–62.

12. Olff M, Amstadter A, Armour C, Birkeland MS, Bui E, Cloitre M, et al. A decennial review of psychotraumatology: what did we learn and where are we going? *Eur J Psychotraumatol* 2019; 10: 1672948.

13. Stancombe J, Williams R, Drury J, Collins H, Lagan L, Barrett A, et al. People's experiences of distress and psychosocial care following a terrorist attack: interviews with survivors of the Manchester Arena bombing in 2017. *BJPsych Open* 2022; 8: e41.

14. Drury J, Stancombe J, Williams R, Collins H, Lagan L, Barrett A, et al. The role of informal social support in recovery among survivors of the 2017 Manchester Arena bombing. *BJPsych Open* 2022; 8: e124.

15. Stancombe J, Williams R, Drury J, Hussey L, Gittins M, Barrett A et al. Trajectories of distress and recovery, secondary stressors, and social cure processes in people who used the resilience hub after the Manchester Arena bombing. *BJPsych Open* 2023; 9: e143.

16. Naldi A, Vallelonga F, Di Liberto A, Cavallo R, Agnesone M, Gonella M, et al. COVID-19 pandemic-related anxiety, distress and burnout: prevalence and associated factors in healthcare workers of North-West Italy. *BJPsych Open* 2021; 7: e27.

17. Williams R, Kemp V, Alexander D. The psychosocial and mental health of people who are affected by conflict, catastrophes, terrorism, adversity and displacement. In *Conflict and Catastrophe Medicine* (eds J Ryan, A Hopperus Buma, C Beadling, A Mozumder, DM Nott): 805–49. Springer, 2014.

18. Norris FH, Friedman MJ, Watson PJ. 60,000 disaster victims speak: Part II. Summary and implications of the disaster mental health research. *Psychiatry* 2002; 65: 240–60.

19. Gabriel R, Ferrando L, Cortón ES, Mingote C, García-Camba E, Liria AF, et al. Psychopathological consequences after a terrorist attack: an epidemiological study among victims, the general population, and police officers. *Eur Psychiatry* 2007; 22: 339–46.

20. DiGrande L, Neria Y, Brackbill RM, Pulliam P, Galea S. Long-term posttraumatic stress symptoms among 3,271 civilian survivors of the September 11, 2001, terrorist attacks on the World Trade Center. *Am J Epidemiol* 2011; 173: 271–81.

21. Kessler RC, Aguilar-Gaxiola S, Alonso J, Benjet C, Bromet WJ, Cardoso G, et al. Trauma and PTSD in the WHO World Mental Health Surveys. *Eur J Psychotraumatol* 2017; 8 (suppl5):1353383.

22. Bonanno GA, Brewin CR, Kaniasty K, Greca AM. Weighing the costs of disaster: consequences, risks, and resilience in individuals, families, and communities. *Psychol Sci Public Interest* 2010; 11: 1–49.

23. Dyb G, Jensen TK, Nygaard E, Ekeberg Ø, Diseths TH, Wentzel-Larsen T, et al. Post-traumatic stress reactions in survivors of the 2011 massacre on Utøya Island, Norway. *Br J Psychiatry* 2014; 204: 361–7.

24. Smith EC, Burkle FM. Paramedic and emergency medical technician reflections on the ongoing impact of the 9/11 terrorist attacks. *Prehosp Disaster Med* 2019; **34**: 56–61.

25. Cockeram A, Cockeram J, eds. *Glimpses of the Falklands War.* British Modern Military History Society, 2022.

26. Williams R, Ntontis E, Alfadhli K, Drury J, Amlôt R. A social model of secondary stressors in relation to disasters, major incidents and conflict: implications for practice. *Int J Disaster Risk Reduct* 2021; **63**: 102436.

27. Lock S, Rubin GJ, Murray V, Rogers MB, Amlôt R, Williams R. Secondary stressors and extreme events and disasters: a systematic review of primary research from 2010–2011. *PLoS Curr* 2012; **4**. Available from: https://doi.org/10 .1371/currents.dis.a9b76fed 1b2dd5c5bfcfc13c87a2f24f.

28. Cyhlarova E, Knapp M, Mays N. Responding to the mental health consequences of the 2015–2016 terrorist attacks in Tunisia, Paris and Brussels: implementation and treatment experiences in the United Kingdom. *J Health Serv Res Policy* 2020; **25**: 172–80.

29. Mennecier D, Hendrick S, De Mol J, Denis J. Experience of victims of Brussels' terrorist attacks: an interpretative phenomenological analysis. *Traumatology* 2020. Available from: https://doi.org/10 .1037/trm0000249.

30. Stene LE, Wentzel-Larsen T, Dyb G. Healthcare needs, experiences and satisfaction after terrorism: a longitudinal study of survivors from the Utøya attack. *Front Psychol* 2016; **7**: 1809.

31. Goldmann E, Galea S. Mental health consequences of disasters. *Annu Rev Public Health* 2014; **35**: 169–83.

32. Department of Health. *NHS Emergency Planning Guidance: Planning for the Psychosocial and Mental Health Care of People Affected by Major Incidents and Disasters: Interim National Strategic Guidance.* Department of Health, 2009.

33. NATO Joint Medical Committee. *Psychosocial Care for People Affected by Disasters and Major Incidents: A Model for Designing, Delivering and Managing Psychosocial Services for People Involved in Major Incidents, Conflict, Disasters and Terrorism.* NATO, 2009.

34. Brewin CR, DePierro J, Pirard P, Vazquez C, Williams R. Why we need to integrate mental health into pandemic planning. *Perspect Public Health* 2020; **140** : 309–10.

35. Bowman C, Branjerdporn G, Turner K, Kamara M, Tyagi N, Josen N, et al. The impact of viral epidemics and pandemics on acute mental health service use: an integrative review. *Health Psychol Rev* 2021; **15**: 1–33.

36. Pierce M, McManus S, Hope H, Hotopf M, Ford T, Hatch SI, et al. Mental health responses to the COVID-19 pandemic: a latent class trajectory analysis using longitudinal data. *Lancet Psychiatry* 2021; **8**: 610–19.

37. Leung TT, Wong H. Community reactions to the SARS crisis in Hong Kong: analysis of a time-limited counseling hotline. *J Hum Behav Soc Environ* 2005; **12**: 1–22.

38. Hopkins JS, Russell D. The mental health effects of coronavirus are a 'slow-motion disaster'. Mother Jones, 2020 (www.motherjones .com/coronavirus-updates/2020/ 04/the-mental-health-effects-of-coronavirus-are-a-slow-motion-disaster/).

39. Red Cross Red Crescent Reference Centre for Psychosocial Support (PS Centre). *'The Greatest Need Was to Be Listened To': The Importance of Mental Health and Psychosocial Support during COVID-19. Experiences and Recommendations from the International Red Cross and Red Crescent Movement.* PS Centre, 2020 (https://pscentre.org/the-greatest-need-was-to-be-listened-to/).

40. World Health Organization (WHO. *Pulse Survey on Continuity of Essential Health Services during the COVID-19 Pandemic: Interim Report, 27 August 2020.* WHO, 2020.

41. Ehrenreich-May J, Halliday ER, Karlovich AR, Gruen RL, Pino AC, Tonarely NA. Brief transdiagnostic intervention for parents with emotional disorder symptoms during the COVID-19 pandemic: a case example. *Cogn Behav Pract* 2021; **28**: 690–700.

42. Johnson S, Dalton-Locke C, San Juan VN, Foye U, Oram S, Papamichail A, et al. Impact on mental health care and on mental health service users of the COVID-19 pandemic: a mixed methods survey of UK mental health care staff. *Soc Psychiatry Psychiatr Epidemiol* 2021; **56**: 25–37.

43. Burton A, McKinlay A, Aughterson H, Fancourt D. Impact of the COVID-19 pandemic on the mental health and well-being of adults with mental health conditions in the UK: a qualitative interview study. *J Ment Health* 2021. Available from: https://doi.org/10.1080/ 09638237.2021.1952953.

44. Rains LS, Johnson S, Barnett P, Steare T, Needle JJ, Carr S, et al. Early impacts of the COVID-19 pandemic on mental health care and on people with mental health conditions: framework synthesis of international experiences and responses. *Soc Psychiatry Psychiatr Epidemiol* 2021; **56**: 13–24.

45. Lai BS, Lewis R, Livings MS, La Greca AM, Esnard A-M. Posttraumatic stress symptom trajectories among children after disaster exposure: a review. *J Trauma Stress* 2017; **30**: 571–82.

46. Williams R, Kemp V. Psychosocial and mental health care before, during and after emergencies, disasters and major incidents. In *Health Emergency Preparedness and Response* (eds C Sellwood, A Wapling): 82–98. CABI, 2016.

47. Kaniasty K, Norris FH. Longitudinal linkages between perceived social support and posttraumatic stress symptoms: sequential roles of social causation and social selection. *J Trauma Stress* 2008; **21**: 274–81.

48. Te Brake H, Dückers M. Early psychosocial interventions after disasters, terrorism and other shocking events: is there a gap between norms and practice in Europe? *Eur J Psychotraumatol* 2013; **4**: 19093.

49. O'Donnell ML, Lau W, Fredrickson J, Gibson K, Bryant RA, Bisson J, et al. An open label pilot study of a brief psychosocial intervention for disaster and trauma survivors. *Front Psychiatry* 2020; **11**: 483.

50. Williams R, Kemp V. Principles for designing and delivering psychosocial and mental healthcare. *BMJ Mil Health* 2020; **166**: 105–10.

51. Allsopp K, Brewin CR, Barrett A, Williams R, Hind D, Chitsabesan P, et al. Responding to mental health needs after terror attacks. *BMJ* 2019; **366**: l4828.

52. Jumbe S, Milner A, Clinch M, Kennedy J, Pinder RJ, Sharpe CA et al. A qualitative evaluation of Southwark Council's public health approach for mitigating the mental health impact of the 2017 London Bridge and Borough Market terror attack. *BMC Public Health* 2021; **21**: 1427.

53. Pirard P, Baubet T, Motreff Y, Rabet G, Marillier M, Vandentorren S et al. Use of mental health supports by civilians exposed to the November 2015 terrorist attacks in Paris. *BMC Health Serv Res* 2020; **20**: 959.

54. NHS England and NHS Improvement. *Responding to the Needs of People Affected by Incidents and Emergencies: Guidance for Planning, Delivering and Evaluating Psychosocial and Mental Healthcare.* NHS England and NHS Improvement, 2021.

Chapter

13

Advances in Pre-Hospital Care

Emir Battaloglu and Keith Porter

The History of Pre-Hospital Care

Ancient History

Methods for the immediate care of the injured and for the care of the sick have been described since the earliest development of written records. Some basic practices date back for millennia, but the subject is continually evolving and developing, and pre-hospital care is now an important medical specialty in its own right.

Early examples of such care include methods for resuscitation, application of field dressings, and emergency transportation to definitive care facilities. Biblical references to such care include Luke 10:34 ('He went to him and bandaged his wounds, pouring on oil and wine. Then he put the man on his own donkey, brought him to an inn and took care of him') and 2 Kings 4:34 ('Then he got on the bed and lay on the body, mouth to mouth, eyes to eyes, hands to hands. As he stretched himself out upon the child, the body grew warm'. In the Islamic world in the early eleventh century Avicenna produced his Canon of Medicine. This work influenced medical practice, including immediate care, for centuries, and his writings were furthered through history by other Persian physicians [1]. In particular, the fifteenth-century court physician Burhan-ud-Din Kermani was the first to describe resuscitation as the combined actions of 'strong movements and massive chest expansion' with 'compression of the left side of the chest' [2].

Military History

The Greek physician Hippocrates decreed that 'War is the only proper school of the surgeon' for the trials and challenges presented to field hospitals and aid stations in conflict zones. Warfare, with its attendant high levels of injury, has always generated advances in the care of the injured. Accounts of the earliest forms of stretcher were recorded in the fourteenth century.

Designs for purpose-made rescue vehicles, beyond the humble donkey, date from the fifteenth century, and the application of vessel ligatures and the use of surgical equipment were also recorded at that time. A major advance in the recovery and transport of the wounded was the development of 'flying ambulances' during the Napoleonic wars by the French surgeon Baron Larrey, who also developed the concept of triage and improved the organisation of field hospitals. Further improvements in the field of pre-hospital and hospital care of the injured resulted from the creation of the Red Cross in the early 1860s, and the adoption of the first Geneva Convention (for the Amelioration of the Condition of the Wounded in Armies in the Field) in 1864. Further major improvements in the recovery of and care for the wounded were made during the two World Wars, and military medicine has continued to provide developments in patient care and pre-hospital treatment, as shown by the important advances in pre-hospital care that were developed during the recent war in Afghanistan.

UK History

A structured approach to pre-hospital care in the UK undoubtedly originated with the efforts of the Royal Humane Society at the end of the eighteenth century, setting up a network of doctors who worked as volunteers to provide immediate medical care at the scenes of accidents, initially in London, following examples from other European cities. Their mandate also included the provision for education in their techniques and activities, spreading general knowledge to develop systems of first aid management. As part of the education programme, guidelines were produced describing acceptable practice for methods of resuscitation, which included:

- warmth
- artificial respiration by mouth to mouth with compression of the abdomen and chest

- fumigation by the introduction of tobacco smoke into the rectum and colon
- rubbing the body
- stimulants
- bleeding
- inducement of vomiting.

Within a few years of its establishment, the Royal Humane Society had set up more than 250 'receiving houses', which were essentially emergency aid stations, and had over 100 medical volunteers. The stations were situated close to lakes and rivers in London. Some were set up in pubs, tents, or workhouses, whereas others were established in purpose-built facilities with wards and staff housing.

An alert system was set up using runners who would advise the medics about incidents. Doctors were recruited by word of mouth, by leaflet campaigns, or through the press. They gained significant experience in both mass gathering and major incident management, notable incidents including the Surrey Gardens Festival in 1856 (when eight people were crushed to death in a large uncontrolled crowd), the Sunderland Magic Show disaster in 1883 (when 183 children were crushed when a crowd was trapped in a stairwell), and the Scotland Yard terrorist bomb in 1884.

As well as delivering clinical care, the Royal Humane Society was involved in research to develop new techniques, and in the development of the necessary equipment for facilitating appropriate first aid and resuscitation. Medical advances during this period included the application of galvanism in an attempt to restart the heart by Gervis and Bowe in 1858, and the introduction of a method of artificial respiration by Henry Sylvester in 1861.

After the Second World War, a notable figure in the development of pre-hospital care in the UK was Dr Kenneth Easton. A general practitioner in Catterick, Yorkshire, he frequently had to deal with the results of road traffic accidents on the A1. In 1967 he set up a Road Accident After Care Scheme (RAACS) in North Riding, Yorkshire, which provided a model for immediate care schemes in the UK. He was a key figure in establishing the British Association for Immediate Care, a charity that brings together people who have an interest in pre-hospital immediate care, and supports and promotes regional and local immediate care schemes across the UK.

A number of medical flying squads were established in the 1950s and 1960s, with the aim of bringing medical and nursing staff, as well as their equipment to the patient in the community. The results of this were variable. Some patients could benefit, but in the case of cardiac arrest the need for very rapid application of cardiopulmonary resuscitation (CPR) and defibrillation meant that flying squads were unlikely to attend in time. In addition, the use of such a squad can deplete the parent department of staff, yet they did have a role to play. The Derbyshire Flying Squad had a significant role in its local area, but it could not save lives on its own without bystander CPR and automatic defibrillation. In general, flying squads varied in their response times and often lacked training or equipment, making them an unreliable resource.

Associations and Organisations

The British Association for Immediate Care (BASICS) was established in 1977, and the membership included doctors, nurses, paramedics, and first aiders. Those who volunteered covered a wide spectrum of clinical activity to form teams with appropriate training and competence to deliver both necessary basic care and enhanced skills. In 1998, BASICS introduced a voluntary accreditation scheme which went some way towards establishing a national minimum standard for medical pre-hospital care responders. This laid the foundation for further development and standard setting.

The model of care that is provided needs to be varied in accordance with geographical and medical requirements. For example, London has a high urban workload but only relatively short distances need to be travelled, whereas a remote part of the Scottish Highlands has a low population density but requires extensive travel. Through the Remote and Rural Areas Resource Initiative (RARARI), standardised training has been given to doctors and nurses in Scotland by BASICS Scotland.

The Faculty of Pre-Hospital Care was established in 1994 and was designed to embrace all pre-hospital care providers. It had clearly defined aims, which included:

- setting and maintaining standards of practice in pre-hospital care
- promoting education in and teaching of pre-hospital care
- initiating technical developments and research in pre-hospital care
- integrating the efforts of all participants in pre-hospital care effectively, and harmonising and

facilitating the onward management of the sick and injured.

The Faculty mission statement states that 'the aim of the Faculty is to promote high standards of teaching and research in pre-hospital care and to set and maintain standards of clinical practice'.

Work undertaken by Dr Brian Steggles and his colleagues within BASICS in the late 1980s, supported by Mr Myles Gibson, the Vice-President of the Royal College of Surgeons of Edinburgh at the time, led to the endeavour to define standards. To this end, the Diploma in Immediate Medical Care was established, complementing the College's established Fellowship in Accident and Emergency Medicine. Candidates came from various parts of the world to sit the exam, which became a 'gold standard' of accreditation for practitioners of pre-hospital care. This has been furthered by the creation of the Fellowship in Immediate Medical Care (FIMC), to recognise the increasing numbers of doctors working with a major commitment within pre-hospital care, such as ambulance service medical directors or those working with helicopter emergency medical services (HEMS).

Recognising the importance of becoming all-encompassing, the Diploma, and subsequently the Fellowship in Immediate Care, was opened to both nurses and paramedics. With the need for advancing medical provision of immediate care, eventually the Postgraduate Medical Education and Training Board (PMETB) recognised pre-hospital emergency medicine as a medical subspecialty.

The Intercollegiate Board for Training in Pre-Hospital Emergency Medicine (IBTPHEM) has subspecialty trainees from anaesthesia, intensive care, acute medicine, and emergency medicine. During training the candidates develop a portfolio of experience, including operational experience, clinical analysis, audit, research, clinical governance, major incident management, mass gathering medicine, and teaching.

In addition to these formal pre-hospital care training programmes, progression to a specialist role in pre-hospital care can be made through a Faculty accreditation route, which includes successfully passing the FIMC.

Public Awareness and First Responders

Individuals who are injured or who develop a critical illness frequently receive their first treatment from bystanders. The value of such treatment has been definitively demonstrated [3], especially in medical cardiac arrest, where good neurological outcome and survival to discharge is correlated with bystander CPR [4]. Public information, education programmes, and access to key equipment items (e.g., defibrillators, haemorrhage control packs) are increasingly available and applied in modern urban environments. CitizenAid, GoodSam, and the Hartford Consensus are all examples of such programmes that advocate for improved knowledge of first aid and availability of life-saving equipment.

Critical Care Teams

Despite the positive association between pre-hospital critical care and the secondary outcome of survival to hospital admission, such care has not been associated with increased rates of survival to hospital discharge [5,6]. Improvement of the latter is the focus of a great deal of research, but so far this has proved a difficult problem to solve [7].

Clinical Advances

There have been a number of important clinical advances that have improved the care that can be offered by those providing pre-hospital care.

Airway

Adjuncts and Airway Devices

Supraglottic airway (SGA) device styles have changed rapidly in recent years, with regard to the shape and material properties of the laryngeal component, cuffed or uncuffed designs, improved positive pressure ventilation profiles, addition of suction ports, and aspiration risk-reduction features (termed second generation), as well as the facility to intubate through the device (termed third generation) [8].

The choice of airway device to be used during the management of cardiac arrest in the pre-hospital environment has been investigated in a number of robust academic studies, with the overall conclusion that there are no significant differences in outcome for patients managed by intubation compared with those managed by SGA [9].

Research into paediatric airway anatomy has questioned earlier designs. As a result, the tolerance of the larynx of paediatric patients for an endotracheal tube without a balloon cuff is being reconsidered.

Uncuffed tubes were thought to have the advantage of exerting less pressure on the walls of the airway than a cuffed tube, with resultant reductions in ischaemic damage and stricture formation. However, these aims were not being met, and the use of cuffed tubes for paediatric intubation has increased in current practice [10].

Monitoring

End-tidal carbon dioxide ($ETCO_2$) monitoring, which is an alternative non-invasive method for determining carbon dioxide levels, has become a well-documented technique and in many settings has been adopted as a gold standard. $ETCO_2$ monitoring has become a key element in resuscitation strategies, airway management, and anaesthesia delivery, and clinical research supports its use in precision targeting of the physiology of individual patients as a guide for resuscitation [11].

Technology

The use of video laryngoscopy (VL) – a fibre-optic camera attached to the end of a traditional laryngoscope blade to aid visualisation of the airway for intubation – has gained popularity recently. However, in the pre-hospital setting, VL has incurred some major problems that have limited its universal application. These include device size, portability, cost, and the difficulties of skill development. Yet multiple studies have demonstrated improved first-pass success rates in a number of contexts, and benefits are likely to be maximised by having robust techniques for overcoming the limitations of VL while harnessing its advantages [12]. VL is certainly likely to lead to advances in pre-hospital airway management practices in the future, with greater portability and improved optical quality. Single-use versions are currently in development.

Spine Trauma

Collars

Cervical collar design and implementation have changed considerably, with the refinement of application patterns and indications, as well as the recognition of the inherent limitations and consequences of application. Due to advances in our understanding of the low incidence of unstable cervical spine injuries, as well as the overall impact on patient outcomes, focused research is needed to evaluate the continued practice of collar application.

Immobilisation

Studies of the spinal movement patterning that occurs with different techniques for extracting the injured patient from the location where injury occurred, as well as the adoption of controlled self-extrication, have modified the approach to spinal stabilisation following injury [13].

Aside from the traditional collar, blocks, and tape, there is increasing evidence that scoop stretchers and/or vacuum mattress devices provide appropriate levels of spinal immobilisation, with the additional benefits of transportation comfort and ease of use [14]. Spine boards for the extrication of patients remain in use, but are no longer recommended as devices for patient transportation, due to their pressure area risk profile and the levels of patient discomfort that they cause [14].

Chest

The availability of modern highly portable equipment has meant that pre-hospital point-of-care ultrasound use is increasing [15]. Improvements in image clarity and better clinical interpretive skills among pre-hospital practitioners have led to advances in the ability to detect intra-thoracic pathology. A similar technological advance has been seen in relation to the use of blood gas analysis, which is of particular value in settings of prolonged field care or transfer medicine.

Tension pneumothorax is commonly treated with needle decompression (ND). The technique has quite a high failure rate, due at least in part to the increased thickness of injured chest walls. The insertion point is usually at the second intercostal space midclavicular line (ICS2-MCL). There is an alternative site at the fifth intercostal space anterior axillary line (ICS5-AAL), but this poses an iatrogenic cardiac risk, and further studies are needed to determine the safety of this alternative site [16]. Bespoke devices for decompression have gained popularity, with increasing evidence for their success rate and reduced complication profile, compared with the simple venous cannula that was used in the past [17].

Simple thoracostomy (also known as finger thoracostomy) for the management of tension pneumothorax has been demonstrated to be a safe and effective intervention for use in the pre-hospital environment [18]. It has been shown to have better success rates than needle decompression, leading to recommendations that it should be the first-line treatment for use by suitably skilled practitioners [19].

The incorporation of venting systems to chest seal devices has been made to minimise the risk of repeated air accumulation and recurrent tension pneumothorax [20]. Vented chest seals have been advocated as the optimal design requirement, and have been adopted into clinical practice over unvented chest seals, as well as three-sided taping of credit cards [21].

The use of tube thoracostomy, or the insertion of a chest drain, in pre-hospital practice is a suitable and appropriate extension of care from the simple thoracostomy [22].

Much attention has been focused on the role of resuscitative thoracotomy – that is, the surgical opening of the chest in order to access the heart. This is because this procedure remains one of the most invasive, yet potentially lifesaving, elements of pre-hospital critical care. Attention has been primarily focused on the crafting of guidelines to define the indications for this treatment, based on the limited but expanding evidence base in the medical literature [23].

Damage Control Resuscitation

Concepts developed from our constantly expanding understanding of trauma physiology have reached a pinnacle with the adoption of damage control resuscitation (DCR). This involves the objective of clinical care of the patient being directed towards management of life- and limb-threatening injuries, direct or secondary, in an expedient and efficient manner in order to minimise the burden of any physiological 'second hit'. The aspects of DCR that are applicable to pre-hospital care are outlined in the following sections.

Haemorrhage Control

With regard to control of haemorrhage, bleeding can be divided into two practical categories – compressible (extremity) haemorrhage and non-compressible (torso) haemorrhage. The increased use of commercial non-pneumatic tourniquets has improved extremity bleeding control, and has also led to the development of devices to manage junctional regions, where compression may potentially be achieved. Junctional tourniquets, for use in the groin or axilla, are effective [24], and the recently developed abdominal tourniquet, which uses external umbilical pressure to compress the abdominal aorta, can provide effective indirect proximal control for pelvic and lower extremity bleeding [25].

Haemostatic wound dressings are another recent addition to the array of treatments available for the control of bleeding in pre-hospital settings. These dressings have two main mechanisms of action – clotting factor activators and adhesive agents [26]. Their haemorrhage control potential is superior to that of standard gauze dressings, and they have been widely adopted [26].

Fracture Splintage, Binders, and Splints

There have recently been improvements in the design and availability of devices for the anatomical alignment and splintage of long bone fractures in order to minimise blood loss and reduce pain (not a novel concept). Modern bespoke traction devices for supporting femoral shaft fractures, along with vacuum splintage of upper limb and leg fractures, are highly effective and are a mainstay of blunt trauma management. A major advance has been the development of pelvic binders, both as a new concept to augment the damage control resuscitation principles, and to stabilise high-energy pelvic fractures. Device designs have improved the practicality and ease of application beyond that of the simple sheet and bandage.

Circulatory Access

Intra-osseous access – insertion of a needle into a bone in order to deliver fluids and medications rapidly – has been widely adopted as a method of circulatory access. The variety of devices, manual or automated insertion techniques, and anatomical location have been expanded to provide versatility. Central venous access in the pre-hospital setting remains little used, but shows potential for use in critical care.

Fluids, Tranexamic Acid, and Blood

As part of the damage-control resuscitation process, permissive hypotension is a bridging technique for supporting the patient during transfer to a site of definitive care. Permissive hypotension maintains vital organ perfusion for bleeding patients by administering a limited volume of fluid, titrated to effect. The aim of this is to stave off the negative physiological impact of shock, while not returning to normal blood pressure with the attendant risk of disrupting fragile clots. This technique has been widely adopted, with the noted relative contraindication of concomitant traumatic brain injury (TBI). The physiological advantages of this approach, compared with large-volume crystalloid administration, have been highlighted by the experience of many practitioners [27]. This paradigm has been recently updated with the experimental concept of hybrid resuscitation, whereby permissive hypotension is limited to the initial 60–90 minutes following injury, after which the aim is to achieve normotension, in order to prevent the sequelae of prolonged hypoperfusion [28].

Tranexamic acid (TXA), a lysine analogue and antifibrinolytic agent, has been shown by large-scale academically robust trials to confer survival advantage for patients with bleeding pathologies. The CRASH-2/3 trial series, the MATTERS trial, and the WOMAN trial have demonstrated the impact of TXA on mortality in a variety of health economies worldwide, leading to its widespread use in pre-hospital practice. However, increasing attention is now being given to which patient populations derive most benefit from TXA administration, and which may be detrimentally affected by it. Severe TBI and gastrointestinal haemorrhage are two diagnoses that are not thought to benefit from TXA administration [29,30].

Resuscitative endovascular balloon occlusion of the aorta (REBOA) is a cutting-edge technique that has been developed from concepts initially described in the 1950s. It is an effective adjunct for the management of the exsanguinating patient, providing a less invasive form of aortic occlusion than that achieved via thoracotomy. Although there are associated complications, especially a higher than 75% incidence of distal arterial thrombus formation [31], the benefit from haemorrhage control is currently being actively explored in a randomised controlled trial within the hospital setting, and the technique will probably be considered for pre-hospital use [31].

Disability

Impact brain apnoea (IBA) is the cessation of breathing following TBI. Recognising the need for urgent basic airway intervention and ventilatory support is a key aspect of managing IBA. TBI patients with IBA also experience cardiovascular system collapse and poorer outcomes, which can often physiologically mimic hypovolaemic shock [32].

Pre-hospital detection of raised intracranial pressure (ICP), typically based on monitoring physiological parameters for Cushing's response, abnormal respiratory patterning, and abnormal pupillary size and reactivity, can result in under-triage of patients [33]. Novel non-invasive technologies for improving rates of detection of raised ICP in TBI include the use of pupillometry, ultrasound measurement of the optic nerve sheath diameter, and transcranial Doppler.

Physiological understanding of TBI, in order to rule out secondary brain injury and optimise outcomes, requires ensuring appropriate airway management, oxygenation, and haemodynamic support to avoid hypoxia and hypotension. In addition, there are brain-specific areas of focus, such as identifying and treating intracranial hypertension, and avoiding seizures and fever, all of which can lead to secondary injury and worsen clinical outcomes.

Prolonged prophylactic hyperventilation, with the deliberate intention of reducing a head injury patient's carbon dioxide levels, is not recommended for controlling ICP, and its use should be reserved for rescue periods for patients with severe TBI. Therapeutic prophylactic hypothermia is also not recommended, due to the lack of robust evidence of benefit.

Medicines

The use of ketamine in pre-hospital care has increased markedly, and it has been widely adopted as the primary agent for analgesic purposes, for providing procedural sedation, and for pre-hospital emergency anaesthesia. Propofol is also commonly used for the control of ICP, but has not demonstrated an improvement in mortality or patient-centred outcomes. In addition, caution is advised, as high-dose propofol has been associated with significant morbidity.

The use of hypertonic saline or mannitol for the control of raised ICP in isolated TBI patients has been advocated [34]. However, multiple high-level studies have concluded that neither of these agents is of significantly more benefit compared with the other, or compared with conventional fluid resuscitation strategies, with regard to long-term patient-centred outcomes. The role of hypertonic saline in TBI is likely to be a key intervention for future large-scale studies.

The use of steroids has repeatedly been investigated as a potential treatment for minimising the neuronal damage exhibited in TBI and spinal cord injury. However, the literature is full of conflicting evidence, and the use of steroids is not currently recommended for improving outcome or reducing ICP. In patients with severe TBI, high-dose methylprednisolone is associated with increased mortality, and is contraindicated [35].

Cardiac Arrest

Cardiac arrest management has been separated to reflect the variation in optimal care between the often distinct entities of medical or traumatic cardiac arrest.

The pathophysiology of and management strategies for medical cardiac arrest are well understood, and early resuscitation measures, including defibrillation, are vital for patient survival.

Traumatic cardiac arrest is attributable to vital organ injury or the physiological sequelae of trauma. It is primarily considered treatable by the reversal of four major abnormalities – the correction of hypoxaemia, relief of tension pneumothoraces or cardiac tamponade, and resuscitation from exsanguination. Modern concepts around the physiological antecedent state before exsanguination have been termed LOST (Low Output State in Trauma), where palpable pulses may be absent due to insufficient circulating volume rather than to true cardiac arrest.

Chest Compressions

Medical cardiac arrest management emphasises high-quality chest compressions in order to prolong the potential survival window for patients to be resuscitated. One recent development has been the availability of mechanical chest compression devices. Although these have not been shown to be superior to manual chest compressions in terms of clinical outcome, they do offer logistic and human resource advantages.

Traumatic cardiac arrest, as an entity, is now defined more formally and receives its own unique physiological understanding. Chest compressions in these circumstances have a more limited role, when combined with the advanced treatment interventions advocated for TCA management. This is most pronounced when exsanguination has occurred and closed chest compressions may have a potentially detrimental effect on the heart and on the ability to regain cardiac contractility. This emphasis on treatment of reversible causes for traumatic cardiac arrest

within dedicated algorithms has led to closed chest compression being de-emphasised, to allow for maximal attention and efficacy [36].

Despite considerable research, the survival rate following TCA remains poor (5–10%). Clearly this is a key area for future studies, especially performance analysis. Progressive application of new technologies such as REBOA, selective aortic arch perfusion, and extracorporeal membrane oxygenation may improve outcomes, but remains experimental at this stage.

Human Factors and Communication

The impact of modern understanding of the factors that can affect performance of tasks when under pressure, the psychological appreciation of mental and physical performance under stress, and the acceptance of the role of interpersonal communication and effective strategies to mitigate the risks of human error, have all played an important role in improving and advancing pre-hospital care. The use of cognitive aids, checklists, aides-mémoire, technological support, and telemedical support to optimise clinical management under pressure or in difficult situations has shown significant non-technical and technical benefits [37].

Telemedicine

Telemedicine is likely to play a large role in future provision of pre-hospital care, with certain services and/or conditions already receiving such support in current practice. An important example is that of the neurologist-supported mobile stroke units, which have shown improvements in care. In addition, the use of telemedicine in austere environment trauma, rural medicine, and military environments has proved successful in achieving high-quality trauma care.

Triage

There has been widespread adoption of triage tools for a variety of conditions that are managed in pre-hospital care, ranging from individualised care pathway selection for time-critical conditions to the role of diagnostics in mass casualty situations. However, significant heterogeneity exists between services and conditions, with few being universally accepted. Refinement of such triage tools will require high levels of data input and outcomes-based analysis, which may be difficult to accomplish.

Within disaster medicine, as well as being used in the management of mass casualty incidents, the triage tools aim to provide classification and prioritization of the injured with increased speed and accuracy. Rapid and accurate triage is vital for the survival of injured people. The optimal use of available resources to increase survival of casualties is one of the important principles of triage systems, and does not conflict with equity in health.

Emergency handover of critical patients is the terminology used to describe the moment of union between pre-hospital and in-hospital health teams. Handover is a complex process, and is affected by human factors, clinician, and patient. Standardisation is a key tactic for enhancing the communication of information and for developing improved practices. One common example is the use of the ATMIST (Age, Time of Injury, Mechanism of Injury, Injury or Illness, Signs, Treatment) mnemonic. The other widely used medical communication tool is the SBAR (Situation, Background, Assessment, Recommendation) mnemonic.

Trauma Networks

The integral role played by pre-hospital care within the establishment of modern trauma networks is considered to be a major advance [38,39]. These services provide the first in a chain of vital links for achieving the best possible neurological and functional patient-centred outcomes. Effective pre-hospital service provision and triage accuracy within established trauma networks are improving these outcomes for injured patients. Similar impacts are seen for cardiac events, including both myocardial infarction and out-of-hospital cardiac arrest, where the trend towards a reduction in time to definitive care hospital transfer, and thus in ischaemia time, is decreasing mortality rates [40].

Clinical Trials

Growing realisation of the need to improve pre-hospital care is demonstrated by the increase in the level of academic focus on this topic that has occurred since the turn of the century. Notable trials which have confirmed positive effects of treatment intervention and influenced pre-hospital care include CRASH-2, PARAMEDIC & PARAMEDIC 2, AIRWAYS-2, ARREST, PART, and PAMPer. In addition, there have been numerous negative trials which have also played a part in the development of improved care. Taken together, these trials highlight the recognition of the field of pre-hospital care as a valid area for the practice of evidence-based medicine.

Training and Knowledge

The range of professionals practising in the pre-hospital environment has also seen a major shift. The clinical role of paramedics has developed significantly over the past century, with an expanding scope of practice entailing timely intervention and enhanced clinical care. An undergraduate degree is a key entry requirement in a number of countries for paramedic practice, and those undertaking postgraduate study to fulfil specialist roles. Paramedics are no longer drivers and stretcher bearers, but clinicians who deliver advanced life-saving interventions, under time-critical pressure and in difficult circumstances.

The level of training and education provided to pre-hospital practitioners is both cause and effect of the increasing development of the clinical medicine delivered.

References

1. Ristagno G, Tang W, Weil MH. Cardiopulmonary resuscitation: from the beginning to the present day. *Crit Care Clin* 2009; **25**: 133–51.

2. Dadmehr M, Bahrami M, Eftekhar B, Ashraf H, Ahangar H. Chest compression for syncope in medieval Persia. *Eur Heart J* 2018; **39**: 2700–701.

3. Oliver GJ, Walter DP, Redmond AD. Prehospital deaths from trauma: are injuries survivable and do bystanders help? *Injury* 2017; **48**: 985–91.

4. Moon S, Ryoo HW, Ahn JY, Lee DE, Do Shin S, Park JH. Association of response time interval with neurological outcomes after out-of-hospital cardiac arrest according to bystander CPR. *Am J Emerg Med* 2020; **38**: 1760–66.

5. von Vopelius-Feldt J, Morris RW, Benger J. The effect of prehospital critical care on survival following out-of-hospital cardiac arrest: a prospective observational study. *Resuscitation* 2020; **146**: 178–87.

6. Hepple DJ, Durrand JW, Bouamra O, Godfrey P. Impact of a physician-led pre-hospital critical care team on outcomes after major trauma. *Anaesthesia* 2019; **74**: 473–9.

7. Michalsen KS, Rognås L, Vandborg M, Erikstrup C, Fenger-Eriksen C. Prehospital transfusion of red blood cells and plasma by an urban ground-based critical care team. *Prehosp Disaster Med* 2021; **36**: 170–74.

8. Sharma B, Sahai C, Sood J. Extraglottic airway devices: technology update. *Med Devices* 2017; **10**: 189.

9. Benger JR, Kirby K, Black S, Brett SJ, Clout M, Lazaroo MJ, et al. Effect of a strategy of a supraglottic airway device vs tracheal intubation during out-of-hospital cardiac arrest on functional outcome: the AIRWAYS-2 randomized clinical trial. *JAMA* 2018; **320**: 779–91.

10. Dalal PG, Murray D, Messner AH, Feng A, McAllister J, Molter D. Pediatric laryngeal dimensions: an age-based analysis. *Anesth Analg* 2009; **108**: 1475–9.

11. Marquez AM, Morgan RW, Ross CE, Berg RA, Sutton RM. Physiology-directed cardiopulmonary resuscitation: advances in precision monitoring during cardiac arrest. *Curr Opin Crit Care* 2018; **24**: 143–50.

12. Savino PB, Reichelderfer S, Mercer MP, Wang RC, Sporer KA. Direct versus video laryngoscopy for prehospital intubation: a systematic review and meta-analysis. *Acad Emerg Med* 2017; **24**: 1018–26.

13. Häske D, Schier L, Weerts JO, Groß B, Rittmann A, Grützner PA, et al. An explorative, biomechanical analysis of spine motion during out-of-hospital extrication procedures. *Injury* 2020; **51**: 185–92.

14. Maschmann C, Jeppesen E, Rubin MA, Barfod C. New clinical guidelines on the spinal stabilisation of adult trauma patients – consensus and evidence based. *Scand J Trauma Resusc Emerg Med* 2019; **27**: 77.

15. van der Weide L, Popal Z, Terra M, Schwarte LA, Ket JC, Kooij FO, et al. Prehospital ultrasound in the management of trauma patients: systematic review of the literature. *Injury* 2019; **50**: 2167–75.

16. Lesperance RN, Carroll CM, Aden JK, Young JB, Nunez TC. Failure rate of prehospital needle decompression for tension pneumothorax in trauma patients. *Am Surg* 2018; **84**: 1750–55.

17. Lubin D, Tang AL, Friese RS, Martin M, Green DJ, Jones T, et al. Modified Veress needle decompression of tension pneumothorax: a randomized crossover animal study. *J Trauma Acute Care Surg* 2013; **75**: 1071–5.

18. Jodie P, Kerstin H. BET 2: pre-hospital finger thoracostomy in patients with chest trauma. *Emerg Med J* 2017; **34**: 419.

19. Hannon L, St Clair T, Smith K, Fitzgerald M, Mitra B, Olaussen A, et al. Finger thoracostomy in patients with chest trauma performed by paramedics on a helicopter emergency medical service. *Emerg Med Australas* 2020; **32**: 650–56.

20. Kotora Jr JG, Henao J, Littlejohn LF, Kircher S. Vented chest seals for prevention of tension pneumothorax in a communicating pneumothorax. *J Emerg Med* 2013; **45**: 686–94.

21. Kuhlwilm V. The use of chest seals in treating sucking chest wounds: a comparison of existing evidence and guideline recommendations. *J Spec Oper Med* 2021; **21**: 94–101.

22. Axtman BC, Stewart KE, Robbins JM, Garwe T, Sarwar Z, Gonzalez RA, et al. Prehospital needle thoracostomy: what are the indications and is a post-trauma center arrival chest tube required? *Am J Surg* 2019; **218**: 1138–42.

23. Lockey DJ, Brohi K. Pre-hospital thoracotomy and the evolution of pre-hospital critical care for victims of trauma. *Injury* 2017; **48**: 1863–4.

24. Schauer SG, April MD, Fisher AD, Cunningham CW, Gurney J. Junctional tourniquet use during combat operations in Afghanistan: the prehospital trauma registry experience. *J Spec Oper Med* 2018; **18**: 71–4.

25. Schechtman DW, Kauvar DS, De Guzman R, Polykratis IA, Prince MD, Kheirabadi BS, et al. Abdominal aortic and junctional tourniquet versus zone III resuscitative endovascular balloon occlusion of the aorta in a swine junctional hemorrhage model. *J Trauma Acute Care Surg* 2020; **88**: 292–7.

26. Welch M, Barratt J, Peters A, Wright C. Systematic review of prehospital haemostatic dressings. *BMJ Mil Health* 2020; **166**: 194–200.

27. Tran A, Yates J, Lau A, Lampron J, Matar M. Permissive hypotension versus conventional resuscitation strategies in adult trauma patients with hemorrhagic shock: a systematic review and meta-analysis of randomized controlled trials. *J Trauma Acute Care Surg* 2018; **84**: 802–8.

28. Midwinter, M. *Fundamentals of Frontline Surgery*. CRC Press, 2021.

29. CRASH-3 Trial Collaborators. Effects of tranexamic acid on death, disability, vascular occlusive events and other morbidities in patients with acute traumatic brain injury (CRASH-3): a randomised, placebo-controlled trial. *Lancet* 2019; **394**: 1713–23.

30. Roberts I, Shakur-Still H, Afolabi A, Akere A, Arribas M, Brenner A, et al. Effects of a high-dose 24-h infusion of tranexamic acid on death and thromboembolic events in patients with acute gastrointestinal bleeding (HALT-IT): an international randomised, double-blind, placebo-controlled trial. *Lancet* 2020; **395**: 1927–36.

31. Lendrum R, Perkins Z, Chana M, Marsden M, Davenport R, Grier G, et al. Pre-hospital resuscitative endovascular balloon occlusion of the aorta (REBOA) for exsanguinating pelvic haemorrhage. *Resuscitation* 2019; **135**: 6–13.

32. Wilson MH, Hinds J, Grier G, Burns B, Carley S, Davies G.

Impact brain apnoea: a forgotten cause of cardiovascular collapse in trauma. *Resuscitation* 2016; **105**: 52–8.

33. Ter Avest E, Taylor S, Wilson M, Lyon RL. Prehospital clinical signs are a poor predictor of raised intracranial pressure following traumatic brain injury. *Emerg Med J* 2021; **38**: 21–6.

34. Miyoshi Y, Kondo Y, Suzuki H, Fukuda T, Yasuda H, Yokobori S. Effects of hypertonic saline versus mannitol in patients with traumatic brain injury in prehospital, emergency department, and intensive care unit settings: a systematic review and meta-analysis. *J Intensive Care* 2020; **8**: 61.

35. Picetti E, Iaccarino C, Servadei F. Letter: *Guidelines for the Management of Severe Traumatic Brain Injury* fourth edition. *Neurosurgery* 2017; **81**: E2.

36. Lott C, Truhlář A, Alfonzo A, Barelli A, González-Salvado V, Hinkelbein J, et al. European Resuscitation Council Guidelines 2021: cardiac arrest in special circumstances. *Resuscitation* 2021; **161**: 152–219.

37. Zhang Z, Brazil J, Ozkaynak M, Desanto K. Evaluative research of technologies for prehospital communication and coordination: a systematic review. *J Med Syst* 2020; **44**: 100.

38. Moran CG, Lecky F, Bouamra O, Lawrence T, Edwards A, Woodford M, et al. Changing the system – major trauma patients and their outcomes in the NHS (England) 2008–17. *EClinicalMedicine* 2018; **2**: 13–21.

39. Moore L, Champion H, Tardif PA, Kuimi BL, O'Reilly G, Leppaniemi A, et al. Impact of trauma system structure on injury outcomes: a systematic review and meta-analysis. *World J Surg* 2018; **42**: 1327–39.

40. Farshid A, Allada C, Chandrasekhar J, Marley P, McGill D, O'Connor S, et al. Shorter ischaemic time and improved survival with pre-hospital STEMI diagnosis and direct transfer for primary PCI. *Heart Lung Circ* 2015; **24**: 234–40.

Chapter

14

The Changing Face of Clinical Medicine in Major Trauma
Lessons from Civilian Practice and Military Deployments

Justine Lee and Keith Porter

Introduction

As we learned in Chapter 13, war is a breeding ground for innovation. Innovations of all kinds, but especially life-saving medical advances at times of war, inspire emotive headlines and have the potential to improve trauma care for the civilian population.

Some practices or interventions were developed from civilian emergency care and were then translated and improved on the battlefield. Others were created in the heat of battle and developed, casualty by casualty, into a product or technique that would go on to improve the chances of survival for many future trauma casualties. Most of these medical advances become associated with war or the military processes able to drive change, but they would probably have come about in time anyway.

Why This Matters

This chapter pays tribute to some of the people, and to medical and technical advances, that have progressed trauma casualty care over the past 30 years. As a result, we should see increasing numbers of civilian major trauma patients with successful outcomes, but their significant trauma sequelae and need for rehabilitation may have impact on many of us, while these survivors integrate back into society and into their workplaces.

Large numbers of severely injured casualties with multiple wounds are the deadly and gruesome reality of war. However, the availability of a large volume of similar casualties within a short period of time enables a process of rapid development and acceleration of medical innovation. Impressive medical advances, such as the discovery of penicillin, antiseptics, modern ambulances, and blood banks, are a legacy of the First and Second World Wars (WWI

and WWII). Medical ultrasound, for example, developed from technology used to detect cracks and defects in the armour plating of WWII tanks. The past 30 years have seen UK armed forces in combat alongside allied forces in Kosovo (Operation Agricola, 1998–2003), Iraq (Operation Telic, 2003–2009) and Afghanistan (Operation Herrick, 2005–2014), and during this time new concepts, equipment, training, capabilities, and governance have been applied in military clinical practice.

However, it must be appreciated that this has not been a comfortable journey. The Strategic Defence Review of 1998 and a post-operational analysis of the Kosovo campaign described the UK's Defence Medical Service (DMS) as severely understaffed and unlikely to be capable of adequately supporting major combat operations [1]. When there is the political will – together with the right social and cultural circumstances – to support transformation, whole system change can occur and, through translation into civilian clinical practice, good practice can continue after the conflict is over.

Emergency medicine was introduced as a new medical specialty in 1994. In 1999, the DMS EM Cadre deployed for the first time in Kosovo [2]. This marked the beginning of a new specialist system of emergency care, aimed at professionally owning patients from the point of wounding to more definitive care in field hospitals. Within 10 years, the survival rate among wounded troops in Afghanistan was over 90% – the highest rate in the history of warfare. The National Clinical Director (NCD) for Trauma Care for National Health Service England (NHSE) told the National Audit Office in 2010 that 'the organisation and facilities of Camp Bastion Field Hospital [Afghanistan] are equivalent to National Health Service best practice for trauma care' ([3] p. 16).

In his final address at the closure of the Bastion Role 3 on 22 September 2014, Lt Col JK Mahan, Commanding Officer of 34 Field Hospital, reflected that the mission in 'Afghanistan has catapulted us to the forefront of battlefield trauma care worldwide'.

At the beginning of the twenty-first century, civilian trauma services within the UK National Health Service (NHS) were also found wanting. In 2007 a report by the National Confidential Enquiry into Patient Outcome and Death, entitled 'Trauma: Who Cares?', together with undesirable evidence from the national surgical institutions, prompted a transformation in trauma care and the development of the national and regional Major Trauma Networks [4]. The UK's network of 32 major trauma centres was launched, and patients with severe injuries are now treated by trauma specialists in specialist hospitals that were specifically established to receive them.

The Influence of Battlefield Trauma Care

Many developments in battlefield trauma care are relevant to civilian trauma practice. If the modern ambulance, antiseptics, and anaesthesia are attributed to WWI, and the development of penicillin and blood banks to WWII, then military operations in Iraq and Afghanistan in the early 2000s are characterised by innovations in treating haemorrhagic shock and traumatic brain injuries as a result of the high incidence of injuries associated with improvised explosive devices (IEDs). The main concepts to be considered in caring for severely injured people include damage control resuscitation (DCR), early administration of blood products, early decision making by senior specialists, and a single coordinated system of trauma care from injury to rehabilitation. Innovations in pre-hospital emergency care (e.g., bone infusion devices, surgical airway kit, chest drain kit), field hospital resuscitation (e.g. platelet apheresis, thromboelastography, recombinant factor VIIa), imaging (e.g., CT scanning, ultrasound scanning, digital X-ray, telemedicine), aeromedical evacuation (e.g., elastomeric pumps for pain relief in transit), and rehabilitation (e.g., limb prosthetics) must also be considered in any exploration of the lessons learned during military conflict [5–7].

Resuscitation

Damage Control Resuscitation

Chapter 13 introduced the concept of DCR. It incorporates damage control surgery (DCS) as part of the resuscitation, rather than the process that occurs after surgery, and is most applicable to trauma casualties at risk of traumatic coagulopathy and death with its aim to address all aspects of the 'lethal triad' of coagulopathy, hypothermia, and acidosis early in the system of trauma care [8].

Several observational studies have shown that around 25% of trauma patients who already have an early coagulopathy on arrival at hospital emergency departments show a fourfold increase in mortality. The assessment of data from the Vietnam War by Ronald Bellamy and his colleagues suggested that acute haemorrhage accounted for 50% of battlefield deaths, and that up to a third of battlefield deaths could be prevented by early management of bleeding limbs [9,10]. The wars in Iraq and Afghanistan were characterised by limb amputation caused by the prolific use of IEDs. Traditionally, the ABC approach to casualty care, which is firmly established in global resuscitation training at all levels, directs addressing any issues of the airway, breathing, and circulation in that order. However, for casualties who are at risk of catastrophic external bleeding, as occurs when there is amputation of limbs by explosion of an IED, massive blood loss is more likely to cause death than is loss of airway, and must be rapidly addressed. In 2006, the UK armed forces introduced the concept of <C>ABC, where <C> or Big C stands for catastrophic haemorrhage, and dictates that self-applied tourniquets and topical haemostatics should be applied first [11–14]. These advances, together with others designed to replace circulatory volume by, for example, intraosseous infusion and consultant-led resuscitation on-scene, have reduced the death rate due to catastrophic external bleeding. Battlefield aid stations were also set up very close to the battle areas, and this saved many lives.

DCR was further developed by the armed forces so that it became a systematic approach to major trauma, combining the <C>ABC paradigm with other clinical techniques from point of wounding to definitive treatment, that minimises blood loss, maximises tissue oxygenation, and optimises outcome [13]. Active measures to stop bleeding and treat coagulopathy are started in pre-hospital settings and extend the time during which patients can receive emergency DCS. Survival outcomes are further improved by limiting surgery during the first trip to the operating theatre, and delaying secondary surgery until the patient's physiology has stabilised [8].

Until 2007, trauma resuscitation in civilian and military practice focused on replacing any blood loss with crystalloid fluids and red blood cell transfusions. Although this may restore blood volume and can increase the oxygen-carrying capacity of the remaining red blood cells to a small extent, it does not address any derangement of coagulation, and may even worsen the patient's physiology [15]. Resuscitation with blood and blood products seems most intuitive, and was supported by Jan Jansen and colleagues, who specified a 1:1 ratio of plasma to red blood cells, supplemented by additional platelets [16]. In 2009, a protocol for resuscitation using a 1:1:1 ratio of plasma to red blood cells to platelets was already being used by the UK armed forces after two studies showed an increase in casualty survival, and use of platelets after every 5 units was suggested.

Since 2008 there has been an increasing effort to optimise transfusion support for each injured person, rather than follow a pre-designated sequence [17]. The thromboelastogram (TEG), which was already being used in elective liver surgery, was developed to monitor the effectiveness of blood and blood products in correcting the coagulopathy of trauma. Later the technology would allow a successful portable TEG device to be used in the field, in a technique known as rotational thermoelectrometry (ROTEM) [18]. One of the benefits of bespoke treatment is minimisation of the unnecessary use of blood components, thereby reducing exposure of donors to risk and also preserving vital blood stocks.

The freshest blood (less than 14 days old) has been shown to be of most benefit in the most severely injured people [19]. This led to the creation of a 5,000-mile blood product supply chain, made possible by a major collaboration between the UK's NHS Blood and Transplant service and the Royal Air Force. However, platelets have a shelf-life of only 3 days, so are much too fragile to make this extraordinary journey. Nevertheless, this knowledge has led to new doctrine, training, and equipment to support platelet apheresis in close proximity to areas where casualties are being treated. This is in effect a donor panel that is established close to a military field hospital, to create its own blood supplies. Apheresis allows plasma and platelets to be collected, while returning the red cells to the donor. This means that donors can give plasma and platelets repeatedly, and it provides a safer pool of donors, who are tested regularly.

Recombinant factor VIIa has also been demonstrated to be lifesaving in exceptional circumstances, but its use is limited due to its cost [20–22]. The studies cited showed that over a period of 12 years, 27% of the UK's casualties required a blood transfusion, with 11% receiving 10 or more units of packed red cells, which is the definition of a massive transfusion. During the whole of 2009, over 3,200 units of blood products were administered as massive transfusions to severely injured UK personnel. This coincided with the peak in the conflict and in numbers of casualties. The mean blood component use per patient was approximately 22 units, and 12% of casualties received more than 100 units of blood and blood products [23]. As soon as control of bleeding is achieved, current practice is to switch to a tailored transfusion, based on clinical and laboratory assessments, including monitoring of each patient's coagulation with continuous point-of-care coagulation testing (i.e., TEG or ROTEM).

Right Turn Resuscitation

Right turn resuscitation (RTR) was named after the route that the most severely ill exsanguinating casualties took in the Role 3 hospital in Camp Bastion, Afghanistan, after arriving in the emergency department [24]. In order to minimise the time to surgical haemostasis as part of their resuscitation, there was no touchdown in the emergency department resuscitation area, and instead these casualties were received directly into the operating theatre. The whole trauma team assembled within the operating theatre to receive these patients. During this initial stage of management, physical examination and investigations were minimised, with no attempt made to define injury beyond identifying the bleeding cavity or limb(s) that needed immediate attention. An immediate definitive airway, a massive blood transfusion, and surgery to 'turn off the tap' was the signature trilogy of initial DCR. Warmed blood could be delivered by rapid transfusers at the rate of 1 unit of blood every 90 seconds. The casualty received further intensive care to correct coagulopathy, hypovolaemia and related acidosis, and hypothermia, and this took place in the operating theatre if the patient was too unstable to be moved, or in the intensive care unit if they improved [25]. Secondary surgery was planned when the patient's physiology had stabilised, and was often undertaken by surgical teams in the Royal Centre for Defence Medicine in Birmingham, which is the UK's Role 4 hospital.

RTR is just one of the measures that have been introduced by the armed forces to improve outcomes. Vital minutes are gained for the most severely injured patients by reconfiguring how teams work together. Critically injured casualties are taken directly from the helicopter into the operating theatre, where anaesthetic, emergency medicine, surgery, and radiology teams conduct complex resuscitation in parallel to improve outcomes.

Translating the Lessons Learned to Civilian Trauma Care

Operating room resuscitation works in the military environment because most military casualties are injured by the effects of an IED blast, penetrating missiles, or fragments. Resuscitative, surgical, and radiological protocols for this pattern of penetrating military injury were established and tested repeatedly. Most civilian studies support computerised tomography (CT) imaging, angiography, and other diagnostics in blunt civilian trauma, but not in penetrating trauma. CT imaging was not deployed in a land-based field hospital until 2004. However, its incorporation as a screening tool in severe blast injury positively informed the process of resuscitation, and led to the UK's Royal College of Radiology publishing its own version of the CT Whole Body (Bastion Protocol) for use in civilian major trauma patients [26]. Once a time-consuming process with significant risk to unstable patients, the CT Whole Body is now an essential part of civilian trauma management. The UK's Trauma Audit and Research Network (TARN) expects that trauma patients who meet the polytrauma criteria will receive a CT scan within 30 minutes of arrival at an emergency department, unless there is a good reason for not achieving this target [27].

The use of medical ultrasound imaging is also well established on military medical deployments. In the early twentieth century, ultrasound scanning (USS) technology was developed by engineers who used pulsed hypersonic echoes to identify flaws in the metal hulls of tanks and naval vessels. By the time of the deployment of UK armed forces to Kosovo in 1999, portable ultrasound devices were available for use in the emergency department to detect free blood in the abdomen and to support the decision to operate. Only radiographers were trained to use USS at that time, but it has since gained popularity as an immediate diagnostic and decision making tool in torso trauma. Today, emergency medicine doctors are often capable of completing a FAST (Focused Assessment using Sonography in Trauma) examination to detect blood in the chest or abdomen, and this takes place in the resuscitation room as an adjunct to the primary survey. Ultrasonography not only assists in identifying trauma pathology, but also supports clinicians' reliable placement of lines such as central access lines, arterial lines, peripheral venous access lines, suprapubic urinary catheters, and nerve catheters for effective delivery of regional analgesia.

Blast Casualties

A significant number of the blast injuries sustained by UK armed forces personnel result in these casualties experiencing severe limb trauma, and they are at risk of breakthrough pain and compartment syndrome during their journey to definitive care in the UK. Regional analgesia for limb trauma with prophylactic fasciotomies was provided before casualties left Afghanistan for the UK [28]. The most commonly used technique was a lumbar epidural (41%), followed by femoral and then sciatic nerve blocks.

Pain and Mental Health

The link between pain and mental health is significant and not straightforward [29]. The military mental health team works closely with the military pain team based at the Royal Centre for Defence Medicine (RCDM), which was an integral part of the support given to military casualties and veterans. Often casualties are conscious at the time of initial resuscitation, so it is important that they have the ability to use tourniquets and to apply their own first field dressings or administer their own morphine from an autoinjector pen before the arrival of trained medical assistance.

The new field dressing was introduced in 2005, along with self-applied arterial tourniquets. The first field dressing had not changed much since the days of WWI, but the new dressing was improved by the addition of a stretchy elastic bandage and chitosan – a non-exothermic novel haemostatic agent derived from crushed shellfish. From 2010 a similar product, known as Celox™ Gauze, was issued. This can be easily packed into large irregular wounds and is available in a number of different preparations, including a field dressing and a pliable ribbon gauze. Novel haemostatic agents could aid the management of external bleeding from junctional wounds, such as wounds in the groin, axilla, or neck, where tourniquets are ineffective or contraindicated and thus effective haemorrhage control had been difficult to achieve.

Tourniquets

Tourniquet use has been somewhat controversial in civilian practice, but at the time of writing is currently in favour in the UK, due to well-supported public trauma campaigns such as Citizen Aid and the Daniel Baird Foundation [30]. In 2007, strong international evidence confirmed the contribution that tourniquets had made to saving soldiers' lives, and they were added to the first aid training programmes of all UK soldiers. A study that reviewed 4½ years of continuous UK military experience in Iraq and Afghanistan in 2003–2007 analysed the impact of application of 107 tourniquets to 70 patients during first aid [31]. Most applications (64 out of 70 patients) occurred after 2006, from which time tourniquets were issued to individual soldiers. It was found that 87% (61 out of 70 soldiers) survived their injuries with a combination of multiple limb amputation, physiological evidence of critical hypovolaemia, and a requirement for massive transfusion at hospital. These unexpected survivors received tourniquets at the point of wounding, and their immediate survival to reach hospital was attributed to this. There were reversible complications in three patients, none of which contributed to unnecessary limb loss [31].

Medical Emergency Response Teams

During Operation Agricola in Kosovo in 1999, the Immediate Response Team (IRT) was responsible for retrieving casualties from the point of wounding. This developed into the Medical Emergency Response Team (MERT) and MERT-Enhanced (MERT-E) Team around 2006. The MERT-E ambulance had the highest capability, delivered by a medical officer, two paramedics, and an emergency department nurse. The medical officer was either a consultant or a senior specialist registrar in emergency medicine or anaesthetics, and was despatched to deliver advanced resuscitative care as close to the time of wounding as possible, and to continue that care during transfer to the next level of trauma care. Helicopters were used to evacuate patients from the point of wounding and, often with the firefight still in progress, with the team attempting to perform critical care interventions in the air, rather than prior to transfer [32].

Approximately 10% of casualties required rapid sequence induction (RSI) of anaesthesia and advanced airway management with controlled ventilation, and some required ongoing cardiopulmonary resuscitation (CPR) in the air. These interventions were of most significant benefit to casualties with severe traumatic brain injury (TBI), and were shown to increase their survival [33]. Other advanced interventions depended on the exact composition and skill set of the team, but included the ability to deliver a surgical airway, chest drainage, intraosseous access, and blood and blood product administration (doctors only), in addition to RSI and intubation.

Venous Access

Many patients cannot be given blood and medications because there is inadequate access to peripheral veins, and the resuscitation process is delayed. Central venous access using the Seldinger technique has largely replaced the venous cutdown approach to vascular access, but cannulation of the internal jugular vein (IJV) is often challenging because of cervical spine immobilisation and limited access to the neck in the trauma environment. Intraosseous infusion was first documented just after WWI, and by WWII was widely used to resuscitate casualties in haemorrhagic shock. However, its use then waned until the early 2000s, when a new cutting needle and battery-powered introducer system was developed. The resulting EZ-IO system was introduced into the UK armed forces in 2006, having already been approved by the UK's Resuscitation Council in 2005 for use with children [34]. Most operators can insert an IO access in less than 10 seconds, usually into the tibial tuberosity or into the lateral aspect of the humeral head or iliac crest. It must not be inserted into a fractured bone or through infected tissue.

Vascular access in a peripherally shut-down polytrauma patient is difficult, and can take up precious time that could be used for fluid resuscitation and drug administration. Therefore, to avoid delay in initiating resuscitation, the IO approach should be the first-line vascular access in casualties with severe trauma, to be augmented by two large-bore peripheral venous cannulae or an 8.5Fr central venous catheter in the subclavian vein when possible. The subclavian vein is large and can still be located despite significant hypovolaemia, unlike the IJV, which often collapses in severe hypovolaemia and increases the risk of carotid puncture (as 54% of IJVs overlie the carotid artery).

Survival after a traumatic cardiac arrest is an exceptional outcome, but when a MERT team can intervene immediately after an arrest using advanced procedures (drugs, airway and surgical skills, and blood transfusion) there is a small window of opportunity. Early access to CPR by soldiers and by the team medic in addition to advanced resuscitation reduces the clinical timeline from wounding to emergency surgery. In a subset analysis, the survival rate following cardiac arrest as a result of trauma was 24% in the military deployed trauma system [35]. This is more than three times higher than the best recorded survival to hospital discharge in UK civilian practice, namely 7.5% in over 10 consecutive years with the London Helicopter Emergency Medical Service (HEMS) [36]. In total, 88% of the unexpected military survivors had their outcome attributed to the advanced resuscitation strategies used by the armed forces to arrest and treat catastrophic haemorrhage after combat trauma. It would be misleading to assume that those people who suffer cardiopulmonary arrest on the battlefield and receive CPR from their buddy have a 24% chance of survival; the difference is made when there is the capacity to sustain the patient and avoid cardiac arrest prior to the arrival of specialist medical support.

The MERT is only on-scene for an average of 2 minutes, because of the hostile environment. This is quite different to the civilian setting; most UK prehospital services tend to 'scoop and run' when there are limited skills, or 'stay and play' if advanced interventions and early intervention are considered advantageous for survival [37]. All of these considerations, combined with direct admission to operating theatre on arrival in hospital, support the achievement of lifesaving interventions within the 'Platinum 10 Minutes' and surgery within the 'Golden Hour' [38].

Surgery

Surgical techniques developed during this time are beyond the scope of this chapter, except to consider the remarkable work, research, and courage of the military and civilian trauma surgeons who work in challenging environments.

The principles of managing high-energy combat wounds have changed little over the last 50 years, and still consist of early debridement, irrigation, prevention of infection, and delayed closure. One of the main

techniques to have changed compared with earlier conflicts has been the use of topical negative pressure (TNP) dressings to manage large high-energy traumatic limb wounds. In addition to having some therapeutic advantage, TNP dressings provide a method of managing large stump wounds efficiently while optimising the potential for limb salvage. Amputated stumps may require serial debridement and significant reconstruction before they start to heal and can be touched. Before TNP dressings became available, patients often reported that the odour of their saturated dressings was very distressing, in addition to experiencing significant pain associated with wounds adhering to the bed sheets and dressings. Topical negative pressure avoids the need for the patient's wounds to remain in contact with soiled dressings for many hours, and this has had a significant impact on patient wellbeing. In 2007, normal civilian practice was to change the TNP dressing every 48 hours. However, the military decided to change the dressings as dictated by the patient's physiology and need, which meant that some dressings were left unchanged for up to 8 days, although the average was 2–3 days. Total time in TNP was usually up to 2 weeks [39].

Data Collection

How did the armed forces demonstrate that all of their efforts were justified, and how were they able to claim that trauma care in the military was a marked improvement over that in the NHS? The answer is by collecting data. Prior to 1997, the UK armed forces did not collect data that allowed any comparison or analysis of trauma system performance. Although its civilian equivalent, TARN, was established in Manchester in the 1980s, it was not until the formation of the major trauma networks in 2010–2012 that funds were identified to support data collection by the major trauma centres. TARN is now a data powerhouse. Back in 2000, the aim of the UK military healthcare system was to provide as near to NHS best practice as was achievable within operational constraints. The assumption was that deployed care was likely to be below the standard of care achieved in the NHS. At first, standards of care appeared to be similar on military operations and in the NHS. However, since 2003 the RCDM trauma audit programme and the Joint Theatre Trauma Registry (JTTR) have comprehensively collected and collated data on all injured military casualties [40]. A key contributor to the success of this endeavour was a dedicated team of trauma nurse coordinators who were deployed to collect data during resuscitation, surgery, and intensive care in field hospitals, and about patients as they were transferred to Role 4, in Birmingham, UK.

An unexpected benefit of the JTTR data was the ability to link patterns of injury with the protective clothing worn and the seating position in vehicles. The trend towards genital injuries was recognised, and this led directly to the development in 2009 of the informally named 'Combat Codpiece', which is a scoop-shaped piece of body armour made of Kevlar, worn to prevent genital injury. Overnight, the devastating genital injury pattern that had been seen previously disappeared. JTTR is a key source for DSTL's continued development of protection, which has been credited with saving soldiers' lives in Afghanistan and Iraq.

The UK armed forces achieve comprehensive coordinated training by training everyone in combat casualty care.

Guidelines

Battlefield Advanced Trauma Life Support (BATLS)

The 2006 edition of the BATLS manual delivered the launch of the <C>ABC and other resuscitation concepts [12]. It introduced condensed clinical assessment if circumstances did not permit a complete trauma team assessment (i.e., the Tactical Rapid Primary Survey, TRaPs) and a standardised patient summary, the MIST Message (Mechanism, Injuries, Signs, Treatment). MIST was adopted within the North Atlantic Treaty Organization (NATO) standardised message requesting casualty evacuation on operations. It was adapted by the National Ambulance Resilience Unit (NARU) as ATMIST, adding to the message Age of patient and Time of injury. Attendance on the Military Operational Surgical Training (MOST) course is mandatory for all surgeons who are due to deploy within the next 6–12 months. All of this training contributes to a sophisticated and blended stepwise trauma system from point of wounding to definitive care, and this is the overarching reason for the demonstrably high rate of unexpected survivors [9,10,41,42].

Clinical Guidelines for Operations

In 2007, Clinical Guidelines for Operations (CGOs) were released, which used the <C>ABC concept as a common starting point for every emergency in medicine [43]. This was a further departure from civilian practice, which compartmentalises how an emergency is approached in terms of trauma, cardiac, environmental, toxicology (poisons, including radiation and chemical agents), and paediatrics. Uniquely, the military concept of CGOs facilitates cross-boundary clinical problem solving designed to be used by any member of the military who is seeking medical assistance.

MIMMS

Before 1992, there was no systematic approach to managing multiple casualty events. On 2 November 1991, the military wing of Musgrave Park Hospital, Belfast, was bombed by the IRA. The medical officer on duty that day was the current Surgeon General, and he acted as the medical commander during the incident, improvising a casualty clearing station, coordinating the evacuation of inpatients, and establishing the treatment of injured people [44]. This led directly to the development of the Major Incident Medical Management and Support (MIMMS) programme in partnership with the Advanced Life Support Group (ALSG) in Manchester [45]. The first MIMMS course ran in Manchester in 1993 and has been adopted globally [46]. Subsequently it has been adapted for the military as the NATO standard in 2004, and for use in hospitals (H-MIMMS).

Further examples of civilian application of military communication tools include:

1. the CSCATTT (Command, Safety, Communications, Assessment, Triage, Treatment, and Transport) approach to mass casualty management
2. the METHANE message (Major Incident- declared, E – Exact location, T – Type of Incident, H – Hazards present or suspected, N – Numbers, type, severity of casualties, E – Emergency Services present and those required), which was adapted from the ETHANE communication tool used in Iraq [34]
3. Sieve and Sort triage, which was developed to prioritise patients for treatment and transfer from a disaster scene, and has been adopted around the world, although in the NHS it has recently been replaced by the new national Major Incident Triage Tool (MITT), which is a universal triage tool for adults and children [47].

The Future

The so-called Forever War in Afghanistan finally came to an end on 30 August 2021, as UK and US troops rapidly evacuated from Afghanistan. During the conflict, many military personnel survived injuries of such severity that they would have been fatal at any other time in history. Because the long-term health outcomes of such injuries are unknown, the ADVANCE (ArmeD serVices trAuma rehabilitatioN outComE) study is researching the long-term physical and psychosocial outcomes of battlefield casualties in the UK armed forces following deployment to Afghanistan between 2002 and 2014 [48]. A total of 1,200 personnel have been recruited to the study, and they will be followed up for a period of 20 years.

Preliminary evidence from retrospective studies has identified an association with a wide variety of long-term health outcomes, including cardiovascular disease, hypertension, diabetes, and adverse mental health outcomes, such as post-traumatic stress disorder (PTSD), anxiety, and depression. The study is also collecting data on physical function, pain, mental health, and socioeconomic outcomes, and conducting research into the impact of injury on behavioural changes such as decreased physical activity, weight gain, substance abuse, and sleep disturbances [48].

It is estimated that 22% of UK military personnel and veterans who deployed to Iraq and Afghanistan have common mental health conditions. US studies report a rise in these conditions in injured military populations, with ranges of 10–46% for depression and 16–36% for anxiety disorders (excluding PTSD) [49]. The prevalence of PTSD in UK military populations is often quoted as lower than in US military veterans. However, the rate of PTSD in the UK cohort rose from 4% in studies in 2006 and 2010 to around 6% in 2018 [50]. In UK injured personnel, a wide rate of 2–59% associated with PTSD clearly demonstrates the need for the mental health of this cohort to be monitored and studied alongside other important long-term outcomes, such as all-cause mortality, physical function, drug and alcohol abuse, hearing loss, suicide ideation and attempts, quality of life, and social and employment outcomes. Research into

these associations may inform future strategies for preventing and intervening after injury, for both military and civilian populations [46].

The importance of identifying conceptual differences in military experiences of care for personnel with traumatic injury compared with civilian pre-hospital care lies with managing expectations of transferring excellent outcomes from the contemporary military operational environment to the civilian home base in the UK. When first deployed in the 1990s, the UK military medical teams aimed to deliver care to the same standards as UK NHS hospitals. However, these standards were soon surpassed, and the military came to set the standards of trauma care for the UK. In particular, the areas where the evidence is strongest lie in the contrast of the seniority of trauma team leaders; inadequate pre-hospital, physician-delivered airway management and supervision of ongoing case management. Only 40% of NHS cases were reviewed by a consultant within 12 hours, compared with all field hospital cases, which are managed by an integrated military consultant team from the outset [8,47].

The future needs to be planned. Medical learning, training, and research are likely to have an impact on UK civilian healthcare as the military and the NHS work far more closely than has ever happened in the past. It is imperative that the UK military medical services effectively transfer excellent outcomes and organisational learning to the NHS trauma care, and that military research into the long-term sequelae of physiological and anatomical disruption has an impact on future trauma knowledge. The future should see joint military and NHS ventures and investments in healthcare research to develop predictive treatment algorithms, future transfusion strategies, total wound care, telemedicine, and the use of augmented reality and virtual reality in treatment delivery and training. We should not be surprised if these technologies could then be used to achieve good outcomes in any future civilian mass casualty events, military conflicts, and global pandemics.

References

1. Houses of Common. *Defence Committee Second Report*. House of Commons, 2000.

2. Hodgetts T, Kenward G, Masud S. Lessons from the first operational deployment of emergency medicine. *J R Army Med Corps* 2000; **146**: 134–42.

3. National Audit Office. *Major Trauma Care in England*. National Audit Office, 2010.

4. McMonagle M. *Trauma: Who Cares?* National Confidential Enquiry into Patient Outcome and Death, 2007.

5. Hodgetts T, Russell R, Russell M, Mahoney P, Kenward G. Evaluation of clinician attitudes to the implementation of novel haemostatics. *J R Army Med Corps* 2005; **151**: 139–41.

6. Mahoney P, Hodgetts T, Russell R, Russell M. Novel haemostatic techniques in military medicine. *J R Army Med Corps* 2005; **151**: 176–8.

7. Fear N, Jones E, Groom M, Greenberg N, Hull L, Hodgetts T, et al. Symptoms of post-concussional syndrome are non-specifically related to mild traumatic brain injury in UK Armed Forces personnel on return from deployment in Iraq: an analysis of self-reported data. *Psychol Med* 2009; **39**: 1379–87.

8. Hodgetts T, Mahoney P, Kirkman E, Midwinter M. Damage control resuscitation. *J R Army Med Corps* 2007; **153**: 299–300.

9. Bellamy RF. The causes of death in conventional land warfare: implications for combat casualty care research. *Mil Med* 1984; **149**: 55–62.

10. Bellamy RF, Maningas PA, Vayer JS. Epidemiology of trauma: military experience. *Ann Emerg Med* 1986; **15**: 1384–8.

11. Hodgetts T, Mahoney P, Clasper J. *Battlefield Advanced Trauma Life Support* 4th ed. Joint Service Publication, 2008.

12. Hodgetts T, Mahoney P, Evans G, Brooks A. Battlefield advanced trauma life support: 3. *J R Army Med Corps* 2006; **152**(suppl); 4.

13. Hodgetts TJ, Mahoney PF, Russell MQ, Byers M. ABC to <C>ABC: redefining the military trauma paradigm. *Emerg Med J* 2006; **23**: 745–6.

14. Hodgetts T, Russell R, Russell M, Mahoney P, Kenward G. Evaluation of clinician attitudes to the implementation of novel haemostatics. *J R Army Med Corps* 2005; **151**: 139–41.

15. Kirkman E, Watts S, Hodgetts T, Mahoney P, Rawlinson S, Midwinter M. A proactive approach to the coagulopathy of trauma: the rationale and guidelines for treatment. *J R Army Med Corps* 2007; **153**: 302–6.

16. Jansen JO, Thomas R, Loudon MA, Brooks A. Damage control resuscitation for patients with major trauma. *BMJ* 2009; **338**: b1778.

17. Wright C, Mahoney P, Hodgetts T, Russell R. Fluid resuscitation: a Defence Medical Services Delphi study into current practice. *J R Army Med Corps* 2009; **155**: 99–104.

18. Jackson G. Ashpole K. Yentis S. The TEG vs the ROTEM thromboelastography/thromboelastometry systems. *Anaesthesia* 2009; **64**: 212–15.

19. Koch CG, Li L, Daniel I, Sessler DI, Figueroa, P, Hoeltge GA, et al. Duration of red-cell storage and complications after cardiac surgery. *N Engl J Med* 2008; **358**: 1229–39

20. Kenet G, Walden R, Eldad A, Martinowitz U. Treatment of traumatic bleeding with recombinant factor VIIa. *Lancet* 1999; **354**: 1879.

21. Williams D, McCarthy R. Recombinant activated factor VII and perioperative blood loss. *Lancet* 2003: **361**: 1745.

22. Hodgetts T, Mahoney P, Kirkman E, Russell R, Thomas R. UK Defence Medical Services guidance for use of recombinant factor VIIa in the deployed military setting. *J R Army Med Corps* 2007; **153**: 307–9.

23. Mercer S, Tarmey N, Woolley T, Wood P, Mahoney P. Haemorrhage and coagulopathy in the Defence Medical Services. *Anaesthesia* 2013; **68**(suppl 1): 49–60.

24. Tai N, Russell R. Right turn resuscitation: frequently asked questions. *J R Army Med Corps* 2011; **157**(suppl 1): s310–14.

25. Blackbourne LH. Combat damage control surgery. *Crit Care Med* 2008; **36**(suppl): s304–10.

26. The Royal College of Radiologists. *Standards of Practice and Guidance for Trauma Radiology in Severely Injured Patients*. National Institute for Health and Care Excellence, 2015 (www.rcr.ac.uk/system/files/publication/field_publication_files/bfcr155_traumaradiol.pdf).

27. Trauma Audit and Research Network (www.tarn.ac.uk).

28. Clasper JC, Aldington DJ. Regional anaesthesia, ballistic limb trauma and acute compartment syndrome. *J R Army Med Corps* 2010; **156**: 77–8.

29. Iversen A. Greenberg N. Mental health of regular and reserve military veterans. *Adv Psychiatr Treat* 2009; **15**: 100–106.

30. Lee C, Porter K, Hodgetts T. Tourniquet use in the civilian pre-hospital setting. *Emerg Med J* 2007; **24**: 584–7.

31. Hodgetts T, Mahoney P. The military tourniquet: a response. *J R Army Med Corps* 2007; **153**: 10–15.

32. McLeod J, Hodgetts T, Mahoney P. Combat 'Category A' calls: evaluating the pre-hospital timelines in a military trauma system. *J R Army Med Corps* 2007; **153**: 266–8.

33. Breeze J, Bowley DM, Harrisson SE, Dye J, Neal C, Bell RS, et al. Survival after traumatic brain injury improves with deployment of neurosurgeons: a comparison of US and UK military treatment facilities during the Iraq and Afghanistan conflicts. *J Neurol Neurosurg Psychiatry* 2020; **91**: 359–65.

34. Cooper B, Mahoney P, Hodgetts T, Mellor A. Intra-osseous access (EZ-IO) for resuscitation: UK military combat experience. *J R Army Med Corps* 2007; **153**: 314–16.

35. Russell R, Hodgetts T, McLeod J, Starkey K, Mahoney P, Harrison K, et al. The role of trauma scoring in developing trauma clinical governance in the Defence

Medical Services. *Philos Trans R Soc Lond B Biol Sci* 2011; **366**: 171–91.

36. Lockey D, Crewdson K, Davies G. Traumatic cardiac arrest: who are the survivors? *Ann Emerg Med* 2006; **48**: 240–44.

37. Hoejenbos M, McManus J, Hodgetts T. Is there one optimal medical treatment and evacuation chain for all situations: 'scoop-and-run' or 'stay-and-play'. *Prehosp Disaster Med* 2008; **23**: s74–8.

38. Cowley RA. A total emergency medical system for the State of Maryland. *Md State Med J* 1975; **24**: 37–45.

39. Penn-Barwell J, Roberts S, Midwinter M, Bishop J. Improved survival in UK combat casualties from Iraq and Afghanistan: 2003–2012. *J Trauma Acute Care Surg* 2015; **78**: 1014–20.

40. Russell R, Hodgetts T, Ollerton J, Massetti P, Skeet J, Bray I, et al. The operational emergency department attendance register: a new epidemiological tool.

J R Army Med Corps 2007; **153**: 244–50.

41. Hodgetts T, Mahoney P, Evans G, Brooks A. Battlefield advanced trauma life support: 1. *J R Army Med Corps* 2006; **152**(suppl); 5–72.

42. Hodgetts T, Mahoney P, Evans G, Brooks A. Battlefield advanced trauma life support: 2. *J R Army Med Corps* 2006; **152**(suppl); 4.

43. Hodgetts T, ed. *Clinical Guidelines for Operations*. Joint Defence Publication 4-03.1. Development, Concepts and Doctrine Centre, 2009.

44. Hodgetts TJ. Lessons from the Musgrave Park Hospital bombing. *Injury* 1993; **24**: 219–21.

45. Hodgetts T, Mackway-Jones K. *Major Incident Medical Management and Support: The Practical Approach*. BMJ Publishing, 1995.

46. Hodgetts T. Training for major incidents: evaluation of perceived ability after exposure to a systematic approach. *Pre-Hosp Immed Care* 2000; **4**: 11–16.

47. Malik NS, Chernbumroong S, Xu Y, Vassallo J, Lee J, Bowley DM, et al. The BCD Triage Sieve outperforms all existing major incident triage tools: comparative analysis using the UK national trauma registry population. *EClinicalMedicine* 2021; **36**: 100888.

48. Bennett AN, Dyball DM, Boos CJ, Fear NT, Schofield S, Bull AMJ, et al. Study protocol for a prospective, longitudinal cohort study investigating the medical and psychosocial outcomes of UK combat casualties from the Afghanistan war: the ADVANCE Study. *BMJ Open* 2020; **10**: e037850.

49. Inoue C, Shawler E, Jordan CH, Jackson CA. *Veteran and Military Mental Health Issues*. StatPearls Publishing, 2023.

50. Dyball D, Bennett AN, Schofield S, Cullinan P, Boos C, Bull A, et al. Mental health outcomes of male UK military personnel deployed to Afghanistan and the role of combat injury: analysis of baseline data from the ADVANCE cohort study. *Lancet* 2022; **9**: 547.

Chapter

15

The Changing Face of Traumatic Injury
Increasing Experiences of Penetrating Gun and Knife Injuries and Their Treatment

Thomas König

Introduction

Blunt trauma remains the most common mechanism of injury in the civilian setting, but in some parts of the world and, particularly in war zones, penetrating trauma is a significant cause of morbidity and mortality [1].

Penetrating wounds are most commonly the result of wounding by sharp knives or weapons such as guns. Knife wounds are typically low-velocity injuries with low-energy transfer to the tissues in the line of the track of the knife. Gunshot wounds range from low-velocity handgun injuries to high-velocity injuries that are the result of bullets fired from more powerful rifles and assault weapons typically used in war. These higher-velocity injuries cause greater tissue destruction, as a result of the greater energy transfer from the projectile to the soft tissues. Both are also associated with fracture of underlying bone that may also result in local tissue damage. In addition, the passage of the projectile may be associated with injury from a blast wave around it. Secondary blast injuries are the result of penetration by bomb fragments or debris. These wounding patterns, more commonly seen in war and terrorist attacks, complicate an already complex wounding pattern [2].

Trauma management principles of reception, assessment, investigation, and treatment may be similar for both blunt and penetrating injury, and the management of penetrating injuries and wounds may follow similar generic principles to blunt injury patterns, but some salient differences do exist.

These differences include management of the wound and underlying organ injury, triage of the injured patient, resuscitation before and in hospital, management of the physiological response to bleeding and injury by damage control/haemostatic resuscitation, evacuation and transfer from the scene, investigation and diagnosis, emergency-room management, operative intervention, and wound management. All of the direct patient care is then further wrapped in an enveloping delivery of care that involves trauma systems, education, governance, audit, quality improvement, assurance, training, and injury prevention.

Penetrating wounds in the UK are rare in low-density population areas such as the countryside and suburbs, whereas there is a higher prevalence in the inner cities. Increases in penetrating trauma rates are being seen, and are being reported in the press. The subtle differences in wounding and its sequalae between penetrating and blunt trauma requires a change in the medical response provided to trauma patients. Improvements in care and in particular access to damage control resuscitation (DCR) and damage control surgery (DCS) to control bleeding may be required. Technological advances and innovation are also needed to help to make inroads into patient care now and in the future.

Wounding Mechanisms

The velocity of the penetrating implement results in variable injury to local tissues depending on the amount of energy transferred. Stab wounds tend to be linear in nature, and therefore possible underlying injury can to a large degree be predicted by the site and direction of the skin wound. Higher-velocity injuries may well result in some degree of blast injury. This is particularly the case for bullets passing through solid organs and gas-filled organs, such as the liver, lung, and bowel. Bullets are also capable of striking tissues such as bone, then fragmenting, and thereafter taking an altered course that may result in the projectile coming to rest in an area remote from the line of trajectory. Bone fragments are also capable of causing multiple surrounding soft tissue injuries that may need to be addressed [3].

Immediate Management

Tissue Injury and Wound Management

Initial management of a patient with penetrating injury is often based on the management of the superficial wound that can be readily accessed (to reduce further bleeding and minimise contamination and potential mortal consequences), but the potential deeper injuries also need to be considered carefully. It is not enough to simply place a large blast-like dressing bandage over a wound and expect this to control bleeding. Local pressure is required to tamponade bleeding vessels. This is then augmented by local wound pressure to promote clot formation and decrease flow into damaged arteries and veins. Wound management also needs to be augmented by systemic management of the physiological consequences and effects of wounding, the most severe of which are bleeding, hypothermia, and coagulopathy.

The most damaging early consequences are haemorrhage (from the neck, thorax, abdomen, junctional areas, or upper and lower limbs), tension pneumothorax (from injury to the thorax and underlying lung with build-up of air around the lung), and cardiac tamponade (build-up of blood around the heart, often as a result of simple stab wounds to the anterior chest). Understanding of the mechanism of injury, timely assessment, injury recognition, and immediate management are therefore vital for a good outcome [4].

Bleeding

Bleeding remains a cause of early death in penetrating trauma patients. There is no safe place to be stabbed. People continue to die on the streets of many cities as a result of low-velocity penetrating trauma to the upper and lower limbs. These peripheral limb wounds with injury to major named vessels are the cause of considerable bleeding, but are also amenable to simple methods of proximal vascular control as well as local wound management. Hard signs of an underlying vascular injury are also evident at an early stage. These include pale pulseless cold paralysed limbs, in addition to signs of significant blood loss on-scene and deranged physiology [5].

We know that pre-hospital clear fluid administration is not required and may in fact be detrimental. We may find that plasma and whole blood will make up the mainstay of early volume replacement during or after vascular control. Synthetic substances that are capable of clotting blood and carrying oxygen may also be regularly used in the future.

Care from Bystanders

Care from bystanders, often with advice from emergency medical services (EMS) call handlers and dispatchers, is aimed at local wound management. Bystanders may be asked to provide pressure and elevation to the wound, but can also be asked to give information about the geographical location, to provide early efforts at scene management, and to give reassurance to the patient and some oversight of care. The aim of this is not to delay the ambulance response but merely to optimise the response by achieving incremental gains in care. Positioning of a patient to permit ready access and evacuation to hospital is also vitally important. Efforts to educate and train the public through 'Stop the Bleed' campaigns and the 'Citizen Aid' scheme aim to promote early care by those present before the emergency services arrive [6,7].

Management of Wounds and Bleeding (Tourniquet, Haemostatic Dressing, and Needle Decompression)

EMS teams, fire and rescue services, and police services are now becoming more routinely equipped with tourniquets, haemostatic dressings, and devices for safely performing chest needle decompression to relieve tension pneumothorax. These tools were traditionally used on the battlefield, but are now being increasingly applied in civilian settings. The Combat Application Tourniquet is simple to place and use, topical haemostatic dressings that promote local clot formation are undergoing modification so that they also place directed pressure over the wound, and bespoke decompression needles that minimise the risk of iatrogenic injury to underlying lungs, heart, and vessels are safer and easier to use. All of these advances ensure early treatment, removing the requirement for prolonged on-scene time and thereby enabling early evacuation to hospital.

The three-sided chest dressing, which often consisted of a flimsy covering and three sides of adherent tape, has now been replaced by bespoke dressings that readily adhere to diaphoretic (sweaty) skin, permit ongoing release of air and blood under pressure, and also prevent the entrainment of air into the thoracic cavity.

Thoracostomy is often performed to prevent the development of tension pneumothorax after intubation and positive pressure ventilation, which is particularly hazardous in the hypovolaemic patient with reduced venous pressure, as increased thoracic pressure may result in reduced venous return and reduced cardiac output. Only when a haemothorax is large are intercostal pleural drains placed in the field. Early autotransfusion of whole blood would be enabled by pre-hospital salvage of warm freshly donated blood and a patient's own blood. This is important when blood stocks are in short supply [8].

Physician-Led/Advanced Paramedic Teams

Helicopter emergency medical services (HEMS), physician-led pre-hospital care teams, and paramedics with advanced skills and experience are capable of delivering a number of advanced procedures aimed at managing severe penetrating injury. Management of the team, procedures, and timely evacuation by personnel experienced in dealing with penetrating trauma ensure that marginal gains are achieved.

Airway management and surgical airway for penetrating neck injury protect the airway in the swelling neck and prevent aspiration of blood in combined tracheal and vascular injury.

Resuscitative thoracotomy by bilateral anterolateral incision permits access to the heart, lungs, and chest wall to relieve tamponade, repair myocardial injury, and control local and general bleeding from the lung and packing of the chest wall. Centrally placed right atrial appendage access permits resuscitation with warmed blood and blood components and correction of altered biochemistry. All of this occurs on-scene or during transfer to hospital before further surgery in the form of DCS or definitive surgery [9].

Administration of blood (to transport oxygen), blood components, tranexamic acid and warming (to promote blood clotting), and calcium and bicarbonate (electrolytes to promote clotting and prevent acidosis), allows haemostatic resuscitation that optimises the patient before surgical intervention on-scene, during evacuation, or in hospital – in essence making the patient fit for surgery. The ABC approach (airway, then breathing, then circulation) of the Advanced Trauma Life Support (ATLS) guidelines of the American College of Surgeons has evolved to <C>ABC, where <C> represents the management of catastrophic haemorrhage before the management of airway and breathing [10].

With all the technological and management advances available to the modern EMS team, it is on occasion important to remember that expeditious intervention and rapid transfer to a higher level of care with more personnel and resources may be required. Simple procedures such as wound bandaging and elevation should not be forgotten or overlooked in favour of more invasive interventions.

Managing the Scene

Military pre-hospital care focuses on 'winning the firefight' in order to prevent further casualties before rendering definitive aid to an injured soldier. There is some reliance on self-aid and 'buddy–buddy' aid before trained medical care becomes available in this environment, and for this reason soldiers, sailors, and airmen are trained to provide self-care. Evacuation from the battlefield may be by land, air, or sea, and care is often delivered during transfer. Civilian EMS systems are also in a position to provide care on-scene and during transfer. We should move towards a model of 'scoop and play' and away from the old concepts of 'stay and play' or 'scoop and run'. On-scene times should be as short as possible, and often in volatile 'forensic' scenes resulting from an altercation this is the preferred course of action. It is also particularly important during mass casualty scenarios, to avoid bottlenecks and the overwhelming of forward casualty areas before arriving in hospital.

Triage

Those patients in extremis may be triaged immediately to a Major Trauma Centre (MTC) and cared for by a pre-alerted team with the experience and skills necessary to perform DCR and DCS. Massive transfusion protocols ensure timely delivery of blood and blood components to the patient for early transfusion. Some trauma triage protocols advise ambulance services as to which centres patients should be taken to. This may result in very sick patients being taken a short distance to a Trauma Unit (TU) to receive immediate care and transfusion to stop bleeding, before onward transfer to a Major Trauma Centre or indeed the TU's own operating theatre in extremis when immediate lifesaving surgery is required and intervention cannot wait until transfer to the MTC. This paradoxical nature of care requires an inclusive network that is capable of providing timely assistance and governance to those with less experience and training in an effort to ensure good outcomes [11].

Timely activation of the emergency department team and indeed the wider hospital will ensure that all personnel are ready, blood is warmed, ultrasound machines are plugged in, operating theatre staff are mobilised, and theatres are ready and warming to ensure that the patient journey is as swift and seamless as possible. Designating these trauma call responses as 'code red'/'advanced'/REBOA/OP Vampire, etc. aims to help this process.

Care in Emergency Departments

Primary survey, secondary survey, plain radiograph imaging supported by ultrasonography, and arterial blood gases (looking at base deficit and lactate levels) allow estimation of injury burden and physiological derangement. Early ultrasound imaging of the pericardium and the heart aims to rule out pericardial tamponade in the patient with a precordial stab wound to the anterior chest in the 'cardiac box'. Abdominal ultrasound scanning – FAST (Focused Assessment by Sonography in Trauma) scanning – looking for evidence of blood within the peritoneal cavity triages patients for intervention or further investigation by cross-sectional imaging such as computerised tomography (CT) scanning if they are physiologically well enough. If the patient is FAST positive (i.e., there is evidence of fluid and/or blood within the abdominal cavity), they may be triaged straight to the operating theatre for early intervention to reduce bleeding and minimise contamination.

'Straight to CT' imaging and investigation has developed as a concept in early management of certain patients on their arrival in emergency departments. Strict protocols are required to select suitable patients to avoid incorrectly triaging them and to separate them from those who are better suited to being taken straight to the operating theatre. Trauma systems are marked on their ability to record data, and CT scanning is important to highlight injuries. Therefore injury scoring has developed significantly. It is also being used more frequently in diagnosing injuries post-mortem [12].

Damage Control Surgery

The aim of DCS is to restore physiological normality, correct coagulopathy, and normalise abnormal electrolyte imbalance and warming. Surgically, this is done by controlling bleeding and minimising contamination. It is not aimed at restoring normal anatomy in the first instance. Damage control begins as early as possible, ideally at the point of wounding and even before arrival in hospital.

Damage control as a concept has its roots in the management of damaged naval ships during battle. Damage control teams are tasked with controlling breaches in the hull by local damage management, closing watertight compartments, and fighting fires around the ship. This is similar in principle to the management of blood loss and contamination from damaged organs.

Early surgery allows the surgeon to acquire information directly by sight about the injury pattern and burden, while at the same time delivering therapy and treatment to minimise blood loss and contamination. A decreased reliance on imaging and greater use of clinical acumen and experience is an advantage for surgeons operating in more austere environments, who may not have the luxury of these imaging modalities. The evolution of surgical specialists has resulted in a downgrading of surgeons who are capable of early and timely decision making (on occasion being asked to make decisions without all the necessary information and without the support of prolonged pre-surgical work-up and multidisciplinary decision making) and maximal intervention. One type of surgical specialist who is coming to the fore is the general 'visceral' trauma surgeon, who is also capable of carrying out temporary or definitive vascular surgical techniques, has experience of paediatric and obstetric care, and when deployed in the military environment is able to perform plastic surgery, burns surgery, neurosurgery, ear, nose, and throat (ENT) surgery, and orthopaedic surgery.

Thoraco-abdominal wounds and junctional areas are termed non-compressible areas (regions where pressure cannot be easily applied to prevent and control ongoing blood loss), and require other methods of wound management. Timely recognition of these patients, and an understanding and acknowledgement that little definitive or indeed temporary can be done in the pre-hospital arena or outside the operating theatre, should encourage early transfer from the scene through the resuscitation room to the operating theatre for cavity access and temporary control of haemorrhage (so-called CATCH procedures). These procedures may involve vascular control by pressure or clamp placement [13].

Bleeding vessels may then by ligated in extremis or shunted to restore some distal perfusion before definitive repair by bypass or interposition grafting. Contamination control by clamp, staple, or pack (e.g., to control leakage of bowel contents from injured segments of bowel) and irrigation of contaminated cavities and drainage are used as part of the DCS procedures available. The concept of DCR is slowly becoming more complex than the surgery it was designed to support and, in essence, intensive care should be delivered in the operating theatre for a more prolonged time before movement to the dedicated intensive care unit. The previous paradigm involved surgery, followed by a period of resuscitation and intensive care, followed by relook surgery to restore anatomy, remove packs, and undertake definitive reconstruction. This has evolved into early haemostatic resuscitation and correction of coagulopathy being performed before, during, and after surgery, before ongoing intensive care in the operating theatre or intensive care unit, before later return to theatre for relook and reconstructive surgery. 'Shock' rooms and operating theatre suites capable of providing resuscitation (supported by near-patient testing and blood transfusion), cross-sectional imaging or interventional radiology and DCS, and then intensive care remove the requirement for patient movement around the hospital, and allow care to be centred in one area. All of these advances aim to reduce morbidity and mortality and improve outcome [14].

Some innovative procedures have evolved in an attempt to reduce bleeding and support central perfusion by attaining proximal control of traditionally non-compressible vessels and areas of injury. These include the placement of tamponade balloons along neck wound tracks that compress the subclavian artery against the underside of the clavicle using Foley catheters or the balloon of an endotracheal tube. Bespoke designs have been postulated that deliver a balloon along the length of a track that then temporarily seals it and controls bleeding (similar to the Sengstaken–Blakemore tubes that are used in oesophageal varices, and that when inflated compress the bleeding vessels). Others have involved syringe-like wound track delivery of haemostatic granules, but these have relied on wound tracks being large enough to accommodate the device, and in knife injuries this may prove difficult. Other advances have included expanding abdominal foam that fills the peritoneal space and reduces bleeding by a tamponade effect. The Abdominal Aortic Junctional Tourniquet placed around the abdomen at the level of the umbilicus is designed to compress the distal aorta (and also the inferior vena cava) and reduce intra-abdominal, pelvic, and lower limb bleeding. All of these and more are similar to the anti-shock trousers that were used in the past, with variable effects on outcome. The timely and well-trusted method of local anaesthetic (with or without adrenaline, but with volume) and simple wound closure and targeted pressure by appropriate pressure dressings should not be forgotten, and should always be considered in the stepwise response [15].

The use of intraluminal aortic balloons and resuscitative endovascular balloon occlusion of the aorta (REBOA) has evolved in recent years. Atraumatic balloons that are easily placed in the common femoral artery and migrated proximally to the thoracic or distal aorta are capable of gaining proximal aortic control and thereby minimising distal bleeding and also improving afterload and optimising myocardial and cerebral blood flow. They have moved resuscitation along and prompted early invasive arterial monitoring augmented by balloon inflation if required to permit control while transfusion is undertaken. Distal ischaemia and local vessel injury are not uncommon sequelae that need to be managed by staged reperfusion and direct vessel repair. The alternative thoracotomy and aortic cross clamp is a considerably more morbid alternative [16].

Wounds, particularly high-velocity penetrating wounds encountered during war, traditionally required extensive debridement and laying open of wounds, elliptical excision of the skin wounds, irrigation, and delayed primary closure. Early closure of wounds risks infection and abscess formation if devitalised and necrotic tissue becomes infected. These wounds should not be closed primarily under any circumstances. Civilian management of gunshot wounds has evolved, and uncomplicated wounds are now simply left alone to heal by secondary intention.

Non-Operative Management

High-volume centres have a number of patients who have benefited from selective non-operative management of their penetrating wounds. It is important to rule out intracavity injury by imaging, admission may follow, and the patient should be monitored closely for a period of time that depends on the nature of their injury. They can then be discharged safe in the knowledge that invasive surgery was not required [17].

Laparoscopy

Laparoscopic surgery in trauma permits inspection of the abdominal cavity and repair of the injured spleen and small bowel with drain placement. It has a role in the patient with normal physiology, but many find laparotomy the preferred method of investigation and therapy in those patients who are temporary responders or non-responders to resuscitation. This requires surgeons to be competent laparoscopists capable of performing both diagnostic and interventional laparoscopic techniques.

Video-assisted thorascopic surgery (VATS) is a minimally invasive method of washing out a hemithorax and treating retained haemothoraces and empyema.

Trauma Systems

The vast majority of Major Trauma Centres in the UK see a low volume of penetrating trauma. However, in the inner cities this volume is increasing, which has resulted in growing experience of and familiarity with penetrating trauma management. In these centres, teams are used to dealing with patients who have been injured minutes, rather than hours, before they are seen. This provides challenges when there is little time to warn and assemble responding trauma teams. Consultant surgeons may be at home and need travel time to attend. It may be more prudent in the future to have these surgeons already in the hospital 24 hours a day. Penetrating trauma patients may also self-present or be brought by friends to their nearest hospital. Without much warning, these incredibly sick patients may present at units not scaled for this response, so timely decisions about treatment and transfer may need to be made. It may be necessary to utilise the assets of the regional pre-hospital care system, such as a helicopter emergency medical service (HEMS) unit, for secondary transfers. Use of telemedicine may assist these smaller units in their decision making and management by permitting oversight from the MTC trauma surgeon who is then in the operating theatre with them. All activity within a region should continue to be under an umbrella of governance and peer review which is steered by standard operating procedures, local and regional teaching, and robust data collection and review to ensure that high-quality care is delivered wherever possible [18].

Education and Training

Teams that manage both penetrating and blunt trauma patients should regularly undergo simulation training and bespoke courses. Surgeons dealing with vascular injury should be familiar with the techniques for attaining proximal vascular control, dissection of vessels, and revascularisation of limbs. High-fidelity models, cadavers (fresh frozen and 'reanimated' and reperfused cadavers that bleed), and live tissue courses are proven methods of improving the care that is given. Individual training is complemented by team training at every level.

Injury Prevention

Protective equipment in the military setting (e.g., eye protection, helmets, body armour, blast underwear) is utilised to protect combatants on the battlefield. There are anecdotal examples of civilians wearing body armour and even placing their own tourniquets. Overall, primary injury prevention is the preferred method of preventing mortality and morbidity from injury. The causes of trauma are many and varied, and all of us who care for trauma patients have an obligation to notify those in leadership positions when laws and legislation need to change to prevent further loss of life. Socioeconomic status is linked to violent crime and personal injury, and efforts to change this will have some bearing on decreasing the rate of violent crime, injury, and mortality rates from homicide.

Future Advances

DCS and DCR are being pushed to the limits on a daily basis. The more experienced we become, the better we get at every stage of care. In some instances, we are managing patients who a number of years ago would not have arrived in hospital, let alone survived to hospital discharge. However, despite these efforts, some patients continue to die of their injuries. More needs to be done.

The stunned heart in myogenic shock after cardiac repair may require a period of rest and organ support, so extracorporeal membrane oxygenation (ECMO) may be considered.

Selective aortic arch perfusion is aimed at preserving blood flow to the heart and the brain – the two organs that must ensure optimal blood flow. It may be that this will be the treatment considered early on for people suffering from haemorrhage-induced traumatic cardiac arrest.

Suspended animation and intentional cooling of the body and its organs while damaged tissues, vessels, and organs are repaired over a more prolonged period may be considered.

Will we still be using large incisions to enter cavities when small nanobots that are targeted to find the injury, repair it, and then degrade will do the work for us? Will these nanobots deliver themselves to the patient's side or will they be delivered by drone, before the patient is evacuated in an autonomous vehicle capable of care in flight?

A bespoke cocktail of blood, blood component therapy, and other products may be tailored to the future victim of penetrating trauma, depending on their genetic makeup and measurement of biomarkers at the time of injury, or indeed prior to injury and then kept in storage for the day when they fall victim to injury.

Summary: Top Tips

General Principles That Emerge from the Science

The principles of management for the majority of penetrating trauma patients remain that less (intervention) is more. The patient should be moved along from the point of wounding to intervention as quickly as possible, with an increasing number of interventions, if required, being implemented as they move along this journey. Damage control principles of resuscitation and surgery should be implemented. Wounds should be optimally treated while the physiological state is supported, to ensure that the patient is fit for the next stage of intervention.

Short-, Medium-, and Long-Term Impacts

We need to continue to do what we do, but do it better. In the short term we must ensure that the basics are done well and practised often. Only when those patients are treated optimally can we then move to those with the severest injuries. We must learn to walk before we can run, and before we can fly!

Implications for Intervention

The increasing number of procedures available to clinicians may lead to greater intervention at an earlier and earlier stage. We may need to forego some interventions in favour of others. For instance, for haemorrhagic truncal bleeding it may be appropriate to simply place a large-bore cannula in the vein of the antecubital fossa, while placing a 4Fr sheath in the common femoral artery and monitoring invasive blood pressure while resuscitating, and carrying this out while en route to hospital or in the lift to the operating theatre. If the patient fails to respond to filling, then upsize the sheath and place a REBOA balloon at the appropriate level in the aorta and restore afterload and central perfusion while trying to promote clot formation in the injured zone.

Practical Aspects of Implementing the Principles

Although it is important that we move forward with advances in care, it must be remembered that, for some injuries, expedited transfer to a facility and team that are capable of providing operative intervention and direct control of bleeding and contamination is important. We should 'scoop and play' from scene to operating theatre, and consider moving the operating theatre closer to the patient rather than having it hidden away in a remote location in the hospital. Future advances that will help to keep the sickest trauma patients alive will require resources, experience, training, technological input, innovation, and blue sky thinking. Care has to be provided within an all-encompassing trauma system that keeps the patient at the centre of everything it does.

References

1. World Health Organization (WHO). *Injuries and Violence: The Facts.* WHO, 2014.

2. Penn-Barwell J. Blast injuries. In *Trauma Care Manual* 3rd ed. (eds I Greaves, K Porter, J Garner): 386–95. CRC Press, 2022.

3. Penn-Barwell J. Firearms, ballistics and gunshot wounds. In *Trauma Care Manual* 3rd ed. (eds I Greaves, K Porter, J Garner): 372–85. CRC Press, 2022.

4. Glen J, Constanti M, Brohi K and Guideline Development Group. Assessment and initial management of major trauma: summary of NICE guidance. *BMJ* 2016; 22: 353.

5. Barker T. Vascular trauma. In *Trauma Care Manual* 3rd ed. (eds I Greaves, K Porter, J Garner): 259–76. CRC Press, 2022.

6. Stop The Bleed (www.stopthebleed.org).

7. citizenAID (www.citizenAID.org).

8. Lee C, Revell M, Porter K, Steyn R. The pre-hospital management of chest injuries: a consensus statement. Faculty of Pre-Hospital Care, Royal College of Surgeons of Edinburgh. *Emerg Med J* 2007: 24: 220–24.

9. Lockey DJ, Brohi K. Pre-hospital thoracotomy and the evolution of

pre-hospital critical care for victims of trauma. *Injury* 2017; 48: 1863–4.

10. Hodgetts TJ, Mahoney PF, Russell MQ, Byers M. ABC to <C> ABC. Redefining the military trauma paradigm. *Emerg Med J* 2006; 23: 745–6.

11. Moran C, Lecky F, Bouamra O, Lawrence T, Edwards A, Woodford M, et al. Changing the system – major trauma patients and their outcomes in the NHS (England) 2008–17. *EClinicalMedicine* 2018; 1: 13–21.

12. Sharpe D. Patient assessment. In *Trauma Care Manual* 3rd ed. (eds I Greaves, K Porter, J Garner): 63–77. CRC Press. 2022.

13. Khan MA. Damage control surgery. In *Trauma Care Manual* 3rd ed. (eds I Greaves, K Porter, J Garner): 169–78. CRC Press, 2022.

14. Hodgetts TJ, Mahoney PF, Kirkman E. Damage control resuscitation. *J R Army Med Corps* 2007; 153: 299–300.

15. Handford C, Parker P. The potential use of the abdominal aortic junctional tourniquet® in a military population: a review of requirement, effectiveness, and usability. *J Spec Oper Med* 2019; 19: 74–9.

16. Lendrum R, Perkins Z, Chana M, Marsden M, Davenport R, Grier G, et al. Pre-hospital resuscitative endovascular balloon occlusion of the aorta (REBOA) for exsanguinating pelvic haemorrhage. *Resuscitation* 2019; 135: 6–13.

17. Coccolini F, Montori G, Catena F, Kluger Y, Biffi W, Moore EE, et al. Splenic trauma: WSES classification and guidelines for adult and paediatric patients. *World J Emerg Surg* 2017; 12: 40.

18. Williams O. Trauma systems, centres and teams. In *Trauma Care Manual* 3rd ed. (eds I Greaves, K Porter, J Garner): 47–62. CRC Press, 2022.

Chapter 16

Lessons from History and the Epidemiology of Severe Epidemics and Pandemics

Plague, Cholera, Influenza, Viral Haemorrhagic Fevers, and Coronaviruses

Tim Healing

Introduction

Severe epidemics and pandemics have probably affected human populations since humankind ceased being wholly nomadic, started to farm, developed technologies, gathered in communities, and began to trade. Domestication of animals brought humans into close contact with a wide range of novel pathogens. Concentrations of people and dwellings together with food stores and poor hygiene allowed for the ready transfer of infections and the evolution of vector species. Larger human communities made it possible for epidemics to occur, and also allowed the maintenance of infections in endemic form. Separation between communities increased the likelihood of variations in organisms due to local mutations, and trade, especially by water, allowed the transfer of infections (or the vectors of infections) between communities.

Regardless of the types of organisms that cause epidemics and pandemics, certain themes are common to all with regard to the outcomes of the outbreaks and the measures used in attempts to control these events. Most of the impacts seen today as a result of the COVID-19 pandemic, and the measures being used to try to control the outbreak, were described centuries ago. Changes in society, technology, and healthcare have altered or added details or altered the importance and the balance of the various factors, and the nature of the causative organisms and the illnesses caused can have similar effects. The themes that will be examined in this chapter include impacts on health, society, the economy, and politics and legal matters. The measures necessary to control pandemics and epidemics will be discussed.

Table 16.1 lists the major pandemics that have occurred in recorded history. It does not list all pandemics, but does include those that caused high levels of morbidity and mortality or were of particular historical significance.

Pandemic Organisms

A pandemic is defined as 'an epidemic occurring worldwide, or over a very wide area, crossing international boundaries and usually affecting a large number of people' [1]. Pandemics occur due to the emergence of a new disease capable of infecting humans, or due to the re-emergence of a disease not seen in human populations for many years. In order for the organism to precipitate a pandemic it must be readily transmissible and sustainable in the human population, it must have mechanisms to allow it to spread in the human population, the populations affected must be wholly susceptible to the organism, and the organism must not be too rapidly lethal.

Most of the organisms that have caused the pandemics listed in Table 16.1 are zoonoses – infections of animals that are transmissible to humans. Cholera is primarily passed from human to human, but there is some evidence of a zoonotic origin. Most zoonotic organisms are not potential causes of pandemics, although they may be able to cause serious local epidemics, as in most instances the animal hosts or the vectors of the organism are limited in their geographical distribution. However, such barriers can be overcome, often due to human activities, and there have been many occasions when the activities of humans have served to spread hosts and vectors widely. Plague, which probably originated in Asia [2], spread throughout the known world due to traders carrying with them one of its rodent hosts, the black rat (*Rattus rattus*), and its vector, the rat flea (*Xenopsylla cheopis*). In more recent times, dengue fever and the Zika virus have spread widely as their vectors, mosquito species of the genus *Aedes*, have been spread by human activity [3].

Table 16.1 Some important pandemics

Name	Date	Location	Estimated mortality
Unknown aetiology			
Antonine Plague (Plague of Galen)	165–180 CE	Asia Minor, Egypt, Greece, Italy	5–10 million
Plague of Cyprian	*c.* 249–262 CE	North Africa, Europe	Unknown (> 1 million?)
Plague (*Yersinia pestis*)			
First pandemic (Plague of Justinian)	541–544 CE	West Africa, Middle East	25 million
Second pandemic (Black Death, 1346–1353)	1346 – early 1800s	Worldwide	75–200 million
Third pandemic	1894–1959	Worldwide	> 12 million
Cholera (*Vibrio cholerae*)			
First pandemic	1817–1824	India, Asia, and south-eastern Europe	Unknown (> 1,000,000?)
Second pandemic	1826–1837	North Africa, Europe, USA, and Canada	Unknown (*c.* 250,000?)
Third pandemic	1846–1860	North Africa, Russia, UK, North and South America, and Asia	> 1.5 million
Fourth pandemic	1863–1875	India, Mediterranean region, Europe, and USA	*c.* 600,000
Fifth pandemic	1881–1896	India, Europe, Asia, and South America	> 300,000
Sixth pandemic	1899-1923	Egypt, Arabian Peninsula, Persia, India, Philippines, and eastern Europe	> 800,000
Seventh pandemic	1961–1975	Indonesia, India, Pakistan, southern Europe, Russia, and Japan	*c.* 100,000
Influenza			
Spanish flu (H1N1)	1918–1920	Worldwide	20–100 million
Asian flu (H2N2)	1957–1958	Worldwide	2 million
Hong Kong flu (H3N2)	1968–1969	Worldwide	1 million
Russian flu (H1N1)	1977–1979	Worldwide	700,000
Swine flu (H1N1)	2009–2010	Worldwide	284,500
Coronavirus			
SARS	2003	Asia, Canada	774
MERS-CoV	2012 –	Middle East, Africa, Asia, Europe, and North and South America	*c.* 900
COVID-19	2019 –	Worldwide	5,666,064 (as at 2 February 2022)
Other			
HIV/AIDS	1980s onwards	Worldwide	> 36 million

Bacteria

Bacteria were major causes of pandemics in the past, and remain potential and actual causes of epidemics. Two bacteria have caused major pandemics in the past, namely plague (*Yersinia pestis*) and cholera (*Vibrio cholerae*). Several bacterial species that were originally thought to be the cause of pandemics are now known to cause secondary infections which may increase the severity of the pandemic. For example, *Haemophilus influenzae* (Pfeiffer's bacillus) had been thought at the time to be the causative organism of the Spanish influenza of 1918–1920. In fact it was not, although it was probably a major cause of the high mortality during that pandemic [4,5].

Viruses

Viruses are important causes of pandemics and epidemics, and have been the leading causes of these throughout the twentieth century and into the twenty-first century.

All three groups of viruses listed in Table 16.1 are RNA viruses that are capable of frequent mutation [6]. This ability makes them prime candidates for causing epidemics and pandemics. An example is the Ebola virus. This usually caused quite small and localised outbreaks in tropical Africa. Recently, however, there have been much larger outbreaks in West Africa and in the Democratic Republic of the Congo (DRC) (see Chapters 17 and 18). Studies of the genetics of the viruses involved have shown that in these outbreaks the virus mutated to forms with increased transmissibility between humans [7,8]. The transmission of the Ebola virus requires close contact between people and contact with infected bodily fluids, so changes in behaviour to reduce such contacts proved to be an effective way of controlling the disease (see Chapters 17 and 18).

Influenza viruses have caused many pandemics, particularly during the last century. Transmitted by the respiratory route and very infectious, influenza viruses mutate frequently. These changes are usually small (antigenic drift), but occasionally larger genetic changes occur (antigenic shift), resulting in novel variants of the virus that can cause pandemics. One of the most damaging pandemics in history was the so-called Spanish Flu of 1918–1920, which is discussed in more detail later in this chapter.

The HIV/AIDS pandemic, which is still ongoing, is also caused by an RNA virus, and has been one of the most serious pandemics, with a very large number of fatalities.

The most recent additions to the collection of pandemic RNA viruses are the coronaviruses. SARS, MERS-CoV, and now SARS-CoV-2 are all quite recent arrivals on the scene. SARS was rapidly controlled by international collaboration and active control measures [9,10], and MERS-CoV has caused relatively few cases, although these are geographically widespread and the disease has a high lethality [11]. SARS-CoV-2 has caused a pandemic which, at the time of publication of this book, is still uncontrolled over much of the world, its ability to mutate allowing it to produce new and more transmissible variants that have made control very difficult. Like the influenzas, these coronaviruses are spread by the respiratory route.

Pandemics as Agents of Social and Historical Change

Pandemics have always exerted major effects on the societies affected, although, in recent times, medical, technological, social, and political advances have made it possible to reduce their impact. Several serious pandemics affected the Roman Empire and may have contributed to its decline. The Antonine Plague (165–180 CE) is estimated to have killed up to one-third of the affected population in some areas (mainly around the Mediterranean), and devastated the Roman army. The Plague of Cyprian (249–262 CE) weakened the army and damaged food production ([12], cited in [13,14]). The Plague of Justinian (541–549 CE, the beginning of the first plague pandemic) may have killed more than 15 million people and exerted a major effect on the histories of Europe and Christendom, although this is disputed by some authors [12,15]. It has been suggested that it weakened the Byzantine Empire at a critical point, preventing the reunification of the core of the Western Roman Empire with the Eastern Roman Empire [16].

The Black Death

The second plague pandemic, the first part of which was known at the time as the 'Great Pestilence' or the 'Great Mortality', but is now called the 'Black Death', probably originated in China in 1331 [2]. It came to the Crimea with an invading Tartar army that besieged a Genoese trading town on the Black Sea in

1347. Genoese traders fleeing the siege carried the disease to Sicily, where the European part of the pandemic began [17]. It reached Spain, France, and Germany during 1348, and England at the end of that year, Norway in 1349, and Eastern Europe in 1350 [18]. Factors such as war, famine, and bad weather contributed to the severity of the pandemic.

The pandemic was probably the worst ever to hit humankind, and the initial and most serious outbreak (1346–1353) was followed by severe outbreaks throughout the remainder of the fourteenth century, with very heavy loss of life. It returned with varying levels of severity until the early nineteenth century. It is estimated that, as a result of the initial outbreak (the 'Black Death'), the population of Europe decreased by about 25% between 1347 and 1350, and that a further 20% was lost in a second major epidemic in 1361 (the *Pestis Secunda*) [16]. The actual numbers who died in the first part of the pandemic may in fact have been lower than the numbers who were lost in the Spanish flu pandemic (discussed later), but the population of the world was smaller in the fourteenth century, so the proportional loss was probably much greater [19]. By 1430, Europe's population was smaller than in 1290, and would not return to pre-pandemic levels until the sixteenth century [17].

The Black Death led to major social change. It contributed to a series of religious, social, and economic upheavals, which had major effects on the course of the history of the world, with Britain being no exception. The seigneurial system began to break down, shortages of labour resulted in the expansion of a wage-based economy that increasingly replaced the feudal labour system, populations became more mobile, and land became relatively plentiful. Divisions between the upper and lower classes broke down and a middle class began to emerge [19–21].

The wages of many labourers rose over the 25 years following the outbreak, but there was also serious inflation, so that real wages fell [22]. Governments attempted to control wages. In England, for example, two pieces of legislation – the Ordinance of Labourers 1349, and the Statute of Labourers 1351 – were designed to restrict wage increases and relocation of workers. Both were extremely unpopular and are thought to have contributed to the Peasants' Revolt of 1381 [23].

The church had been a dominating force before the pandemic, and in the early stages of the pandemic many turned to religion for comfort and support. However, many priests died and were replaced with less suitable or well-trained people, and the church began to fall into disrepute. Its influence was damaged, people's beliefs were undermined, and they became disillusioned. The power and influence of the church began to decline, and the outbreak is suggested to have contributed to the Reformation. Lack of confidence in the church led to the emergence of bizarre alternatives to the established order (for example, the Flagellants, a religious movement that sought redemption through mortification of the flesh). Such sects were frequently intolerant and encouraged attacks on minorities such as Jews, lepers, and foreigners [19].

The plague had a major effect on art and literature and is credited by some with being an important factor in the Italian Renaissance [24]. It was chronicled by famous writers, philosophers, and rulers such as Boccaccio and Petrarch [25]. Several themes persisted, especially those dealing with the frailty of life and the triumph of death.

Cholera

Cholera was the major cause of pandemics during much of the nineteenth century [26], with the disease being spread through improved transportation systems [27]. It is a bacterial infection caused by a Gram-negative bacterium, *Vibrio cholerae*, which is found in brackish or salt-water environments where it lives attached to planktonic crustacea and some shellfish [28]. Where it is endemic, most infections are mild, but in populations not previously exposed to it (or under immunological stress due to famine or war) the organism can cause a severe and life-threatening infection, with profuse watery diarrhoea leading to severe dehydration and death within hours or days. The disease can be treated by rehydrating the patient and giving antibiotics; this reduces mortality from as high as 60% to below 1%. It is estimated that there are still up to four million cases of cholera a year worldwide, with possibly over 140,000 deaths [29].

Five cholera pandemics affected Europe during the nineteenth century, and a sixth began at the end of that century and ended in the 1920s. The seventh pandemic began in 1961. Although some considered that it ended in 1975, the persistence of the strain involved has led the World Health Organization (WHO) to consider the pandemic to be ongoing. Each pandemic caused serious morbidity and mortality but did lead to major improvements in hygiene and public health. During the third pandemic, in the middle of the nineteenth century, concerns and fears about the disease, together with the impact of the 'Great Stink' caused by the heavily polluted River Thames, led to the movement to clean up London and its river [30]. Major engineering works were undertaken under the direction of Sir Joseph Bazalgette to provide London with a proper sewage system. Social reforms were put in place, led by pioneers such as Sir Edwin Chadwick, whose self-financed 'Report on the Sanitary Condition of the Labouring Population of Great Britain' of 1842 was a key document in the recognition of the need for reform [31]. Another important outcome of the third pandemic was the beginning of the science of epidemiology. Dr John Snow, an anaesthetist practising in London, was interested in cholera and undertook a detailed investigation of an outbreak in Soho in 1854. He used mapping to identify the source of the outbreak, which was a particular well with a pump. His subsequent investigations of outbreaks confirmed the link between cholera and contaminated water [32].

The discovery by Filippo Pacini in 1854 and independently by Robert Koch in 1884 that cholera was caused by a microorganism and not by 'miasmas', and the understanding of the nature and epidemiology of that organism, led to the realisation that cholera could be prevented by disinfection of potable water [33,34]. This, combined with the recognition that what killed cholera patients was dehydration, led to the current recommendations for the prevention and treatment of the disease. These are effective but can easily break down. For example, there have been several outbreaks of cholera in the Yemen in recent years because of the civil war in that country [35].

Influenza

Influenza, a highly infectious respiratory disease, has probably been an important cause of morbidity and mortality for millennia, but the first pandemic of the disease is thought to have occurred in 1510 [36].

The Spanish Flu

An influenza pandemic began in 1918, during the last year of the First World War, caused by an H1N1 influenza A virus. It was one of the deadliest pandemics ever recorded, and is estimated to have infected about one-third of the population of the world (c. 500 million people) and to have led to between 20 million and 100 million deaths, although it has recently been suggested that the latter figure is probably an overestimate [37]. The origin of the outbreak is unknown, but the first documented cases occurred in Kansas in the USA in March 1918 [5]. By April it had spread to the other main combatants in the war (Britain, France, and Germany). Wartime censorship largely prevented reports of the disease in the combatant nations, and the first widely distributed reports came from neutral Spain, which led to the linking of the pandemic to that nation [5].

The ability of the medical profession to combat the pandemic was very limited. The initial assumption that it was caused by Pfeiffer's bacillus (*Haemophilus influenzae*) led to extensive efforts to produce an antiserum. However, this organism was actually a cause of secondary infections, and attempts to combat it were of little value. Some doctors suspected that the cause was a 'filter-passing organism' (a virus), but the virus that causes flu remained unknown throughout the Spanish Flu pandemic and was only identified in 1931. Some good results were obtained by the transfusion of serum from recovered patients, but the great majority of cases could only be treated symptomatically [5].

Attempts to control the spread of the disease were largely limited to social distancing measures, including isolation and quarantine, banning of mass gatherings (e.g., closure of sports grounds, schools, universities, theatres, and places of worship), limiting use of public transport, and personal protective measures such as wearing masks. Disinfectants were used extensively to try to limit spread in public places. Strict maritime quarantine procedures were put in place by many nations [5].

Every aspect of human activity was affected by the pandemic, although it can be difficult to disentangle its effects from those caused by the war itself [5]. The pandemic may have helped the Allied forces to bring the war to an earlier conclusion because it hit the Central powers earlier than the Allies, and morbidity and mortality were higher (partly due to reduced health in the Central powers nations, due to food shortages caused by the Allied blockade). The economic impact was varied, and in most instances the negative impact was quite short (but hit hardest where control measures were put in place late or not at all) [5].

Influenza can affect all age groups, but is usually only highly dangerous to the very young and the elderly. However, the Spanish Flu proved unusually lethal to young adults, and the losses among this age group were particularly severe. The men in this age group in the nations at war had already been hit hard by losses in battle, and many were in poor health. The loss of even more people in this group (just when they had survived the conflict) had a profound psychological impact on the nations that were affected [5].

It is difficult to determine the long-term impact of the pandemic [5]. The interwar years were a period of great change, and it is difficult to disentangle the impacts of the war and of the pandemic on this process. The post-war years saw much change in the fields of health and medical science. In specialties such as surgery, infection control, and infectious disease the war had accelerated progress towards understanding the control of problems and of the nature, prevention, and treatment of infection. There was also an upsurge in alternative medicine and healthcare.

There were some less well-defined impacts that did not become obvious until many years later. One group, some of whose members were adversely affected, consisted of people who had been *in utero* during the pandemic. Douglas Almond, writing in 2006, noted that 'Cohorts in utero during the pandemic displayed reduced educational attainment, increased rates of physical disability, lower income, lower socioeconomic status, and higher transfer payments received compared with other birth cohorts' [38].

Controlling Epidemics and Pandemics

It was realised centuries ago that it was possible to prevent or at least limit the spread of communicable disease by reducing or eliminating the likelihood of transmission from one person to another. There are several ways in which this has been attempted over the years:

1. preventing contact between people:

   a. isolating the sick to prevent contact with the healthy

   b. quarantining those who have been exposed to a disease, but whose infection status is unknown, to prevent contact with the healthy

   c. restricting population movements and social activities

2. maintaining physical separation between people who do meet

3. using mechanical protection (e.g., masks, hand hygiene, ventilation) to reduce the risk of transmission of an infection.

With the advent of modern medicine, additional weapons for fighting pandemics are now available.

1. Vaccination aims to create an immunological barrier to the spread of a disease, and to reduce the impact of the infection on individuals.

2. The development of successful treatments for a disease can reduce morbidity and mortality due to the disease and thereby reduce its impact to acceptable levels. This can complement or take the place of the other measures mentioned.

All of these techniques require wholehearted support from and compliance of the majority of the members of the affected societies if they are to work.

Non-Pharmaceutical Measures
Preventing Contact Between People
Social Distancing

The non-pharmaceutical disease control measures that have been used during the COVID-19 pandemic to prevent (or at least reduce) contact between individuals are based on centuries of accumulated knowledge and experience of many pandemics and disease outbreaks, and are now collectively known as social distancing. They involve both reducing how often people come into close contact with each other, and maintaining a physical distance between people when they do so. They include closing workplaces, schools, and higher education colleges, cancellation of mass gatherings, closure of places of worship and entertainment, the isolation of the sick, the quarantining of contacts, and restricting the movement of the population. The WHO has suggested that 'physical distancing' is a preferable term to 'social distancing', because it is physical separation that prevents transmission; technology allows people to remain socially connected.

Individual people who have the disease but are not ill enough to require hospitalisation need to isolate themselves for the duration of the infection, and those who have been exposed to infected people but are not showing symptoms of the infection need to quarantine themselves until they are past the known incubation period of the disease. People who are particularly at risk of serious disease or death due to underlying conditions need to quarantine themselves as well (this is known as self-shielding).

Isolation and Quarantine

Isolation and quarantine are not simple concepts. Isolation involves separation of people suffering from a communicable disease from those who are healthy, whereas quarantine involves restriction of the movement of healthy people who may have been exposed to a disease, to prevent the spread of the disease to the healthy. Both are disease control and preventive measures that are a legacy of the many epidemics and pandemics that have occurred over the centuries. However, they go much further than the medical and clinical, epidemiological, and public health aspects of preventing disease transmission, as they imply forced restriction of the movements of the people or populations involved. Taken together with the other social distancing measures described in this chapter, these have constitutional, political, economic, social, behavioural, psychological, ethical, and moral implications [10].

The need to separate the sick from the well to prevent the spread of disease has been recognised for centuries. In the Bible (Leviticus 13:45–46) it states that 'Anyone with such a defiling disease must wear torn clothes, let their hair be unkempt, cover the lower part of their face and cry out, Unclean! Unclean! As long as they have the disease, they remain unclean. They must live alone; they must live outside the camp'. In the Ṣaḥīḥ al-Bukhārī (one of the Kutub al-Sittah, six major Hadith collections of Sunni Islam, compiled by the Persian scholar Muhammad al-Bukhari) it states: 'If you hear of an outbreak of plague in a land, do not enter it; but if the plague breaks out in a place while you are in it, do not leave that place'. In 549 CE the Byzantine Emperor Justinian enacted a law to hinder and isolate people from plague-infected regions after a devastating outbreak of what was probably bubonic plague [39], and in the seventh century CE China had a policy of detaining plague-stricken people arriving in its ports.

Quarantine as a control measure began to be developed and codified during the second plague pandemic (the Black Death). In 1348, to prevent the spread of the disease, the Venetian authorities closed the city's waters to suspect vessels, and subjected travellers and ships to 40 days of isolation. (The word quarantine is derived from a Venetian dialect form of the Italian *quaranta giorni*, meaning 40 days.) For more than five centuries this was accepted across Europe as the only real defence against the spread of plague, and a major industry developed to manage and enforce quarantine, particularly in the Mediterranean, including a complex of health passports, ships' bills of health, quarantine guards, and lazarettos [40].

By the end of the nineteenth century a better understanding of infectious disease, combined with factors such as much more rapid travel, improved communications, and more perishable cargoes requiring rapid transport to their destination led to the replacement of maritime quarantine by port health inspection. This remains in operation for goods and passengers carried by sea (Free Pratique), but became impractical for goods and people travelling by air. In 2005, the current version of the International Health Regulations (IHR) was published with the aim of 'preventing, protecting against, controlling and providing a public health response to the international spread of disease in ways that are commensurate with and restricted to public health risks and avoid unnecessary interference with international traffic and trade' [41]. The IHR is an international instrument that is legally binding on 194 of the 195 countries in the world, including all of the WHO Member States (see Chapter 17) .

In modern times, social distancing measures have been successfully implemented in several epidemics. A feature of these measures is that they need to be applied as soon as possible and maintained until the risk has decreased to manageable proportions. Martin Bootsma and Neil Ferguson examined the effect of public health measures on the 1918–1920 influenza pandemic (the Spanish flu) in cities in the USA, and noted that 'the timing of public health interventions had a profound influence on the pattern of the autumn wave of the 1918 pandemic in different cities. Cities that introduced measures early in their epidemics achieved moderate but significant reductions in overall mortality' [42].

The drawbacks of physical and social distancing for people can include loneliness, loss of jobs, reduced productivity, and the loss of other benefits associated with human interaction, although some of these can now be partly mitigated by technology. In terms of societies, the economic impacts can be very large, and changes in some types of behaviour (e.g., a shift to online shopping) can have long-term economic impacts.

Other Control Measures (Mechanical Protection)

Spacing measures can be combined with other activities, such as the use of masks, hand washing/sanitisation, and ventilation of enclosed areas, to interrupt chains of infection and keep the numbers of cases as low as possible, thus reducing the pressures on the healthcare services and on society, and reducing the numbers of deaths. The lockdowns imposed in the early stages of the COVID-19 pandemic were based on these concepts. The title of the 'Hands, Face, Space, Fresh Air' campaign established by Public Health England summarises the essential activities required.

The successful application of these measures relies on compliance by the affected population. If they are to work, they need to be accompanied by educational activities to persuade people of the social value of observing such behaviours, and if persuasion fails, measures to enforce observance have to be considered. Unfortunately, measures designed to control disease, which on the face of it are wholly sensible, can all too easily become the tools of unscrupulous politicians and others, and used to manipulate public opinion. A simple and effective measure such as requiring the wearing of masks, which both limit transmission of respiratory organisms from infected people and reduce the risk of infection of uninfected people, has sometimes been characterised as an attack on individual freedom. This has been seen repeatedly during the COVID-19 pandemic, but is not new. During the 1918–1920 influenza pandemic an anti-mask league was set up in San Francisco to protest an ordinance that required people in the city to wear masks [43,44].

Treating Cases

Developing effective treatments for a disease can dramatically reduce the impact of the disease on the individual and on society. For example, using corticosteroids such as dexamethasone markedly reduced mortality due to infection with the SARS-CoV-2 virus. This, combined with other drugs that reduce morbidity and mortality (e.g., the antiviral drug Paxlovid), has gone a long way towards reducing the dangers of the infection for the susceptible, and hence the fear of the infection itself.

Vaccination

The non-pharmaceutical measures described earlier in the chapter can be useful in two ways. First, by reducing morbidity, they reduce demands on healthcare services and also reduce pressures on other activities that maintain society (e.g., transport, security, infrastructure, food distribution). Second, they can protect those people who are most vulnerable to the disease due to age or pre-existing medical conditions. However, these are essentially stop-gap measures designed to reduce rates of transmission of infection. Ultimately, a pandemic or outbreak will not end until a sufficient proportion of the population has a reasonable level of immunity to the disease. In the ideal situation, at this point the R_t value (the effective reproduction number – that is, the average number of new infections caused by a single infected individual at time t in the partially susceptible population) cannot rise above a value of 1, and the uncontrolled spread of the disease ceases. The term used to describe population immunity is herd immunity, although this term has a variety of meanings [45,46]. Herd immunity can be developed in two ways – by a sufficient proportion of the population catching the disease and developing immunity, or by developing an effective vaccine and vaccination programme. In both cases, distancing measures can be used to try to keep the impact of the disease at a level that ensures that society will not be overwhelmed before herd immunity develops. In the case of a disease such as COVID-19, which has a high mortality among certain risk groups, developing herd immunity by natural infection carries with it the risk of an unacceptably high mortality rate. In such a situation, and in the absence of effective treatments, vaccination is the only method by which herd immunity can be achieved without unacceptable losses, and the non-pharmaceutical measures described earlier are a vital part of the control programme.

Not all vaccines provide complete immunity to infection. For example, the vaccines against influenza and those initially developed against COVID-19 do provide a good level of protection against the development of serious illness, and greatly reduce the risk of dying of the disease. However, they do not necessarily protect against catching the disease. This also appears to be true with regard to the resistance to re-infection that is conferred by naturally acquired infections (especially with COVID-19). Some vaccinated people, and some who have previously been infected, may develop asymptomatic infections, which also occur in people with a first infection, particularly younger people, with the attendant transmission risks. This is why there is a need to continue with non-pharmaceutical protective measures.

Much of our understanding of the workings of vaccines and the altered dynamics of infections in the presence of effective vaccines comes from vaccination programmes in wealthy countries with high vaccine coverage and regular boosters. Sadly, however, the distribution and availability of vaccines against COVID-19 have been far from equitable, with many low- and low-middle income countries receiving far too few doses to cover their populations effectively. This failure to ensure equitable distribution and availability of vaccines has left a large proportion of the world's population at risk of the disease, and has not reduced the risk of the emergence of new variants of the disease. Vaccine inequity has also increased resentment directed at wealthy nations that have cornered the market in the available vaccines and failed to support worldwide distribution.

Reluctance to accept vaccination can greatly hinder control of a pandemic. Some countries have reacted to such behaviour during the COVID-19 outbreak by introducing coercive measures. Vaccination programmes therefore need to be accompanied by active information campaigns to ensure that populations have access to the facts. The spread of false propaganda by those who are against vaccination (for whatever reason) needs to be countered firmly.

In the early phases of the COVID-19 pandemic the majority of serious infections and deaths occurred in the elderly and in some younger people with underlying conditions that increased the severity of the infection. Now the combination of effective vaccines and successful treatments has meant that, even among the elderly and other higher-risk individuals, the risk of serious disease and death is much lower, and most infections in younger people seem to be milder. This, in combination with the ending of lockdowns and other social restrictions, has led many to assume that the problem is at an end, and that life can return to what is seen as normality. At the time of publication of this book, people seem to see no further need to adopt measures such as masking, spacing, and ventilation.

A growing problem associated with COVID-19 is that although most people recover fully from the acute infection, some patients continue to experience a range of effects for months. This condition is called post-COVID syndrome (or Long COVID), and is likely to present a major challenge to physical and mental healthcare in the coming years (see Chapter 17).

Conclusion

History has shown that controlling a pandemic requires a very high level of worldwide national and international collaboration in all relevant fields, active and effective epidemiological and public health systems, high-grade medical care and facilities, collaborative research, an understanding of the organism, and development of vaccines/treatments. It requires effective support by wealthy nations of lower-income countries where health services are poor and funds are scarce. It demands social responsibility by national populations, prevention of social breakdown, and the acceptance of actions to reduce transmission, including lockdown, isolation, quarantine, and non-pharmaceutical control measures. An unimpeded flow of accurate information is required both within and between nations to inform the public and to neutralise rumours, fake news, and conspiracy theories. Skilful politicians are needed to maintain the difficult balance between control measures and economic and social needs, and for populations to accept the measures needed to control disease transmission in the period before vaccines can exert their full effect.

The whole range of appropriate non-pharmaceutical health and public health interventions needs to be deployed during a pandemic. Epidemiological investigation and surveillance, the detection, isolation, and treatment of cases, and quarantine of contacts demand an active and effective test and trace system. Encouragement of home nursing and minimising use of medical facilities by those who can be cared for at home both contribute to preventing health services from being overwhelmed. Reducing demands on medical and healthcare services due to the pandemic itself is not only vital for control of the pandemic, but is also essential to prevent increases in morbidity and mortality due to other medical conditions which go untreated due to the demands of the outbreak. For example, during the Ebola outbreak in West Africa in 2013–2016 it is estimated that the increased mortality due to untreated malaria, tuberculosis, and HIV/AIDS was similar to the mortality due to the outbreak itself [47]. In the UK, the number of people awaiting treatment for conditions other than COVID-19 increased from the low thousands to several million during the first years of the pandemic [48,49].

Given the frequency with which people are exposed to novel infections and the readiness with which some organisms can mutate, the need for preparedness to combat pandemics on a worldwide basis is paramount. Nations in low- or middle-income countries or with poor healthcare need to be supported by wealthier nations, if only as a matter of self-interest. Failure to control a disease, in whatever type of country is involved, can allow the emergence of mutated varieties of the pathogen which may be less susceptible to vaccines or treatments and/or more readily transmitted than earlier strains (this has been seen on a number of occasions during the COVID-19 outbreak). To quote the UN Secretary General António Guterres, speaking at the launch of a report on the socioeconomics of COVID-19 on 31 March 2020, 'Let us remember that we are only as strong as the weakest health system in our interconnected world'.

References

1. Porta M, ed. *A Dictionary of Epidemiology* 6th ed. Oxford University Press, 2016.

2. Morelli G, Song Y, Mazzoni CJ, Eppinger M, Roumagnac P, Wagner D et al. *Yersinia pestis* genome sequencing identifies patterns of global phylogenetic diversity. *Nat Genet* 2010; 42: 1140–43.

3. Tatem AJ, Rogers DJ, Hay SI. Global transport networks and infectious disease spread. *Adv Parasitol* 2006; 62: 293–343.

4. Morens DM, Taubenberger JK, Fauci AS. Predominant role of bacterial pneumonia as a cause of death in pandemic influenza: implications for pandemic influenza preparedness. *J Infect Dis* 2008; 198: 962–70.

5. Spinney L. *Pale Rider: The Spanish Flu of 1918 and How It Changed the World*. Jonathan Cape, 2017.

6. Duffy S. Why are RNA virus mutation rates so damn high? *PLoS Biol* 2018; 16: e3000003.

7. Diehl WE, Lin AE, Grubaugh ND, Carvalho LM, Kim K, Kyawe PP, et al. Ebola virus glycoprotein with increased infectivity dominated the 2013–2014 epidemic. *Cell* 2016; 167: 1088-98.

8. Urbanowicz RA, McClure CP, Sakuntabhai A, Sall AA, Kobinger G, Muller MA, et al. Human adaptation of Ebola virus during the West African outbreak. *Cell* 2016; 167: 1079-87.

9. World Health Organization. *SARS: How a Global Epidemic Was Stopped*. WHO Western Pacific Region, 2006.

10. Tognotti E. Lessons from the history of quarantine, from plague to influenza A. *Emerg Infect Dis* 2013; 19: 254–9.

11. World Health Organization (WHO). *Middle East Respiratory Syndrome Coronavirus (MERS-CoV): Key Facts*. WHO, 2019.

12. Harper K. *The Fate of Rome: Climate, Disease, and the End of an Empire*. Princeton University Press, 2017.

13. Huremović D. Brief history of pandemics (pandemics throughout history). *Psychiatry Pandemics* 2019; 16: 7–35.

14. Haldon J, Elton H, Huebner SR, Izdebski A, Mordechai L, Newfield TP. Plagues, climate change, and the end of an empire. A response to Kyle Harper's *The Fate of Rome* (2): Plagues and a crisis of empire. *History Compass* 2018; 16: e12506.

15. Mordechai L, Eisenberg M, Newfield TP, Izdebski A, Kay JE, Poinar H. The Justinianic Plague: an inconsequential pandemic? *Proc Natl Acad Sci USA* 2019; 116: 25546–54.

16. Rosen W. *Justinian's Flea: Plague, Empire and the Birth of Europe*. Jonathan Cape, 2007.

17. Frith J. The history of plague – Part 1. The three great pandemics. *J Mil Veterans Health* 2012; 20: 11–16.

18. Twigg G. *The Black Death: A Biological Reappraisal*. Batsford Academic and Educational, 1984.

19. Cantor NF. *In the Wake of the Plague: The Black Death and the World It Made*. The Free Press, 2001.

20. Zeigler P. *The Black Death*. The History Press, 1969.

21. Dyer C. *Everyday Life in Medieval England*. Hambledon and London, 2000.

22. Munro J. *Before and After the Black Death: Money, Prices, and Wages in Fourteenth-Century England*. Working Paper No. 24. Department of Economics and Institute for Policy Analysis, University of Toronto, 2004 (www.economics.utoronto.ca/public/workingPapers/UT-ECIPA-MUNRO-04-04.pdf).

23. Dyer C. *Making a Living in the Middle Ages: The People of Britain 850–1520*. Yale University Press, 2009.

24. Tuchmann B. *A Distant Mirror*. Knopf, 1978.

25. Bennett JM, Hollister CW. *Mediaeval Europe: A Short History*. McGraw-Hill, 2006.

26. Thomas AJ. *Cholera: The Victorian Plague*. Pen & Sword Books Ltd, 2015.

27. Tatem AJ, Rogers DJ, Hay SI. Global transport networks and infectious disease spread. *Adv Parasitol* 2006; 62: 293–343.

28. Lutz C, Erken M, Noorian P, Su S, McDougald D. Environmental reservoirs and mechanisms of persistence of *Vibrio cholerae*. *Front Microbiol* 2013; 4: 375.

29. World Health Organization (WHO). *Cholera Fact Sheet*. WHO, 2022.

30. Halliday S. *The Great Stink of London: Sir Joseph Bazalgette and the Cleansing of the Victorian Metropolis*. The History Press, 2013.

31. Chadwick E. *Report on the Sanitary Condition of the Labouring Population of Great Britain*. 1842.

32. Snow J. *On the Mode of Communication of Cholera*. John Churchill, 1855.

33. Bentivoglio M, Pacini P. Filippo Pacini: a determined observer. *Brain Res Bull* 1995; 38: 161–5.

34. Howard-Jones N. Robert Koch and the cholera vibrio: a centenary. *Br Med J (Clin Res Ed)* 1984; 288: 379–81.

35. Qadri F, Islam T, Clemens JD. Cholera in Yemen – an old foe rearing its ugly head. *N Engl J Med* 2017; 377: 2005–7.

36. Morens DM, Taubenberger JK, Folkers GK, Fauci AS. Pandemic influenza's 500th anniversary. *Clin Infect Dis* 2010; 51: 1442–4.

37. Spreeuwenberg P, Kroneman M, Paget J. Reassessing the global mortality burden of the 1918 influenza pandemic. *Am J Epidemiol.* 2018; 187: 2561–7.

38. Almond D. Is the 1918 influenza pandemic over? Long-term effects of in utero influenza exposure in the post-1940 U.S. population. *J Polit Econ* 2006; 114: 672–712.

39. Drews K. 2013. A brief history of quarantine. *Virginia Tech Undergrad Hist Rev* 2013; 2. Available from: https://doi.org/10.21061/vtuhr.v2i0.16

40. Booker J. *Maritime Quarantine: The British Experience, c.1650–1900*. Routledge, 2016.

41. World Health Organization (WHO). *International Health Regulations (2005)* 3rd ed. WHO Publications, 2016.

42. Bootsma MCJ, Ferguson NM. The effect of public health measures on the 1918 influenza pandemic in U.S. cities. *Proc Natl Acad Sci USA* 2007; 104: 7588–93.

43. Crosby AW. *America's Forgotten Pandemic: The Influenza of 1918* 2nd ed. Cambridge University Press, 2003.

44. University of Michigan Center for the History of Medicine: Influenza Encyclopedia San Francisco, *California and the 1918–1919 Influenza Epidemic.* (www.influenzaarchive.org/cities/city-sanfrancisco.html#).

45. Topley WWC, Wilson GS. The spread of bacterial infection: the problem of herd immunity. *J Hyg (Lond)* 1923; 21: 243–9.

46. Fine P, Eames K, Heymann DL. Herd immunity: a rough guide. *Clin Infect Dis* 2011; 52: 911–16.

47. Parpia AS, Ndeffo-Mbah ML, Wenzel NS, Galvani AP. Effects of response to 2014–2015 Ebola outbreak on deaths from malaria, HIV/AIDS, and tuberculosis, West Africa. *Emerg Infect Dis* 2016; 22: 433–41.

48. O'Dowd A. NHS waiting list hits 14 year record high of 4.7 million people. *BMJ* 2021; 373: n995.

49. Mahase E. Covid-19: Omicron is 'battering' the NHS and causing 'untold suffering' for patients, say doctors. *BMJ* 2022; 376: o45.

Chapter

17

The Health Aspects of Epidemics and Pandemics

Andrew D Green and Sharon Irvine

Introduction

Infectious diseases have shaped human history and have had significant impacts on the way that societies have developed and later crumbled (see also Chapters 7 and 16). In many cases they were related to geographical locations, often associated with vector-borne transmission, and some came from animals (zoonoses). Diseases that affect domesticated animals were and are also important.

Before the twentieth century, the movement of infectious diseases from one part of the world to another was affected by the means available for transport as well as by economic and agricultural pressures, including slavery, natural disasters, conflicts, and invasions. Although means of long-distance transport were slow, with infected travellers either recovering or dying before reaching home or their destination, the movement of large groups of people resulting from those other pressures often meant the associated large-scale movement of infectious diseases. Examples include the beginning of the second plague pandemic, which was associated with conflict in Asia and Europe in the fourteenth century (a pandemic that lasted for centuries and included the Black Death), the introduction of smallpox into South America by European invaders in the sixteenth century, and the introduction of yellow fever from Africa into South America due to the slave trade.

The term pandemic was first used in the early nineteenth century, to describe a large cholera outbreak affecting wide geographical areas. Termed the first pandemic, it spread from the Bay of Bengal region of India to affect the entire world within 3 years. Although cholera had been recognised for millennia, this was the first time that rapid global spread had occurred. This was attributed to the expansion in overland trade and shipping routes [1].

Many pandemics of different infectious diseases have since been reported. Global pandemics may have

a rapid onset, such as the current SARS-CoV-2/COVID-19, which spread worldwide in a few weeks. They can also be insidious, with slow global spread – for example, HIV/AIDS has a long incubation period, is difficult to recognise in the early stages, and worldwide transmission probably occurred for decades before the disease was recognised [2].

The detailed epidemiology varies according to the routes of transmission and the clinical features of the disease, but the patterns seen in the late twentieth and early twenty-first centuries have been greatly influenced by rapid low-cost international travel, particularly by air. In 2019, before COVID-19, over 4.5 billion people travelled by air annually, with the number projected to grow to over 10 billion by 2040 [3]. Each passenger could circumnavigate the world within the incubation period of any infectious disease, and rapid disease spread is now inevitable.

We support the need to establish robust systems that allow early identification of such events both locally and globally, with proportionate response mechanisms in place. National and international resilience requires investment of money and resources, and redundancy of capacity to allow rapid responses. However, in times of economic stress, prioritisation of efforts to mitigate the unquantifiable theoretical possibility of a disease event may be difficult for governments to justify, and many nations remain ill prepared.

New and Emerging Infectious Diseases

Medicine rode a wave of optimism in the mid-twentieth century. 'The war against infectious diseases has been won' stated the US Surgeon General, William H Steward, in May 1967.

There was an endless supply of new antimicrobials apparently capable of treating all infectious diseases. Vaccines against common infections and insecticides to control insect disease vectors were widely available, and the World Health Organization (WHO) was providing international leadership for global control and eradication of infectious diseases. The US Surgeon General's statement in 1967 simply expressed what was regarded as common knowledge.

The next decade produced unexpected challenges. Antimicrobial resistance was reported for many pathogens [4,5], and malaria was resurgent, as the harmful effects of insecticides were recognised and vector control programmes ceased [6]. No new immunisations were developed and introduced into the UK between 1970 (rubella, measles) and 1988 (combined measles, mumps, and rubella) [7].

The international impact of uncontrolled global spread of infectious diseases came into sharp focus in the early 1980s. In 1981, in the Bay Area of California, a series of new infections were reported in previously healthy individuals. This was eventually recognised as HIV/AIDS.

The appearance of multiple new infections during the 1980s led to rapid investment in resources for infectious disease surveillance, research into basic microbiology and diagnostics, therapeutics, vaccine development, and patient management facilities, including an expansion in specialist hospital capacity. Better descriptive epidemiology and new diagnostic technologies were needed to identify new disease patterns and biological agents associated with other previously unrecognised diseases, not simply those related to HIV/AIDS. A review by an expert group of the National Institutes of Health (NIH) in the USA, which was published in 1992, described the issues in detail and made recommendations about national planning responses [8]. It included a definition of emerging infectious diseases that remains in common use today:

- outbreaks of previously unknown infectious diseases
- known infectious diseases that have rapidly increased in incidence or geographic range in the last two decades
- persistence of infectious diseases that cannot be controlled.

Twelve months after the NIH Report was published there was a high-profile outbreak of hantavirus, a zoonotic virus endemic in rodents, with a different clinical picture of human disease, hantavirus pulmonary syndrome, to that seen before, haemorrhagic fever with renal syndrome, that seemed to affect Native American people disproportionately [9]. This generated national and international interest and catalysed action. A journal was established in 1995 by the Centers for Disease Control (CDC) in the USA, which focused on emerging infectious diseases (EID) [10]. In parallel, the National Center for Emerging and Zoonotic Infectious Diseases (NCEZID) was created at CDC, and there was expansion of the National Institute of Allergy and Infectious Diseases (NIAID).

The potential direct and indirect effects of worldwide large-scale outbreaks attracted the attention of politicians and those concerned with national and international security. In 1996, President Bill Clinton established a national policy to address threats posed by EID, describing areas of work including domestic and international surveillance, prevention, and response measures [11]. This coincided with revised threat assessments by American intelligence agencies, and led to a report being published in 2000 by the US National Intelligence Council (NIC), which identified infectious diseases as a major threat to global stability in the following 20 years [12].

As if to reinforce these warnings, an outbreak of a novel vector-borne zoonosis that caused encephalitis occurred in 1999 in New York City. This was due to West Nile virus, which is transmitted from birds to humans by mosquitoes, and within 5 years it had spread across the continent and killed over 500 people [13]. President Clinton also initiated significant investment to respond to the deliberate release of biological agents (i.e., bioterrorism), developing a programme that became known as Project BioShield [14]. In 2001 the 9/11 terrorist attacks in the USA were followed by the deliberate release of anthrax spores via the US Postal Service. This provoked a funding increase within the USA for strengthening all aspects of detection and responses to biological events. This investment in resources, training, and education soon showed the difficulties posed by infectious diseases. A national threat assessment, which was conducted in 2001 after 9/11 and indicated that there was a risk of smallpox release on American soil, led to widespread vaccination of military personnel and first responders [15]. In May 2003, exposure to rodents imported from West Africa caused an outbreak of monkeypox across six Midwest states, affecting at least 71 people. Despite the training of health providers, and anxiety about bioterrorism and possible smallpox release, the diagnosis of monkeypox was mostly missed or delayed, despite having clinical features typical of orthopoxvirus infection [16]. This disease has recently reappeared, with cases being reported from many countries at the time of publication of this book, and the outbreak declared by the WHO as a Public Health Emergency of International Concern (PHEIC) under the International Health Regulations [17].

In the UK in 2002, the Chief Medical Officer produced a report entitled 'Getting Ahead of the Curve', which highlighted infectious diseases and a strategy for combating the challenges presented by them [18]. It was similar to the strategy outlined 10 years earlier by the NIH in the USA, emphasising improved surveillance, laboratory support, investigation and management of incidents and outbreaks, and investment in vaccine research. It led to the formation of the Health Protection Agency, which brought together several agencies (including the Public Health Laboratory Service), the establishment of Expert Committees to monitor different aspects of infectious diseases and their control, a restructuring of laboratory networks, and a change in the management and control of healthcare-associated infections in the UK [19].

The severe acute respiratory syndrome (SARS) outbreak in 2003 further focused planning and response in the UK. Cross-government-department studies, commissioned by the Government Chief Scientist, resulted in the publication in 2006 of the Foresight Report, entitled 'Infectious Diseases: Preparing for the Future'. Although wide-ranging in its scope and recommendations, particularly regarding disease detection, surveillance, and management, unlike the NIH report it was only partially implemented, having not received the necessary support from central government. As the report itself commented, 'The project does not seek to tell stakeholders what they should or must do. Rather, its findings are provided for policy makers and stakeholders to consider and to interpret within the context of their own situation and their own policy development processes' [20].

An outbreak of influenza in 2009 caused international concern. Named swine flu, it was related to a minor change (a so-called drift) in the antigenic structure of the H1N1 strain of influenza virus, rather than to a major change (a so-called shift) such as usually precedes a flu pandemic. The WHO initially described the incident as an outbreak, and then later as a PHEIC under the International Health Regulations [17]. The outbreak did not meet the then current WHO description of an influenza pandemic – that is, 'when a new influenza virus appears against which the human population has no immunity, resulting in several simultaneous epidemics worldwide with enormous numbers of deaths and illness'. There was international confusion and misunderstanding, which handicapped the global response [21]. It also made the WHO wary about early declarations of pandemics or PHEICs, and arguably led to the delay in the international reaction to the West Africa Ebola outbreak in 2014–2015, which inaction ultimately caused increased numbers of deaths [22].

In the UK, significant effort was directed into pandemic preparedness for influenza. A national strategy, published in 2011, was later recognised to be highly disease-specific, focused only on health responses as opposed to wider considerations across other sectors, and was unsuited to infectious disease challenges other than flu [23]. Individual government departments each developed their own strategy for an influenza pandemic, without an overarching strategic direction or integration.

Continuing concerns about the global impacts of infectious diseases led to a security review in the USA being conducted by the NIC in 2012. This anticipated scenarios that could create worldwide disruption and might occur before 2030. It concluded that a severe pandemic of an infectious disease was one of the greatest potential Black Swan events, possibly leading to a global crisis [24], on a par with nuclear war, collapse of a global superpower, and climate change [25]. The National Security Strategy for the UK in 2011 identified pandemic disease as a 'tier-1' security risk (the highest level), and deliberate release of biological agents as a 'tier-2' risk [26].

A study conducted in 2013 examined possible effects on wider UK society and security outside purely health-related impacts of major infectious disease outbreaks or pandemics, other than those due to influenza or to deliberate release. It concluded that a review of national resilience to inform National Risk Assessments and the National Risk Register should be undertaken with respect to emerging and persistent infectious diseases (EPID). It recommended examination across government departments of challenges to health, security, operational capability, and business continuity by operational analysis using infectious disease modelling. It made recommendations with regard to the effects of interventions to mitigate outcomes, and it recommended that existing surveillance

Table 17.1 Statements from the Emerging and Persistent Infectious Diseases (EPID) Workshop Report. Ulaeto et al. 2014. [28] © Crown Copyright 2014. Reproduced under the terms of the Open Government Licence.

1. Public responses to the appearance of a novel infectious disease will be significantly influenced by the perception of immediate short-term risk to individuals and their close families, which may differ from the actual risk. These short-term perceptions could indirectly result in longer-term social and economic consequences

2. Communications are critically important at all stages, and when done effectively should reduce public anxiety and encourage mitigating behaviour. Preparation of a proactive response plan may be more effective than reactive communications as a result of an incident

3. Public understanding of a disease and its effects may be best achieved by advance long-term education, and provision of accurate and timely information. Confidence is most likely to be undermined by a failure to acknowledge that there are limits to understanding a new disease, and that knowledge will increase over time. So information and advice to the public will change over time

4. New technologies will directly influence the response to an outbreak. These include novel diagnostic tests (including over-the-counter diagnostics) which may or may not be validated, new forms of communication and social networking, and new information technology (e.g., software programmes, mobile phone applications)

5. Existing surveillance systems for infectious diseases in humans and animals within the UK appear robust and would probably lead to early recognition of a novel infectious disease. Similar systems do not exist in all countries, and it is likely that the first introduction into the UK would be from a previously unrecognised source overseas

6. Infectious disease modelling can be highly sophisticated and can produce detailed outputs. Expert interpretation is essential and needs to be communicated to policy makers in a clear and unambiguous way

7. Long-term consequences of an EPID event are difficult to predict, since immediate responses may vary and there may be unexpected outcomes. Planning should take account of the risk of unforeseen consequences through flexibility of response and redundancy in capacity

systems be reviewed with respect to their ability to detect novel infections, and what enhanced surveillance methods were needed [27]. In 2014, further cross-government work explored potential scenarios. The subsequent report included statements that resonate with events later seen with SARS-CoV-2 [28] (see Table 17.1).

In 2016, a national emergency planning exercise involving health and social care and central and local government examined the impact of pandemic influenza on the UK. This was Exercise Cygnus. The findings were published in May 2020, when COVID-19 had already had a significant impact on the UK. Some findings were specific to pandemic influenza, but others were equally applicable to other diseases, and some proved important during COVID-19. Examples included the impact on social care, the vulnerability of care homes to infectious diseases, and the additional pressure that might be posed by staff sickness in the health sector and elsewhere [29].

The Ebola outbreak in West Africa in 2014–2016 led to an international effort to restrict the spread of the disease. The response was poorly coordinated, lacked strategic direction, and many nations developed local policies as opposed to synchronised efforts to support those nations that were most severely affected. Where targeted support was given to specific countries, there was criticism that the aid provided was not necessarily relevant or appropriate to local needs [30]. One troubling area that was exposed during this outbreak was the behaviour of some individual people and groups of people delivering healthcare who conducted research in unethical ways. The WHO urgently issued revised guidance on ethical conduct in such events [31].

After that outbreak, several collaborative initiatives were announced to try to address the issues identified and to move towards global health security for all nations by delivering support networks and surge capacity from affluent economies to support under-resourced countries. As so often happens, the proposals were soon amended or halted as political and economic issues assumed greater importance [32].

To confound international disease control efforts further, several global leaders and much of the international HIV/AIDS community announced in 2018 that 'an end to the AIDS pandemic is imminent', despite clear evidence to the contrary. A review of that approach later concluded that this was further evidence of an international focus on disease-specific matters, rather than a 'pluripotential strategy that might allow development of robust systems that were flexible and could respond to as yet unknown agents which might cause future pandemics' [33].

Almost inevitably, a new disease with epidemic potential appeared. Cases of infection with a novel coronavirus (subsequently named severe acute respiratory syndrome coronavirus 2, or SARS-CoV-2) were identified in Wuhan in China in late 2019. The virus is thought to be a zoonosis, but the route by which it entered the human population is uncertain. It is readily transmissible from person to person by the respiratory route, with a basic reproduction number (R_o) estimated to be as high as 6.1 [34], which is much higher, for example, than that of the influenza virus involved in the outbreak of 1918, which was estimated to have an R_o value of 1.8 [35]. It spread rapidly, initially in China, but within weeks there were cases being reported around the world. The outbreak was declared a PHEIC by the WHO in January 2020, and was officially named COVID-19 in February of that year. At the time of publication of this book, the pandemic is continuing.

It rapidly became clear that people of all ages were susceptible to the infection, and that although younger people rarely became seriously ill, older people and those with comorbidities were far more likely to develop severe and possibly life-threatening illnesses.

COVID-19 can affect virtually all of the organs of the body [36]. Symptoms usually appear 4–5 days after exposure, and commonly include cough, fever, and loss of the sense of smell and taste, but other symptoms, including headaches, nasal congestion, muscle pain, and sore throat, can occur. As the pandemic has progressed, as the virus has evolved, and as increasing numbers of people have developed at least some immunity through infection or vaccination, the spectrum of symptoms has changed; for example, many sufferers now report experiencing severe lethargy. Most symptomatic cases are only mildly ill, but about 14% need hospital admission and about 5% need intensive care due to respiratory failure, septic shock, or multiorgan dysfunction. At least 30% of those infected are asymptomatic but can still spread the disease.

Most people recover fully from the acute infection, although up to 80% may have some effects for more

Box 17.1 Post-COVID syndrome: WHO clinical case definition

Post-COVID-19 syndrome occurs in individuals with a history of probable or confirmed SARS-CoV-2 infection, usually 3 months from the onset, with symptoms that last for at least 2 months and cannot be explained by an alternative diagnosis. Common symptoms include, but are not limited to, fatigue, shortness of breath, and cognitive dysfunction, and generally have an impact on everyday functioning. Symptoms might be new onset following initial recovery from an acute COVID-19 episode, or persist from the initial illness. Symptoms might also fluctuate or relapse over time.

Box 17.2 Post-COVID syndrome: UK Office for National Statistics definition

Symptoms persisting for more than 4 weeks after the first suspected coronavirus (COVID-19) infection, that were not explained by something else.

than 2 weeks [37], but long-term organ damage has been described and some patients continue to experience a range of effects for months. The UK Office for National Statistics (ONS) estimated that about 14% of people who tested positive for SARS-CoV-2 experienced one or more symptoms for longer than 3 months [38], and a study of over 250,000 survivors of COVID-19, mainly in the USA, showed that about 37% of them experienced one or more symptoms between 3 and 6 months after diagnosis [39].

This condition is called post-COVID syndrome or Long COVID, and is characterised by symptoms persisting or appearing after the normal convalescence period. There is no single definition of the condition, but the WHO has produced a clinical case definition (see Box 17.1). The definition used by the UK Office for National Statistics is shown in Box 17.2.

Sufferers from post-COVID syndrome display a wide range of symptoms, commonly including fatigue, post-exertional malaise, and cognitive dysfunction [40]. Other symptoms include muscle weakness, headaches, shortness of breath, loss or distortion of the sense of smell, and low fever [37]. A Scottish study of 159 patients who had been hospitalised with COVID-19 and who were followed for 1 year showed that they had a number of continuing health conditions, including 'persisting cardio-renal inflammation, lung involvement, haemostatic pathway activation and impairments in physical and psychological function' [41].

The pandemic has caused considerable concerns and problems with regard to mental health. Lockdowns, bereavements, job losses, furloughs, and business failures have caused psychosocial problems in some people. Others have been badly affected by extended hospitalisations and the stresses associated with serious illness and treatments such as intensive care, or due to the development of post-COVID syndrome. Serious concerns have been expressed about damage to the development of children, due to reduced interaction with other children and adults and to interruptions to schooling.

There is evidence for substantial neurological and psychiatric morbidity resulting from COVID-19 infection itself, which suggests that survivors are at increased risk of psychiatric sequelae and that these risks are greatest in, although not limited to, those people who have had a severe infection [42]. Encephalopathy is common in hospitalised patients with SARS-CoV-2 infection, and serious neurological manifestations, including meningitis/encephalitis, stroke, and seizure, also occur [43]. There have been reports of cognitive decline following COVID infection, particularly among older patients [44].

Initial attempts to control the pandemic involved non-pharmaceutical interventions suitable for any outbreak of a respiratory disease (see Chapter 16), including lockdowns, banning of mass gatherings, use of masks, spacing between people, hand washing, and room ventilation. These helped to slow the spread of infection and limited the exposure of many susceptible people; they are still used as the main weapon against the infection in many countries. However, observance of such controls can be almost impossible in poorer countries, where the need to earn means that even basic control measures cannot be observed by many (see Chapters 7 and 16).

At the time of publication of this book, wealthier nations continue to try to return to pre-pandemic normality. This ignores the risks posed by the continuing pandemic, including the possible emergence of new and more deadly or less treatable variants. However, living with the disease is becoming an ever greater possibility, especially in higher-income countries, due to access to vaccinations and effective treatments. Novel technologies have produced COVID-19 vaccines in unusually short periods of time, and research has identified drugs that effectively reduce mortality and morbidity. However, there is great inequity throughout the world with regard to access to these developments, and even to basic therapeutic items such as oxygen, especially affecting people who live in low- and lower-middle income countries.

Although the final course of the pandemic remains uncertain, the fact that such an event can occur, and that global healthcare could come close to being overwhelmed in the absence of detailed planning and resource allocation, has once again provoked discussion and proposals for future preparedness by both health professionals [45] and political leaders [46].

References

1. Selwyn S. Cholera old and new. *Proc R Soc Med* 1977; 70: 301–2.

2. De Cock KM, Jaffe HW, Curran JW. Reflections on 40 years of AIDS. *Emerg Infect Dis* 2021; 27: 1553–60.

3. International Civil Aviation Organization (ICAO). *Annual Report 2019. The World of Air Transport in 2019*. ICAO, 2019 (www.icao.int/annual-report-2019/Pages/the-world-of-air-transport-in-2019.aspx).

4. Duckworth G. 40 years of methicillin resistant *Staphylococcus aureus*. *BMJ* 2001; 323: 644–5.

5. Murray JF, Schraufnagel DE, Hopewell PC. Treatment of tuberculosis – a historical perspective. *Ann Am Thorac Soc* 2015; 12: 1749–59.

6. Cohen JM, Smith DL, Cotter C, Ward A, Yarney G, Sabot OJ, et al. Malaria resurgence: a systematic review and assessment of its causes. *Malar J* 2012; 11: 122.

7. Public Health England. *Vaccination Timeline Table from 1796 to Present*. Public Health England, 2019 (www.gov.uk/government/publications/vaccination-timeline/vaccination-timeline-from-1796-to-present).

8. Lederberg J, Shope RE, Oaks SC, ed. *Emerging Infections: Microbial Threats to Health in the United States*. National Academies Press (US), 1992.

9. Centers for Disease Control and Prevention. Outbreak of acute illness – southwestern United

States, 1993. *MMWR Morb Mortal Wkly Rep* 1993; 42: 421–4.

10. Satcher D. Emerging infections: getting ahead of the curve. *Emerg Infect Dis* 1995; 1: 1–6.

11. Clinton WJ. *Presidential Decision Directive NSTC-7: Emerging Infectious Diseases*. The White House, 1996.

12. National Intelligence Council. *The Global Infectious Disease Threat and Its Implications for the United States*. NIE 99-17D. National Intelligence Council, 2000.

13. Roehrig JT. West Nile virus in the United States — a historical perspective. *Viruses* 2013; 5: 3088–108.

14. The White House. *Project BioShield: Progress in the War on Terror*. The White House Archives, 2004 (https://georgewbush-whitehouse.archives.gov/infocus/bioshield/index.html).

15. Wharton M, Strikas RA, Harpaz R, Rotz LD, Schwartz B, Casey CG, et al. Recommendations for using smallpox vaccine in a pre-event vaccination program. *MMWR Recomm Rep* 2003; 52: 1–16.

16. Sejvar J, Chowdary Y, Schomogyi M, Stevens J, Patel J, Karem K, et al. Human monkeypox infection: a family cluster in the midwestern United States. *J Infect Dis* 2004; 190: 1833–40.

17. World Health Organization (WHO). *Fifty-Eighth World Health Assembly. Resolution WHA58.3: Revision of the International Health Regulations*. WHO, 2005 (www.who.int/gb/ebwha/pdf_files/WHA58/WHA58_3-en.pdf).

18. Department of Health. *Getting Ahead of the Curve: A Strategy for Combating Infectious Diseases (Including Other Aspects of Health Protection)*. Department of Health, 2003.

19. The Health Foundation. *Infection Prevention and Control: Lessons from Acute Care in England*. The Health Foundation, 2015.

20. Foresight. *Infectious Diseases: Preparing for the Future. Executive Summary*. Government Office for Science, 2006.

21. Doshi P. The elusive definition of pandemic influenza. *Bull World Health Organ* 2011; 89: 532–8.

22. Moon S, Sridhar D, Pate MA, Jha AK, Clinton C, Delauney S, et al. Will Ebola change the game? Ten essential reforms before the next pandemic. The report of the Harvard-LSHTM Independent Panel on the Global Response to Ebola. *Lancet* 2015; 386: 2204–21.

23. Department of Health. *UK Influenza Pandemic Preparedness Strategy*. Department of Health, 2011.

24. Taleb NN. *The Black Swan: The Impact of the Highly Improbable*. Penguin, 2007.

25. National Intelligence Council. *Global Trends 2030: Alternative Worlds*. National Intelligence Council, 2012 (www.dni.gov/nic/globaltrends).

26. HM Government. *A Strong Britain in an Age of Uncertainty: The National Security Strategy*. The Stationery Office Limited, 2011.

27. Biggins PDE, Barnett A, Foot VJ, Gillard, Green AD, Ulaeto DO, et al. Emerging and persistent infectious diseases (EPID) and the implication for defence and national security: a scoping study. 2013.

28. Ulaeto D, Irving D, Barnett A. *Emerging and Persistent Infectious Diseases (EPID): Workshop Report*. Defence Science and Technology Laboratory (Dstl), Porton Down, 2014 (https://researchonline.lshtm.ac.uk/id/eprint/1680755).

29. Pegg D. What was Exercise Cygnus and what did it find? The 2016 simulation of a pandemic found holes in the UK's readiness for such a crisis. *The Guardian*, 7 May 2020 (www.theguardian.com/world/2020/may/07/what-was-exercise-cygnus-and-what-did-it-find).

30. Scott V, Crawford-Browne S, Sanders D. Critiquing the response to the Ebola epidemic through a Primary Health Care Approach. *BMC Public Health* 2016; 16: 410.

31. World Health Organization (WHO). *Guidance for Managing Ethical Issues in Infectious Disease Outbreaks*. WHO, 2016 (apps.who.int/iris/handle/10665/250580).

32. Ravi SJ, Snyder MR, Rivers C. Review of international efforts to strengthen the global outbreak response system since the 2014–16 West Africa Ebola Epidemic. *Health Policy Plan* 2019; 34: 47–54.

33. Bekker L-G, Alleyne G, Baral S, Cepeda J, Daskalaksis D, Dowdy D, et al. Advancing global health and strengthening the HIV response in the era of the Sustainable Development Goals: the International AIDS Society—Lancet Commission. *Lancet* 2018; 392: 312–58.

34. Ke R, Romero-Severson E, Steven Sanchea S, Hengartner N. Estimating the reproductive number Ro of SARS-CoV-2 in the United States and eight European countries and implications for vaccination. *J Theor Biol* 2021; 17: 110621.

35. Biggerstaff M, Cauchemez S, Reed C, Manoj G, Finelli L. Estimates of the reproduction number for seasonal, pandemic, and zoonotic influenza: a systematic review of the literature. *BMC Infect Dis* 2014; 14: 480.

36. Puelles VG, Lütgehetmann M, Lindenmeyer MT, Sprehake JP, Wong MN, Allweiss L, et al. Multiorgan and renal tropism of SARS-CoV-2. *N Engl J Med* 2020; 383: 590–92.

37. Lopez-Leon S, Wegman-Ostrosky T, Perelman C, Sepulveda R,

Rebolledo PA, Cuapio A, et al. More than 50 long-term effects of COVID-19: a systematic review and meta-analysis. *Sci Rep* 2021; 11: 16144.

38. Office for National Statistics. *Prevalence of Ongoing Symptoms Following Coronavirus (COVID-19) Infection in the UK: 30 March 2023*. Office for National Statistics, 2023.

39. Taquet M, Derco Q, Luciano S, Geddes JR, Husain M, Harrison PJ, et al. Incidence, co-occurrence, and evolution of long-COVID features: a 6-month retrospective cohort study of 273,618 survivors of COVID-19. *PLoS Med* 2021; 20: e1003773.

40. Lopez-Leon S, Wegman-Ostrosky T, Perelman C, Sepulveda A, Rebolledo PA, Cuapio A, et al. More than 50 long-term effects of COVID-19: a systematic review and meta-analysis. *Sci Rep* 2021; 11: 16144.

41. Morrow AJ, Sykes R, McIntosh A, Kamdar A, Bagot C, Bayes HK, et al. A multisystem, cardio-renal investigation of post-COVID-19 illness. *Nat Med* 2022; 28: 1303–13.

42. Taquet M, Geddes JR, Husain M, Luciano S, Harrison PJ. 6-month neurological and psychiatric outcomes in 236,379 survivors of COVID-19: a retrospective cohort study using electronic health records. *Lancet Psychiatry* 2021; 8: 416-27.

43. Cervantes-Arslanian AM, Venkata C, Anand P, Burns JD, Ong CJ, LeMahieu AM, et al. Neurologic manifestations of severe acute respiratory syndrome coronavirus 2 infection in hospitalized patients during the first year of the COVID-19 pandemic. *Crit Care Explor* 2022; 4: e0686.

44. Liu Y-H, Chen Y, Wang Q-H, Wang L-R, Jiang L, Yang Y, et al. One-year trajectory of cognitive changes in older survivors of COVID-19 in Wuhan, China: a longitudinal cohort study. *JAMA Neurol* 2022; 79: 509–17.

45. Wilensky GR. 2020 revealed how poorly the US was prepared for COVID-19 – and future pandemics. *JAMA* 2021; 325: 1029–30.

46. Alvis S, Macon-Cooney B, Said J. *Global Coordination Requirements for COVID-19 and Future Pandemics*. Tony Blair Institute for Social Change, 2020 (institute.global/tony-blair/world-was-not-prepared-covid-19-we-should-learn-lessons-and-change).

Chapter

18

Challenges in Managing Epidemics and Pandemics Illustrated by Ebola and COVID-19
A Case Study Perspective

Claire Bayntun

Introduction

Several pandemics and major outbreaks caused by viruses occurred at the end of the twentieth and the beginning of the twenty-first centuries (see Chapters 16 and 17). Sadly, lessons learned from these outbreaks were not always remembered or translated into global and national policies for coping with future outbreaks. This chapter examines two of these outbreaks, Ebola in West Africa (2013–2015) and the COVID-19 pandemic. The lessons identified are compared and contrasted.

General Principles That Emerge from the Public Health and Social Sciences Perspective

Ebola: Experience from the 2013–2015 West Africa Outbreak

Control of communicable disease outbreaks demands a thorough knowledge of the way the disease is transmitted. The transmission dynamics of the Ebola virus are well documented [1,2]. Communicating these details to the affected populations was vital, and as the outbreak progressed, effective and appropriate public health messaging ensured that people knew that the infection was spread by contact with body fluids. However, persuading people to limit practices involving such contact was slow to develop. The World Health Organization (WHO) and Médecins sans Frontières (MSF) attempted to produce suitable messages by consulting academic anthropologists, but this side-lined local sources and expertise and led to ineffective messaging across a broad spectrum of public health communications and response management activities, arguably with disastrous consequences. The effects of this were particularly serious with regard to traditional burial practices. Insensitive

management of cadavers, and delays in producing a socially acceptable alternative, led to traditional burials being practised 'underground', which resulted in localised Ebola outbreaks [3].

As part of the control programme, households with an Ebola patient were quarantined, frequently without effective provision for meals, income, and medical care, and this quarantine was enforced by local military personnel. A quarantined household in a community stigmatised those in the household and the whole community, acting as a disincentive to report cases, and undermining the quarantine system, contact tracing efforts, and the collection of data to direct the response. To try to improve the situation, students were enlisted to carry out contact tracing, but the outcomes reflected the poorly resourced training, and management of, this important task. MSF recognised the issues in late 2014 and developed an informal system of local Aunty Networks in Freetown to improve contact tracing, parallel to the official avenues.

The outbreak spread widely and rapidly in urban settings, in contrast to earlier outbreaks that mainly occurred in more isolated rural communities, where the virus burned out before it could spread significantly. In the West African outbreak, spread was greatest along trading routes and into cities. Major efforts were made to limit this spread, which occurred in all of the three countries most severely affected – Sierra Leone, Guinea, and Liberia – but with limited success. By contrast, three countries that saw only a few cases linked to the main outbreak – Mali, Nigeria, and Senegal – showed excellent locally led rapid responses, effective contact tracing, and successful breaking of transmission chains. However, these countries knew about the outbreak and had full resources ready on stand-by.

Several organisations attempted to identify and map health facilities in the affected countries, aiming to record up-to-date information about supplies and staff available to manage patients with Ebola and other health conditions. This became critical as many local health facilities closed, partly due to staff morbidity and mortality, but also as violence was directed against health facilities and personnel due to mistrust of the authorities. Staff felt unsafe, were poorly trained, lacked personal protective equipment (PPE), and had few medicines and equipment to manage Ebola patients. Staff reductions, and closure of some facilities, together with a widespread reluctance by patients to attend health centres due to fear of contracting Ebola, meant that all healthcare activities were affected. Increased morbidity and mortality were recorded in some localities for diseases such as malaria, tuberculosis, and HIV/AIDS, and there were also increases in maternal and infant morbidity and mortality [4–7].

Digital tools enabled responders to identify hotspots through increases in internet searches for symptoms and treatments. Interactive apps drawing on the health facility mapping data supported disease surveillance, advised users about red areas (i.e., outbreak hotspots), and offered guidance on what to do and where to go for care. Mobile phones were widely used, but digital skills varied, resulting in inequalities of access to accurate information. The spread of misinformation through social media fuelled mistrust, as well as violence towards responders and authorities.

COVID-19

It is important to recognise how much was known about the virus and its transmission dynamics early in the pandemic, due to research in China [8]. In particular, early release of gene-sequencing data allowed rapid vaccine development so that within less than 1 year after the virus was first identified, some populations were receiving internationally approved vaccines.

Non-pharmaceutical measures can help to control the spread of respiratory viruses both in the absence of a vaccine and as adjuncts to vaccination programmes (see Chapter 16). However, public health management strategies using these measures were, and are, quite diverse across populations around the world. The effectiveness of different strategies and the outcomes varied significantly, in large part due to how the use of knowledge played out in specific political, social, cultural, behavioural, and climate/

seasonal environments [9]. In addition, many of the actions needed to reduce transmission of a disease such as COVID-19 (e.g., personal distancing, lockdowns), are impossible for many people in urban poverty, who live in crowded and poorly ventilated dwellings and need to work daily outside their homes (see Chapter 7) [10].

Home-working and home-schooling have been possible for much of the population of countries with modern infrastructures and well-developed communications and digital services. Enhanced technologies have also enabled coordination of systems on a large scale, offering data capture and analytics to support decision making and the transfer of knowledge. At the same time, inequalities have been exacerbated due to differences in access to reliable digital technology, the internet, and appropriate home-working conditions and space.

Opportunities emerged to strengthen the global community from the shared experience of living through the pandemic, with effective yet remotely operated partnerships developed for collaboration, as well as digital tools and apps supporting surveillance, contact tracing, and vaccine delivery. Sadly, these have also enabled increases in cybercrime, including risks of abuse for children who are studying and spending more time online. There has been an explosion of hacking and fraud, with vulnerable groups (e.g., older people, people who are less internet literate) being disproportionately affected. The WHO declared the infodemic to be a major concern with regard to the management of the pandemic [11], with misinformation fuelling confusion, adding to fears, and generating mistrust of authorities, treatments, and vaccines.

The widespread use of surveillance and contact tracing tools, as well as the imposition of isolation and quarantine, infringed civil liberties in some situations [12]. Different cultures reacted in different ways and voiced varying levels of concern about restrictions and surveillance, related to societal norms and ideologies.

A Description of the Short-, Medium-, and Long-Term Impacts

Impacts of Ebola

Short-term issues that affected the initial outbreak response in West Africa centred on uncertainty about the epidemiological situation. Poor disease surveillance meant that accurate information was not available, leading to confusion about the need for intervention and the amount of intervention required, slow decision making, and delayed local and international responses, allowing the outbreak to spread rapidly. These delays and failings also led to a mistrust of authorities, and allowed conspiracy theories to grow unchecked.

In the medium term, the numbers of organisations involved in supporting the management of the response increased. Most lacked experience in managing this type and scale of outbreak, leading to challenges in coordination and cooperation in response efforts, both within and between organisations.

The long-term impacts are best reviewed through consideration of what happened at local, regional, and global levels. Local economic impacts were mixed; there was serious damage to internal agriculture and trade, and promised international investment and donations never materialised [13].

At the regional level, the picture is also mixed. Although public health system infrastructure and expertise remain under-developed across the affected countries and their regional neighbours, disease surveillance systems improved in West Africa overall, and other coordination and collaboration initiatives have developed successfully. Of great value was the creation in 2017 of Africa Centres for Disease Control and Prevention (Africa CDC) and other disease management entities which now offer vital coordination, collaboration, and training roles in the COVID-19 response.

Among the many global platforms and organisations involved in disease management, important lessons and recommendations emerged from the Ebola outbreak. Not all benefited from the investment or change envisioned in the immediate aftermath, but a positive example is the Coalition for Epidemic Preparedness Initiative (CEPI). This has played a significant role in the COVID-19 pandemic as part of the COVAX initiative, accelerating collaborative research and development responses.

Impacts of COVID-19

The short-term impacts of the COVID-19 pandemic have been experienced differently around the world, reflecting the degree of spread, the range of transmission rates, and the varied responses of governments, with impacts varying with prior cultural norms and societal experience with respiratory outbreaks.

Specifically, there was a range of responses to the government-enforced lockdowns that extended for months for some populations. The impacts were more manageable for certain populations, with systems providing services and resources for those in isolation, whereas others suffered greater impacts on mental health and wellbeing. For example, one multinational study showed that diagnosis of anxiety increased across all age groups [14], which was widely predicted given the situation and the uncertainties.

As lockdown and general social distancing became entrenched in the medium term, businesses closed and unemployment increased. There were efforts to manage these impacts, with some governments subsidising the costs of employment (e.g., through the staff furlough schemes in the UK). There has been an exacerbation of inequalities within and across societies, with poorer households facing food and housing insecurity, and increased reports of domestic abuse affecting both adults and children [15].

A long-term problem has been the accumulation of patients not treated for conditions other than COVID-19, a problem that is likely to affect healthcare worldwide for years. A significant additional long-term challenge is the management of patients who have post-COVID syndrome or Long COVID, with sequelae of the infection persisting for months, or longer, after the original infection (see Chapters 16 and 17).

The pandemic resulted in a global economic recession [16], although there are signs of recovery in some sectors [17]. There is a recognition that although some industries will not return to pre-pandemic production and trade levels, there are opportunities for new industries to emerge. At the time of publication of this book, the conflict in the Ukraine is compounding the damage to the world economy and recovery.

The vulnerability of the global trading system to the impacts of a pandemic (e.g., reliance on just-in-time deliveries of critical goods and services) may result in increased investment in nationally independent solutions. However, governments borrowed to manage the impacts of the pandemic, resulting in debts that are affecting long-term recovery, as well as the risks of additional inequalities among populations due to cuts in services and increased prices.

The longer-term social impacts of the COVID-19 pandemic are becoming clearer, and it is challenging to understand the extent to which there will be new norms in how populations live. For example, the desire for, and acceptance of, travel have changed due to the risks and uncertainties around contracting the virus. Many people have concerns about rapid national policy changes with regard to items such as quarantine on returning from areas where upsurges in cases have occurred, or new variants have appeared. The cost, availability, and ease of holiday and business travel have also changed. There is a sector-wide shift in recognising the impacts on climate that are associated with travel, and opportunities to conduct business remotely have received investment, becoming widely embedded and normalised. For many businesses, home-working and reduced commuting seem likely to continue.

Although many people are now happy to attend mass-gatherings (e.g., football matches, music festivals), attitudes to other forms of gathering seem to have changed, with the expectation that training, business, entertainment, and even some social events should be available to join remotely, not least to widen their accessibility and to reduce environmental impacts of mass travel. In many sectors, greater awareness and consideration are shown for people with dependants, mobility concerns, travel time and distance concerns, and mental health and wellbeing concerns. Further innovation and investment will focus on offering effective hybrid technology to support events and meetings, with some people attending in person and others joining remotely.

The use of masks is increasingly endorsed and accepted in societies where this practice was previously unusual. Other interventions, such as physical distancing and ventilation, may become part of routine social and business activities, and people may isolate at home when unwell. However, there is a widespread desire to return to pre-COVID-19 normality, and the rapidity with which populations in countries such as the UK have abandoned the use of masks and observance of social distancing, and are willing to attend mass gatherings, despite continued high COVID-19 incidence levels, raises concerns about the willingness of populations to observe basic preventive measures in the long term (see Chapter 16).

Although there were large costs associated with responses to the pandemic, it is not clear whether sustained investment will be available for development of public health systems, to prepare for and prevent future health challenges. This is a particular concern given the competition for diminished government resources and the need for investment to stimulate economic recovery.

There has been a greater recognition of how crises increase inequalities, and the fact that the vulnerable suffer the greatest impacts. Research and investments are required to address inequalities within and across populations, in order to understand the complex issues and address the upstream determinants appropriately.

The strain on health systems has affected the education and training of health professionals. Many were diverted into caring for COVID-19 patients, interrupting their studies and careers to do so. On the positive side, there has been an increase in training delivered through remote systems, supporting communities of health professionals both in terms of the COVID-19 response (e.g., the continent-wide training provided by Africa CDC for health workers and for personal and professional development). These changes to online and remote activities have also flourished for clinical consultations, supported by the development of new tools and apps. There are rich opportunities for fresh thinking and technological innovation to support national and international health sector development.

Furthermore, there has been an increased awareness of global issues, such as the need to focus investment on sustainable development, supporting the international health agenda, and recognising the inter-dependencies of global communities. There is a burgeoning of new global initiatives, such as COVAX and the ACT accelerator. There are plans to improve mechanisms of disease management and governance, through the revision of the International Health Regulations (IHR), and the agreement for a Treaty on Pandemics. Importantly, there are opportunities to ensure that the world is better positioned to deal with such crises in the future (e.g., through the launch of the WHO Hub for Pandemic and Epidemic Intelligence).

The Implications for Intervention: Prevent, Prepare, Respond, And Recover

Ebola

There was no preparation for an outbreak of Ebola in West Africa, as this disease was not recognised as a problem in that region. There was serological evidence that Ebola occurred in human populations in the area [18,19], but this material dated from the 1980s and was not routinely referenced by those working on viral haemorrhagic fevers in the region, a programme that focused mainly on Lassa fever.

Human and financial resources for managing existing health threats in the West African region were minimal at the time of the outbreak, with no immediate possibility of an adequate internal response. In addition, worldwide there were few Ebola experts. Previous outbreaks occurred in Eastern and Central Africa, and most of the expertise was concentrated in those areas. Globally, a few individuals, mainly working for MSF and the WHO, had such experience.

In addition to clinical, microbiological, and public health knowledge, outbreak management requires an understanding of culture and political history specific to localities and ethnic groups, so that the response is sensitive to local needs. There must be an awareness of any mistrust of authorities in the affected areas. Understanding these factors is critical if accurate epidemiological data are to be collected, and to prevent unreported disease transmission. Early in the Ebola outbreak, these aspects of surveillance and data gathering were inadequately managed, and the data were unreliable. Informal channels (e.g., MSF's Aunty Networks) became valuable information sources.

Response decision making was initially uncoordinated, with multiple actors failing to cooperate effectively. Leaders of the affected countries worried that national sovereignty was being ignored, while others reported that too much time was being spent on diplomacy, rather than on developing the capacity for an effective nationally led response.

The International Health Regulations require that the WHO is notified of occurrences such as an Ebola outbreak [20]. However, many argue that countries lack incentives to declare an outbreak due to concerns about impacts on trade, travel, the economy, and the country's long-term reputation. Delays during the Ebola outbreak may be attributable to this reticence. The WHO was accused of delaying declaring a Public Health Emergency of International Concern (PHEIC), in part due to the lack of reliable surveillance data, but also because it had been accused of over-reacting when it had declared the first PHEIC for the swine flu H1N1 pandemic in 2009.

Although the influx of international agencies was vital, there were significant challenges in achieving collaboration and cooperation in response management. Each agency had different experience, expertise, and training that was not always aligned to the local context, and they were accountable to different funders with different agendas. Inefficiencies and cultural misunderstandings resulted in poor cooperation in the early stages of the international response. Once the Sierra Leone National Ebola Response Centre (NERC) was established, competition between organisations was better managed [21], but the issues around research, regulations for data collection and sharing, permission to take samples out of the affected countries, consent and ethics all remained inadequately controlled (see Chapter 17).

Communications management was patchy, with new products and services being developed in competition with each other, and with varied levels of effectiveness. Management of misinformation and mistrust proved complex, and was poorly handled by both local and international agencies.

Crises may require military assistance to help to manage logistics, provide security, and support the interventions. MSF called for military support in the outbreak, via a statement to the UN in September 2014, recognising that the health services and other organisations on the ground were unable to cope. Unfortunately, this was at a time when military intervention in the region was mistrusted and created fear due to recent civil conflicts in the area. Despite this, military support was vital to the outbreak programmes.

The promised international investment to support the recovery of the health systems and the wider economies of the affected nations has not materialised [22]. Unfortunately, despite hopes that the legacy of systems developed in response to the outbreak, such as laboratories, would provide long-term benefits, few examples of infrastructure and training have translated into sustainable benefits to the affected health systems.

COVID-19

In the years following the Ebola outbreak, international and national attempts at prevention and preparedness planning for outbreaks, epidemics, and pandemics did not translate into an adequate capability to respond in practice. Influenza was considered to be the greatest pandemic threat, and preparations focused on that disease. Countries that had achieved high scores on pandemic preparedness and IHR evaluation checklists, as well as undertaking multi-agency simulation exercises and stockpiling critical resources such as PPE, failed to translate this into effective management of the COVID-19 pandemic. Nations that were considered to have the most advanced public health systems and highest levels of expertise in tackling outbreaks (e.g., the UK and the USA) failed to mitigate the impacts of the COVID-19 pandemic, and experienced some of the highest rates of morbidity and mortality. By contrast, Asian countries with experience of infectious disease outbreaks, and particularly the original severe acute respiratory syndrome (SARS) coronavirus outbreak in 2003, were better at recognising the need to mitigate community and economic harm through rapid control measures. Western countries were cautious about implementing restrictions, and perhaps there was a false sense of security as it was assumed that checklist scores would translate into an effective response.

As a result, responses differed across countries and regions. Despite warnings and guidance from the WHO early in the outbreak, governments made their own response decisions. Delays in implementing WHO guidance resulted in higher rates of transmission, increased levels of morbidity and mortality across societies, irrelevance of preparedness checklist status, and ultimately greater negative economic impacts [23]. By contrast, countries that adopted non-pharmaceutical interventions (NPIs) early were better protected.

Some cultures have ideological challenges, with interference by the state in personal liberties. Western societies are typically more self-oriented and less community-oriented. For example, the wearing of masks principally protects others by preventing transmission of infection from the wearer, but in Western societies, individuals were more likely to wear a mask if they considered that it would protect them from infection.

In order to implement recommended public health measures, support systems were needed to enable adherence. To do so effectively, a state needs sufficient infrastructure and resources to provide basic needs and services such as food, income, and accommodation. For some societies there were risks of actual and perceived autocratic abuse, as well as police and military brutality.

Global collaboration in the response was also important. There were extreme examples of political nationalism – for example, in relation to the procurement of PPE, access to test systems and reagents, and

the production and sharing of vaccines and treatments. At the same time, there were notable successes in regional cooperation across Asia and Africa [24].

In general, the science and medical communities cooperated better than the politicians, with important outcomes in terms of the understanding and characterisation of the virus and the disease, as well as the development and production of treatments and vaccines. There are important examples of global solidarity, such as the ACT accelerator/COVAX initiatives, strengthening global collaboration for the long-term benefit of science, research, and medicine.

The nature of recovery from the COVID-19 pandemic has yet to be determined.

Practical Aspects of Implementing the Principles: Now and Looking Forwards

There will be many national and international commissions and numerous studies by academic bodies to analyse and assess the management of the COVID-19 pandemic and identify lessons learned. This was the case following the Ebola outbreak in West Africa.

Often in crises, with examples from across the world, the national responses are centrally led. Although this can offer benefits in terms of consistency of responses, and economies in resource management, the approach is hampered by a limited ability to consider the insights held by those with long-term involvement in local service provision. Successful responses require familiary with the demographics, languages, history, vulnerabilities, and needs of the communities involved.

The WHO has evolved with each major health crisis, reviewing current tools and developing new systems and structures to improve future preparedness and response. The WHO Emergency Programme, developed following the Ebola outbreak in West Africa, played a leading role throughout COVID-19. The recently launched WHO Hub for Pandemic and Epidemic Intelligence, born of the experience with COVID-19, recognises the need for a focus on data, information, and knowledge collation and management during health crises.

The role of the IHR [20] is being reviewed. Official notification is associated with disincentives, and the COVID-19 pandemic has shown that, in practice, the IHR checklist scores do not relate well to success or failure in the management of outbreaks and a pandemic. Political leaders are calling for an international pandemic treaty [25,26].

The findings of the reviews may highlight the opportunity for the ACT Accelerator/COVAX initiatives to be established to manage the coordination and collaboration structure for treatments and vaccines for other infectious diseases, including those with epidemic and pandemic potential.

Such platforms of collaboration across the world can help to swing the pendulum that has been moving towards nationalistic agendas back towards an ethos of global solidarity. The pandemic highlights the nature of humankind as an inter-dependent global community; strengthening this is critical as we prepare for and manage future epidemics, pandemics, and other planet-wide crises.

References

1. Dowell SF, Mukunu R, Ksiazek TG, Khan AS, Rollin PE, Peters CJ, et al. Transmission of Ebola hemorrhagic fever: a study of risk factors in family members, Kikwit, Democratic Republic of the Congo, 1995. *J Infect Dis* 1999; 179(suppl 1): S87–91.

2. Suresh R, Dashrath M. Transmission of Ebola virus disease: an overview. *Ann Glob Health* 2014; 80: 444–51.

3. Shah JJ. The dead bodies of the West African Ebola epidemic: understanding the importance of traditional burial practices. *Inquiries J* 2015; 7: 1–4.

4. Walker PGT, White MT, Griffin JT, Reynolds A, Ferguson NM, Ghani AC, et al. Malaria morbidity and mortality in Ebola-affected countries caused by decreased health-care capacity, and the potential effect of mitigation strategies: a modelling analysis. *Lancet Infect Dis* 2015; 15: 825-832.

5. Ribacke KJB, Saulnier DD, Eriksson A, von Schreeb J. Effects of the West Africa Ebola Virus Disease on health-care utilization – a systematic review. *Front Public Health* 2016; 4: 222.

6. Vygen S, Tiffany A, Rull M, Ventura A, Wolz A, Jambai A, et al. Changes in health-seeking behavior did not result in increased all-cause mortality during the Ebola outbreak in Western Area, Sierra Leone. *Am J Trop Med Hyg* 2016; 95: 897–901.

7. Mæstad O, Shumbullo EL. *Ebola Outbreak 2014–2016: Effects on Other Health Services*. Chr. Michelsen Institute, 2020.

8. Xiang Y-T, Li W, Zhang Q, Jin Y, Rao W-W, Zeng L-N, et al. Timely research papers about COVID-19 in China. *Lancet* 2020; 395: 684–5.

9. Kennedy DS, Vu V, Ritchie H, Bartlein R, Rothschild O, Bausch DG, et al. COVID-19: identifying countries with indicators of success in responding to the outbreak. *Gates Open Res* 2021; 4: 62.

10. Du J, King R, Chanchani R. *Tackling Inequality in Cities is Essential for Fighting COVID-19*. World Resources Institute, 2020 (www.wri.org/insights/tackling-inequality-cities-essential-fighting-covid-19).

11. World Health Organization (WHO). *Let's Flatten the Infodemic Curve*. WHO, undated (www.who.int/news-room/spotlight/let-s-flatten-the-infodemic-curve).

12. Civil Liberties Union for Europe. *Demanding on Democracy: Country & Trend Reports on Democratic Records by Civil Liberties Organisations Across the European Union*. European Union, 2020 (dq4n3btxmr8c9.cloudfront.net/files/AuYJXv/Report_Liberties_EU2020.pdf).

13. UN Development Group (UNDG)–Western and Central Africa. *Socio-Economic Impact of Ebola Virus Disease in West African Countries: A Call for National and Regional Containment, Recovery and Prevention*. UNDG–Western and Central Africa, 2015 (reliefweb.int/sites/reliefweb.int/files/resources/ebola-west-africa.pdf).

14. COVID-19 Mental Disorders Collaborators. Global prevalence and burden of depressive and anxiety disorders in 204 countries and territories in 2020 due to the COVID-19 pandemic. *Lancet* 2021; 398: 1700–12.

15. Stiglitz J. *Conquering the Great Divide*. International Monetary Fund, 2020.

16. World Bank. *COVID-19 to Plunge Global Economy into Worst Recession since World War II*. World Bank, 2020 (www.worldbank.org/en/news/press-release/2020/06/08/covid-19-to-plunge-global-economy-into-worst-recession-since-world-war-ii).

17. World Bank. *The Global Economy: On Track for Strong but Uneven Growth as COVID-19 Still Weighs*. World Bank, 2021 (www.worldbank.org/en/news/feature/2021/06/08/the-global-economy-on-track-for-strong-but-uneven-growth-as-covid-19-still-weighs).

18. Knobloch K, Albiez EJ, Schmitz H. A serological survey on viral haemorrhagic fevers in Liberia. *Ann Virol (Inst Pasteur)* 1982; 133: 125–8.

19. Van der Waals FW, Pomeroy KL, Goudsmit J, Asher DM, Gajdusek DC. Hemorrhagic fever virus infections in an isolated rainforest area of central Liberia. Limitations of the indirect immunofluorescence slide test for antibody screening in Africa. *Trop Geogr Med* 1986; 38: 209–14.

20. World Health Organization (WHO). *International Health Regulations (2005)* 3rd ed. WHO, 2016.

21. Ross E. Command and control of Sierra Leone's Ebola outbreak response: evolution of the response architecture. *Philos Trans R Soc Lond B Biol Sci* 2017; 372: 20160306.

22. Ravi SJ, Snyder MR, Rivers C. Review of international efforts to strengthen the global outbreak response system since the 2014–16 West Africa Ebola Epidemic. *Health Policy Plan* 2019; 34: 47–54.

23. Kompas T, Grafton RQ, Che TN, Chu L, Camac J. Health and economic costs of early and delayed suppression and the unmitigated spread of COVID-19: the case of Australia. *PLoS One* 2021; 16: e0252400.

24. Centers for Disease Control and Prevention (CDC). *Africa CDC Launches Continent-Wide Response.* CDC, 2020 (www.cdc .gov/globalhealth/ healthprotection/fieldupdates/fall-2020/africa-cdc-covid.html).

25. Global Health Centre. *Options for a Global Pandemic Treaty.* BMJ, 2021 (www.bmj.com/global-pandemic-treaty).

26. European Council. *An International Treaty on Pandemic Prevention and Preparedness.* European Council, 2022 (www .consilium.europa.eu/en/policies/ coronavirus/pandemic-treaty/).

Chapter

19

The Role of the Public: Understanding Group Processes in Emergencies, Incidents, Disasters, and Disease Outbreaks

John Drury

What is the Role of the Public in Emergencies, Major Incidents, and Disasters?

In the past, the authorities have often seen the public as a problem in relation to the official response to emergencies, incidents, terrorist events, disasters, disease outbreaks and conflicts (EITDDC). Supposedly, the public either fail to act, and are therefore wholly dependent on the professionals, or they act in the wrong way, actively obstructing or overburdening the professionals. In each case, in the context of an EITDDC, the rational person of everyday life apparently gives way to a form of collective vulnerability, or even pathology, to which people in the role of authority are somehow immune.

Today, the discourse of community resilience and similar frameworks is a formal recognition of the value, and indeed the necessity, of public involvement in emergency preparedness, resilience, and response (EPRR). However, some residue of the older pathologising representations still exists. In addition, our understanding of the psychological underpinnings of collectively resilient responses in the public has progressed significantly in recent years, although it is still developing. It is important, therefore, to continue to document the evidence, and to develop theory adequate to this evidence, of adaptive public responses in EITDDC. Key questions include the following. What are the variables that determine the extent to which the public response is adaptive or resilient in major incidents? Do different kinds of major incident have different effects on the public's capacity for resilient behaviour? Also, what is the role of the professionals and authorities in facilitating and avoiding undermining resilient responses in the public?

In this chapter, I first summarise how understandings of the role of the public in emergencies have changed over time. Then I outline a conceptual framework, the social identity approach, that has proved fruitful for understanding how the public responds in these events. The focus here, and in the other chapters in this section of the book, is on behaviour. However, social identity processes also have implications for mental health, both via behaviour and directly. The chapter explains these connections and points to the other chapters that elaborate on these arguments, with empirical examples.

Representations of Public Behaviour in Emergencies and Disasters: From Mass Pathology to Collective Resilience

Early accounts of public responses to EITDDC suggested that a threat coupled with only limited opportunity for escape would lead to collective panic, defined as overreaction and impulsive and competitive behaviour, caused by fear [1]. Being in a crowd was said to magnify these effects through 'contagion'. In addition, in the aftermath of EITDDCs, survivors were said to be pathologically helpless and dependent – too stunned and passive to care for themselves [2]. There was also the notion that criminal behaviour, particularly in the form of looting, is inevitable in the wake of emergencies and disasters [3]. Chapter 8 in Section 1 of this book considers these and other common myths and misinterpretations.

These were not simply academic accounts. They grew from attempts to address practical problems, in particular the problem of troop disarray when under attack [4]. The concern that the public is likely to panic has been cited by authorities as a reason to vindicate withholding information about threats [5]. Expecting public passivity rationalises top-down command and control. Perceiving survivors' actions as disorderly and criminal justifies a coercive rather than humanitarian response [6].

These representations were problematised from relatively early in the history of scholarly accounts of behaviour. Thus Enrico Quarantelli has made the important point that there is no flight in many disasters, with the opposite reaction being the reality, with people often remaining in place or even approaching the threat [2]. Where there is flight, it cannot always be described as panic. And Charles Fritz noted the common occurrence of what he called 'therapeutic communities' [7]. Reversing the assumed roles of professionals and public, he stated 'Most of the initial search, rescue, and relief activities [following a disaster] are undertaken by disaster victims before the arrival of organized outside aid' ([7] p. 10).

Some public responses were found to be more adaptive than others; in some evacuations, people competed, whereas they cooperated in others [2]. What the early accounts missed were the key variables that made a difference. One of the major determining factors was the official response itself. Emergency response strategies based on assumptions of inherent vulnerability among the public could *create* this vulnerability that the authorities perceive as inherent in the public. For example, withholding information from the public increases public anxiety, distress, and even helplessness [8].

Representations of adaptive public response had long existed alongside accounts of collective pathology, at least in popular discourse. The 'Blitz spirit' is a well-known example; and 'Britain can take it' is another example from the Second World War (one which was rejected by its subjects when it was used by the authorities as an excuse for not providing support). However, in the UK there was a step change in recognising in policy the public's capacity for resilient behaviours in the 2000s. The Civil Contingencies Act 2004 (as amended) included legislating for a programme of 'community resilience'. Community resilience in the official guidance is defined as 'public empowered to harness local resources and expertise to help themselves and their communities to:

- Prepare, respond and recover from disruptive challenges, in a way that complements the activity of Category 1 and 2 emergency responders;
- Plan and adapt to long term social and environmental changes to ensure their future prosperity and resilience' [9].

The Civil Contingencies Act 2004, and the enhanced recognition of 'resilience' in the public, followed a series of major incidents – a fuel crisis, an outbreak of foot-and-mouth disease, serious flooding, and fears of pandemic flu. An important focus, however, was the threat of terrorism following the 9/11 attacks in the USA in 2001. In these cases and others anticipated in the future, the UK government understood that professional responders might not be able to get to the scene of the major incident in sufficient time or numbers. The public had to fill the gap. In the new approach, therefore, the public were not just 'victims' or even simply 'survivors', but potentially active participants in preparedness, response, and recovery [6,10].

There are three points to make about resilient communities and their official recognition. The first point is that at the core of this public involvement is the social support – 'help', in the official language – that people provide for each other during and after major incidents. Research has identified the different forms that such support can take. Thus Krzysztof Kaniasty and Fran Norris distinguish between informational, emotional, and practical/tangible support [11]. Different forms of support have different effects or functions. From the perspective of disaster risk reduction, it is practical support that is crucial for recovery (e.g., [12]). From the perspective of psychology and mental health, research shows that perceived support (belief in the availability of support) contributes more than received support (actual receipt of help) to wellbeing (see Chapter 20). This suggests that people's perception of support matters. Indeed, practical support is interpretable as feeling cared for, which means that it has a dimension of emotional support, and this contributes to mental health and recovery.

The second point is that 'therapeutic communities' have temporal limits. Even the most 'prepared' communities have finite emotional and practical resources. In Chapter 21, Kaniasty suggests that levels of support provided decline as the continuing need for support surpasses its availability. In addition, chronic distress and the potential for conflict eventually erode supportive relationships. After a flood, for example, continued struggles to claim insurance and rebuild one's home are significant secondary stressors, but the new sense of community, and hence sources of support, may have declined months earlier [13]. Communities can be sustained or re-created, but this is difficult and requires conscious effort and organisation, rather than being 'spontaneous' like the 'therapeutic community' that emerged in the response phase (see Chapters 23 and 24).

The third point is that, despite the progress in theory and in policy, tensions continue to exist in the authorities' recognition and understanding of the role of the public in responses to major incidents. References to 'panic' in official guidance have declined, but they still coexist with representations of an adaptive public in some guidance documents [10]. Where the public is represented as having qualities of psychosocial resilience in recent official guidance, it has tended to be in the form of individual people, even as the guidance refers to 'communities', *collective* entities, as the necessary basis for resilience. Despite the fact that social support among members of the public takes place in crowds and arises from crowd processes (see Chapters 22 and 23), the 'crowd' as a positive force is absent from the guidance. Where 'the public' and 'the community' are depicted as having resilient qualities, they are still subordinate to the emergency services and the other relevant formal organisations. Thus, although some scholarly accounts of the role of the public use terms such as 'civilian first responders', 'zero responders', and 'the fourth emergency service' (see Chapter 22) [6], the public is also reduced to being a recipient of 'services'.

From Social Identity to Social Cure

The varieties, contingencies, and tensions in the meaning of 'community resilience' mean that there is still a need to disseminate and to understand the psychology underlying public responses in EITDDC. The chapters in Section 4 of this book provide a theoretical framework for that underlying psychology, as well as a substantial body of research evidence. The main focus here is on the variables that shape the extent to which the people who are affected by an emergency provide support for each other, as well as the form of that support. Those people closest to the threat are the ones most at risk, but they are also the people most able to provide support. They have a personal stake in trying to escape rather than helping others, but, surprisingly often, they remain at the scene and try to support others, including strangers. Over time, people outside the immediate area of an emergency may also provide support, and it is important to understand whether this response is shaped by the same psychological processes as in the case of the behaviour of 'survivors'. In each case – that is, survivors' behaviour and wider solidarity – understanding the process can inform and improve policy and practice.

The modern theory of groups in social psychology is known as the social identity approach [14]. The earliest theories depicted groups as psychologically regressive, and the dominant theories until the 1980s reduced groups to interpersonal processes. By contrast, in the social identity approach, groups are understood as based on shared cognitive representations, or self-categories, which are neither inferior nor reducible to personal psychology. As well as our personal identities, we can define ourselves according to group memberships (e.g., English, Manchester City supporter, teacher). Where these group memberships matter to us, they operate as social identities, and act as drivers of cognition, emotion, and behaviour. Specifically, as identity shifts from 'I' to 'we', so the norms, values, and interests through which we understand the world, and which shape our behaviour, shift from our personal ones to those associated with the group. Different groups have different group norms, which can explain why the same person behaves very differently in one context (e.g., at a football match) compared with another (e.g., in an ambulance crew).

Seeing those around us as a 'we' or 'us' has consequences for how we relate to them [15]. We feel greater trust and care towards them if they are part of the 'we' than if they are not. We assume that these others see the world as we do and share our goals. We also have greater expectations of support from them. All this translates into greater intimacy in behaviour, more interaction, more mutual social influence, and more support given.

Furthermore, shared interests, norms, goals and expectations of support mean that coordination becomes easier. People can act as one because, psychologically, they *are* one [4].

These principles have been applied to make sense of a series of group phenomena, including ingroup preference, collective action, hostility and harmony between groups, group productivity, conformity, minority influence, and crowd behaviour [16]. In organisational settings, the social approach has helped to explain effective leadership, organisational citizenship, and successful and unsuccessful mergers [16].

Since the late 2000s, the most significant development in the social identity approach, and perhaps the most significant development in social psychology in this period, has been the application of these principles to health and wellbeing [14]. Across a range of health and mental health conditions, social identity processes have been found to mitigate experiences and outcomes. The core mechanisms whereby social identity can enhance wellbeing and reduce ill-health are connectedness, meaning, social support, and efficacy [14]. In Chapter 20 in this book, Orla Muldoon provides a powerful example, showing how social identity processes can interact with post-traumatic stress following an earthquake. Among participants, social identity resources were associated with less distress, and group efficacy was associated with post-traumatic growth.

Our understanding of behavioural responses of the public to EITDDC has developed through a combination of social identity/social cure principles with findings from studies of crowd behaviour. In this approach, shared social identity, which includes that based on the sense of common fate that people experience when they are affected by an emergency, provides motives to support others who are affected. Shared social identity also creates expectations that these other people are likely to provide support for oneself. Expected support, in turn, is the basis of psychological outcomes such as group efficacy and wellbeing [17]. This approach has now helped to explain public behaviour across a wide variety of major emergencies and incidents, including earthquakes, floods, fires, terrorist attacks, and sinking ships [4], and it has helped to explain behaviour both in the immediate response (see Chapter 22) and in the recovery phase (see Chapter 23) after emergencies. In events such as these, membership of psychological groups is typically adaptive: group membership can help people to escape, survive and recover. Acting as an individual person in these situations is often less adaptive: think of people competing as they try to evacuate through a doorway.

If social identity is a driver of the support and cooperation needed among members of the public in an emergency, then it is understandable that people who are active in community groups set up to respond to the emergency consciously invoke shared identity as they try to mobilise others. The need for such a strategy becomes more important over time as the situational affordances (i.e., common fate) that led people spontaneously to see themselves as a group ebb during the recovery period. Chapters 22 and 23 illustrate this strategic dimension of social identity in the case of floods and COVID-19 mutual aid groups, respectively.

In addition, shared social identity can help to explain why members of the public who are not affected by the emergency or major incident also try to offer solidarity. Here, too, organisers of solidarity campaigns can consciously invoke common fate or common identity as a way of demonstrating the relevance of a disaster to others outside the emergency or disaster (see Chapter 26).

The value of the social identity approach is evidenced by its ability to generate practical recommendations for facilitating effective public participation in EPRR. Practical recommendations based on the social identity approach have been employed in the NATO guidelines on psychosocial care [18], Department of Health guidance, event safety training [4], and UK guidance produced in response to the COVID-19 pandemic. In each case the key ideas include recognising and facilitating social identity through communication in particular. Perhaps the most successful example of the translation of social identity principles into guidance and training for emergency response is Holly Carter's work on mass casualty decontamination following CBRN incidents (see Chapter 25) [19]. Here a programme of research provided evidence that effective communication with the public could significantly increase the efficiency of the decontamination process. This has led to a change in perspective when training responders, from regarding casualties as passive recipients of healthcare, to be controlled or coerced, to recognising the public as an invaluable resource or partner to be engaged and informed.

Caveats and Conclusions

Practical need and modern psychological theory agree that the public has the capacity to be proactive in EPRR. In emergencies, members of the public have the psychological capability, and often the motivation, to provide each other with the practical and emotional support needed to reduce distress, to protect each other from further harm, to treat injuries, and to save lives. But are they partners to, equals with, or subordinate to the professionals? There are different perspectives on this question [10], and indeed even when there is an emphasis on the capability of the public this is not necessarily without problems – at least for the authorities.

First, there is the problem of 'convergence' [20]. This manifests itself in people, usually not survivors themselves, offering assistance that is not needed or appropriate, and indeed which may be obstructive (e.g., donations that are unsuitable and which volunteers then have to spend valuable hours sorting through) [6]. Second, collective resilience of the public is a double-edged sword for the authorities. The more independent and empowered members of the public become, the greater is the possibility that they are able to act upon purposes and aspirations which the authorities did not anticipate or wish for, including operating without a need for the authorities [21]. A final caveat concerns the concept of 'resilience' itself. The idea of a public that can withstand attacks and privation has in the past been used as an excuse for government neglect, as referred to earlier in this chapter (e.g., the attitude that 'Britain can take it'

during the Second World War) [22]. We should continue to beware of its usage by the authorities.

The research evidence shows that public participation in response to emergencies is common and should be expected. Its expression is in forms of social support. This chapter argues that the basis of this adaptive response is largely in group processes of shared identity. Although there may be some problems and risk inherent in public participation in the responses made to emergencies, because of its typicality and overall benefit it is important that the authorities plan for it, work with it, and harness and facilitate it where possible. The chapters in this section of the book apply these principles to different types of major incident and explain the implications for responders, authorities, and the public.

References

1. Quarantelli EL. The sociology of panic. In *International Encyclopedia of the Social and Behavioural Sciences* (eds NJ Smelser, PB Baltes):11020-3. Pergamon Press, 2001.

2. Quarantelli EL. Images of withdrawal behavior in disasters: some basic misconceptions. *Soc Probl* 1960; **8**: 68–79.

3. Alexander DE. Misconception as a barrier to teaching about disasters. *Prehosp Disaster Med* 2007; **22**: 95–103.

4. Drury J. The role of social identity processes in mass emergency behaviour: an integrative review. *Eur Rev Soc Psychol* 2018; **29**: 38–81.

5. Proulx G, Sime JD. To prevent 'panic' in an underground emergency: why not tell people the truth? *Fire Safety Sci* 1991; **3**: 843–52.

6. Drury J, Carter H, Cocking C, Ntontis E, Tekin Guven S, Amlôt R. Facilitating collective psychosocial resilience in the public in emergencies: twelve recommendations based on the social identity approach. *Front Public Health* 2019; **7**: 141.

7. Fritz CE. *Disasters and Mental Health: Therapeutic Principles Drawn from Disaster Studies.* Disaster Research Center, 1996.

8. Glass TA, Schoch-Spana M. Bioterrorism and the people: how to vaccinate a city against panic. *Clin Infect Dis* 2002; **34**: 217–23.

9. HM Government. *Community Resilience Development Framework.* HM Government, 2019 (www.gov.uk/government/publications/community-resilience-development-framework).

10. Drury J, Novelli D, Stott C. Representing crowd behaviour in emergency planning guidance: 'mass panic' or collective resilience? *Resilience* 2013; **1**: 18–37.

11. Kaniasty K, Norris FH. In search of altruistic community: patterns of social support mobilization following Hurricane Hugo. *Am J Community Psychol* 1995; **23**: 447–77.

12. Dinh NC, Ubukata F, Tan NQ, Ha VH. How do social connections accelerate post-flood recovery? Insights from a survey of rural households in central Vietnam. *Int J Disaster Risk Reduct* 2021; **61**: 102342.

13. Williams R, Ntontis E, Alfadhli K, Drury J, Amlôt R. A social model of secondary stressors in relation to disasters, major incidents and conflict: implications for practice. *Int J Disaster Risk Reduct* 2021; **63**: 102436.

14. Haslam C, Jetten J, Cruwys T, Dingle GA, Haslam SA. *The New Psychology of Health: Unlocking the Social Cure.* Routledge, 2018.

15. Hopkins N, Reicher S, Stevenson C, Pandey K, Shankar S, Tewari S. Social relations in crowds: recognition, validation and solidarity. *Eur J Soc Psychol* 2019; **49**: 1283–97.

16. Haslam SA. *Psychology in Organizations* 2nd ed. Sage, 2012.

17. Ntontis E, Drury J, Amlôt R, Rubin GJ, Williams R, Saavedra P. Collective resilience in the disaster recovery period: emergent social identity and observed social support are associated with collective efficacy, well-being, and the provision of social support. *Br J Soc Psychol* 2020; **60**: 2075–95.

18. NATO/EAPC. *Psychosocial Care for People Affected by Disasters and Major Incidents: A Model for Designing, Delivering and Managing Psychosocial Services for People Involved in Major*

Incidents, Conflict, Disasters and Terrorism. NATO/EAPC, 2009.

19. Carter H, Drury J, Rubin GJ, Williams R, Amlôt R. Applying crowd psychology to develop recommendations for the management of mass decontamination. *Health Secur* 2015; **13**: 45–53.

20. Fritz CE, Mathewson JH. *Convergence Behavior in Disasters: A Problem in Social Control.* National Academy of Sciences-National Research Council, 1957.

21. Solnit R. *A Paradise Built in Hell: The Extraordinary Communities That Arise in Disaster.* Penguin, 2009.

22. Williams R, Kaufman KR. Narrative review of the COVID-19, healthcare and healthcarers thematic series. *BJPsych Open* 2022; **8**: e34.

Chapter

20

Social Identity and Traumatic Stress in the Context of an Earthquake and a Pandemic

Understanding the Roles of Shared and Isolating Social Experiences

Orla Muldoon

Introduction

The robust cross-cultural and historical evidence that exposure to extremely traumatic events can trigger extreme psychological distress stands in direct contrast to a growing awareness that experience of traumatic events does not always lead to adverse social and psychological outcomes [1]. Extreme psychological distress, which manifests with symptoms such as psychological numbing, experiencing of the trauma, and altered cognitions and mood, is often referred to as post-traumatic stress disorder (PTSD) [2]. However, this is only one outcome of traumatic experience. Resilience in the face of extreme stress is also commonplace [3], as is post-traumatic growth – a sense of personal strength or enhancement that arises from surviving adversity [4]. We are remarkably poor at predicting who is likely to be adversely affected by trauma [5], and psychological interventions to support people affected have limited efficacy [6,7]. In this chapter, I review how trauma is structured by group life and consider the role that social identity-based resources may play in explaining trauma trajectories.

Despite its regular usage, there is limited clarity about the definition of trauma. Valery Krupnik delineates two definitions [8]. One tends to be very narrow and is located within the DSM-5 PSTD diagnosis. The second broader definition proposed by Krupnik grounds trauma within general theories of stress [8]. Similarly, in line with Krupnik, I here use the term trauma to refer to a process that is part of a wider stress response. One element of this process consists of the traumatic experiences that are a form of extreme stress. This understanding of stress is grounded in the integrated social identity model of stress, which places groups and social identities at the heart of response [9]. Although my interest here is in

traumatic responses such as mental health and well-being generally, and post-traumatic stress (PTS) symptoms and resilience specifically [2], this view moves away from seeing traumatic experiences as a source of psychopathology. Rather it highlights trauma as a process that may result in psychological changes in response to extreme experiences or adverse social conditions.

Researchers from a range of disciplines, including psychology, epidemiology, and political science, have observed that health risks are not equally distributed. Members of some groups are much more likely to be at risk for trauma and poor health outcomes than are members of other groups [10,11]. However, these unequal health risks have typically been studied by focusing on the demographics of a population, rather than on psychological group memberships as studied by social identity theorists [12]. Using a social identity approach to reimagine trauma as a collective phenomenon requires more than coding social and demographic factors. It highlights that traumatic experiences can arise from 'mere categorisation'. The risks associated with certain group memberships, such as being born in a war-torn nation, or gender at birth, as well as affecting risk, shape the available resources for dealing with the trauma. In so doing these groups memberships also shape group members' ability to subsequently manage their experiences [13]. Typically identification with groups involves trade-offs. Low-status groups, for example, are disadvantaged by their social position, but their minoritised position can result in greater identification with similar people, who in turn become an important source of social support [14]. I conclude the chapter by thinking about the implications of these forces for facilitating those negotiating trauma and adversity.

Table 20.1 Mean post-traumatic stress (PTS), experience, and social identity resource scores by ethnic group in a study of Nepali earthquake survivors (n = 399)

*Ethnic/caste group	Chhetri	Brahim	Janajati	Dalit	Other
Mean number of earthquake loss experiences (Scale 0–5 events)	2.34	2.44	2.84	2.57	2.84
PTS cases within each group (%)	47.3	45	59.8	57.8	66.2
Sense of shared experience (measured from 1 ('not at all') to 7 ('very much') on a Likert scale)	5.08	5.04	5.20	5.63	5.52
Collective efficacy (measured from 1 ('not at all') to 7 ('very much') on a Likert scale)	4.78	4.81	4.57	4.38	4.19
Community identification (measured from 1 ('not at all') to 7 ('very much') on a Likert scale)	5.68	5.61	5.75	5.74	5.32
N	26	49	72	11	47

* Note: Chhetri and Brahim are considered high-status groups, whereas Janajati, Dalit, and others are seen as lower-status groups in Nepal.

Traumatic Experiences Are Structured by Group Life

Our experiences of trauma are shaped by collective sociocultural forces [13,15,16]. We only need to think of the experience that various groups of people have had over the course of the COVID-19 pandemic to illustrate this point. Despite the public health emphasis on solidarity and 'being in it together', research shows that experience of the pandemic has varied systematically. Those groups that cannot afford the luxuries of social distancing, self-isolation, or even running water and soap are made infinitely more vulnerable to the pandemic [17]. These groups have felt the worst of the pandemic, and their experience has been compounded by inequality of access to healthcare and vaccines across the globe as the pandemic has continued [18]. Nations in the Global South that can be thought of as populations or groups with little access to vaccines and healthcare have been brutalised by COVID-19. Nations in the Global North with better vaccine and healthcare infrastructure have been offered meaningful medical support and containment. In short, in this pandemic, national group membership matters and those who are citizens of poorer nations are affected by the disease at a greater rate and pace than the general population because of the material circumstances of their lives [18].

As well as seeing this patterned risk of trauma across nations, within-nation differences are also evident [13,16]. For example, being a member of a socio-economically deprived group within a nation also adds to trauma risk. In our work in Nepal, we have shown how ethnic group membership, sometimes still referred to as 'caste', was linked to experience of trauma and loss as a consequence of the earthquake in 2015 [19]. In a study of 399 people living and working in villages close to the epicentre of the quake, it was apparent that ethnic/cast group membership had a significant main effect on reported personal injury and loss experiences. As a consequence, those people in the lowest-status ethnic and caste groups were more likely to report symptoms indicative of clinically significant PTSD (see Table 20.1) [19]. Traumatic experience is profoundly bound up with our group memberships. This is a widespread phenomenon. Less powerful groups are, on average, more likely to be at risk of political violence, gendered violence, the effects of natural hazards such as earthquakes, and pandemics. This applies to national, ethnic, and caste group membership, as well as to gender and class, all of which relate to risk of traumatic experience.

Trauma, Status, and Group Resources

There is growing awareness that experience of traumatic events does not always have long-lasting negative implications for mental health [5]. The majority of people who encounter extreme and distressing events prove to be resilient to their impact [20]. For many people, the pandemic fits the definition of a traumatic event in so far as it threatens their lives and the lives of others whom they care about. Yet there is also evidence of considerable psychological resilience across time in those people tasked with responding to pandemics [21]. Indeed resilience is the main response to the range of adversities that people experience because of war, political violence, rape, sexual assault, accidents, and disaster. For example, although 50% of people in Northern Ireland have been exposed to more than one traumatic incident as a consequence of political violence [22], only 1 in 10 people show symptoms severe enough to warrant a diagnosis of PTSD [23]. Accordingly, understanding the basis of psychological resilience to trauma is no less important than understanding vulnerability.

Perhaps because trauma experience has been understood at the level of individual people in much of the existing literature, the direct impact of the traumatic experience on PTS symptoms is well documented. However, traumatic experience also changes relationships within groups and group members' definitions of themselves. Returning to our survey of people affected by the earthquake in Nepal, this study also examined the link between experience of trauma and people's understanding of group resources such as identification with their community ($r = 0.204$, $p < 0.001$) and their sense of shared social relations with others affected by the earthquake ($r = 0.114$, $p < 0.01$) [19]. Those people who reported greater experience of the earthquake were also more likely to have increased identification with their community and a better sense of shared social relations with others similarly affected. Similarly, John Drury and colleagues in another study of earthquake survivors found that identities emerged in its aftermath that could facilitate social support. In this way we can see that experience of trauma involves trade-offs [24]. Although traumatic experience during disasters is clearly a cause of distress, it can also result in stronger group-based connections to people who are similarly affected (see Chapter 22). Also, of course, strong supportive group relationships and increased identification with people who are similarly affected are an important part of understanding resilience to trauma [9,21].

Alexander Haslam believes that status is centrally important to understanding identities [25]. In general, minority identities are more likely to be chronically salient [26], and this brings with it an awareness on the part of group members of their positionality in society as a minority. Majority or dominant group members, on the other hand, are often less mindful of intergroup relations in ways that make them less aware of their identity position vis-à-vis others [27]. Indeed majority identities can be so

ubiquitous that group members have difficulty appreciating them as 'social' identities [28]. For this reason, majority and minority group members approach and adapt to trauma differently in part because their group status affects psychological accessibility of the group-based social identity resources.

Minorities or low-status groups typically have more interdependent models of agency [29]. Such models of agency tend to support interconnection and reliance on others, and are likely to promote action where it is normative to respond to the expectations and influence of others [30]. Returning to our work in Nepal, then, we see that social identity resources associated with ethnic/caste group membership (see Table 20.1) are relevant for negotiating trauma. Indeed, consistent with greater interdependence of low-status groups, the members of the low-status Dalit, Janajati, and other groups had significantly higher levels of community identification and a significantly stronger sense of shared experience than the high-status groups during the earthquake. These identity resources also offer strong protection against PTS in the face of trauma [19]. On the other hand, collective efficacy – the sense that the collective can overcome the situation – did not appear to mitigate PTS symptoms. Perhaps because the situation was so uncontrollable and unpredictable, higher collective efficacy amplified PTS symptoms [19]. This attribute was more in evidence in higher-status groups, and although it was associated with greater distress it was also associated with stronger post-traumatic growth.

We also examined the effects of group status on people's responses to the COVID-19 crisis in recently completed studies in Ireland and the UK [31]. Here again we found that social identity resources interacted with group status. Minority group members who saw themselves as less prototypical of their national group reported comparatively lower solidarity with the national community at the time of the emergence of the COVID-19 crisis. As public health advice in Ireland and the UK was often framed with reference to the nation, this had a knock-on effect on people's willingness to engage with the COVID-19 health advice. In this way it would appear that as well as the material realities that have affected minority group members' risk of contracting COVID-19 during the pandemic, group status affects health via prototypicality and solidarity available to minority groups. In short, social identity-based solidarity is an important resource for health, resilience, and adjustment during times of stress and as people negotiate trauma [32].

Conclusion

Our analysis of the value of a social identity lens for understanding trauma highlights a number of guiding principles that emerge from the available research. Current practice places emphasis on what is often termed *interpersonal* support, such as psychotherapy or counselling [33]. Among other things, this focuses on working to facilitate supports within existing families and dyads. I agree that families can offer interpersonal support, but also note that they are important proximal groups. An important guiding principle emerging from the available research is an orientation to trauma support that also considers broader groups and social identities, beyond families and dyads, that can provide similar support in the aftermath of trauma. It will often be important, for example, to protect the integrity of broader social identities such as those associated with work, religion, or ethnic groups. Access to these group memberships represents an important resource as people negotiate trauma. In reality this means that efforts to keep those affected by trauma nested within existing supportive occupational, community, religious, or ethnic groupings are imperative.

In practice, implementing this guidance is not straightforward. Those people most affected by trauma are often on the margins, and/or made marginal, by their experience. Traumatic events often threaten people's tangible and psychological resources (see Chapter 54) [34]. Resource loss after trauma can compound socioeconomic disadvantage, sparking a downward spiral of loss [35]. Trauma can displace people and force their removal from valued social groups. The COVID-19 pandemic has brought this issue into sharp relief. Concern regarding disease spread has separated many people from their networks of support. Moreover, the tendency for powerless or low-status groups to be affected by trauma means that their sense of collective efficacy in the aftermath of trauma is often depleted. A final principle arising from this analysis is that traumatic experience can be disempowering, and this is particularly likely to be the case for low-status groups. In an ontologically insecure world, our own positionality can mean that there is comfort in pathologising those adversely affected by trauma [36], and in our eagerness to help and alleviate individual suffering we can inadvertently disempower marginal groups. All actions to support groups affected by trauma need to promote the group's sense of empowerment and agency, as this is the central resource from which people draw strength.

The trajectories through trauma include PTS, resilience, and growth. Although symptoms of stress may often emerge first, it is important to remember that other outcomes may also co-emerge and even coexist with PTS symptoms. Medium- and longer-terms outcomes such as resilience and growth can follow distress. PTS-based distress may even be a necessary precursor to post-traumatic growth [37]. Moreover, because trauma can have an impact on social identity resources, it may also have longer-term impacts. For example, we have shown how traumatic experience can affect feelings of identity-based threat in Northern Ireland and adversely affect attitudes to peace and reconciliation [22]. In addition, in work with survivors of gender-based violence, we offer preliminary evidence that trauma can result in identity-based activism and psychological resilience [38]. There is no denying that working with marginal groups can be very challenging. However, the social identity analysis offered here attends to the interplay of the social and the psychological, and this offers an approach to empowered support for even the most marginal groups that are negotiating trauma [39].

References

1. Summerfield D. The invention of post-traumatic stress disorder and the social usefulness of a psychiatric category. *BMJ* 2001; 322: 95–8.

2. American Psychiatric Association. *Diagnostic and Statistical Manual of mental disorders: DSM-5.* American Psychiatric Association, 2013.

3. Charuvastra A, Cloitre M. 2008. Social bonds and posttraumatic stress disorder. *Annu Rev Psychol* 2008; 59: 301–28.

4. Tedeschi RG, Calhoun L. Posttraumatic growth: a new perspective on psychotraumatology. *Psychiatric Times* 2004; 21: 58–60.

5. Nemeroff CB, Bremner JD, Foa EB, Mayberg HS, North CS, Stein MB. Posttraumatic stress disorder: a state-of-the-science review. *J Psychiatr Res* 2006; 40: 1–21.

6. Bisson JI, Roberts NP, Andrew M, Cooper R, Lewis C. Psychological therapies for chronic post-traumatic stress disorder (PTSD) in adults. *Cochrane Database Syst Rev* 2013; 2013: CD003388.

7. Borek AJ, Abraham C, Smith JR, Greaves CJ, Tarrant M. A checklist to improve reporting of group-based behaviour-change interventions. *BMC Public Health* 2015; 15: 963.

8. Krupnik V. Trauma or adversity? *Traumatology* 2019; 25: 256.

9. Haslam SA, Reicher S. Stressing the group: social identity and the unfolding dynamics of responses to stress. *J Appl Psychol* 2006; 91: 1037.

10. Marmot M. The health gap: the challenge of an unequal world. *Lancet* 2015; 386: 2442–4.

11. Wilkinson RG, Pickett KE. Income inequality and population health: a review and explanation of the evidence. *Soc Sci Med* 2006; 62: 1768–84.

12. Haslam C, Jetten J, Cruwys T, Dingle GA, Haslam SA. *The New Psychology of Health: Unlocking the Social Cure*. Routledge, 2018.

13. Muldoon OT, Lowe RD, Jetten J, Cruwys T, Haslam SA. Personal and political: post-traumatic stress through the lens of social identity, power, and politics. *Polit Psychol* 2021; 42: 501–33.

14. Schmitt MT, Branscombe NR, Postmes T, Garcia A. The consequences of perceived discrimination for psychological well-being: a meta-analytic review. *Psychol Bull* 2014; 140: 921.

15. Muldoon OT, Lowe RD. Social identity, groups, and post-traumatic stress disorder. *Polit Psychol* 2012; 33: 259–73.

16. Muldoon OT. Understanding the impact of political violence in childhood: a theoretical review using a social identity approach. *Clin Psychol Rev* 2013; 33: 929–39.

17. Chung RY, Dong D, Li MM. Socioeconomic gradient in health and the covid-19 outbreak. *BMJ* 2020; 369: m1329.

18. Atchison C, Bowman L, Eaton J, Imai N, Redd R, Pristera P. et al. *Report 10: Public Response to UK Government Recommendations on COVID-19: Population Survey, 17–18 March 2020*. Imperial College London, 2020.

19. Muldoon OT, Acharya K, Jay S, Adhikari K, Pettigrew J, Lowe RD. Community identity and collective efficacy: a social cure for traumatic stress in post-earthquake Nepal. *Eur J Soc Psychol* 2017; 47: 904–15.

20. Agaibi CE, Wilson JP. Trauma, PTSD, and resilience: a review of the literature. *Trauma Violence Abuse* 2005; 6: 195–216.

21. Killgore WD, Taylor EC, Cloonan SA, Dailey NS. Psychological resilience during the COVID-19 lockdown. *Psychiatry Res* 2020; 291: 113216.

22. Schmid K, Muldoon OT. Perceived threat, social identification, and psychological well-being: the effects of political conflict exposure. *Polit Psychol* 2015; 36: 75–92.

23. Muldoon OT, Downes C. Social identification and post-traumatic stress symptoms in post-conflict Northern Ireland. *Br J Psychiatry* 2007; 191: 146–9.

24. Drury J, Brown R, González R, Miranda D. Emergent social identity and observing social support predict social support provided by survivors in a disaster: solidarity in the 2010 Chile earthquake. *Eur J Soc Psychol* 2016; 46: 209–23.

25. Haslam SA. *Psychology in Organizations*. Sage, 2004.

26. Wang K, Dovidio JF. Perceiving and confronting sexism: the causal role of gender identity salience. *Psychol Women Q* 2017; 41: 65–76.

27. Schmitt MT, Davies K, Hung M, Wright SC. Identity moderates the effects of Christmas displays on mood, self-esteem, and inclusion. *J Exp Soc Psychol* 2010; 46: 1017–22.

28. DiAngelo R. *White Fragility: Why It's So Hard for White People to Talk About Racism*. Beacon Press, 2018.

29. Jay S, Muldoon OT. Social class and models of agency: independent and interdependent agency as educational (dis) advantage. *J Commun Appl Soc Psychol* 2018; 28: 318–31.

30. Stephens NM, Fryberg SA, Markus HR, Johnson CS, Covarrubias R. Unseen disadvantage: how American universities' focus on independence undermines the academic performance of first-generation college students. *J Pers Soc Psychol* 2012; 102: 1178–97.

31. Foran AM, Roth J, Jay S, Griffin, SM, Maher, PJ, McHugh C, et al. Solidarity matters: prototypicality and minority and majority adherence to national COVID-19 Health Advice. *Int Rev Soc Psychol* 2021; 34: 25.

32. Kearns M, Muldoon OT, Msetfi RM, Surgenor PW. Darkness into light? Identification with the crowd at a suicide prevention fundraiser promotes well-being amongst participants. *Eur J Soc Psychol* 2017; 47: 878–88.

33. Lee E, Bowles K. Navigating treatment recommendations for PTSD: a rapid review. *Int J Ment Health* 2023: 52: 4–44.

34. Hobfoll SE. The influence of culture, community, and the nested-self in the stress process: advancing conservation of resources theory. *Appl Psychol* 2001; 50: 337–421.

35. Heath NM, Hall BJ, Canetti D, Hobfoll SE. Exposure to political violence, psychological distress, resource loss, and benefit finding as predictors of domestic violence

among Palestinians. *Psychol Trauma* 2013; 5: 366–76.

36. Kinnvall C. Globalization and religious nationalism: self, identity, and the search for ontological security. *Polit Psychol* 2004; 25: 741–67.

37. Muldoon OT, Haslam SA, Haslam C, Cruwys T, Kearns M, Jetten J. The social psychology of responses to trauma: social identity pathways associated with divergent traumatic responses. *Eur Rev Soc Psychol* 2019; 30: 311–48.

38. Haslam C. Latilla T, Muldoon,O, Cruwys T, Kearns M. Multiple group membership supports resilience and growth in response to violence and abuse. *J Commun Appl Soc Psychol* 2021; 32: 241–57.

39. Jay S. Winterburn M, Jha J, Sah, AK, Choudhary R, Muldoon OT. A resilience building collaboration: a social identity empowerment approach to trauma management in leprosy-affected communities. *Psychol Trauma* 2022; 14: 940–47.

Chapter

21

Mobilisation and Deterioration of Social Support Following Disasters Resulting from Natural and Human-Induced Hazards

Krzysztof Kaniasty and Beata Urbańska

Introduction

Disasters resulting from natural hazards and/or human activity cause substantial and enduring psychological and social harm. People who have experienced disasters may show a myriad of psychological problems, including symptoms of post-traumatic stress, grief, depression, anxiety, stress-related health costs, and other declines in psychological and social wellbeing. However, severe levels of these problems are typically observed in a minority of exposed people. Indeed many empirical studies that examine people's mental health after disasters have documented impressive resilience among the majority of survivors [1]. Indisputably, numerous psychological and social resources guard people against deleterious impacts of calamities and empower them to recover successfully and show resilience. Chief among them is the personal and communal capacity to protect, maintain, and augment in times of adversity survivors' perceptions of being supported and belonging to a cohesive social group and community. People's efforts to cope with the oppressive forces of catastrophic events become a shared responsibility and cooperative action. In the end, success or failure in coping with collective crises depends to a large extent on interpersonal and social functioning.

Research on public responses to disasters often speaks of two very different, and at times conflicting, interpersonal and social dynamics that routinely emerge in the aftermath of disasters. Immediately after the impact, communities of survivors, professional supporters, and empathic witnesses rush into action, become resources for each other, and engage in high levels of mutual helping. Often, however, this heroic and compassionate post-disaster sense of togetherness is short-lived, and inevitably it ceases. The sense of unity in shared suffering is frequently surpassed by a gradual realisation of depletion of resources, competition, fatigue, and solitude during the arduous recovery. It may seem a paradox that the milieu of post-disaster dynamics is a juxtaposition of contrasting processes of mobilisation and deterioration of interpersonal and community resources.

One way of empirically capturing interpersonal and community dynamics of disasters has been strongly influenced by the literature on social support. Social support has been routinely referred to as interpersonal connections that provide people with *actual help* and *embed them* into a web of social relationships that are *perceived* as caring and readily available in times of need [2]. This broad definition of social support is useful because it clearly identifies three distinct operational and measurable facets of social support – received social support (i.e., being actually helped by others in times of need), social embeddedness (i.e., types and frequency of interpersonal and community connections), and perceived support (i.e., the belief that help would be available if needed). Empirical examinations offer a wealth of evidence documenting that a path of post-disaster mobilisation of resources emerges instantaneously in the domain of *received support*, whereas the path of a lingering sense of deterioration of resources occurs in the domains of *perceived support* and *social embeddedness* [3].

Mobilisation of Received Social Support After Disasters

Post-disaster mobilisation of received social support epitomises both the proverbial alarm reaction stage and the fundamental human expectation that, if help is needed, supporters will provide it. Abundance of mutual helping engrossing whole communities in the aftermath of disasters has been described with numerous heartening labels (e.g., democracy of distress, post-disaster utopia, universal equanimity), with the notion of 'altruistic community' being the most defining [4]. Frequent features of such collectives are heightened internal solidarity, a sense of unity, disappearance of community conflicts, utopian mood, an overall sense of altruism, and heroic action. Class, ethnic, and social barriers may disappear, but only temporarily [3].

There are rules and patterns governing mobilization of social support after disasters. The rule of relative needs gives priority to survivors who experience the greatest disaster exposure, operationalised as tangible losses and experience of trauma e.g., [5,6]. Yet altruistic communities are not governed in the most egalitarian ways and cannot escape pre-existing and emerging societal and/or local stratifications of inclusion and exclusion. In receiving support, the rule of relative advantage or disadvantage typically favours people who are younger, female, married, more educated, and have access to larger support networks, or exhibit greater comfort with regard to help-seeking e.g., [5–7]. A strong sense of common identity of shared suffering thrusts survivors into prosocial behaviour; regrettably, however, its scope may be narrowed to in-groups based on salient categorizations related to economic status, ethnicity and nationality, and other social and political status-quo entitlements e.g., [8]. These rules and patterns (i.e., interactions of the extent of disaster exposure with advantages/disadvantages in support receipt that are reflected in patterns of neglect or patterns of concern) of informal and formal aid distribution saliently underscore the austere reality that not all survivors are fully included in post-disaster altruistic communities e.g., [5,9].

Historically, the literature on disasters asserts that the increased benevolence and community cohesion post crisis carry with them 'therapeutic features' that might result in an 'amplified rebound' effect [10]. In other words, these intensified expressions of communal concern and support for each other may alleviate the adverse social and psychological consequences of disasters (hence another label – therapeutic community). Consistently with the spirit of therapeutic communities, research has found that receipt of post-disaster social support is positively associated with a subsequent sense of community solidarity [11], and other favourable appraisals of interpersonal (e.g., perceived social support) and community relationships (e.g., community cohesion, beliefs in the benevolence of people, efficacy of mutual helping) [12]. Ultimately, from the viewpoint of general social support theory and research, the therapeutic value of actually receiving social support would be empirically supported if greater amounts of received help after disasters were protective of the psychological wellbeing of survivors. Recent years have brought an increase in the number of investigations examining people's receipt of social support after disasters. Greater amounts of received social support were shown to exert a salutary direct effect on the mental health of survivors e.g., [9,11,13], and/ or most benefited those people who experienced greater exposure to the destructive forces of disasters (i.e., they had a stressor-buffering effect) e.g., [14–16]. It should be noted, however, that there are limits to these affirmative effects because they are often circumscribed by the type of social support received, the respondents' characteristics, or assessed outcomes. For example, Jonathan Platt and colleagues showed that only emotional received support was associated with lower levels of post-traumatic stress, whereas tangible and informational received support yielded null effects [13]. More strikingly, Damodar Suar and colleagues reported that received emotional support protected tsunami survivors from greater levels of symptoms of post-traumatic stress disorder (PTSD), whereas greater quantities of received help that was tangible and informational were associated with more distress [9,13]. Outcomes of this kind are not uncommon in the empirical literature on social support received following disasters e.g., [17], as well as in other contexts, but they are not necessarily perplexing (e.g., psychological suffering constitutes a clear cue for social networks to mobilise their supportive efforts). The complexities of the available findings concerning received social support following disasters call for newer approaches that go beyond simple enumerations of the quantity of acts of receiving help, and additionally consider other parameters of social support exchanges (e.g., appraisals of its effectiveness [18], equity in receiving and providing support [19]).

Deterioration of Perceived Social Support and Social Embeddedness After Disasters

Assessments of perceived social support in studies of survivors of disasters are definitely more frequent, and their findings are generally more straightforward, than investigations examining receipt of social support after disasters [3]. As expected, based on the voluminous literature documenting the advantages of beliefs of being reliably connected to others, studies typically found that higher levels of perceived support are directly associated with better psychological health and/or that perceptions of social support moderate the link between disaster exposure and distress. The evidence is strong because some of the researchers were afforded rare opportunities to investigate these relationships using prospective longitudinal designs that controlled for levels of survivors' functioning before the disaster e.g., [20,21]. Of course, given the abundance of examinations of perceived social support, there are also null or contradictory findings in the literature. Yet their presence should not threaten our overall confidence in the benefits of perceived social support for survivors of disasters. These exceptions to the rule may inspire more in-depth explanations and invite more complex investigations.

Although part of the variance in perceptions of social support can be attributed to relatively stable personal characteristics (e.g., attachment styles, personality traits, social skills), it would be naive to consider this important psychological resource as a static phenomenon. A closer inspection of correlation tables of many quantitative studies of people affected by disasters, as well as a careful reading of survivors' accounts offered by insightful qualitative investigations, frequently suggest that disastrous events lead to erosion in people's appraisals of the availability of social support e.g., [6,20–22]. People's perceptions of social support decline because survivors' expectations, which are relatively high for most people, cannot be sustained within the reality of recovery after disasters. It is highly probable that within survivors' social networks are people who are also survivors – hence they may not be able to engage in routinely expected roles as support providers. Lower levels of perceived social support may reflect the simple fact that the need for support among all affected surpasses its availability. Downturns in appraisals of availability of social support post disaster could be veridical assessments of current circumstances. In fact, studies documenting clear mental health benefits of perceived social support also registered a deterioration in social support after disasters [20–22]. It seems reasonable to suggest that deterioration of perceived social support after disasters may act as one of the most plausible mediators linking the extent of disaster exposure and its consequences for people's psychological distress. More direct investigations are needed into the

model of deterioration of perceived social support post disaster [20,22], given that other studies offer only partial support of it [11,23].

The great majority of the research presented in this chapter is based on the fundamental premise that resources that offer social support are critical antecedents to wellbeing, and their presence or absence contributes to psychological recovery of survivors of disasters. Although the social causation framework (i.e., resource disadvantages increase the risk of subsequent mental ill health) has dominated the field, longitudinal cross-lag studies assessing viability of the alternative framework of social selection (i.e., ill mental health undermines resource attainment) are becoming more frequent. Krzysztof Kaniasty and Fran Norris report a four-wave study of survivors of floods and mudslides (from 6 to 24 months afterwards), which showed that the salutary effect of perceived social support on distress in the earlier phase of coping reflected the social causation mechanism [24]. At the midpoint of the study both causation and selection processes contemporaneously emerged as significant causal paths, whereas in the final phase of the assessments the eroding impact of distress on subsequent perceptions of support reflected the social selection mechanism. Through a study of children after Hurricane Katrina, Betty Lai and colleagues offered support for a social selection model indicating that post-traumatic distress undermined perceived social support [25]. The study by Platt and colleagues, mentioned earlier in this chapter, which investigated received social support in the aftermath of Hurricane Ike concluded that social causation and selection were both present post disaster, but were restricted to emotional social support [13]. Recognising reciprocal relationships between social resources and psychological wellbeing is essential, as both social causation and selection processes are important in advancing theory, research, and practice in the topic of disaster health.

It could be said that both received support and perceived support serve only as proxy assessments of a variety of social dynamics after disasters, whereas social embeddedness captures the breadth and assortment of interpersonal connectedness and sense of community. Studies show that both increases and decreases in engagement in community activities occur after disasters, and either may be an asset or a liability. Frederick Weil, Matthew Lee, and Edward Shihadeh used three waves of data collection covering an 18-month period after Hurricane Katrina, and documented that, initially, more socially embedded people exhibited greater psychological difficulties but had better psychological functioning than less embedded people at later times [26]. Higher levels of social participation post disaster were associated with lower psychological distress following an earthquake in Japan [27]. Moderate levels of group participation led to decreased frequencies of symptoms of PTSD among residents in Australia who were affected by bushfires, whereas people's low or high involvement in social activities was associated with poorer outcomes [28]. Greater levels of collective efficacy in a sample of health workers exposed to a hurricane resulted in a lower likelihood of their having PTSD [29]. Interpersonal and community animosities and disagreements after experiencing a disaster were predictive of lower levels of perceived social support and community cohesion, and greater withdrawal from interpersonal contacts [12]. Likewise, Hung Wong and colleagues [30] showed that exposure to an earthquake had a negative impact on survivors' subjective appraisals of social capital availability. Nevertheless, perceptions of sense of community, connectedness, and mutual trust protected their psychological wellbeing. Frankly, all social support resources offer both advantages and disadvantages.

A few final observations are necessary about challenges to social support in the context of human-induced catastrophes. Disasters caused by natural hazards typically adhere, in Kai Erikson's words, to Aristotle's rules of dramatic narrative, with an unambiguous beginning, middle, and end [31]. On the other hand, many human-induced disasters, which are catastrophes with varied doses of human culpability for their occurrence and/or mitigation (e.g., toxic contamination, chemical spills, or technological/industrial accidents), more often than not 'violate all the rules of plot' because their impact is frequently slowly evolving, vague, and not readily perceptible. These kinds of disasters are characterised by a lack of consensus about appraisals of their origin and severity, an overabundance of misinformation, mistrust of authorities, diminished social capital, and bitter polarisation and anatomisation of community. Despite a few instances to the contrary (see Chapter 26), survivors of such protracted disasters commonly face their predicaments and interminable sense of collective uncertainty without the benefits of altruistic communities. The post-disaster social milieu of communities victimised by

disasters resulting from technological failures and environmental contamination is ridden with deterioration of social support and erosion of sense of community. In fact, the terms toxic or corrosive communities have been used to describe the socio-psychological fallout of these events [32]. Liesel Ritchie and colleagues examined community and psychological functioning after a major environmental contamination, and documented that disruptions of personal relationships and community involvement were associated with higher levels of distress [33]. Rebecca Cline and colleagues investigated a slowly evolving exposure to amphibole asbestos and empirically supported a model tracing how greater community conflict spilled into greater family disagreements that placed constraints on discussing the disaster's health consequences, and ultimately resulted in a perceived sense of failed social support and poorer psychological functioning [34]. In a study of the lasting impact of a coastal oil spill, Vanessa Parks and colleagues showed that perceived social support protected most people's mental health in the affected region, but it was positively associated with distress among people whose livelihoods were dependent on a healthy environment (i.e., fishers) [35]. Complexities loom in the dynamics of social support in the wake of all disasters.

We hasten to add, however, a necessary qualification to this brief outline of social support and community processes in the aftermath of human-induced catastrophes. Public reactions to undoubtedly malicious and premeditated acts of terrorism, violence, and destruction generally have their patriotic stages of collective resolve and determination. The human history of trauma offers many examples of how communities faced with oppression have bonded together in a sense of common outrage, fearless drive to survive, and communal purpose in recovery [32].

Recommendations

Recommendations for Studies of Communities Recovering from Disastrous Events

Research attempting to uncover the multilayered realities of people and communities coping with disasters is very difficult. Disasters defy geographical, social, and cultural boundaries. They defy time limits as various phases of disaster recovery imprint themselves on every aspect of life. Adding to the complexity, disasters are often very different, and each may beget unique demands and create very specific needs. Likewise, summarising disaster studies in the search for coherent and replicable patterns is difficult and could be untenable. Nevertheless, from the perspective of investigations focusing on social support processes post disaster, the following may augment the potential usefulness of our research for practice.

- Clear operational definitions of social support measures are essential; distinctions among different facets of this umbrella construct do matter.
- Assessing social support with one or two items aiming to tap good or bad social relationships is no longer sufficient; studies should include established instruments with known psychometric properties.
- It is imperative to explicitly specify in manuscripts how long after the event the data were collected; more importantly, timeframes to which respondents refer when answering social support items should be clearly identified.
- Investigations of social support actually received/ provided post disaster are still outnumbered by studies of perceived social support, the context of actual social support exchanges (quality, reciprocity, equity, transparency) is most relevant.
- Assessments of the role of economic, social, and cultural factors should become an inherent part of analyses; these characteristics of survivors and communities too often prevent an egalitarian access to post-disaster assistance and social support.
- Null and contradictory findings call for in-depth evaluations that explain them not only as emerging from the idiosyncrasies of a disaster context; inconsistencies of available findings may inspire novel research questions, and in turn would improve and strengthen theoretical frameworks and recommendations for practice.
- The adage that 'nothing is as practical as a good theory' [36] is not just a truism; it is a path leading disaster research beyond the routine conclusion that social support is a critical resource for people recovering from collective disastrous events.

Recommendations for Interventions Within Communities Recovering from Disastrous Events

'A disaster is defined as a basic disruption of the social context within which individuals and group function' [10, p. 651]. Hence, from this perspective, the key issue is how to prevent deterioration of social support that evolves over time in so many milieus after disasters. Interventions after disasters should be rooted in coordinated efforts that aim to maintain and augment survivors' perceptions of being supported and belonging to a cohesive social group and community.

- All types of social support are needed by disaster survivors, regardless of the disaster's cause; emotional support may be most readily offered, and hence abundant, but both tangible and informational support may have more impact.
- '*Help smarter, not harder*'; efficacious and sensitive delivery of support is more important than its sheer quantity.
- A swift return to routine activities and social roles is imperative; commonplace social interactions offer the best forums for sharing experiences, feelings, and information.
- It is empowering for survivors to be able to help each other; local communities should be assisted to make mutual social support exchanges easier and lasting beyond the initial, and often short-lived, experience of solidarity and altruistic behaviour.
- It must be recognised how social stratifications prevent many survivors from accessing disaster assistance and social support offered by *altruistic communities*; socially, politically, morally, and religiously sanctioned patterns of inequality may fuel discrimination and deprivation of certain subgroups post crisis.

Acknowledgement

Preparation of this chapter was supported by Grant OPUS⊠19 grant No. 2020/37/B/HS6/02957 awarded to Krzysztof Kaniasty from the Polish National Science Centre (Narodowe Centrum Nauki).

References

1. Bonanno GA, Brewin CR, Kaniasty K, Greca AML. Weighing the costs of disaster: consequences, risks, and resilience in individuals, families, and communities. *Psychol Sci Public Interest* 2010; **11**: 1–49.

2. Hobfoll SE, Stokes JP. The process and mechanics of social support. In *The Handbook of Research in Personal Relationships* (eds S Duck, DF Fray, SE Hobfoll, B Ickes, B Montgomery): 497–517. Wiley, 1988.

3. Kaniasty K, Norris FH. Distinctions that matter: received social support, perceived social support, and social embeddedness after disasters. In *Mental Health and Disasters* (eds Y Neria, S Galea, FH Norris): 175–202. Cambridge University Press, 2009.

4. Barton AM. *Communities in Disaster*. Doubleday, 1969.

5. Kaniasty K, Norris FH. In search of altruistic community: patterns of social support mobilization following Hurricane Hugo. *Am J Community Psychol* 1995; **23**: 447–77.

6. Norris FH, Baker CK, Murphy AD, Kaniasty K. Social support mobilization and deterioration after Mexico's 1999 flood: effects of context, gender, and time. *Am J Community Psychol* 2005; **36**: 15–28.

7. Kaniasty KI, Norris FH. Help-seeking comfort and receiving social support: the role of ethnicity and context of need. *Am J Community Psychol* 2000: **28**: 545–81.

8. Vezzali L, Versari A, Cadamuro A, Trifiletti E, Di Bernardo GA. Out-group threats and distress as antecedents of common in-group identity among majority and minority group members in the aftermath of a natural disaster. *Int J Psychol* 2018; **53**: 417–25.

9. Suar D, Sekhar Das S, Alat P, Kumar R. Exposure, loss, and support predicting the dimensions of posttsunami trauma. *J Loss Trauma* 2017; **22**: 427–39.

10. Fritz CE. Disasters. In *Contemporary Social Problems* (eds RK Merton, RA Nisbet): 561–94. Harcourt, 1961.

11. Littleton H, Haney L, Schoemann A, Allen A, Benight C. Received support in the aftermath of Hurricane Florence: reciprocal relations among perceived support, community solidarity, and PTSD. *Anxiety Stress Coping* 2022; **35**: 270–83.

12. Kaniasty K. Predicting social psychological well-being following trauma: the role of postdisaster social support. *Psychol Trauma* 2012; **4**: 22–33.

13. Platt JM, Lowe SR, Galea S, Norris FH, Koenen KC. A longitudinal study of the bidirectional relationship between social support and posttraumatic stress following a natural disaster: postdisaster social support and traumatic stress. *J Trauma Stress* 2016; **29**: 205–13.

14. Arnberg FK, Hultman CM, Michel P-O, Lundin T. Social support moderates posttraumatic stress and general distress after disaster: buffering role of social support. *J Trauma Stress* 2012; **25**: 721–7.

15. McGuire AP, Gauthier JM, Anderson LM, Hollingsworth DW, Tracy M, Galea S, et al. Social support moderates effects of natural disaster exposure on depression and posttraumatic stress disorder symptoms: effects for displaced and nondisplaced residents: social support moderates natural disaster effects. *J Trauma Stress* 2018; **31**: 223–33.

16. Warner LM, Gutiérrez-Doña B, Villegas Angulo M, Schwarzer R. Resource loss, self-efficacy, and family support predict

17. Hall BJ, Sou K, Chen W, Zhou F, Chang K, Latkin C. An evaluation of the buffering effects of types and sources of support on depressive symptoms among natural disaster-exposed Chinese adults. *Psychiatry* 2016; **79**: 389–402.

18. Shang F, Kaniasty K, Cowlishaw S, Wade D, Ma H, Forbes D. The impact of received social support on posttraumatic growth after disaster: the importance of both support quantity and quality. *Psychol Trauma* 2022; **14**: 1134–41.

19. Pandit A, Nakagawa Y. How does reciprocal exchange of social support alleviate individuals' depression in an earthquake-damaged community? *Int J Environ Res Public Health* 2021; **18**: 1585.

20. Kaniasty K, Norris FH. A test of the social support deterioration model in the context of natural disaster. *J Pers Soc Psychol* 1993; **64**: 395–408.

21. Lowe SR, Chan CS, Rhodes JE. Pre-hurricane perceived social support protects against psychological distress: a longitudinal analysis of low-income mothers. *J Consult Clin Psychol* 2010; **78**: 551–60.

22. Norris FH, Kaniasty K. Received and perceived social support in times of stress: a test of the social support deterioration deterrence model. *J Pers Soc Psychol* 1996; **71**: 498–511.

23. Shiba K, Yazawa A, Kino S, Kondo K, Aida J, Kawachi I. Depressive symptoms in the aftermath of major disaster: empirical test of the social support deterioration model using natural experiment. *Wellbeing Space Soc* 2020; **1**: 100006.

posttraumatic stress symptoms: a 3-year study of earthquake survivors. *Anxiety Stress Coping* 2015; **28**: 239–53.

24. Kaniasty K, Norris FH. Longitudinal linkages between perceived social support and posttraumatic stress symptoms: sequential roles of social causation and social selection. *J Trauma Stress* 2008; **21**: 274–81.

25. Lai BS, Osborne MC, Piscitello J, Self-Brown S, Kelley ML. The relationship between social support and posttraumatic stress symptoms among youth exposed to a natural disaster. *Eur J Psychotraumatol* 2018; **9**(suppl 2): 1450042.

26. Weil F, Lee MR, Shihadeh ES. The burdens of social capital: how socially-involved people dealt with stress after Hurricane Katrina. *Soc Sci Res* 2012; **41**: 110–19.

27. Matsuyama Y, Aida J, Hase A, Sato Y, Koyama S, Tsuboya T, et al. Do community- and individual-level social relationships contribute to the mental health of disaster survivors? A multilevel prospective study after the Great East Japan Earthquake. *Soc Sci Med* 2016; **151**: 187–95.

28. Gallagher HC, Block K, Gibbs L, Forbes D, Lusher D, Molyneaux R, et al. The effect of group involvement on post-disaster mental health: a longitudinal multilevel analysis. *Soc Sci Med* 2019; **220**: 167–75.

29. Ursano RJ, McKibben JBA, Reissman DB, Liu X, Wang L, Sampson RJ, et al. Posttraumatic stress disorder and community collective efficacy following the 2004 Florida hurricanes. *PLoS One* 2014; **9**: e88467.

30. Wong H, Huang Y, Fu Y, Zhang Y. Impacts of structural social capital and cognitive social capital on the psychological status of survivors of the Ya'an earthquake. *Appl Res Qual Life* 2019; **14**: 1411–33.

31. Erikson K. *A New Species of Trouble: The Human Experience of Modern Disasters.* W.W. Norton & Company, 1994.

32. Kaniasty K, Norris FH. Social support in the aftermath of disasters, catastrophes, and acts of terrorism: altruistic, overwhelmed, uncertain, antagonistic, and patriotic communities. In *Bioterrorism: Psychological and Public Health Interventions* (eds R Ursano, A Norwood, C Fullerton): 200–29. Cambridge University Press, 2004.

33. Ritchie LA, Gill DA, Long MA. Factors influencing stress response avoidance behaviors following technological disasters: a case study of the 2008 TVA coal ash spill. *Environ Hazards* 2020; **19**: 442–62.

34. Cline RJW, Orom H, Chung JE, Hernandez T. The role of social toxicity in responses to a slowly-evolving environmental disaster: the case of amphibole asbestos exposure in Libby, Montana, USA. *Am J Community Psychol* 2014; **54**: 12–27.

35. Parks V, Slack T, Ramchand R, Drakeford L, Finucane ML, Lee MR. Fishing households, social support, and depression after the Deepwater Horizon oil spill. *Rural Sociol* 2020; **85**: 495–518.

36. Lewin K. Psychology and the process of group living. *J Soc Psychol* 1943; **17**: 113–31.

Chapter

Collective Responses to Terrorist Attacks

Chris Cocking and Anne Templeton

Introduction

Studies of public behaviour during disasters stretch back over 50 years [1,2], with an increased interest in terrorist attacks since the attacks on September 11, 2001, in the USA. Evidence from these incidents shows that, contrary to common views about the irrationality of crowd behaviour, mass panic is a myth that is not supported by detailed evidence of what happens (see Chapter 8 for more information) [3]. For instance, although there was significant disruption and destruction from the aerial bombing campaigns of the Second World War, the civilian populations affected were nonetheless remarkably resilient, and the authorities' fears of a breakdown of the wider societal fabric in the face of these attacks were rarely justified [4]. However, despite the lack of evidence for mass panic, emergency planning guidelines are often influenced by the fear of needing to manage widespread 'irrational' behaviour in mass emergencies [5].

Social psychology has been applied to studying terrorist attacks and identifies the mechanisms behind public responses, as well as explaining the processes behind people's behaviour [6]. It does this by exploring the relationship between individuals and groups through the concepts of social identities, social norms and social influence, and collective behaviour – all of which occur during terrorist attacks. Social psychological approaches also emphasise how shared identities and social norms produce social influence and mutual social support to enhance effective responses to such incidents. Furthermore, because terrorist attacks are collective events with multiple actors and social groups, it is important to go beyond accounts that focus on an individual person's behaviour and understand also how people behave collectively in groups.

Group Responses to Emergencies

Classical irrationalist models suggested that people lose behavioural control in crowds, and panic can spread through the crowd via automatic contagion [7]. They assert that, when people in a crowd experience an emergency, their perceptions become less accurate, causing fear to become exaggerated, which leads to irrational and competitive behaviour [8]. In contrast, recent research on the psychology of crowd behaviour in terrorist attacks and other mass casualty incidents (MCIs) has developed the notion that crowds behave more cooperatively than is assumed by earlier irrationalist models [6,9,10]. Social networks usually endure following emergencies. However, recent psychological perspectives have examined how social networks can be created by the incidents themselves and often emerge during the acute phase of emergencies [6]. Therefore they can also help to explain the psychological mechanisms that make cooperative behaviour possible – this emergent shared identity creates social bonds that encourage cooperative, rather than selfish, behaviour. Consequently, people not only support others, but also expect to be supported themselves, thus creating cooperative social norms that influence others. In other words, these emergent cooperative social norms can happen not just *despite* an incident, but also *because* of it.

Research using social identity theory [11], and self-categorisation theory [12] suggests that, when crowd members shift from being individuals to seeing themselves as part of a group, they can respond collectively to events. This can be important for terrorist attacks intended to cause harm in crowded spaces. In these novel situations, the common fate of those who are attacked can lead people who were previously strangers to unite as a group. Thus there is a cognitive transformation from personal to social identity that creates a united psychological crowd, wherein others facing the emergency are seen to be part of one's group.

People unifying into a group can be seen in the responses of crowd members during terrorist attacks, such as the bombings in London on 7 July 2005 (or

7/7), when 56 people, including the four terrorists, were killed by bombs on three underground trains and a bus [9]. Analyses of interviews with survivors about their experiences, and of archive material relating to 7/7, show how people who previously did not have any sense of connection with others around them, because they were commuters on a crowded train during rush hour, quickly developed a common identity from a shared sense of fate once the incident started [13]. This resulted in survivors providing emotional and practical support, such as providing first aid, passing round water, assisting with evacuation, and comforting the casualties.

This emergent identity can also create more generalised cooperative social norms, and recent research with earthquake survivors has found that seeing others provide support is linked to people engaging in such cooperative behaviour themselves [14]. The Social Identity Model of Collective Psychosocial Resilience (SIMCPR) was developed from this body of work to provide a theoretical explanation for cooperation in these circumstances [6]. Primarily, the SIMCPR proposes that mass emergencies can create a shared sense of fate ('we're all in this together') that encourages cooperation via the new identity that those people affected share with others in the same incident.

Social Influence in Terrorist Attacks

In stressful situations, crowd members often collectively coordinate responses guided by their group membership, and ingroup members can become reference points who influence others' perceptions and behaviour [13,14]. There are multiple possible responses during a terrorist attack, such as escaping,[1] confronting the attacker(s),[2] or providing support to other people [9,10]. In these uncertain moments, crowd members look to ingroup members for information about how to respond. They are more likely to be influenced by the behaviour of people they think are ingroup members, because these people are judged to be more competent and trustworthy than outgroup members. Research from social appraisal theory provides insights into how assessments of situations are shaped by the emotional responses of others [15]. In uncertain and/or stressful situations,

people are likely to use social appraisal – that is, their perceptions of how others are emotionally responding to the situation – to make sense of their environment [16]. This is especially the case when a person is viewed as a competent judge of the situation. So, for instance, an interview study of social influence processes used during 7/7 suggested that prototypical leader figures who crowd members identified with were more influential than those who were not prototypical [13]. This is illustrated by the following survivor comparing the influence of two different leader figures who emerged after one of the explosions:

> PARTICIPANT: There was a girl . . . standing on the seats and saying 'right everybody don't panic, it's going to be all right, we don't know what's happened, but people know we're here . . . they will come and get us . . . let's all keep calm' . . . this woman who was trying to direct things was keeping people safe. . . . There was a stupid man . . . who also thought he was very self-important. The other woman was just good at taking control and calming people down, keeping a calm atmosphere, and he was going 'we've got to get out of here!'
>
> INTERVIEWER: Did you notice any difference in the way people listened to either of them?
>
> PARTICIPANT: I think people seemed to be glad that there was somebody like the . . . woman taking some kind of control. . . . I think people looked to that . . . and she had a good strong voice, she was sensible, she commanded some kind of respect and authority if you like and what she was saying was very sensible, so people were taking note . . . the bloke he was just a bit of a pompous ass and I don't think people were really taking much notice of him (Participant 88).

The prototypical leader is the one with a shared identity with crowd members. Here it seems that the woman who was calm (like the other survivors) was perceived by group members as best exemplifying the group definition and goals [17]. Coordinated crowd action often ensues from these social influence processes.

Other research demonstrates how an emergent shared social identity can have numerous benefits for people in emergencies. For example, crowd members feel safer when they are with ingroup members, they are less likely to exhibit competitive behaviours towards ingroup members during emergency evacuations [9,10], and are more likely to help those people whom they perceive to be ingroup members compared with those outside their group

---

[1] www.bbc.co.uk/news/world-europe-34827497
[2] www.bbc.co.uk/news/uk-england-london-50608315

[17]. Crucially for coordinating safety, social identification with others in an emergency can lead to people expecting support from ingroup members, which is associated with providing coordinated social support for others and feeling more able to effectively respond to the emergency [18,19]. Research on 7/7 shows that, where help was not provided for others, this was often attributed to people being physically unable to provide help, such as not being near other survivors or being physically injured and/or in shock themselves. This mutual support among survivors prevailed even when they did not know if another bomb was going to be detonated, with some putting themselves at risk by returning to the wreckage to help others evacuate.

Similar findings of shared social identity leading to mutual aid and support can be seen in a variety of other emergencies, such as fires, sinking cruise ships, tower block evacuations, and train accidents and floods [10] (see Chapter 23 in this latter regard). Research has consistently found that emergent shared social identities are common and lead to supportive behaviours and cohesive coordination in the immediate aftermath of emergencies [5], and that prosocial behaviour among crowds can possibly reduce the number of casualties in emergencies [20]. Even in incidents in which initial confusion and crowd flight occur, these actions are often quickly superseded by social cohesion and supportive behaviour among crowd members [21]. Finally, support of this nature can continue in a long-term context through people creating and maintaining mutual support groups of survivors after disasters [22].

Crowd Members as Zero Responders

The practicalities of emergency response mean that it is usually the public who are first on the scene at MCIs [23]. Terrorist attacks often target crowded areas to maximise disruption and casualties. Therefore many members of the public may be in the vicinity when incidents begin, and so are likely to intervene before the arrival of emergency responders. Indeed more lives can be saved by members of the public than by professional responders in MCIs, and bystanders can intervene up to 70% of the time before professional emergency services arrive [24]. Sometimes bystanders even confront attackers in active shooter incidents [25]. These kinds of interventions can bring direct and quantifiable health benefits, and increased public involvement in emergencies can lead to increased

survival rates, quicker casualty evacuation, and better incident management. This spontaneous public involvement in emergencies has been described as 'zero responders', as they are present before the arrival of professional first responders [26].

There have been calls for emergency planning protocols to accommodate crowd members' desire to help in emergencies and use them as a potential additional resource [26,27]. Current UK guidelines do not tend to consider public intervention to the extent that this involvement could then be incorporated into practical advice for first responders. Therefore an opportunity to draw upon extra resources is potentially being missed. This is because, however efficient response times by emergency responders are, they will never be instantaneous, and there will always be a delay between an incident happening and first responders arriving on scene. Furthermore, although large events in the UK often have crowd management and first-aid-trained personnel deployed on site, it would not be feasible to deploy sufficient resources of first responders at each event in the case of a major incident.

In the case of terrorist attacks, emergency responders may also face delays before being deployed. This is because counter-terrorism protocols require that safe zones are established to minimise risks to responders, meaning that there can be delays in entering 'hot zones' of potential ongoing terrorist activity. An example is the Manchester Arena bombing in 2017, although excessive delays have been strongly criticised by the public inquiry into this major incident [27]. During delays, the public can become the key source of emergency aid, as they may already be in the 'hot zone' and are likely to be present in larger numbers before any organised responder groups have arrived. Any delay in attending to casualties at MCIs can have serious consequences. For instance, at recent major incidents in the UK, such as 7/7 and the 2017 Manchester Arena attack, the first ambulances arrived within 10–15 minutes, but survivors who have catastrophic injuries can bleed to death in less than 10 minutes. Thus the Manchester Arena attack saw members of the public providing emotional and practical support for casualties, including comforting people who were distressed, dressing people's wounds, and staunching blood flow before the emergency services arrived. The Kerslake Report into the Manchester Arena bombing made explicit reference to the concept of zero responders in its recommendations for improving response to future incidents [27]. Thus there is now acknowledgement that crowd members can be a powerful immediate resource in emergencies, by providing support and enhancing safety in dangerous and uncertain circumstances.

Conclusion

Terrorist attacks by their very nature are intended to cause mass disruption and fear in civilian populations. It is an open question as to whether these attacks engender qualitatively different public responses compared with other emergencies, incidents, disasters, and disease outbreaks. In other words, does knowing that outside actors are intent on harming crowd members create more fear and/or panicked behaviour among the people who are affected? This is a topic worthy of potential future research. Nevertheless, assumptions of public vulnerability are often overstated, and the notion of mass panic in incidents is not supported by evidence. Instead, people affected behave much more resiliently than is often expected, and crowd members can be an important asset. They provide valuable practical and emotional support and can save lives through their coordinated response. However, the benefits that crowds can provide are often overlooked in emergency planning because their reactions are assumed to be problematic. This can lead to less efficient responses to terrorist attacks and contribute to future negative relations between crowds and emergency responders. Therefore we end this chapter with some recommendations for improving responses to terrorist attacks by recognising and accommodating the potential for more resilient public responses than was assumed in outdated panic models of human behaviour in emergencies.

Recent practical recommendations for professionals suggested encouraging community resilience in mass emergencies by supporting behaviours that will help the public to 'develop and maintain their own capacity for such resilience' [28]. Overall, these recommendations draw largely from research evidence on the shared sense of adversity that emerges in those affected by terrorist attacks, resulting in a shared common identity that promotes cooperative behaviour before the emergency services arrive. Current emergency planning and response guidelines and practice tend to deny, or at least downplay, the public's agency

and ability to actively help in emergencies. However, MCIs such as the Manchester Arena bombing in 2017 have seen examples of public intervention in the acute stages of the incident before emergency responders arrived. The benefits of embedding these 'zero responders' within emergency planning and response guidelines are twofold – first, it helps to democratise emergency planning and response, and second, it provides valuable resources that could be harnessed by emergency planners using this potential force multiplier in their responses to MCIs.

The emergent social identities that stem from the shared fate of experiencing terrorist attacks can have enduring benefits when the immediate threat recedes. Given the substantial impact that terror-related emergencies can have on people who experienced the incident, it is important to look at how the immediate support in an emergency can continue and be harnessed to increase resilience and wellbeing in the longer term. Numerous enduring grass-roots social groups have emerged from high-profile terrorist emergencies [22]. Survivors' involvement in community support groups after emergencies has been associated with increased self-efficacy and collective efficacy in response to danger [29] (see Chapter 23). Moreover, feeling part of a group with the community can be associated with positive psychological outcomes after a disaster, such as efficacy and greater compassion for others. However, these support groups are largely led by survivors and are not always a substantial part of planning for recovery after emergencies. Moving forward, we recommend that emergency planning should include measures to support and provide resources for survivor-led groups to facilitate longer-term recovery and resilience. The value of these endeavours is demonstrated in Chapters 5, 12, 27, and 28 of this book. Overall, if there was greater recognition within official planning and response guidelines of the public's potentially positive and helpful collective responses to terrorist attacks, this could help to reduce the disruption and casualties that these attacks can cause.

Key Points

1. General Principles That Emerge from the Science

This chapter helps to further develop the novel theoretical notion of collective psychosocial resilience in the face of danger, whereby emergent cooperation can happen not just *despite* a terrorist incident, but also *because* of it.

2. A Description of the Short-, Medium-, And Long-Term Impacts

Given the decreased likelihood of MCIs during COVID-19 lockdown, the immediate short-term impact is that emergency planners can revisit their emergency planning protocols to consider the possibility of zero-responder involvement at future MCIs. More medium-term impacts include the further development and increased democratization of emergency planning protocols to incorporate increased public intervention. The longer-term impacts include creating plans to sufficiently resource survivor-led support groups to support long-term resilience.

3. The Implications for Intervention

The involvement of 'zero responders' could mean that a valuable potential resource and force multiplier could be harnessed by emergency planners in their responses to MCIs.

4. Practical Aspects of Implementing the Principles

The possible benefits of intervention by the public at MCIs can be overlooked in emergency planning, because their reactions are often assumed to be problematic. Therefore greater understanding of this phenomenon by professional first responders and practical strategies for optimising such intervention need to be encouraged.

References

1. Aguirre BE. Emergency evacuations, panic, and social psychology. *Psychiatry* 2005; 68: 121–9.

2. Fritz CE *Disasters and Mental Health: Therapeutic Principles Drawn from Disaster Studies*. University of Delaware, Disaster Research Center, 1961/1996 (http://udspace.udel.edu/handle/19716/1325).

3. Quarantelli EL. Panic, sociology of. In *International Encyclopedia of the Social and Behavioural Sciences* (eds NJ Smelser, PB Baltes): 11020–23. Pergamon Press. 2001.

4. Jones E, Woolven R, Durodie B, Wessely S. Civilian morale during the Second World War: responses to air-raids re-examined. *Soc Hist Med* 2004; 17: 463–79.

5. Drury J, Novelli D, Stott C. Representing crowd behaviour in emergency planning guidance: 'mass panic' or collective resilience? *Resilience* 2013; 1: 18–37.

6. Drury J. The role of social identity processes in mass emergency behaviour: an integrative review. *Eur Rev Soc Psychol* 2018; 29: 8–81.

7. Le Bon G. *The Crowd: A Study of the Popular Mind* (trans. FT Unwin). Dover Publications Inc., 2002.

8. Freud S. Mass psychology and the analysis of the I. In *Mass Psychology and Other Writings* (ed. S Freud): 15–100. Penguin Books, 2004.

9. Drury J, Cocking C, Reicher SD. The nature of collective resilience: survivor reactions to the 2005 London bombings. *Int J Mass Emerg Disasters* 2009; 27: 66–95.

10. Drury J, Cocking C, Reicher SD. Everyone for themselves? A comparative study of crowd solidarity among emergency survivors. *Br J Soc Psychol* 2009; 48: 487–506.

11. Tajfel H, Turner JC. An integrative theory of intergroup conflict. In *The Social Psychology of Intergroup Relations* (eds WG Austin, S Worchel): 33–7. Brooks/Cole, 1979.

12. Turner JC, Hogg MA. Oakes PJ, Reicher SD, Wetherell MS. *Rediscovering the Social Group: A Self-Categorization Theory*. Basil Blackwell, 1987.

13. Cocking C. The role of 'zero-responders' during 7/7: implications for the emergency services. *Int J Emerg Serv* 2013; 2: 79–93.

14. Drury J, Brown R, González R, Miranda D. Emergent social identity and observing social support predict social support provided by survivors in a disaster: solidarity in the 2010 Chile earthquake. *Eur J Soc Psychol* 2016; 46: 209-223.

15. Manstead ASR, Fischer AH. Social appraisal: the social world as object of and influence on appraisal processes. In *Appraisal Processes in Emotion: Theory, Research, Application* (eds KR Schere, A Schorr, T Johnstone): 221–32. Oxford University Press, 2001.

16. Bruder M, Fischer A, Manstead ASR. Social appraisal as a cause of collective emotions. In *Collective Emotions* (eds C von Scheve, M Salmela): 141–55. Oxford University Press, 2014.

17. Hogg MA. A social identity theory of leadership. *Pers Soc Psychol Rev* 2001; 5: 184–200.

18. Alnabulsi H, Drury J. Social identification moderates the effect of crowd density on safety at the Hajj. *Proc Natl Acad Sci USA* 2014; 111: 9091–6.

19. Levine M, Prosser A, Evans D, Reicher S. Identity and emergency intervention: how social group membership and inclusiveness of group boundaries shape helping behaviour. *Pers Soc Psychol Bull* 2002; 34: 443–53.

20. Bartolucci A, Casareale C, Drury J. Cooperative and competitive behaviour among passengers during the Costa Concordia disaster. *Safety Sci* 2021; 134: 105055.

21. Cocking C. Crowd flight in response to police dispersal techniques: a momentary lapse of reason? *J Invest Psychol Offender Profil* 2013; 10: 219–36.

22. Eyre, A. The value of peer support groups following disaster: from Aberfan to Manchester. *Bereave Care* 2019; 38: 115–21.

23. Cabinet Office. *National Risk Register 2020*. HMSO, 2020.

24. Faul M, Aikman SN, Sasser SM. Bystander intervention prior to the arrival of emergency medical services: comparing assistance across types of medical emergencies. *Prehosp Emerg Care* 2016; 20: 317–23.

25. Blair JP, Martaindale MH. *United States Active Shooter Events From 2000 to 2010: Training and Equipment Implications*. Texas State University, 2013.

26. Lemyre L. *Public Communication of CBRN Risk in Canada: Research, Training and Tools to Enable*. Paper presented at the PIRATE Project Stakeholders Workshop. Health Protection Agency, 2010.

27. Drury J, Carter H, Cocking C, Ntontis E, Tekin Guven S, Amlôt R. Facilitating collective psychosocial resilience in the public in emergencies: twelve recommendations based on the social identity approach. *Front Public Health* 2019; 7: 141.

28. Kerslake RW. *The Kerslake Report: An Independent Review into the Preparedness for, and Emergency Response to, the Manchester Arena Attack on 22nd May 2017*. The Kerslake Arena Review, 2018 (www.kerslakearenareview.co.uk/media/1022/kerslake_arena_review_printed_final.pdf).

29. Hobfoll S, Watson P, Bell C, Bryant R, Brymer M, Friedman M, et al. Five essential elements of immediate and mid-term mass trauma intervention: empirical evidence. *Psychiatry* 2007; 70: 283–315.

Chapter

23

Collective Psychosocial Resilience as a Group Process Following Flooding

How It Arises and How Groups Can Sustain It

Evangelos Ntontis and Meng Logan Zhang

Introduction

In this chapter we discuss the social psychology of how communities respond to flooding. We argue that collective psychosocial resilience – that is, people's capacity to spontaneously form groups, coordinate, mobilise, and expect solidarity and social support – is a function of shared social identity [1]. We demonstrate the significance of flooding in terms of its potential widespread and long-term impact on infrastructure and health. We discuss one of the key strategies used to mitigate the effects of flooding and climate change in general, which is developing community resilience. Existing policy and practice relating to community resilience emphasise the role of social capital (i.e., social networks, community trust, and cohesion). However, this concept cannot account for the dynamic emergence of social groups in disasters or the underlying psychosocial processes of community responses to extreme events.

Drawing on experimental, survey, and interview data from major floods in England and Ireland, we discuss the processes through which shared social identity emerges at the onset of flooding and becomes the basis of collective psychosocial resilience. Considering the potentially prolonged impact of flooding and the importance of community cohesion and solidarity in the aftermath of disasters, we examine why shared social identity endures or declines over time. Overall, we argue that the social identity approach can support the realisation of the community resilience agenda by providing a dynamic framework through which to understand collective behaviour in extreme events.

Flooding and Community Resilience

Flooding is the most common weather-related major incident worldwide [2]. Since the 1980s, flooding has killed more than 200,000 people and affected around 2.8 billion people globally [2,3]. The prevalence and intensity of floods are likely to increase due to the effects of climate change, with dire consequences for infrastructure, security, livelihoods, and physical and mental health [3,4]. In terms of the mental health impacts of flooding, an increased prevalence of anxiety, post-traumatic stress, and depression has been observed among people affected 1 or even 2 years after the incident [5,6]. Crucially, flooding affects people not only directly through primary stressors (e.g., injuries, floodwater) but also indirectly through secondary stressors. Secondary stressors are rooted either in people's life circumstances and social factors (e.g., policies, practices, organisational arrangements) that exist prior to a disaster, or in societal responses to a disaster; both factors can interact with a disaster and become sources of distress over and above the impact of primary stressors [7]. In the case of flooding, people can be affected by secondary stressors (e.g., relationship problems, additional work pressure, worrying about children's wellbeing and education) and this may result in psychosocial problems and morbidity [8].

Governments, and international and national institutions target developing community resilience to protect people from the immediate and long-term effects of flooding and climate change [3,4,9]. A range of definitions of community resilience has been offered over time [10,11], but for the purposes of this chapter we follow Fran Norris and her colleagues, who define community resilience as 'a process linking a set of adaptive capacities to a positive trajectory of functioning and adaptation after a disturbance' [10, p. 130]. According to Norris and her colleagues, community resilience should not be treated as merely an outcome or a static, stable, and unchanging element; rather, it is best described as an active *process*, which is dependent on various capacities that can be developed and harnessed [11].

Treating community resilience as a process allows us to explore the capacities that can facilitate it. Norris and her colleagues reflect on various capacities, such as economic development, channels of communication and information, social capital, and community competence [10]. Social capital is the most widely used psychosocial concept upon which community resilience policy is built [12, p. 87]. One of the definitions of social capital is 'the aggregate of the actual or potential resources which are linked to possession of a durable network of more or less institutionalised relationships of mutual acquaintance and recognition' [13, p. 21]. The argument posed by the social capital approach is that dense social networks and social bonds between community members are the basis of trust and norms of reciprocity that can lead to more effective community responses to and recovery from disasters [14]. Daniel Aldrich presents examples whereby communities with stronger social networks and ties did not disperse after disasters; they mobilised resources and social support effectively, coordinated collectively, and provided informal insurance to those affected [14].

However, scholars have pointed to various limitations of the social capital concept. Despite emphasising the importance of social networks, social capital does not explain the psychosocial processes through which such networks are mobilised and operate, such as community competence and collective efficacy [15,16]. Moreover, disasters are often characterised by the emergence of social groups that lack pre-existing bonds [17] (Chapters 5, 21, and 27 relate to these observations). Due to its focus on pre-existing bonds, social capital cannot explain the psychosocial processes whereby social bonds and networks are formed, often spontaneously, leading to empowerment and community resilience [18]. Therefore we next present a model and set of concepts based on the social identity approach that can explain the aforementioned processes in a dynamic manner.

Social Identity, Collective Psychosocial Resilience, and Flooding

According to the social identity approach in social psychology, our self-concept comprises both personal identities (e.g., personal characteristics) and social identities (e.g., community identity, gender identity, national identity, professional identity) [19,20]. Social identities depend on the groups to which we belong and with which we identify. Different social identities are associated with different social norms, interests, patterns, and expectations of behaviour, and which of

our identities is salient and guides our thinking and behaviour varies depending on the social contexts in which we find ourselves [19,20].

The Social Identity Model of Collective Psychosocial Resilience (SIMCPR) argues that emergence of groups in disasters in the absence of pre-existing bonds is a function of shared social identity [1,21]. When a disaster strikes, a sense of common fate experienced by the people affected can cause them to perceive each other as more similar and as psychologically closer to one another. In other words, the shared experience of that disaster can transform people's perspectives of themselves from the individual ('me') to the collective ('us'). The emergence of shared social identities (e.g., perceiving one another as fellow community members) can facilitate cognitive, emotional, and behavioural changes. People are motivated, for example, to act in terms of the collective interests of the group, express solidarity and provide social support for ingroup members, and trust and expect support from fellow ingroup members. The other chapters in this section of this book have all used these constructs. These processes can lead to a range of positive outcomes, such as increased wellbeing, perceptions of collective efficacy, and empowerment (see Figure 23.1). Convergent empirical evidence for the model comes from experiments and from a range of real incidents, including bombings, earthquakes, fires, stadium crushes, and sinking ships [21].

The SIMCPR has also expanded our understanding of community resilience in flooding. As we said earlier, a limitation of the social capital approach is that it cannot account for how groups emerge in the absence of pre-existing bonds or explain the psychological principles that underpin their mobilisation [18]. Additionally, despite the fact that the impact of flooding can be prolonged and does not stop when the waters recede [6], emergent groups and the camaraderie that often characterises the early stages of disasters often decline at a time when this support is most important [17] (Chapter 21 considers these matters in detail). Thus, since the social support that social groups make available can be crucial for community resilience, we need a way of understanding the dynamic nature of group formation as well as of groups' endurance or decline following a disaster.

Therefore we summarise next the empirical evidence from studies conducted by us in Ireland and England after the major floods in 2009 and in late

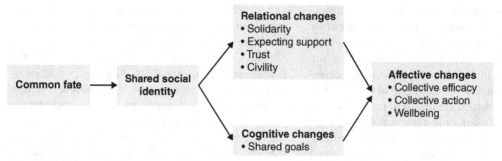

Figure 23.1 The social identity model of collective psychosocial resilience [1].

2015/early 2016, respectively. Our first question concerned whether there was evidence of collective behaviour and of spontaneous groups emerging, and whether the concept of shared social identity could explain these observations. Our second question focused on how emergent groups and collective behaviour might change over time, and how these changes might be explained by social identity processes.

Social Identity Processes in the Early Stages of Flooding

Both of us have conducted studies that explored how communities responded to a flood disaster, and whether social identity could account for collective behaviours. Evangelos Ntontis visited York, UK in February 2015, almost 2 months after the flood, and interviewed an opportunity sample of 17 residents, of whom 4 were flooded, 5 were disrupted (i.e., they resided in the surrounding area but no water entered their homes), and 8 were not flooded. Both affected and unaffected participants reported that they did not experience any connectedness before the incident, but the social boundaries that were present between people before the disaster had dissolved and given rise to an emerging sense of community and of feeling that they were members of one group when the flood occurred. Unaffected or disrupted residents reported feeling concerned about fellow community members because of the damage that the latter experienced, either because of the perceived inadequacy of the official responses, or due to experiencing common secondary stressors (e.g., looting). People also reported providing practical support and information for those who were affected, or reaching out to other survivors to provide them with emotional support despite having had no previous connection with them [22]. Throughout the interviews,

participants used language that suggested shared social identity (e.g., 'your fellows', 'community spirit', 'everybody coming together'). Similarly, in 2018, Meng Logan Zhang visited a village in Ireland that had flooded in 2009, and interviewed 18 residents. Nine participants had experienced flooding, whereas 9 had not. In his analysis, Zhang reports similar findings to those volunteered in York, whereby a clear pattern of shared identity among both flooded and unaffected residents emerged. Widespread provision of social support for the people affected and very few reports of selfish behaviours were also documented [23].

In contrast to the study by Ntontis and his colleagues [22], in which participants mentioned the lack of a community spirit before the flood, Zhang's participants referred to the strong social capital (i.e., pre-existing social bonds) that characterised the village before the flood, and which might have also contributed to the community's response to help the people who were affected. Zhang complemented his findings through two experimental studies that explored how the severity of the flood (severe vs. mild) and pre-existing unity (unity vs. no unity) might affect emergent shared social identity and helping behaviour, as well as how observing a unified community can mobilise prosocial behaviours through the effect of a shared social identity. The results showed that perceiving the flood as more severe was associated with increased prosocial behaviour, and this effect was mediated by shared social identity. Importantly, these effects were moderated by perceptions of pre-existing unity, showing that emergent identification with the community was lower when people perceived their community as cohesive in the pre-disaster context. In addition, Zhang and his colleagues showed that observing a unified and cohesive community was associated with a range of prosocial behaviours, and this relationship was mediated by perceptions of shared social identity [23].

Overall, both studies emphasise the importance of social connectedness in how communities respond to flooding. However, there seems to be an important interaction between social capital (i.e., pre-existing networks and cohesion) and emergent social identity. When there is no history of connectedness between the people affected (e.g., in the case of bombings in tube trains or shopping centres [24], or in the case of urban areas in which there are low levels of social connectedness), social capital is likely to play no role in defining collective behaviour. Rather it is much more likely that collective behaviour is facilitated through an emergent social identity. However, in spaces with existing social capital (i.e., a history of social connectedness), such as in villages or rural areas, pre-existing networks are likely to be mobilised and offer support to community members in need with less evidence of new disaster communities emerging [14]. Thus it might be the presence or absence of prior connectedness due to the nature of the settings where the flooding incidents took place (village vs. city) that could potentially explain differences in how communities mobilised in the studies by Zhang and Ntontis, respectively.

Social Identity Processes in the Aftermath and Recovery Periods That Follow Flooding

Emergent groups do not endure indefinitely after the impact of an incident or disaster [25]. Often, old problems reappear and the social support that characterised the early stages of disasters may disappear [17]. Chapter 21 discusses empirical research on the support mobilisation and deterioration paths. However, the continued support that emergent communities mobilise can be very important for people affected by disasters [26], especially when we consider that the effects of flooding can persist for a long time after the waters have receded [6].

We conducted a series of studies that examined whether social identity processes continue to operate during the recovery period, as well as the factors associated with the endurance or decline of emergent shared social identities. Ntontis conducted a questionnaire survey study with samples collected from York, UK at 8, 15, and 21 months after the flood to further explore the extent to which social identity processes

persist during the recovery period [27]. In line with the SIMCPR, common fate was associated with shared social identity in the months that followed the flooding incident. Moreover, shared social identity predicted people's expectations of support, sharing goals with others, higher perceptions of collective efficacy, and increased wellbeing. These findings were complemented by experimental and qualitative evidence to further unpack the dynamics of social identity processes in the recovery phase, which we summarise next.

Experimental findings from Zhang suggested that shared social identity within a community hit by a disaster was stronger when participants perceived the disaster as having occurred more recently than when they perceived it as having occurred in the more distant past. Interview data from Zhang's participants showed that the duration of shared social identity was short-lived, and disappeared when the floodwaters had receded [23] (again this reflects the contents of Chapter 21). Similarly, Ntontis revisited York, UK in 2017, 15 months after the flooding incident, and interviewed 19 residents [28]. Sixteen residents had been flooded and 3 were disrupted. Analysis showed that 11 participants reported experiencing a shared social identity 15 months after the flood, whereas 8 did not. Explaining the decline of shared social identity, some participants reported a lack of common fate and a return to personal concerns and priorities – that is, the absence of a unifying factor caused a return to the status quo before the disaster and a decline in perceived community identity. However, other participants in Ntontis' study reported that the emergent community spirit that they had experienced during the early stages of the flooding disappeared when they received unequal treatment from the authorities. Another reason for a perceived decline was related to people no longer considering themselves in terms of being 'flood victims', and dissociating themselves from the incident. Importantly, some participants reported a persisting shared social identity that was related to experiencing a common fate with others in the past, the ongoing provision of social support that made them feel cared for by their community, or persisting secondary stressors. Other participants reported strategically and intentionally sustaining and affirming their community identity by gathering to commemorate the disaster and their collective response to it [28].

Conclusions

1. General Principles That Emerge from Science

In line with Norris and her colleagues [10], we view community resilience as a process dependent on various resources, and we argue that social identity is one such resource that should be taken into account within community resilience policy and practice [29]. The social identity approach [19] can help us to understand the psychosocial mechanisms that underlie the spontaneous emergence of groups during flooding, the mobilisation of solidarity and social support, and their endurance or decline in the aftermath of the disaster [21]. Importantly, as we highlighted earlier, the dynamics of community responses vary depending on whether there is a history of social connectedness in the affected communities or not. In view of the fact that extreme weather events will become even more prevalent and more severe in the future because of climate change, a firmer grasp of the underlying psychosocial dynamics of community mobilisation is necessary. We hope that the theoretical model and the empirical evidence provided in this chapter are a step in this direction.

2. The Implications for Intervention

Any successful intervention should:

1. recognise the importance of emergent groups in facilitating a successful response to and long-term recovery from flooding
2. provide emergent groups with the resources that allow them to operate (e.g., meeting hubs, tasks that can be carried out by their members) and potentially solidify in the long term
3. recognise and enable groups to express their identity (e.g., through commemorations and official acknowledgement)

4. reduce inequality and inequities in how people are treated in the recovery periods after disasters, which can erode their emergent social identity
5. understand and operate in line with the norms and values of emergent groups, rather than against them
6. have knowledge about the history and nature of the communities affected, because the response of different communities to a disaster depends, among a number of factors, on the pre-existing or emergent social relations among community members and between community members and the authorities.

3. Practical Aspects of Implementing the Principles

Seeing the potential of communities to demonstrate resilience in the face of adversity recognised in official guidance is a step in the right direction. However, these behaviours should not be treated as a given, and should not be treated as a panacea for tackling the effects of climate change in a decontextualised manner. For example, in times of extreme capitalism, neoliberal politics, and financial cuts to public services, claims regarding the resilience of people at the individual and collective levels may be misused by politicians to justify austerity cuts, to minimise public spending, and to bypass governmental responsibilities for supporting communities materially and financially [30]. As Fran Norris and colleagues [10] and Rebecca Wickes and colleagues [15] argue, economic prosperity and physical infrastructure are also crucial for community resilience. Thus, apart from social bonds, effective policies for community resilience can benefit from effective flood defences as well as investment in community spaces that allow pre-existing social bonds to endure, and emergent social bonds to solidify.

References

1. Drury J, Carter H, Cocking C, Ntontis E, Guven ST, Amlot R. Facilitating collective psychosocial resilience in the public in emergencies: twelve recommendations based on the social identity approach. *Front Public Health* 2019; 7:141.

2. Jakubicka T, Vos F, Phalkey R, Marx M. *Health Impacts of Floods in Europe: Data Gaps and Information Needs from a Spatial Perspective. A MICRODIS Report.* Centre for Research on the Epidemiology of Disasters, 2010 (www.preventionweb.net/files/19820_healthimpactsoffloodsineurope1.pdf).

3. Menne B, Murray V, eds. *Floods in the WHO European Region: Health Effects and Their Prevention.* WHO Regional Office for Europe, 2013.

4. UN Office for Disaster Risk Reduction (UNDRR). *Sendai Framework for Disaster Risk Reduction 2015–2030.* UNDRR, 2015.

5. Waite TD, Chaintarli K, Beck CR, Bone A, Amlôt R, Kovats S, et al. The English national cohort study of flooding and health: cross-

sectional analysis of mental health outcomes at year one. *BMC Public Health* 2017; 17: 129.

6. Jermacane D, Waite TD, Beck CR, Bone A, Amlôt R, Reacher M, et al. The English National Cohort Study of Flooding and Health: the change in the prevalence of psychological morbidity at year two. *BMC Public Health* 2018; 18: 330.

7. Williams R, Ntontis E, Alfadhli K, Drury J, Amlôt R. A social model of secondary stressors in relation to disasters, major incidents, and conflict: implications for practice. *Int J Disaster Risk Reduct* 2021; 63: 102436.

8. Tempest EL, English National Study on Flooding and Health Study Group, Carter B, Beck CR, Rubin GJ. Secondary stressors are associated with probable psychological morbidity after flooding: a cross-sectional analysis. *Eur J Public Health* 2017; 27: 1042–7.

9. HM Government. *Community Resilience Development Framework*. Cabinet Office, 2019 (assets.publishing.service.gov.uk/ government/uploads/system/ uploads/attachment_data/file/ 828813/20190902-Community_ Resilience_Development_ Framework_Final.pdf).

10. Norris FH, Stevens SP, Pfefferbaum B, Wyche KF, Pfefferbaum RL. Community resilience as a metaphor, theory, set of capacities, and strategy for disaster readiness. *Am J Community Psychol* 2008; 41: 127–50.

11. Patel S, Rogers M, Amlôt R, Rubin G. What do we mean by 'community resilience'? A systematic literature review of how it is defined in the literature. *PLoS Curr* 2017; 9. Available from: https://doi.org/10.1371/ currents.dis.db775aff25efc5 ac4f0660ad9c9f7db2.

12. Twigger-Ross C, Brooks K, Papadopoulou L, Orr P, Sadauskis R, Coke A, et al. *Community Resilience to Climate Change:*

An Evidence Review. Joseph Rowntree Foundation, 2015.

13. Bourdieu P. The forms of capital. In *Handbook of Theory and Research for the Sociology of Education* (ed. JG Richardson): 241–58. Bloomsbury, 1986.

14. Aldrich DP. The importance of social capital in building community resilience. In *Rethinking Resilience, Adaptation and Transformation in a Time of Change* (eds W Yan, W Galloway): 357–64. Springer, 2017.

15. Wickes R, Zahnow R, Taylor M, Piquero AR. Neighborhood structure, social capital, and community resilience: longitudinal evidence from the 2011 Brisbane flood disaster. *Soc Sci Q* 2015; 96: 330–53.

16. Shreve C, Fordham M. Mobilising resources for resilience. In *Framing Community Disaster Resilience: Resources, Capacities, Learning, and Action* (eds H Deeming, M Fordham, C Kuhlicke, L Pedoth, S Schneiderbauer, C Shreve): 27–42. Wiley-Blackwell, 2019.

17. Quarantelli EL. *Disaster Related Social Behavior: Summary of 50 Years of Research Findings*. University of Delaware Disaster Research Center, 1999.

18. Uekusa S. Rethinking resilience: Bourdieu's contribution to disaster research. *Resilience* 2017; 6: 181–95.

19. Tajfel H, Turner JC. An integrative theory of intergroup conflict. In *The Social Psychology of Intergroup Relations* (eds WG Austin, S Worchel): 33–7. Brooks/ Cole, 1979.

20. Turner JC, Hogg MA, Oakes PJ, Reicher S, Wetherell M. *Rediscovering the Social Group: A Self-Categorisation Theory*. Blackwell, 1987.

21. Drury J. The role of social identity processes in mass emergency behaviour: an integrative review. *Eur Rev Soc Psychol* 2018; 29: 38–81.

22. Ntontis E, Drury J, Amlôt R, Rubin GJ, Williams R. Emergent social identities in floods: implications for community psychosocial resilience. *J Community Appl Soc Psychol* 2018; 28: 3–14.

23. Zhang ML. The antecedents, consequences and trajectories of shared identity in emergencies and disasters. Unpublished PhD thesis, University of St Andrews, 2020. Available from: https://doi .org/10.17630/sta/25.

24. Drury J, Cocking C, Reicher SD. The nature of collective resilience: survivor reactions to the 2005 London bombings. *Int J Mass Emerg Disasters* 2009; 27: 66–95.

25. Fritz C, Williams H. The human being in disasters: a research perspective. *Ann Am Acad Polit Soc Sci* 1957; 309: 42–51.

26. Solnit R. *A Paradise Built in Hell: The Extraordinary Communities That Arise in Disaster*. Penguin Books, 2009.

27. Ntontis E, Drury J, Amlot R, Rubin GJ, Williams R, Saavedra P. Collective resilience in the disaster recovery period: emergent social identity and observed social support are associated with collective efficacy, well-being, and the provision of social support. *Br J Soc Psychol* 2021; 60: 1075–95.

28. Ntontis E, Drury J, Amlôt R, Rubin GJ, Williams R. Endurance or decline of emergent groups following a flood disaster: implications for community resilience. *Int J Disaster Risk Reduct* 2020; 45: 101493.

29. Ntontis E, Drury J, Amlôt R, Rubin GJ, Williams R. Community resilience and flooding in UK guidance: a review of concepts, definitions, and their implications. *J Contingencies Crisis Manag* 2018; 27: 2–13.

30. Furedi F. From the narrative of the Blitz to the Rhetoric of vulnerability. *Cult Sociol* 2007; 1: 235–54.

Chapter

24

Facilitating the Public Response to COVID-19
Group Processes and Mutual Aid

John Drury, Evangelos Ntontis, Maria Fernandes-Jesus, and Guanlan Mao

Introduction

Active community engagement with the public health response is critical in successful responses to disease outbreaks [1]. In the case of the global COVID-19 pandemic, actions by members of the public have been central to combating the spread of the virus. Physical distancing, working from home, face coverings, and self-isolation were crucial from the beginning of the pandemic, and continued to be important during the vaccine rollout [2]. The purpose of this chapter is to understand the psychological facilitators of this public involvement.

The first part of the chapter summarises research on the key psychological predictors of engagement in protective behaviours in the COVID pandemic. We show that, in some cases, practical factors are more important than psychological ones. In the second part, the main focus of the chapter, we describe how mutual aid groups have helped people to shield and self-isolate during the pandemic, and we summarise research on the factors that have sustained these groups over time. We draw out the general principles and the policy and practice implications that emerge from the research on this topic. Our focus is largely on evidence from the UK, although many of the points covered in this chapter apply equally to the situation in other countries. Group processes such as social identification are important in public responses to the pandemic, both for personal engagement and for people's involvement in mutual aid groups. However, material and practical support are necessary for people to act on these psychological motivations. Therefore we recommend that authorities should provide the material resources to support social solidarity as an essential part of the response in disease outbreaks.

Understanding Public Engagement with Protective Behaviours in the COVID-19 Pandemic

By 22 May 2021, the Public Health England Behavioural Science Reference Cell Literature Report had recorded over 2,400 publications on COVID and behaviour, which gives a sense of the sheer volume of research on the role of psychology in the pandemic [3]. Here we focus on the research on predictors of physical distancing, as an example, before broadening this discussion out to other predictive behaviours. We note that although many governments use the term 'social distancing', the World Health Organization (WHO) recommends the term 'physical distancing' to refer to the 1- or 2-metre rules for interaction [4].

Most of the studies on physical distancing in the COVID-19 pandemic have been in the form of cross-sectional surveys, with a smaller number of panel studies, experiments, and observational studies. Most have been carried out in Western Europe or North America. Across the different designs and subject populations there are clear patterns in terms of common predictors of health-related behaviours [5]. Thus people's perception of risk has an impact on their level of adherence [6], as does their belief that physical distancing is effective in providing protection [7]. In addition, there are three types of predictor that relate to *social identity* or *group processes*. First, strength of identification with a relevant valued category, such as national identification [8], or identification with one's family [9], has been found to enhance self-reported adherence to physical distancing regulations. Second, relationships with others, including wider solidarity [10], empathy with vulnerable groups [11], and, negatively, low trust in government, also predict adherence [12]. Third, the group process that seems to be most important is social norms [13] (i.e., the perceived behaviour of others, particularly where there is a shared identity with these other people) [14].

In the UK, regular surveys routinely showed that adherence to physical distancing and other protective behaviours was self-reported as generally at high levels throughout the pandemic (i.e., 2020–2021) [15]. There were two key variations in this overall pattern. The first variation was temporal. Levels of adherence varied over time, in particular in relation to certain national events and announcements. For example, as restrictions were introduced (including lockdowns and laws about face coverings), so levels of adherence increased, and as restrictions were eased, so levels of adherence, particularly around distancing, decreased [16].

The second variation was in terms of the particular protective behaviours. Levels of adherence were high for hand cleansing, physical distancing, and wearing face coverings [15], whereas adherence to self-isolation was low [17]. An obvious difference between these various protective behaviours is that whereas hand cleansing, physical distancing, and wearing face coverings were relatively low-cost and easy for each person to perform, isolating at home was both high-cost and required significant support from other people.

Self-isolation poses significant financial and practical challenges. In the UK, notification of a positive test result for COVID or contact with someone who had tested positive required self-isolation at home for 10 days. The financial challenge that this created for people is evident in the fact that adherence was lowest among the lowest paid people, and that financial reasons were among the most significant reported in surveys [17]. In terms of the practical challenges, in some countries (e.g., Taiwan) healthcare systems provided wrap-around support for those people who were self-isolating, which included necessities such as grocery shopping [18]. In the UK, as in many other countries, however, practical support for people who were self-isolating was left to the community. This meant relying on families, friends, neighbours, and the many mutual aid or community support groups that were formed in response to these and other needs during the pandemic. Next, we examine the role of mutual aid groups in the pandemic and discuss the

psychological principles that led to their emergence and operation.

How Mutual Aid Groups Have Supported People During the COVID-19 Pandemic

In response to the pandemic there was a sharp rise in volunteering and supportive behaviours among the public. Over 750,000 people signed up to volunteer with the National Health Service (NHS) [19]. Office for National Statistics (ONS) surveys reported a rise in informal volunteering [20]. Provision of support, which was offered and provided, was reflected in public perceptions of support. For example, the ONS survey for 7 May 2020 reported that 'feelings of community have increased over the past few weeks' and that '8 in 10 adults said they thought people were doing more to help others since the coronavirus pandemic' [21]. Similar patterns were observed in other countries (e.g., [22]).

As well as formal volunteering and ad hoc support from individual people, support came from the many local mutual aid groups that sprang up in response to the pandemic. In the UK, the first COVID mutual aid or community support groups were set up in March 2020, shortly before the first lockdown, to support the most vulnerable people who were shielding at home [23]. As the numbers infected rose sharply – the UK 7-day average in April 2020 was close to 5,000 – the main focus of mutual aid groups shifted to assisting people who were self-isolating. By July 2020, estimates suggested that over 4,000 such local groups had formed over the course of the pandemic, in addition to many existing groups that had changed their functions, with as many as 3 million participants involved [24].

Mutual aid groups were an essential part of the public response to the COVID-19 pandemic in the UK [24]. Provision of grocery shopping for people who were self-isolating was perhaps their main contribution, but these groups were also involved in collecting prescriptions, dog walking, postal and library services, emotional and informational support, and providing entertainment/leisure, among others [25].

In the UK, after a decline in infections in summer 2020, the need for support for people who were in self-isolation rose again steeply in the autumn; the 7-day average for positive tests in October 2020 reached as high as c. 22,000. By this time, most of the mutual aid groups had been operating for 8 months. A key challenge for these groups in meeting needs was not only how to support those people who were self-isolating, but also how to sustain themselves. Spontaneous community support is common in the wake of disasters [26], but typically it declines within a few months as energy and resources decline (e.g., [27]) (see also Chapters 21 and 23 for more information about the support mobilisation and deterioration pathways). In the case of COVID mutual aid groups, their activity is largely unpaid, it can be physically and emotionally demanding, volunteers themselves risk becoming infected, resources are often limited, and it may be difficult to maintain volunteers' morale [25]. There is therefore a need to understand what sustains COVID mutual aid groups. In the remainder of this section we summarise recent research that has addressed this question.

A rapid review of 27 articles on volunteering in the UK during the pandemic [25] identified several factors as important in sustaining effective volunteering, including established networks among residents and good relationships with existing organisations. Factors identified by groups as being important in retaining volunteers included having clear boundaries (i.e., not asking people to engage in activities with which they were uncomfortable), providing social rewards, fostering good relationships with the volunteers, and valuing volunteers' contributions [28].

One factor that might help to keep volunteers involved would be the extent to which the activity provides them with wellbeing. In his classic account of therapeutic communities, Fritz suggested that participating in post-disaster support could have mental health benefits [26]. The social cure approach in psychology complements this suggestion by proposing mechanisms through which psychological group membership can bolster wellbeing, including offering connectedness, support, efficacy, and meaning [29]. Based on these models, we carried out an interview study to explore the possible consequences of participation in mutual aid groups for participants' mental health and wellbeing [30]. The interviewees were 11 volunteers in mutual aid groups aligned to a housing campaign organisation, ACORN. The sample comprised a mixture of people who had previously been involved in ACORN's campaigning and those who had joined recently to get involved in COVID mutual aid. Activities included door-to-door food delivery, administration support, post collection, social calls, and assisting at a foodbank.

Our analysis suggests that participation in the mutual aid group provided participants with wellbeing in different ways, including positive emotional experiences, increased sense of engagement in life, improved social relationships, and a greater sense of control. These findings build on previous research showing that volunteering can benefit participants' wellbeing through social cure processes such as contributing to a sense of belonging [31]. Our findings add to this previous research by showing how these processes can operate in a COVID setting in which there is potential risk to participants.

Identities and framings of the activities were important for the people we interviewed. Those who viewed their participation through the lens of their political identity were able to experience additional benefits, such as feelings of empowerment. Those people who possessed a more apolitical shared identity linked this to new feelings of connectedness and camaraderie [30].

In a second study, we interviewed 32 organisers of COVID mutual aid and community solidarity groups in the UK between September 2020 and January 2021 to examine (a) the strategies they employed to keep the groups going and (b) any experiences or other factors found to be important in keeping volunteers involved. By speaking to organisers we intended to get evidence on what worked, and by interviewing people across the UK and in different types of mutual aid groups (some political and some not, some working with local authorities and some not) we hoped to get a range of views and experiences.

Two types of factor appeared to be foundational in sustaining the groups over time. First, access to and use of *resources* in the local area were critical. Mutual aid groups were highly dependent on small donations and local volunteers. Local businesses and companies donated food and other grocery items. Charities and food banks offered donations or made their resources (e.g., vans) available. Community centres opened their kitchens so that groups could cook and distribute hot meals. Local printers donated leaflets and posters that were then distributed by local volunteers. Volunteers used their own vehicles, laptops, phones, and other personal resources. Second, *trust* and hence positive relations at different levels, with existing organisations, with other support groups, and with people in the community, was essential.

In addition to these foundational factors, organisers employed a number of strategies to keep volunteers engaged and motivated. Twenty interviewees said that they actively tried to keep the communication regular within the group, including by asking volunteers about their needs regularly, and trying to respond to their needs, thereby creating a culture of care in the group. Indeed the importance of caring for and supporting group members was explicitly mentioned by 22 participants. Interviewees developed guidelines to protect volunteers and avoid the risk of spreading the virus when providing support for other people. Interviewees also mentioned the importance of ensuring that no volunteer got overloaded, that the workload was distributed fairly, and that emotional support was provided for volunteers when necessary. Participants used WhatsApp and Facebook groups, as well as regular telephone calls, to facilitate internal communication. Most of the groups organised regular meetings. Although most meetings were online, some groups had the opportunity to meet outdoors. The structure of the group seemed to matter. Although there was often a division of labour between organisers, interviewees suggested that an open or horizontal organisation helped to sustain others' engagement.

A sense of being a part of the group was something that organisers sought to foster among volunteers. In fact, a sense of belonging to or identification with the group or with the local community was also an emergent experience reported by many – that is, it was something that arose spontaneously from participation and served to motivate people to continue participation. Other positive experiences common among interviewees that drove further involvement included group efficacy, perceived support, positive emotion, and wellbeing. People maintained their commitment to the groups when they felt that they were making a difference, they learned new skills, and they enjoyed the activity. Some of these findings have been echoed by other researchers who have shown that identification is a predictor of mutual aid participation [32], and that the mental health benefits of mutual aid participation are predicted by a sense of unity and community identification [33].

Conclusions

General Principles That Emerge from the Research

Group processes, which include identification, relations with other groups, and group norms and influence, are not the only psychological predictors of the public engaging with the public health response to the COVID-19 pandemic. However, they have been shown to be important in their own right, and as prisms for other key predictors such as risk perception. For example, adherence decreases where risk is framed in terms of personal outcomes and people define themselves as fit, young, and healthy. It is worth noting that identification has been found to be a predictor of overall compliance in panel studies [34], and that it plays a role in other relevant behaviours, such as people engaging with infection testing. Identification also interacts with trust in authority [35].

It is important to understand, however, that in many cases the ability of the public to act upon these psychological motivations required sufficient practical and material support. In the case of self-isolation, surveys show that people's financial situation was a key predictor of adherence to the rules, and that intentions to self-isolate were higher than reported self-isolation [17]. This evidence suggests that willingness to adhere was not always matched by sufficient financial capacity to do so. In our studies of mutual aid groups, we found that groups were able to sustain themselves because they had access to the resources they needed to perform their tasks, namely people's availability to participate and access to goods and funds. The ability to mobilise resources in the long term is a challenge faced by many groups, especially those working with marginalised groups and in a socioeconomically deprived area [36]. Clearly, without resources and with insufficient volunteers, groups are likely to lack efficacy and those members who remain are at risk of burnout.

Understanding low levels of engagement with protective behaviours during the pandemic as psychological weakness or selfishness is the wrong psychology. Far from 'fatiguing', the public were willing to endure sacrifices for the greater good [16]. Changes in levels of engagement reflected changes in official communication, and sometimes became less clear, and information on the efficacy of behaviours was only believed where there was trust in the authorities, which varied with different social groups. However, the 'weakness' and 'selfishness' explanations did have a function, despite lacking supportive evidence. This was to blame the public for their own illness (see Chapter 19) and to absolve the authorities of culpability. The analysis presented in this chapter is not only an evidence-based alternative to this approach, but also offers the basis for actionable practical recommendations.

Policy and Practical Implications of the Research

A first recommendation is to use the psychological principles described here to maintain the public's engagement with the protective behaviours that are required in the pandemic. A motivation to 'do it for our community', whether this involves wearing a face covering or volunteering, requires a sense of being part of that community. Forms of communication from the public health authorities can convey that sense of shared identity simply through the language used (e.g., using the term 'we' instead of 'you'). However, more fundamentally, the structure of the relationship between these authorities and the public matters, too. Employing principles of coproduction for interventions means that the public are involved from the outset, own the aims, and can act as ambassadors for the measures to others in their community.

A second recommendation is a simple one. In order to fix the biggest gap in areas of public engagement with protective behaviours, those people who are self-isolating should be given sufficient financial support so that staying at home does not mean that they lose money.

Given the importance of resources in sustaining COVID-19 mutual aid groups, the third recommendation is that practical and financial support should be provided for COVID-19 mutual aid groups. However, this should be done without constraining or interfering in their actions, decisions, or activities, so that these groups are still attractive to people who want to support their communities without bureaucracy, and even campaign against wider injustices.

Our knowledge of the factors that have facilitated the public response to COVID-19 is growing. The aim is to take this knowledge back to those members of the public who are active in order to help them to sustain the most demanding and difficult actions, such as running COVID mutual aid groups. A repository of case studies, examples of what works, and lessons learned can be found at www.sussex.ac.uk/research/projects/groups-and-covid/community-support-and-mutual-aid

Acknowledgments

This work was supported by the UK Research and Innovation/Economic and Social Research Council (grant reference number ES/V005383/1), with assistance from Sanj Choudhury.

References

1. Costello A. *A Social Vaccine for Ebola. A Lesson for the Democratic Republic of Congo.* Anthony Costello, 2018 (www.anthonycostello.net/2018/05/20/a-social-vaccine-for-ebola-a-lesson-for-the-democratic-republic-of-congo/).

2. Independent SAGE. *Maintaining Adherence to Protective Behaviours During Vaccination Roll-Out.* Independent SAGE, 2021 (www.independentsage.org/wp-content/uploads/2021/01/Adverse-behavioural-effects-of-vaccines-7.1.pdf).

3. Public Health England. *Finding the Evidence: Coronavirus.* Public Health England, 2021 (https://phelibrary.koha-ptfs.co.uk/coronavirusinformation/).

4. World Health Organization (WHO). *COVID-19 Press Conference.* WHO, 2020 (www.who.int/docs/default-source/coronaviruse/transcripts/who-audio-emergencies-coronavirus-press-conference-full-20mar2020.pdf?sfvrsn=1eafbff_0).

5. British Psychological Society. *Behavioural Science and Disease Prevention: Psychological Guidance for Optimising Policies and Communication.* British Psychological Society, 2020 (www.bps.org.uk/coronavirus-resources/professional/behavioural-science-disease-prevention-psychological-guidance).

6. Folmer RC, Kuiper ME, Olthuis E, Kooistra EB, de Bruijn AL, Brownlee M, et al. *Maintaining Compliance When the Virus Returns: Understanding Adherence to Social Distancing Measures in the Netherlands in July 2020.* PsyArXiv, 2020 (https://psyarxiv.com/vx3mn/).

7. Clark C, Davila A, Regis M, Kraus S. Predictors of COVID-19 voluntary compliance behaviors: an international investigation. *Glob Transit* 2020; **2**: 76–82.

8. Van Bavel JJ, Cichocka A, Capraro V, Sjåstad H, Nezlek JB, Alfano M, et al. *National Identity Predicts Public Health Support during a Global Pandemic: Results from 67 Nations.* PsyArXiv, 2020 (https://psyarxiv.com/ydt95/).

9. Vignoles VL, Jaser Z, Taylor Z, Ntontis E. Harnessing shared identities to mobilize resilient responses to the COVID-19

pandemic. *Polit Psychol* 2021; **42**: 817–26.

10. Liekefett L, Becker J. Compliance with governmental restrictions during the coronavirus pandemic: a matter of personal self-protection or solidarity with people in risk groups? *Br J Soc Psychol* 2021; **60**: 924–46.

11. Pfattheicher S, Nockur L, Böhm R, Sassenrath C, Petersen MB. The emotional path to action: empathy promotes physical distancing and wearing of face masks during the COVID-19 pandemic. *Psychol Sci* 2020; **31**: 1363–73.

12. Nivette A, Ribeaud D, Murray A, Steinhoff A, Bechtiger L, Hepp U, et al. Non-compliance with COVID-19-related public health measures among young adults in Switzerland: insights from a longitudinal cohort study. *Soc Sci Med* 2021; **268**: 113370.

13. Van Lissa CJ, Stroebe W, van Dellen M, Leander P, Agostini M, Gutzkow B, et al. *Early Indicators of COVID-19 Infection Prevention Behaviors: Machine Learning Identifies Personal and Country-Level Factors.* PsyArXiv, 2020 (https://psyarxiv.com/whjsb/).

14. Tuncgenc B, El Zein M, Sulik J, Newson M, Zhao Y, Dezecache G, et al. Social influence matters: we follow pandemic guidelines most when our close circle does. *Br J Psychol* 2021; **112**: 763–80.

15. Office for National Statistics. *Coronavirus and the Social Impacts on Great Britain: 30 April 2021.* Office for National Statistics, 2021 (www.ons.gov.uk/peoplepopulationandcommunity/healthandsocialcare/healthandwellbeing/bulletins/coronavirusandthesocialimpactsongreatbritain/30april2021#main-indicators).

16. Drury J. *Mitigating the New Variant SARS-CoV-2 Virus: How to Support Public Adherence to Physical Distancing.* Crowds and Identities, 2020 (https://blogs.sussex.ac.uk/crowdsidentities/2020/12/27/mitigating-the-new-variant-sars-cov-2-virus-how-to-support-public-adherence-to-physical-distancing/).

17. Smith LE, Potts HWW, Amlôt R, Fear NT, Michie S, Rubin GJ. Adherence to the test, trace, and isolate system in the UK: results from 37 nationally representative surveys. *BMJ* 2021; **372**: n608.

18. Patel J, Fernandes G, Sridhar D. How can we improve self-isolation and quarantine for covid-19? *BMJ* 2021; **372**: n625.

19. Butler P. A million volunteer to help NHS and others during Covid-19 outbreak. *The Guardian*, 13 April 2020 (www.theguardian.com/society/2020/apr/13/a-million-volunteer-to-help-nhs-and-others-during-covid-19-lockdown).

20. Office for National Statistics. *Executive Summary: Community Life COVID-19 Re-Contact Survey 2020.* Office for National Statistics, 2020 (www.gov.uk/government/statistics/community-life-covid-19-re-contact-survey-2020-main-report/executive-summary-community-life-recontact-survey-2020).

21. Office for National Statistics. *Coronavirus and the Social Impacts on Great Britain: 7 May 2020.* Office for National Statistics, 2020 (www.ons.gov.uk/peoplepopulationandcommunity/healthandsocialcare/healthandwellbeing/bulletins/coronavirusandthesocialimpactsongreatbritain/7may2020#how-relationships-are-changing-and-community-support-networks).

22. Solnit R. 'The way we get through this is together': the rise of mutual aid under coronavirus. *The Guardian*, 14 May 2020 (www.theguardian.com/world/2020/may/14/mutual-aid-coronavirus-pandemic-rebecca-solnit).

23. Booth R. Community aid groups set up across UK amid coronavirus crisis. *The Guardian*, 16 March 2020 (www.theguardian.com/society/2020/mar/16/community-aid-groups-set-up-across-uk-amid-coronavirus-crisis).

24. Tiratelli L, Kaye S. *Communities vs. Coronavirus: The Rise of Mutual Aid.* New Local, 2020 (www.newlocal.org.uk/publications/communities-vs-coronavirus-the-rise-of-mutual-aid/).

25. Mao G, Fernandes-Jesus M, Ntontis E, Drury J. What have we learned about COVID-19 volunteering in the UK? A rapid review of the literature. *BMC Public Health* 2021; **21**: 1470.

26. Fritz CE. *Disasters and Mental Health: Therapeutic Principles Drawn from Disaster Studies.* Disaster Research Center, 1961 (http://udspace.udel.edu/handle/19716/1325).

27. Kaniasty K, Norris FH. The experience of disaster: individuals and communities sharing trauma. In *Response to Disaster: Psychosocial, Community, and Ecological Approaches* (eds R Gist, B Lubin): 25–61. Brunner/Maze, 1999.

28. McCabe A, Wilson M, Paine AE. *Stepping Up and Helping Out: Grassroots Volunteering in Response to COVID-19.* Local Trust, 2020.

29. Haslam C, Jetten J, Cruwys T, Dingle GA, Haslam SA. *The New Psychology of Health: Unlocking the Social Cure.* Routledge, 2018.

30. Mao G, Drury J, Fernandes-Jesus M, Ntontis E. How participation in Covid-19 mutual aid groups affects subjective well-being and how political identity moderates these effects. *Anal Soc Issues Public Policy* 2021; **21**: 1082–112.

31. Gray D, Stevenson C. How can 'we' help? Exploring the role of shared social identity in the

experiences and benefits of volunteering. *J Community Appl Soc Psychol* 2020; **30**: 341–53.

32. Wakefield J, Bowe M, Kellezi B. Who helps and why? A longitudinal exploration of volunteer role identity, between-group closeness, and community identification as predictors of coordinated helping during the COVID-19 pandemic. *Br J Soc Psychol* 2022; **61**: 907–23.

33. Bowe M, Wakefield J, Kellezi B, Stevenson C, McNamara N, Jones B, et al. The mental health benefits of community helping during crisis: coordinated helping, community identification and sense of unity during the COVID-19 pandemic. *J Community Appl Soc Psychol* 2022; **32**: 521–35.

34. Stevenson C, Wakefield JRH, Felsner I, Drury J, Costa S. Collectively coping with coronavirus: local community identification predicts giving support and lockdown adherence during the COVID-19 pandemic. *Br J Soc Psychol* 2021; **60**: 1403–18.

35. Robin C, Symons C, Carter H. Rapid thematic analysis of community social and online media in response to mass asymptomatic COVID-19 testing in Liverpool, England. [Preprint] 2021. Available from: www.researchsquare.com/article/rs-370851/v1

36. Greater London Authority (GLA). *The Experience of Mutual Aid in London*. GLA, 2020 (https://data.gov.uk/dataset/b8adb6dd-7408-4821-a38e-5b27bdba9b21/the-experience-of-mutual-aid-in-london).

Chapter

25

The Social Psychology of Mass Casualty Decontamination in Chemical, Biological, Radiological, or Nuclear (CBRN) Incidents

Holly Carter, Charles Symons, Dale Weston, and Richard Amlôt

Introduction

Large-scale incidents that involve chemical, biological, radiological, or nuclear (CBRN) material, whether accidental toxic industrial chemical releases, or deliberate chemical terrorism/warfare, remain a high-impact public health threat [1]. Mass casualty decontamination is a critical early intervention involving the rapid removal of hazardous substances from skin and hair to reduce adverse health outcomes. Decontamination is most effective when carried out quickly after the event [2]. In the UK, the recent Initial Operational Response (IOR) programme is a rapidly deployable precursor to specialist decontamination showering, and is designed to facilitate initiating decontamination prior to the arrival of specialist teams [3]. IOR actions include evacuating people from the source of contamination, removing their outer clothing (disrobing), and decontaminating their skin and hair with absorbent materials such as paper towels (dry decontamination), or with clean water if the substance is caustic.

For the sake of casualties' health *and* public health more broadly, it is essential that (a) casualties remain in place until decontamination is complete and (b) they are willing and able to undertake any actions recommended by emergency responders. However, CBRN incidents are inherently unfamiliar and ambiguous, and are likely to be very frightening for members of the public. Additionally, CBRN incidents differ from other types of emergencies in several ways. First, they require members of the public to remain at the scene of the incident in order to undergo decontamination and to avoid secondary contamination of other people and places. This may differ from other types of incident, in which people are likely to leave the scene in order to move away from the threat. Second, they require a unique specialist response that is likely to be unfamiliar to most people. Finally, interventions such as decontamination, which are designed to reduce

the health risk from incidents, may be more frightening for members of the public than the incident itself if they are not managed appropriately [4]. Therefore it is important to understand how the people affected are likely to behave during these types of incident, and to explore ways to optimise public cooperation and compliance with responders' instructions.

In a recent programme of research the social identity approach has been applied to examine the psychosocial aspects involved in the process of decontamination [5,6]. This focuses on the willingness and ability of members of the public to undergo decontamination. This research programme highlights the role of social identity in shaping public behaviour, and affecting public health outcomes, during incidents that involve mass decontamination [7]. When people share an identity it affects the way in which they behave, both with members of their own group and with members of other groups. Therefore the extent to which members of the public identify with each other, and with emergency responders, affects the outcomes from the incident [7]. This approach has previously been applied to understanding behaviour during various types of crowd events, including, but not limited to, riots [8], football matches [9], and crowds in emergencies [10]. In this chapter we describe applying the social identity approach to understanding the behaviour of crowds during incidents that require mass casualty decontamination [7].

The Research

A key finding from this research programme is that the way in which emergency responders manage an incident does affect the nature of the relationship between emergency responders and members of the public. In turn, this affects the behaviour of the public and hence outcomes from that incident [7,11]. Traditionally it has been suggested that the public is likely to behave in a disorderly or irrational way during emergencies, and (as Chapter 8 portrays) that it is likely to panic [12]. This view has been prevalent in planning assumptions for emergencies, including CBRN incidents, and (as outlined in Chapter 19) has led to a focus on controlling members of the public during these incidents [13]. Our research suggests that a shared social identity between responders and members of the public is necessary to enhance public willingness and capacity to engage with the process of decontamination. Emergency planners and responders must shift from regarding members of the public as passive recipients of healthcare, to be controlled or managed, to recognising the public as an important part of the emergency response, who should be engaged and informed before and during situations in which decontamination is required [14]. This relationship between emergency planners and responders and the public should not be confined to the duration of an incident, and should ideally be established in advance of future incidents [14,15].

Crucially, for shared identity to develop, the public should perceive responders as acting in a way that is legitimate, and this includes treating people fairly. However, if responders are perceived to attempt to control members of the public, these actions and attitudes are likely to be experienced as unfair or illegitimate, and could result in members of the public refusing to comply with responders' instructions, thereby producing the very resistance or 'disorderliness' that responders may see as inherent [7]. The rest of this chapter describes the specific actions that responders can take prior to an incident, in the early stages of an incident, and during an incident, to establish and maintain shared identity between themselves and members of the public, and thereby improve health outcomes [7,11,16].

Prior to an Incident

Prior to a CBRN incident occurring, the public should be informed about what to expect, and what actions they can take, in the event that an incident occurs. Not only is this likely to ensure that members of the public know what to do and can take actions quickly [15], but also it helps to foster shared norms and expectations between members of the public and authorities [14,15]. This is likely to help to facilitate the development of shared identity between members of the public and responders, and to make it easier for

responders to communicate with members of the public on arrival at an incident [7].

Increasingly, policymakers recognise the importance of involving the public in planning for disasters and emergencies, and this is included in the 2015–2030 Sendai Framework for Disaster Risk Reduction [17]. Several pre-incident information campaigns have been developed in an attempt to improve public preparedness for major incidents, including the 'Run, Hide, Tell' campaign for marauding terrorist firearms attacks [18], and the 'See it, Say it, Sorted' campaign that is designed to improve awareness on rail networks [19]. When developing these campaigns, it is essential that policymakers work closely with members of the public in order to ensure that they are involved in planning and preparing for emergencies, and that information provided prior to any incident occurring meets their needs; this also helps to foster the development of shared identity [14].

An example of a pre-incident information campaign for incidents that potentially require some form of decontamination is the REMOVE campaign [20]. This campaign is based on the IOR principles, which were described earlier in this chapter [3], and it provides members of the public with actions that they can take to help themselves and others during the early stages of an incident that involves hazardous materials, including CBRN incidents. Early drafts of the REMOVE information were evaluated, using focus groups with members of the public, to assess the participants' perceptions of the efficacy of the information, and to identify areas for improvement [21]. Following positive feedback from these focus groups, a revised version of REMOVE was evaluated using an online survey [16]. The findings showed that participants' knowledge and confidence in taking actions during these types of incidents increased significantly after viewing the REMOVE information. Participants also felt that the information was useful and easy to understand, and said that they would be willing to take the recommended actions. Additionally, there was overwhelming support for providing this type of information to the public, with only 4% of participants stating that they would not want to receive this information prior to an incident [16].

Thus the findings from the REMOVE campaign demonstrate the importance of providing pre-incident information for CBRN incidents that is intended to improve public knowledge and confidence in taking appropriate actions. This is in line with findings from a systematic review, which found that where public information campaigns have been developed for CBRN incidents they have resulted in improved public preparedness [15]. Pre-incident information should therefore (a) include information about the actions that people can take to protect themselves and others, (b) explain why these actions are effective, and (c) be provided using multiple platforms, ensuring consistency of information across each platform. Since information designed to improve preparedness for CBRN incidents constitutes basic first aid actions that also apply to other types of hazardous materials incidents (e.g., accidental chemical spills), this information should be widely distributed in any first aid context. It can also be delivered as a wider public information campaign during times of particularly high risk when, for example, there is a clear and identifiable CBRN-related threat to national security.

The Early Stages of an Incident

It is not sufficient to simply direct or instruct casualties to follow a set of instructions. Casualties need to know *why* decontamination is necessary. They are unlikely to have experienced an incident requiring decontamination before, and so need to understand why decontamination is important, and what it involves. During the early stages of an incident, responders should focus on enhancing casualties' willingness to undertake recommended actions (e.g., disrobing, undergoing decontamination). In order to achieve this, it is crucial that responders communicate with members of the public about the actions they are taking, what actions members of the public can take, and why these actions are effective. Doing so is likely to increase public perceptions of the legitimacy of responders' actions, and thereby foster a shared identity between responders and members of the public, with shared norms developed around undergoing decontamination processes to protect public health [22,23]. This shared identity is crucial for motivating casualties to remain in place (rather than leave to go home, which risks spreading the contaminant) and to adhere to any recommended actions for their decontamination.

As outlined, pre-incident communication is likely to be an effective way of preparing potential casualties

for this situation. In addition, responders should engage with possibly contaminated people as soon as possible after the known or suspected release of a hazardous agent. At this stage, responders should focus on communicating openly and honestly about the nature of the threat, and on explaining to members of the public what actions they can take to protect themselves, and why such actions are effective.

Communicate Honestly About the Threat

Policy and practice for mass decontamination have traditionally been based on assumptions about public behaviour during emergencies, derived from traditional theories of crowd behaviour (e.g., that, as described earlier, people will panic). This has led to a focus on the need to control members of the public, including withholding information from them due to fear that if given that information they will behave irrationally [13,24]. However (as Chapter 8 explains), decades of research now show that panic is rare during emergencies, and that people are much more likely to behave in helpful and cooperative ways [10,25], and (as Chapters 22 and 23 illustrate) may render services that make important contributions to the overall responses. The social identity approach suggests that this is because members of the public are likely to experience a sense of shared identity during such incidents, due to the shared fate they all face, and that it is this shared identity that motivates helpful and cooperative behaviour [10]. Reliance on traditional assumptions about maladaptive behaviour during emergencies is misguided, particularly as lack of information may itself create the anxiety [26] and 'disorderly' behaviour [27] that the people responsible for managing the incident are hoping to avoid. Withholding information is also likely to hinder the development of shared identity between responders and members of the public. If members of the public identify with each other, but not with emergency responders managing the incident, they may unite to challenge responders' authority by, for example, refusing to undergo decontamination [7].

Additionally, far from creating maladaptive public responses, accurate information about the health threat is a key factor in motivating adaptive responses [28]. This proposition is supported by findings from a double-blind randomised controlled experiment, in which participants viewed an immersive virtual reality video depicting a scenario that required IOR [29].

In this experiment, communicating honestly about the severity and likelihood of contamination, rather than withholding information, resulted in participants' greater willingness to comply with recommended actions (i.e., to make an adaptive health response to the threat), and this further highlights the importance of honest communication.

Communicate About Efficacy of Decontamination

Although it is important that responders communicate honestly about the nature of the threat, they must also communicate what actions people should take to reduce their risk, which in this case is decontamination, and explain why these actions are effective. Communicating about a threat, without also communicating about effective actions that can be taken to reduce the risk from that threat, is likely to be less effective and could be counterproductive – for example, it could lead to denial of risk [28]. Conversely, explaining why a recommended action is effective has been shown to result in improved compliance with decontamination procedures [22,29].

Explaining why members of the public are being asked to take certain actions and why such actions are effective is also likely to enhance people's perceptions of responders' legitimacy. In a randomised online experiment [23] and field experiment [22], communication that contained updates about actions being taken by responders and health-focused reasons as to why decontamination was necessary resulted in participants reporting their increased perceptions of responders' legitimacy, which in turn enhanced their shared identification with emergency responders. These increased perceptions of responders' legitimacy and identification with emergency responders subsequently resulted in greater willingness to cooperate with each other and comply with instructions for decontamination.

During the Incident

Provide Sufficient Practical Information

Once members of the public are motivated to undergo decontamination, they need to be provided with sufficient practical information about how to perform decontamination, and be willing to work together to ensure that the process runs smoothly.

Evidence from mass decontamination field exercises and a decontamination field experiment shows that providing sufficient practical information results in reduced confusion among members of the public during the decontamination process [22,26], and improved speed and efficiency of decontamination [22]. Providing practical information can therefore ensure that people know how to protect themselves and others.

Foster Willingness to Work Together

By explaining openly and honestly the actions that members of the public need to take and providing sufficient practical information, responders are likely to enhance public willingness and ability to take protective actions. However, it is also necessary for members of the public to work together to ensure that the decontamination process runs smoothly. Incidents that require decontamination are likely to involve a fairly small number of responders compared with the numbers of members of the public affected. The more that members of the public are willing and able to work together, the more smoothly the process is likely to run [7]. Working together in this context involves two key factors, namely cooperation (e.g., forming an orderly queue to go through decontamination) and active helping (e.g., assisting others to go through the process of decontamination).

People are more likely to work together if they identify with each other [30]. As already noted, shared identity is likely to be experienced by members of the public involved in a CBRN incident, due to the sense of shared fate that they all face [10]. When there is a shared identity among a group of people, this results in (a) greater salience of shared goals (in this case, the goal of undergoing decontamination) [30], (b) a sense of collective agency, which is a belief that the people involved in the incident can work together to achieve shared goals and overcome any challenges they face [31], and (c) motivation to help and cooperate with other group members [30,32]. Evidence suggests that if responders foster shared identity between members of the public and themselves, this can further enhance any shared identity among members of the public by uniting them around shared goals (e.g., decontamination) [22,23,33]. Effective communication from emergency responders, as described earlier, can achieve this by (a) promoting public willingness to work together, by establishing trust, which enhances identification with emergency responders and ensures that undergoing decontamination is accepted as a shared goal, and (b) promoting the public's ability to work together, by providing people with the information that they need in order to know what to do during decontamination.

Demonstrate Respect for Public Needs

Concerns about Privacy

Decontamination involves removing clothing and potentially undergoing a shower in front of a large number of people. Although establishing the need for decontamination as a shared norm, using the actions described earlier, is likely to go some way towards helping people to feel more comfortable. Evidence from real incidents [13], field exercises [13,26,33], and a field experiment [22] reveals that concerns about privacy remain a potential barrier to compliance. To overcome this, responders should try, as far as possible, to ensure that people's needs for privacy are met during decontamination. Responders should explain the reasons why it is not possible to meet privacy needs when this occurs. This demonstrates understanding and respect for the public's needs, and enhances the perceived legitimacy of responders' actions [22,33].

Vulnerable Groups of People

As well as demonstrating respect for public needs for privacy, responders must also understand and demonstrate respect for other personal needs, including understanding the needs of members of vulnerable groups. There are many factors that may make someone more vulnerable during an incident that requires decontamination. For this reason it is helpful to take a functional needs approach, in which the needs that different people may have are considered in terms of how they may affect their ability to undergo decontamination [24]. There are four main areas of functional need that should be considered when planning for decontamination: (a) physical needs, including any factors that may make it difficult for someone to physically undergo decontamination; (b) communication needs, including any factors that may make it difficult for someone to hear, see, or understand responders' instructions; (c) pre-existing health needs, including any factors that may make someone more susceptible to either the decontamination process or

the effects of the CBRN agent; (d) social and cultural needs, including any social or cultural norms that may make it difficult for someone to undertake particular actions.

A review of the literature on the needs of vulnerable groups during decontamination revealed several actions that responders can take to ensure that the needs of all are met [24]. They include (a) implementing a buddy system, whereby a person with additional functional needs during decontamination is paired with another member of the public, (b) providing simple pictorial instructions, (c) allowing individuals to retain any functional aids (e.g., prosthetic limbs, walking aids) where possible during decontamination, and (d) considering ethical, religious, and cultural needs, especially when asking people to disrobe. It is essential that responders treat everyone as an expert in their own needs, and that they work to ensure that, wherever possible, those needs are met. This also demonstrates respect for public needs, enhances the public's perceptions of responders' legitimacy, and increases willingness to comply with responders' instructions [7].

Summary and Recommendations

During incidents that require decontamination, the nature of the relationship between responders and members of the public is likely to play a key part in shaping public behaviour. The way in which responders manage an incident affects the nature of the relationship between members of the public and responders and the way in which members of the public behave, which will affect health outcomes. Effective communication must begin prior to an incident occurring, continuing into the early stages of an incident and throughout the duration of the incident. There are several actions that responders should take at each stage to facilitate smooth running of the decontamination process, and to improve outcomes.

Information provided before the incident occurs should:

- describe the actions that people can take to protect themselves and others in the event of a CBRN incident
- explain why the recommended actions are effective for reducing risk
- be provided using multiple platforms, ensuring consistency of information across each platform.

In the early stages of an incident, responders should:

- communicate openly and honestly with members of the public about the nature of the threat
- inform members of the public about the actions they can take to protect themselves and others
- provide health-focused explanations as to why each recommended action is important, and how it will protect members of the public.

During the incident, responders should:

- provide sufficient practical information to enable members of the public to take the actions recommended
- demonstrate respect for the public's needs, including needs for privacy
- treat each person as an expert in their own needs
- ensure that support is available for people who have additional functional needs.

References

1. Cabinet Office. *Global Britain in a Competitive Age: The Integrated Review of Security, Defence, Development and Foreign Policy*. HM Government, 2021 (www.gov.uk/government/publications/global-britain-in-a-competitive-age-the-integrated-review-of-security-defence-development-and-foreign-policy/global-britain-in-a-competitive-age-the-integrated-review-of-security-defence-development-and-foreign-policy).

2. Chilcott RP. Managing mass casualties and decontamination. *Environ int* 2014; 72: 37–45.

3. Home Office. *Initial Operational Response to a CBRN Incident*. Home Office, 2015 (www.jesip.org.uk/uploads/media/pdf/CBRN%20JOPs/IOR_Guidance_V2_July_2015.pdf).

4. Holloway HC, Norwood AE, Fullerton CS, Engel CC, Ursano RJ. The threat of biological weapons: prophylaxis and mitigation of psychological and social consequences. *JAMA* 1997; 278: 425–7.

5. Tajfel H, Turner J. An integrative theory of intergroup conflict. In *The Social Psychology of Intergroup Relations* (eds WG Austin, S Worchel): 33–47. Wadsworth, 1979.

6. Turner JC, Hogg MA, Oakes PJ, Reicher SD, Wetherell MS. *Rediscovering the Social Group: A Self-Categorization Theory*. Basil Blackwell, 1987.

7. Carter H, Drury J, Rubin GJ, Williams R, Amlôt R. Applying crowd psychology to develop recommendations for the management of mass decontamination. *Health Secur* 2015; 13: 45–53.

8. Reicher S. The St Pauls riot: an explanation of the limits of crowd action in terms of a social identity model. *Eur J Soc Psychol* 1984;14: 1–21.

9. Stott C, Reicher S. How conflict escalates: the inter-group dynamics of collective football crowd violence. *Sociology* 1998; 32: 353–77.

10. Drury J, Cocking C, Reicher S. The nature of collective resilience: survivor reactions to the 2005 London bombings. *Int J Mass Emerg Disasters* 2009; 27: 66–95.

11. Carter H, Drury J, Amlôt R. Social identity and intergroup relationships in the management of crowds during mass emergencies and disasters: recommendations for emergency planners and responders. *Policing* 2020; 14: 931–44.

12. Le Bon G. *The Crowd: A Study of the Popular Mind*. Ernest Benn, 1895.

13. Carter H, Drury J, Rubin GJ, Williams R, Amlôt R. Communication during mass casualty decontamination: highlighting the gaps. *Int J Emerg Serv* 2013; 2: 29–48.

14. Drury J, Carter H, Cocking C, Ntontis E, Tekin Guven S,

Amlôt R. Facilitating collective psychosocial resilience in the public in emergencies: twelve recommendations based on the social identity approach. *Front Public Health* 2019; 7: 141.

15. Carter H, Drury J, Amlôt R. Recommendations for improving public engagement with pre-incident information materials for initial response to a chemical, biological, radiological or nuclear (CBRN) incident: a systematic review. *Int J Disaster Risk Reduct* 2020; 51: 101796.

16. Carter HE, Gauntlett L, Amlôt R. Public perceptions of the 'Remove, Remove, Remove' information campaign before and during a hazardous materials incident: a survey. *Health Secur* 2021; 19: 100–107.

17. UN Office for Disaster Risk Reduction (UNDRR). *Sendai Framework for Disaster Risk Reduction 2015–2030*. UNDRR, 2015. (www.preventionweb.net/files/43291_sendaiframeworkfordrren.pdf).

18. City of London Police. *Run Hide Tell*. City of London Police, 2017 (www.cityoflondon.police.uk/advice-and-support/counteringterrorism/Pages/stay-safe.aspx).

19. British Transport Police. *New National Rail Security Campaign Starts Today: 'See it. Say it. Sorted'*. British Transport Police, 2016 (www.btp.police.uk/latest_news/

see_it_say_it_sorted_new_natio
.aspx).

20. National Ambulance Resilience Unit (NARU). *'Remove, Remove, Remove' – refreshed IOR Messaging Released by NARU.* NARU, 2018 (https://naru.org.uk/remove-remove-remove-refreshed-ior-messaging-is-released-by-naru/).

21. Carter H, Weston D, Symons C, Amlot R. Public perceptions of pre-incident information campaign materials for the initial response to a chemical incident. *Disaster Prev Manag* 2019; 28. Available from: https://doi.org/10.1108/DPM-10-2018-0342.

22. Carter H, Drury J, Amlôt R, Rubin GJ, Williams R. Effective responder communication improves efficiency and psychological outcomes in a mass decontamination field experiment: implications for public behaviour in the event of a chemical incident. *PLoS One* 2014; 9: e89846.

23. Carter H, Drury J, Amlôt R, Rubin GJ, Williams R. Effective responder communication, perceived responder legitimacy, and group identification predict public cooperation and compliance in a mass

decontamination visualization experiment. *J Appl Soc Psychol* 2015; 45: 173–89.

24. Carter H, Amlôt R. Mass casualty decontamination guidance and psychosocial aspects of CBRN incident management: a review and synthesis. *PLoS Curr* 2016; 8. Available from: https://doi.org/10.1371/currents.dis.c2d3d652d9d07a2a620ed5429e017ef5.

25. Clarke L. Panic: myth or reality? *Contexts* 2002; 1: 21–6.

26. Carter H, Drury J, Rubin GJ, Williams R, Amlôt R. Public experiences of mass casualty decontamination. *Biosecur Bioterror* 2012; 10: 280–89.

27. Stott C, Hutchison P, Drury J. 'Hooligans' abroad? Intergroup dynamics, social identity and participation in collective 'disorder' at the 1998 World Cup Finals. *Br J Soc Psychol* 2001; 40: 359–384.

28. Peters G-JY, Ruiter RA, Kok G. Threatening communication: a critical re-analysis and a revised meta-analytic test of fear appeal theory. *Health Psychol Rev* 2013; 7 (suppl 1): S8–31.

29. Symons C, Amlôt R, Carter H, Rubin GJ. Effects of threat and efficacy messages on expected

adherence to decontamination protocols in an immersive simulated chemical incident: a randomized controlled experiment. *J Contingencies Crisis Manag* 2021; 29: 54–76.

30. Drury, J. Collective resilience in mass emergencies and disasters: a social identity model. In *The Social Cure: Identity, Health, and Well-Being* (eds J Jetten, C Haslam, SA Haslam): 195–215. Psychology Press, 2012.

31. Haslam C, Reicher S. Stressing the group: social identity and the unfolding dynamics of responses to stress. *J Appl Psychol* 2006; 91: 1037–52.

32. Drury J, Cocking C, Reicher S, Burton A, Schofield D, Hardwick A, et al. Cooperation versus competition in a mass emergency evacuation: a new laboratory simulation and a new theoretical model. *Behav Res Methods* 2009; 41, 957–70.

33. Carter H, Drury J, Amlôt R, Rubin GJ, Williams R. Perceived responder legitimacy and group identification predict cooperation and compliance in a mass decontamination field exercise. *Basic Appl Soc Psychol* 2013; 35: 575–85.

Chapter

26

Factors That Determine Wider Solidarity Responses After a Major Incident or Disaster

Trevor K James, Selin Tekin, and Hanna Zagefka

Introduction

During and in the aftermath of an emergencies, incidents, terrorist events, disasters, disease outbreaks and conflicts (EITDDC), acts of community support are not only displayed by those people who are directly affected by the events, but can also be supported by 'outsiders' [1]. The focus of this chapter is on the psychological drivers of assistance offered by individuals who are not directly affected by a tragedy. We refer to this as 'intergroup solidarity'. Intergroup solidarity arises when different groups come together in a crisis and work together in the face of adversity.

Intergroup Solidarity

There are three features that delineate intergroup solidarity from related concepts such as intergroup helping and charitable behaviours, which we argue are conceptually different. First, intergroup solidarity can be political in that it is driven by an awareness of social and political inequalities and injustices. Second, we propose that intergroup solidarity is often more enduring, and potentially more costly, than discrete acts of prosociality (e.g., a one-off charitable donation). Third, aid is not restricted to the groups to which we belong (i.e., ingroups), as people from the wider community not directly affected by events (i.e., outgroups) might also show solidarity with survivors and bereaved families [1]. Intergroup solidarity thus consists of allyship from an outgroup member that is manifested in support behaviours. Moreover, it can result in social support through community groups that provide mutual aid [2], as well as meeting people's practical needs for, for example, food, accommodation, and medical supplies [3], or meeting political needs relating to justice [4]. We elaborate on the three defining features of intergroup solidarity that we propose.

The political dimension of intergroup solidarity relates to the fact that disasters disproportionately affect disadvantaged sections of the community [5–7]. Unequal resource distribution prior to a disaster significantly affects people's ability to recover in the aftermath. Therefore working-class and disadvantaged ethnic groups suffer disproportionately due to systemic inequalities and political mismanagement [5–7]. Indeed people often support each other in seeking justice for their perceived mistreatment by authorities [4]. An awareness of social injustices, as well as the political context, is a defining feature in our account of intergroup solidarity.

The second defining feature is that intergroup solidarity is more enduring than short-term helping responses. It implies assistance over a longer period, meaning that it is essential to analyse how support develops along a timeline [8]. Chapter 23 offers support for this proposition based on research on flooding. This lasting support element distinguishes intergroup solidarity from quick one-off acts of helping (e.g., in response to a charitable fundraising appeal).

The third feature is that intergroup solidarity focuses on allyship from outgroup members, defined either in terms of a distinction between those people who are affected by the incident and injustices that led to it compared with people who are not, or in terms of other salient group memberships, such as class or ethnicity. Intergroup solidarity thus entails a sense of 'us' supporting 'them'.

An example of a disaster that gave rise to intergroup solidarity was the Grenfell Tower fire of 2017 in London, England. Grenfell Tower was a 24-storey housing block that contained 120 flats in a mix of social housing and private homes. It was managed by Kensington and Chelsea Tenant Management Organisation (KCTMO) on behalf of the local authority. A fire began on 14 June 2017, and spread rapidly due to the cheap flammable cladding used during initial refurbishment undertaken by KCTMO in 2016 [9]. In total, 72 people died and over 200 were made homeless. Thousands were left traumatised.

It was the worst fire in the UK since the Second World War. Many of the people who died were from working-class backgrounds and/or disadvantaged ethnic groups [10]. Despite residents having raised the issue of fire safety repeatedly in the 4 years preceding the fire, KCTMO did not undertake improvements to safety requirements. In the immediate aftermath of the fire, wider community members – that is, outgroups – came together for mutual support for food and accommodation [11]. These community members also created campaign events to seek justice for the victims. These demands for justice not only related to the needs of Grenfell Tower survivors and bereaved families, but also related to people still at risk due to the unsafe social housing conditions being offered to marginalised groups. Notably, the wider community demonstrated solidarity and attended campaign activities. For example, a monthly Silent Walk was attended by people from wider communities who had not suffered first-hand [4]. The Grenfell Tower fire gave rise to behaviour that can be conceptualised in terms of intergroup solidarity. Helping behaviours were driven by an awareness of political injustices that had been endured over time, and included an intergroup component in the allyship offered by people who were not themselves directly affected by the fire.

Psychological Drivers of Intergroup Solidarity After a Disaster: How Identities Shape Attitudes Towards Helping

Previous research into predictors of support for action against political injustices has identified several key psychological factors. Liga Klavina and colleagues found that anger, group identification, and the perceived likelihood that one's actions will make a difference were key predictors of Latino Americans acting in support of Black Americans [12]. Rim Saab and colleagues found that moral outrage and sympathy in response to a disadvantaged outgroup's suffering had significant impacts [13]. The key roles played by moral outrage and perceived efficacy were also shown by Francesco and colleagues, who studied prosocial actions on behalf of 'poor people' – an outgroup to the study's participants [14]. Furthermore, negative emotions, such as perspective taking and group-based guilt, have also been found to be important [15]. However, although all of these factors play a key role

in understanding collective solidarity more generally, it is worth elaborating on one of the key processes that inform the emergence of intergroup solidarity after a disaster – that is, social identity.

Historically, psychologists have noted that how a person perceives their identity can play an important role in solidarity – for example, with regard to the Second World War and allyship towards the Jewish community against deportation [16] and the 'Blitz spirit' (Chapter 22 describes the latter in more detail). Researchers have focused on how motives associated with group memberships (e.g., a sense of belonging) can amplify intergroup solidarity in order to further understand these helping behaviours. For example, allies from advantaged groups can be driven to help by a wish to bolster and verify an identity that values moral affirmation and acceptance [17]. Similarly, individuals who value being part of a salient group will feel more positive if they behave in a manner that their group values [18]. Therefore if a person perceives that helping after a disaster is normative within their social ingroup and a fundamental aspect of their identity, displays of intergroup solidarity are likely to generate emotional responses that encourage helping, and that person is more likely to engage [19].

Interestingly, this suggests that identification with the group that needs help is not necessary. The identification that matters can be with a group of supporters (e.g., 'I, a Western citizen, identify with other supporters of Syrian refugees', or 'I, a white person, identify with other white people who support the Black Lives Matter movement'). Therefore belonging to a group with a shared sense of common purpose of providing support for other groups can provide psychological benefits, such as a sense of belonging and meaning in life [17] Because of the beneficial psychological effects for the person of belonging to groups acting in solidarity, these actions can be assumed to be self-reinforcing. Those who act in solidarity and in tandem with other people are rewarded with a sense of community, belonging, and purpose, which in turn increases the likelihood of future acts of solidarity. Participants in the Grenfell Silent Walks reported feeling motivated and connected to others as one aspect of their participation, which encouraged renewed participation the following month [4]. Even months and years later, campaigners continued their social support by attending the Silent Walks, and are likely to have benefited psychologically from being members of this support group.

If identity, and specifically group identities, can elicit wider helping, it is worth considering how campaigners can elicit aid through group memberships. Importantly, psychological group memberships can be variably defined. For example, shared group identity can take the form of an existing superordinate category (e.g., humanity) or a new emerging group identity (e.g., all of us affected) [20], depending on what is salient to the individual at the time. For example, members of two European nations might see each other as outgroup members if national membership is salient, or as ingroup members if they think of the superordinate category of the European Union [21]. Salient shared superordinate category membership can thus, in a sense, turn outgroup members into ingroup members, and this kind of shared category membership on the superordinate level is likely to encourage solidarity and increased engagement with helping behaviours [22]. This effect could occur out of a sense of perspective taking and group-based guilt [15], or it could occur through shared identity arising from a sense of common fate (as Chapters 22 and 23 show) [23]. In short, intergroup solidarity can arise out of a sense of commonality between one's ingroup and the victim group at higher levels of abstraction, while maintaining awareness of separateness and distinctiveness at lower levels of categorisation [16,17,20–23].

In summary, the research we have outlined here suggests that perceiving a shared identity can be a powerful factor in creating a sense of commonality even between distinct social groups. For example, the perception that we are all 'in it together' (i.e., have a perceived common fate) in the fight against COVID-19 can turn outgroup members into psychological ingroup members and lead to acts of solidarity [8,23]. In the case of the Grenfell Tower fire, when survivors and bereaved families came together and campaigned against the actions of authorities before and after the fire, they also protested against the current social housing conditions and the flammable type of cladding that was being used in hundreds of buildings around England [9–11]. As a result, this sense of injustice was shared by the wider community that came together during the campaign activities [1]. Furthermore, through working together on a common cause, they generated a shared identity at a superordinate level, which in turn resulted in intergroup solidarity [4].

Practical and Strategic Recommendations for Eliciting Intergroup Solidarity from the Wider Community

The wider community could be a valuable resource for the health services, in terms of both acute emergency care and longer-term care (Chapters 23 and 24 illustrate this point). We propose two distinct leverage points for community interventions, based on identity processes, that could be utilised by campaigners and local authorities. The first is shared identity of outgroup members with the survivors, often at a higher level of categorisation, and the second is shared identity of outgroup members with other non-victim supporters. Figure 26.1 summarises the processes that are involved.

To illustrate, campaigners can increase intergroup solidarity by making salient shared superordinate group memberships that focus on either a sense of common fate or a common identity [8,22,23]. For example, advertising campaigns to encourage prosocial community behaviours might focus on identities unrelated to the large-scale event (e.g., 'in the end, we are all humans' or 'we, the disadvantaged, need to stick together'), or they might focus on commonality that arises from the event itself (e.g., 'even though we

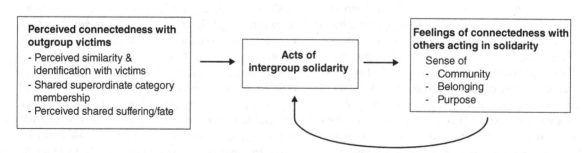

Figure 26.1 Identity processes driving intergroup solidarity after large-scale events.

are members of different nations, we all share the common fate of facing the COVID-19 pandemic together').

The second identity approach is focusing not on shared group membership with people who are directly affected by the major incident, but on commonality with other supporters acting in solidarity. If acts of solidarity create a sense of community, either physically through crowd events such as the Grenfell Silent Walks [4], or via social media using hashtags and Facebook groups, they are likely to further reinforce and encourage future acts of solidarity (see Figure 26.1). Intergroup solidarity is something that is 'done', not only 'felt', and it is done in conjunction with other people. To the extent that actions are designed in such a way that they enhance supporters' wellbeing, by tapping into rewarding psychological mechanisms such as belonging, empowerment, and a sense of purpose, they are more likely to endure over time [8].

However, we note three caveats related to the use of leveraging identity processes to elicit intergroup solidarity. First, campaigns that highlight shared group membership with specific groups may inadvertently result in the exclusion of other groups. This was found in a recent study that investigated help across national boundaries during the COVID-19 pandemic [24]. If shared group membership is used to encourage solidarity, appeals to identity need to be supplemented with clear messaging that discourages the search for external scapegoats, and the associated idea that the ingroup is morally 'exempt' from helping outgroup members.

A second caveat is that emphasising group memberships might not only increase the salience of shared group memberships with victims of a large-scale event, but could also potentially increase the salience of shared group memberships with the alleged perpetrators, which could result in a range of defence mechanisms that discourage prosocial responses [24,25]. In the case of the Grenfell disaster, if wealthy landlords are seen to be responsible for the fire, perhaps due to poor prior financial investment and/or failure to follow health and safety legislation, it could be counterproductive to remind people that they belong to this wealthy group. Individuals may feel pride towards their ingroup, which in turn could lead to a defensive refusal to accept that their group – and by extension they themselves – is responsible for the disaster, thereby shifting blame to others.

A third caveat is that helping behaviours offered by a privileged group may not be trusted, or they may be construed by minoritised groups as disingenuous or due to strategic motives [26,27]. This is because the benefits of psychological group membership are malleable; the same prosocial act can be intergroup or intragroup or interpersonal, depending on the salient level of categorisation in that situation. For example, perceptions of prosocial intentions might differ depending on one's perspective – an act by white allies intending to signal intergroup solidarity towards a disadvantaged ethnic group could be perceived by that group as 'whitewashing' (e.g., inserting white allies into leadership positions) or neo-colonialism (e.g., being paternalistic and offering aid that is not requested). This highlights the importance of considering the perspectives of all actors in an emergency.

A further consideration is whether local authorities, policymakers, and campaigners are interested in short- or longer-term impacts. Major events and disasters often have a long legacy, generating support structures initially that may deteriorate over time [9] (Chapter 23 covers this matter). This merits consideration of how the psychological processes identified might generate intergroup solidarity, not only in the immediate short term (less than 1 year later) but also in the longer term (more than 3 years later). As previously stated, our definition of solidarity is not short-lived, but endures over time. Therefore the identity processes highlighted in this chapter can generate intergroup solidarity in the immediate aftermath and in the long term. Solidarity is likely to prevail if feelings of connectedness with the event's victims and survivors persist and/or if feelings of connectedness with others acting in solidarity persist (i.e., a group consciousness) [28]. Feelings of connectedness with the victims and survivors are likely to endure to the extent that secondary stressors continue to be perceived in collective terms, and if political rhetoric that emphasises inclusive categories supports this mentality [4] (Chapter 9 provides a substantial account of secondary stressors). For example, focusing on blaming specific groups for not following COVID-19 regulations could result in divisiveness that undermines wider cooperative behaviours in both the short and long term [24]. By contrast, feelings of connectedness with other supporters are likely to endure over time if group identification is salient and emphasised, and if such group identification has psychological benefits. If the goal is to have longer-term impacts over several years, then it is essential to adopt a strategic approach that elicits solidarity through shared group membership and that avoids scapegoating specific groups.

We end with an important consideration. It is, which social groups campaigners should focus on when eliciting prosocial behaviours. Earlier we saw that identity processes can be used to mitigate the impacts of major incidents, by encouraging solidarity from the less affected wider community. Practitioners might also ask, if the goal is to elicit aid from the wider community, *which* groups should be targeted. For example, solidarity might be sought and offered by members of privileged groups, or between members of different disadvantaged groups, and both may be effective strategies. However, one barrier for eliciting solidarity from advantaged group members is that they may refuse a call for allyship. This may be because of resistance to acknowledging that the ingroup is relatively privileged or partly at fault. Therefore another strategy may be to elicit aid from disadvantaged groups. Other disadvantaged groups are likely to be disproportionately affected by tragedies, and it might therefore be easier to communicate a sense of shared adversity and the need to work together. For example, Black and Asian communities consist of numerous subgroups, but collectively they are at increased risk of infection with COVID-19 [5]. This suggests that solidarity between different disadvantaged groups is more easily elicited than solidarity from advantaged groups. However, there are two important considerations. First, eliciting intra-minority support places the burden of helping on

disadvantaged groups, who may be less financially able to help. Second, intergroup competition can be a significant barrier to eliciting intergroup solidarity. Although disadvantaged groups have a vested interest in working together, when these groups are engaged in competitive victimhood, arguing that their problems and challenges are more important or deserving of attention is likely to be detrimental [29]. A potential remedy, which may also be effective for more privileged allies, is to focus on critical consciousness [30] by drawing attention to systemic injustices and the underlying factors that cause them. Disadvantaged allies are then more likely to recognise that they share the same systemic barriers, rather than attribute blame. However, we need a public discourse to achieve this more nuanced understanding that focuses on economic and political antecedents, rather than on the blaming and stigmatisation of specific social groups (e.g., in relation to COVID-19) [6].

Conclusion

Research into intergroup solidarity is an exciting new field, and it is fair to say that researchers see solidarity as a complex concept that involves more than merely helping another person in need. It is beyond the scope of this chapter to fully discuss the concept, but we offer what we hope is a useful demarcation and starting point for practitioners and policymakers. Identity processes have the potential to identify leverage points for eliciting intergroup solidarity after large-scale events both in the short term and in the long term.

References

1. Tekin S, Drury J. How do those affected by a disaster organize to meet their needs for justice? Campaign strategies and partial victories following the Grenfell Tower fire. *J Soc Polit Psychol* 2023; 11. Available from: https://doi.org/10.5964/jspp.8567.

2. Bowe M, Wakefield JRH, Kellezi B, et al. The mental health benefits of community helping during crisis: coordinated helping, community identification and sense of unity during the COVID-19 pandemic.

J Community Appl Soc Psychol 2021; 32: 521–35.

3. Solnit R. *A Paradise Built in Hell: The Extraordinary Communities That Arise in Disaster*. Penguin, 2010.

4. Tekin S, Drury J. Silent Walk as a street mobilization: campaigning following the Grenfell Tower fire. *J Community Appl Soc Psychol* 2021; 31: 425–37.

5. Templeton A, Tekin Guven S, Hoerst C, Vestergren S, Davidson L, Ballentyne S, et al. Inequalities and identity processes in crises: recommendations for facilitating

safe response to the COVID-19 pandemic. *Br J Soc Psychol* 2020; 59: 674–85.

6. Drury J, Reicher S, Stott C. COVID-19 in context: why do people die in emergencies? It's probably not because of collective psychology. *Br J Soc Psychol* 2020; 59: 686–93.

7. Iacobucci G. Covid-19: increased risk among ethnic minorities is largely due to poverty and social disparities. *BMJ* 2020; 371: m4099.

8. Ntontis E, Drury J, Amlot R, Rubin GJ, Williams R. Endurance

or decline of emergent groups following a flood disaster: implications for community resilience. *Int J Disaster Risk Reduct* 2020; **45**: 1–9.

9. Renwick D. Organizing in mute. In: *After Grenfell* (eds Bulley D, Edkins J, El-Elnany N): 19–46. Pluto Press, 2019.

10. Bulley D. Everyday life and death in the global city. In *After Grenfell* (eds Bulley D, Edkins J, El-Elnany N): 1–18. Pluto Press, 2019.

11. Charles M. Come unity and community in the face of impunity. In *After Grenfell* (eds Bulley D, Edkins J, El-Enany N): 167–93. Pluto Press, 2019.

12. Klavina L, van Zomeren M. Protesting to protect 'us' and/or 'them'? Explaining why members of third groups are willing to engage in collective action. *Group Processes Intergroup Relat* 2020; **23**: 140–60.

13. Saab R, Tausch N, Spears R, Cheung WY. Acting in solidarity: testing an extended dual pathway model of collective action by bystander group members. *Br J Soc Psychol* 2015; **54**: 539–60.

14. Fattori F, Pozzi M, Marzana D, Mannarini T. A proposal for an integrated model of prosocial behavior and collective action as the expression of global citizenship. *Eur J Soc Psychol* 2015; **45**: 907–17.

15. Mallett RK, Huntsinger JR, Sinclair S, Swim JK. Seeing through their eyes: when majority group members take collective action on behalf of an outgroup. *Group Processes Intergroup Relat* 2008; **11**: 451–70.

16. Reicher S, Cassidy C, Wolpert I, Hopkins N, Levine M. Saving Bulgaria's Jews: an analysis of social identity and the mobilisation of social solidarity. *Eur J Soc Psychol* 2006; **36**: 49–72.

17. Selvanathan HP, Lickel B, Dasgupta N. An integrative framework on the impact of allies: how identity-based needs influence intergroup solidarity and social movements. *Eur J Soc Psychol* 2020; **50**: 1344–61.

18. Roblain A, Hanioti M, Paulis, E, Van Haute E, Green EGT. The social network of solidarity with migrants: the role of perceived injunctive norms on intergroup helping behaviors. *Eur J Soc Psychol* 2020; **50**: 1306–17.

19. Gordijn EH, Yzerbyt V, Wigboldus D, Dumont M. Emotional reactions to harmful intergroup behavior. *Eur J Soc Psychol.* 2006; **36**: 15–30.

20. Ntontis E, Drury J, Amlôt R, Rubin GJ, Williams R. Emergent social identities in a flood: implications for community psychosocial resilience. *J Community Appl Soc Psychol* 2018; **28**: 3–14.

21. Levine M, Prosser A, Evans D, Reicher S. Identity and emergency intervention: how social group membership and inclusiveness of group boundaries shape helping behavior. *Pers Soc Psychol Bull* 2005; **31**: 443–53.

22. Zagefka H. Prosociality during COVID-19: globally focussed solidarity brings greater benefits than nationally focussed solidarity. *J Community Appl Soc Psychol* 2022; **32**: 73–86.

23. Drury J. The role of social identity processes in mass emergency behaviour: an integrative review. *Eur Rev Soc Psychol* 2018; **29**: 38–81.

24. Zagefka H. Intergroup helping during the coronavirus crisis: effects of group identification, ingroup blame and third party outgroup blame. *J Community Appl Soc Psychol* 2020; **33**: 83–93.

25. James TK, Zagefka H. The effects of group memberships of victims and perpetrators in humanly caused disasters on charitable donations to victims. *J Appl Soc Psychol* 2017; **47**: 446–58.

26. Halabi S, Dovidio JF, Nadler A. When intergroup helping helps intergroup relations: the moderating role of trust in the outgroup. *J Exp Soc Psychol* 2021; **95**: 104141.

27. van Leeuwen E, Zagefka H, eds. *Intergroup Helping*. Springer, 2017.

28. Thomas EF, Smith LG, McGarty C, Reese G, Kende A, Bliuc AM, et al. When and how social movements mobilize action within and across nations to promote solidarity with refugees. *Eur J Soc Psychol* 2019; **49**: 213–29.

29. Shnabel N, Noor M. Competitive victimhood among Jewish and Palestinian Israelis reflects differential threats to their identities: the perspective of the needs-based model. In *Social Issues and Interventions. Restoring Civil Societies: The Psychology of Intervention and Engagement Following Crisis* (eds Jonas KJ, Morton TA): 192–207. Wiley Blackwell, 2012.

30. Burson E, Godfrey EB. Intraminority solidarity: the role of critical consciousness. *Eur J Soc Psychol* 2020; **50**: 1362–77.

27

Principles for Intervening with the Wellbeing, Psychosocial, and Mental Health Needs of Mass Casualties

Richard Williams, John Stancombe, and Verity Kemp

Introduction

We begin by setting out the requirements for an appropriately broad framework that spans a sufficient range of conceptual appreciations of people's needs after they are affected by emergencies, incidents, terrorist events, disasters, disease outbreaks and conflicts (EITDDC). Therefore we start by examining the nature of the problems that people endure if they are affected by EITDDC. It is tempting to think that events affect people in very different ways that are particular to what they have experienced or what is occurring. There is some truth in this but, as we continue to discover, there are also similarities. We should consider these similarities because they enable us to make generic plans for emergencies with a view to adapting them to accommodate the particularities of each circumstance, once we have made the initial responses that are essential as soon as each emergency arises. This chapter outlines such a generic approach. It builds on the matters covered in Sections 1 to 3.

The Nature of the Problems Experienced by People Affected by Emergencies, Incidents, and Disease Outbreaks

This chapter draws on a number of sources, including a companion book from Cambridge University Press. One chapter in it was co-written by two of the authors (RW and VK) of this chapter. It is highly relevant to the contents of this chapter [1]. Here we deepen and develop the content offered in that chapter and draw in other material to offer an integrated approach to designing and delivering the various components of comprehensive mental healthcare for people affected by EITDDC events.

In another chapter, by Carol Fullerton, and colleagues, in that book, there is a summary of the impacts of EITDDC that is reproduced here as Figure 27.1 [2].

It provides a simple conception of the psychosocial and behavioural consequences of EITDDC, and emphasises the significance of distress, behaviour changes, and (for some people) mental health disorders. It states that:

> In the immediate aftermath of a disaster, individuals and families and communities may respond in adaptive, effective ways or they may make fear-based decisions, resulting in unhelpful behaviors. The adaptive capacities of individuals and groups within a community are variable, and need to be understood before a crisis in order to effectively identify post-event mental health services required [3].

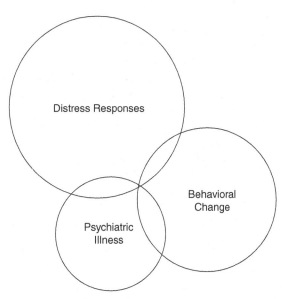

Figure 27.1 A simplified summary of the impacts of EITDDC on people affected [2]. Reproduced with permission from Cambridge University Press.

Table 27.1 Groups of people who have differing mental health needs following disasters [3]. Reproduced under licence CCBY 4.0.

1 People who are at risk of distress, mental health problems, and mental disorders, principally anxiety, depressive, and substance use disorders, consequent on their direct and indirect involvement in events and who present new and additional demands on mental health services

2 People who have continuing needs for mental health services for pre-existing conditions, but whose care is threatened by challenges to the business continuity of pre-existing mental health services consequent on network and community dislocation

3 People whose involvement in an emergency provokes or precipitates the relapse of a pre-existing mental disorder

4 People who are responders and whose mental health might be put at raised risk consequent on their work

Alexander McFarlane and Richard Williams assign the people affected into the four main groups listed in Table 27.1 [3]. They advise that planners should take account of each of these groups when considering the needs for psychosocial and mental health services after EITDDC.

The Inter-Agency Standing Committee (IASC) is formed by the heads of an array of UN and non-UN humanitarian organisations. It has published 'Guidelines on Mental Health and Psychosocial Support in Emergency Settings', which delineate groups of survivors according to the psychosocial and psychiatric consequences that they may experience [4]. The guidelines propose that it is possible to develop a community response and development strategy for use before, during, and after emergencies, thereby enabling a flexible approach that is appropriate to providing care for people in their communities.

In 2012, Wietse Tol and Mark van Ommeren drew attention to the array of emergencies that occur and the array of outcomes that can result [5]. They pointed out that 'mental health practitioners in humanitarian settings frequently encounter people with severe pre-existing neuropsychiatric disorders …'. Thus it is important to consider not only the nature of each emergency, and the primary stressors that it brings, but also the population of people affected and their

unmet needs when planning. Tol and van Ommeren also point out that 'disasters and armed conflicts … impact the social conditions that shape mental health, through increased poverty, threats to human rights, domestic and community violence and changes in social relations'.

The IASC guidelines identify the importance of people experiencing:

1. pre-existing social problems (e.g., extreme poverty) associated with belonging to a group that is discriminated against, marginalised, or politically oppressed; these are usually considered to be secondary stressors (see Chapter 9), and the COVID-19 pandemic has shown the huge importance of conditions of these kinds

2. emergency-induced social problems (e.g., family separation, disruption of social networks, destruction of community structures, resources, and trust, increased gender-based violence)

3. distress, grief, and other psychosocial experiences and needs that are induced by each emergency

4. mental health disorders that may be induced by the emergency, including substance use and substance use disorders, depression and anxiety disorders, post-traumatic stress disorder (PTSD), and sustained personality changes

5. social problems that are induced by provision of humanitarian aid (e.g., undermining of community structures or traditional support mechanisms)

6. psychosocial problems induced by provision of humanitarian aid (e.g., worries due to lack of information about food distribution or due to poor management of the information that is provided)

7. pre-existing mental health or psychiatric problems (e.g., severe mental disorder, alcohol and drug misuse).

Certain populations should be offered particular consideration when planning responses to adverse and untoward incidents. They include people who are at higher risk due to certain specific aspects of gender, children and adolescents, older people, socioeconomically disadvantaged people, minority and marginalised people, people with pre-existing health conditions, and people who are more often exposed to emergencies, including emergency responders [6]. McFarlane and Williams support the use of evidence-informed interventions, including tailored community education aimed at decreasing post-event distress and mental and physical health-related issues, and early intervention to allow screening for more adverse effects. In addition, expert recommendations and case studies should form part of these responses [3].

Thus emergencies, incidents, and disease outbreaks may result in a very wide range of psychosocial and mental health impacts that cover the majority of the spectrum of problems that people may experience. Hence there are conspicuous challenges in deciding how best to define the impacts and delineate the responses that people require. This matter is raised by John Alderdice in Chapter 3 when he points out the complexities and asks how we are to define 'mental health problems'. Readers will note that the several approaches to categorisation summarised thus far are based on pragmatic approaches to understanding what is happening to people or has happened to them, and the mechanisms by which higher than average risks operate (matters that we began to consider in Chapters 5, 6, 10, 11, and 12). They raise some fundamental conceptual issues, and we look at examples next because understanding them is likely to assist us in developing a coherent approach to caring for people who are affected.

The Nature of Distress and People's Needs

Distress

One of the challenges in studying people's experiences of major incidents is agreeing definitions of the terminology used. One example that requires greater clarity is the nature of distress. As we have seen in Chapter 12, there are three approaches to distress that stood out in our research. First, some of the literature refers to distress being comprised of subthreshold symptoms of anxiety, depression, or post-traumatic stress disorder [7] (arguably, Chapter 35 uses terms in this way). However, it seems to us that this approach risks considering distress to consist of collections of mental health symptoms that are, together, insufficient to reach diagnostic thresholds.

The second common use of the term 'distress' is in relation to emergencies, to depict people who have a range of experiences that are anticipated, and usually much broader than symptoms of common mental disorders [8]. The authors' own qualitative research has shown that distress is a highly variable and

heterogeneous set of experiences and emotions that can disrupt everyday life and sometimes interfere with people's functioning. Our findings are that these experiences are broader than sets of symptoms that are often drawn from psychopathological research. This has resulted in some researchers creating inventories of the kinds of experiences that people may have after untoward events, drawn from observing populations of affected people and other approaches to diagnosing mental health problems [9,10]. Some accounts organise these potential experiences into emotional, cognitive, social, and physical domains [9,11]. Often these lists find their way into public-facing leaflets describing the kinds of experiences that people might have. Some of these lists may be examined in epidemiological surveys to identify the frequencies with which common symptoms of disorders occur.

A third approach to defining distress is based on the experiences of people who say that they have been or are subjectively distressed. This is the way in which the term is applied in practice.

Our definition of distress is as follows: 'People are likely to feel stressed in emergencies and incidents. Their experiences are described as distress when they are accompanied by emotions, thoughts, and physical sensations that are upsetting or which affect their relationships and functioning at work or at home'. Thus, in our view, distress is not a diagnosis, but it may also accompany a diagnosed mental health disorder.

Understanding People's Feelings, Behaviour, and Needs Before, During, and After Emergencies, Incidents, Disasters and Disease Outbreaks

As a consequence of the range of impacts on people of their exposure to EITDDC, understanding how people feel and behave and their psychosocial and mental health needs before, during, and after emergencies is crucial to planning and delivering responses. We observe in Chapter 12 that recent studies have demonstrated that qualitative approaches can provide valuable insights into people's lived experience of psychosocial distress and its course – insights that quantitative approaches may lack. We therefore commend mixed methods of approaches to studying the impacts of emergencies, incidents, disasters, and outbreaks of communicable diseases on humans.

Table 27.2 Comparison of biomedical and psychosocial approaches to public education about mental health (© Cromby J, Harper D, Reavey P, 2013 [8], *Psychology, Mental Health and Distress*, Red Globe Press, used by permission of Bloomsbury Publishing Plc).

Biomedical approach	Psychosocial approach
Sees the person's mental health problems as the main problem	Sees barriers in society as the main problem
Sees problems as a symptom of an underlying disease process and illness	Sees problems as an understandable response to adverse life events
Sees societal reactions as due to the stigma attached to having a mental health problem	Sees societal reactions as due to discrimination against a marginalised group (e.g., racism, sexism)
Public education aims to remove perceived blame attached to the individual by 'blaming' the illness rather than the person	Rejects the relevance of notions of 'blame', and aims to promote diversity, reduce fear, and increase empathy and understanding
Key public education slogan: 'Mental illness is an illness like any other'	Key public education slogans: 'I'm crazy – so what?' and 'It's normal to be different'

Another way of considering people's needs is to review the kinds of interventions and treatments from which they may benefit. There are a number of evidence-based treatments that are appropriate for assisting people who develop mental health disorders after emergencies, incidents, and disease outbreaks. In strict medical terms, the evidence for social interventions that are based on the principles of psychological first aid is not substantial, but it is improving. Also, application of psychosocial interventions, which we broadly term psychosocial care, has goals that are broader than seeking a reduction in symptoms, because they also seek improvements in people's social relationships and their better integration into their families and communities, as well as improved functioning [12]. Thus social prescribing is increasingly widely practised in healthcare and is one example of a psychosocial intervention.

This raises a fundamental question about approaches to assisting people after their exposure to adverse events. The treatments for mental health disorders are based on biomedical approaches, whereas the interventions that constitute care for people who have problems that do not reach diagnostic thresholds draw on the psychosocial approach. A comparison of these two approaches is provided in Table 27.2.

In truth, few interventions or treatments lie wholly in one domain or the other, and the contents of Table 27.2 paint these approaches somewhat stereotypically. This means, in our opinion, that a broad and comprehensive approach to providing the

care that people require after experiencing EITDDCs should call on both the biomedical and psychosocial approaches as outlined in Table 27.2. Ideally, these approaches should be well integrated in planning for a broad pattern of interventions and treatments that may be offered based on meeting people's needs.

The Integrated Psychosocial Approach

When we first set out our integrated approach in 2009, we called it the *psychosocial approach* [13,14, p. 82]. However, in the light of possible confusion, because it is clear that other authors use the term psychosocial in a narrower way, we now call our approach the *integrated psychosocial approach*. In essence, it describes:

- distinguishing people who are distressed and do not have indications of a mental health disorder from those people who require biomedical interventions
- basing distinctions between the two sorts of conditions on the trajectories of people's stress levels and dysfunction
- providing assistance for the majority of distressed people through lower-intensity psychosocial care.

This means that planners should recognise that the majority of people are likely to be distressed by what they have witnessed or the events that have involved them, and a much smaller but nonetheless significant proportion of people may develop a mental health disorder. Many members of the large group of people who are distressed are likely to recover reasonably rapidly if given support by their families, friends, and colleagues at work. Some people may find helpful in their recovery contacts with people who were affected by the same incident. They may develop shared social identities and derive considerable comfort, social support, and efficacy from meeting with people who have been similarly affected.

However, the research conducted after the Manchester Arena bombing has drawn greater attention to a group of people who lie between those who are distressed and recover reasonably quickly and those who require mental healthcare. These are people who appear not to have a mental health disorder, but whose distress may continue for several years after the event(s) by which they have been affected. We were surprised to find how large was this group in our cohort of people affected by the Manchester bombing. Their suffering did not appear to be ameliorated solely by the passing of time and receiving comfort and support from families and friends. Many of them suffered secondary stressors. Services for them appeared to be thin on the ground, and, in our experience, are not well integrated with mental healthcare or with services provided by other agencies. Thus a key requirement of our integrated approach is the integration of services delivered by a number of agencies across disciplinary boundaries.

Our integrated approach also means that people who are thought to show the signs of both distress and mental disorder may require elements from both approaches to be combined in the care that they are offered.

Thus the way in which we understand people's needs has real and practical implications for the ways in which responses are developed. For example, research on the Manchester Arena bombing using qualitative and quantitative techniques found that people who are distressed – whether the distress is mild, moderate, or severe – seek open and early access to authoritative sources of information and emotional support. This finding emphasises the importance of planning services to ensure that there is early ease of access to appropriate responses.

A further grouping of people was identified by Lord Dennis Stevenson and Paul Farmer's review of mental health and employers, published in 2017, which included organisations of all types [15]. It identifies three broad groups of staff in any organisation (see Figure 27.2, which has been reproduced from the report). That review considered how employees might

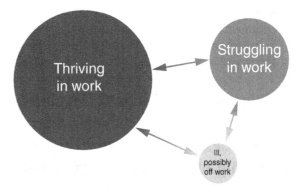

Figure 27.2 Three phases that people experience in work [15])
(© Crown copyright 2017: reproduced under the Open Government Licence v3.0).

be better supported. Although its findings are relevant to staff of organisations that deliver care for other people as their main function, this approach can also be applied to the needs of communities and people within them. The review by Stevenson and Farmer presents three challenges to employers (which are also summarised in Figure 27.2):

- assisting employees to thrive at work
- supporting staff who are struggling
- enabling people who are ill to recover and return to work.

Section 5 of this book focuses on meeting the needs of staff. However, we think that the approach outlined by Stevenson and Farmer applies to everyone. Certainly it makes sense of another confusion in the language often used in relation to people experiencing EITDDC that relates to the terms wellbeing and mental health. Often these terms are used to describe all forms of intervention. However, as we show in the next paragraph, wellbeing and mental health are not equivalent terms. We think that more careful use of language would help us to plan and deliver more effective services.

We conclude by drawing together research and several sources which suggest that it is very important for all of the agencies to come together well before any incident to agree a comprehensive plan, with the intention of:

- sustaining the wellbeing of everyone affected (this is the *wellbeing agenda*)
- identifying and responding to the social and psychological needs for intervention and support of people who are distressed but who do not reach the thresholds for further specialist mental health assessment and treatment (this is the *psychosocial agenda*)

- identifying, assessing, and meeting the needs for treatment of everyone who is identified as potentially having a mental health disorder (this is the *mental health agenda*).

An Approach to Planning and Organising the Services Required by People After Emergencies, Incidents, and Disasters, and During and After Disease Outbreaks

Richard Williams and his colleagues offer a framework that brings together the aforementioned three agendas to meet the needs of groups of people who are at higher risk [16]. People identified as being at higher risk include families, relatives of people who have been directly involved, and other carers at the time when disasters strike and during the recovery phase that follows.

Figure 27.3 shows a model of care that supports a strategy for developing key community leaders, community development, and delivering psychosocial care and mental healthcare that should be planned before events occur so that such care is available during and after incidents. It links the wellbeing, psychosocial, and mental health agendas into a wider plan. This model was developed by the authors to reflect science and people's preferences and needs.

Chapter 28 focuses on how to sustain people and communities by actioning a wellbeing agenda, and how to respond to people who are struggling and/or distressed or otherwise require psychosocial care.

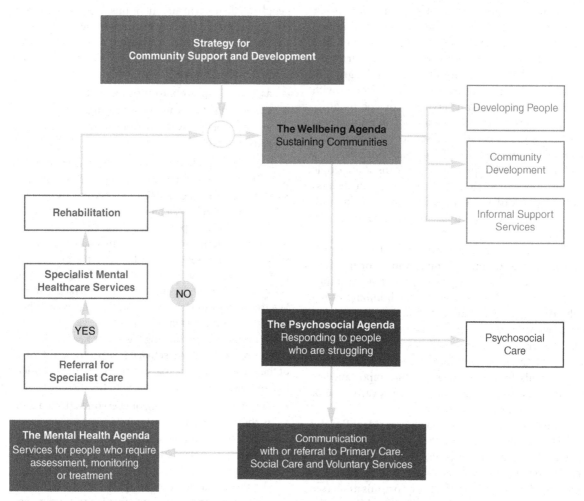

Figure 27.3 A model of care for delivering the wellbeing, psychosocial, and mental healthcare agendas (© R Williams, V Kemp, 2020. All rights reserved).

Table 27.3 The 12 core principles for designing and delivering services for communities [14] (© R Williams, J Bisson, V Kemp, 2015).

The principles	
1	Agree values, ethics, and approaches to human rights
2	Agree definitions of terms
3	Orientate services to families and communities in the cultures in which they live, relate, and work
4	Translate lessons from evidence and experience into plans and frameworks for delivering psychosocial care and mental healthcare
5	Integrate psychosocial care and mental healthcare responses into policies and plans for humanitarian aid, welfare, wellbeing, social care, and healthcare agencies' work
6	Ensure that communications are effective
7	Adopt a balanced approach to designing and delivering psychosocial care and mental healthcare
8	Bring together agencies to create integrated comprehensive psychosocial care and mental healthcare programmes
9	Adopt a strategic stepped model of community care
10	Ensure that psychosocial care and mental healthcare are available for responders and people who intervene
11	Build on existing services and skills to develop and deliver effective responses
12	Work to agreed standards

Chapter 29 covers the mental health agenda for an affected population. Section 5 takes forward the practical approach described here and applies it to rescue, recovery, and healthcare staff, including employees of all the Blue Light Services.

If it is to be coherent, this model of care should incorporate the principles of what is termed emergency planning, resilience, and response (EPRR) in the UK. This is because a model of care is likely to be most effective in response to the needs of communities if it addresses, fits in with, and coordinates with overall emergency response plans at international, national, regional, and local community levels. There are seven core phases in the cyclical process for planning for and managing emergencies, the so-called *management cycle for emergencies*, which is illustrated in Figure 27.4.

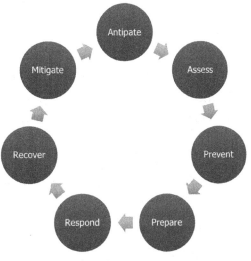

Figure 27.4 Management cycle for emergencies. (© R Williams, V Kemp, 2015, all rights reserved.)

Developing Policy, Service Design, and Service Delivery: Supporting the Development of a Strategy for Delivering the Wellbeing, Psychosocial, and Mental Health Agendas

The authors took the learning from the approaches and sources described earlier and the science to develop *12 core principles for designing and delivering services for communities* in order to underpin a strategy for all three agendas within coherent plans for community responses and development before, during, and after emergencies. The 12 principles appear in the book chapter published in 2017, and are summarised in Table 27.3 and described briefly in the text that follows [1].

Table 27.4 Translating lessons into effective policies, plans, and service delivery (© R Williams, J Bisson, V Kemp, 2015)

Policy level	Nature of action	The intention of the action
1	National and provincial civil administrations set policies that determine the strategic requirements for services	Policies at this level set the overall aims and objectives for responses to disasters
2	Responsible authorities design frameworks for services	Government policies should require the responsible authorities to create strategic plans for and design services by bringing together evidence from research, past experience, and knowledge of the provinces that might be affected, their populations, and risk profiles
3	Responsible authorities create and deliver services nationally, provincially, and locally according to the scale of response required	Plans for delivering psychosocial care and mental healthcare should include how particular services relate to partner services, and how affected populations are guided to and through them. They should be based on the best evidence available and awareness of the preferences of the people who are likely to use them. The authorities should test delivery of services through exercises
4	Responsible authorities create plans for supporting, training, and caring for staff who intervene in order to support good effective clinical practice and best use of slender resources	Plans for good clinical practice concern how clinical staff take account of the needs and preferences of patients, deploy their clinical skills, and work with patients to agree how guidelines, care pathways, and protocols are interpreted in individual cases. They should also include plans for sustaining and intervening with staff
5	Civil administrations and the responsible authorities evaluate the performance of services	Civil administrations and the authorities are responsible for evaluating and managing the performance of psychosocial and mental healthcare against their identified purposes

1. Agree Values, Ethics, and Approaches to Human Rights

In 2015 the Bevan Commission stated that identifying values should be the starting point for defining the purposes of services and the principles that underpin them [17]. Responsible authorities at state, regional, local, and community levels should agree values, ethics, and human rights, and an agreed statement must be at the heart of developing and delivering their responses to emergencies. Doing no further harm would be one value that underpins all plans to protect people from the psychosocial and mental health effects of all emergencies.

2. Agree Definitions of Terms

Agreed cross-agency definitions of terms in frequent use relating to psychosocial and mental health responses for people affected by disasters are important to ensure clarity in developing and delivering services for people affected by emergencies. The authors have observed that an array of terms without clear agreement of definitions can result in uncertainty, poor communications, confusion, and delay.

3. Orientate Services to Families and Communities in the Cultures in which they Live, Relate, and Work

When planning and designing psychosocial and mental healthcare, account must be taken of the needs of families and communities, of their cultures, and of where they live and work. This must be underpinned by taking into account up-to-date knowledge of the risk factors that affect people, communities, and people's needs regardless of age. It must also take into consideration people's preferences.

4. Translate Lessons from Evidence and Experience into Plans and Frameworks for Delivering Psychosocial Care and Mental Healthcare

Table 27.4 summarises how translating lessons learned from research and experience into ethical plans for responses during and after emergencies can become actions. Planning and preparation of psychosocial and mental health programmes are fundamental to ensuring appropriately funded and designed services.

5. Integrate Psychosocial Care and Mental Healthcare Responses into Policies and Plans for Humanitarian Aid, Welfare, Wellbeing, Social Care, and Healthcare Agencies' Work

Integration of medical rescue, immediate physical interventions, continuing physical healthcare, recovery and rehabilitation, business continuity planning for pre-existing programmes for the general population (which may otherwise be depleted as a consequence of disasters), and psychosocial responses and mental healthcare is advised by McFarlane and Williams [3], and should be a component of effective planning prior to emergencies.

6. Ensure That Communications Are Effective

Effective communications between key people are fundamental to ensuring preparation and effective responses to emergencies. This helps people to:

- prepare for a possible threat by helping to manage apprehensions, advise on prudent responses, and ensure as far as possible that the public understand evidence-informed interventions and what might be damaging misinformation
- build resilient people and communities and thereby help to keep people well
- support community and personal self-efficacy
- provide information about care programmes that offer support for people who develop mental health disorders
- ensure that rights are sustained
- ensure that media inquiries are met with positive and cooperative approaches.

7. Adopt a Balanced Approach to Designing and Delivering Psychosocial Care and Mental Healthcare

A cooperative approach by planners, service designers, and providers across agency and disciplinary boundaries is required for planning responses effectively and for recovering from emergencies. This approach is underpinned by a number of actions, four of which are listed here:

1. balancing validation of people's psychosocial experiences with responding to their needs for psychosocial care and mental healthcare
2. balancing top-down with bottom-up approaches
3. recognising, evaluating, and managing the stressors that create psychosocial needs for affected people
4. adopting the integrated psychosocial approach for designing and delivering effective services.

8. Bring Together Agencies to Create Integrated Comprehensive Psychosocial Care and Mental Healthcare Programmes

After an emergency, the majority of people affected are unlikely to require specialist mental healthcare. Providing psychosocial care is recommended by David Forbes and colleagues to meet the needs of the majority of people affected by emergencies [12]. This approach is also likely to ensure that specialist mental health services and practitioners are available for people with diagnosed disorders.

Provider agencies should develop an appropriate range of psychosocial and mental health services that will meet the needs of people affected. Three main types of programmes are needed that:

1. sustain coping and resourcefulness by every community and employer having wellbeing programmes available all the time (the wellbeing agenda)
2. ensure that psychosocial care is available to everyone who requires it (the psychosocial agenda)
3. provide timely access to effective mental healthcare.

In addition, a small proportion of affected people is likely to require long-term mental health services.

Each of these types of programme is characterised by three common features – ensuring good *communications*, restoring *social networks and connectedness*, and ensuring *community support*. However, no one agency is likely to be able to provide all three types of programme, and this is why they must come together to ensure that there is complementarity of what each offers, and that there are no substantial gaps.

9. Adopt a Strategic Stepped Model of Community Care

The authors' approach to providing appropriate responses for people and their communities must take account of their changing needs. It is also important to ensure a balance between wellbeing, psychosocial care, and mental healthcare [13,18].

10. Ensure that Psychosocial Care and Mental Healthcare Are Available for Responders and People Who Intervene

Section 5 of this book covers the needs of people who respond to single-incident, recurring and ongoing EITDDCs. The COVID-19 pandemic has shown that it is imperative that planners take into account the psychosocial and mental health needs of all responders, rescuers, and the staff of aid and healthcare agencies [9,19,20].

11. Build on Existing Services and Skills to Develop and Deliver Effective Responses

Ideally services that deliver psychosocial care and/or mental healthcare should be funded sufficiently so that they have the capacity and capability to respond to emergencies, and they should be capable of responding to an appropriate variety of types of EITDDC.

12. Work to Agreed Standards

A common set of agreed minimum standards should be adopted that are suitable for use in the wake of a range of emergencies. There is a requirement to recognise that a devastating emergency may make it impossible to achieve even the minimum standards. Nonetheless, all agencies that are involved in responding and recovery should agree to work to a common set of standards [16]. Adopting standards contributes powerfully to risk reduction by inspiring well-designed and well-conducted mechanisms for information gathering, research, and evaluation.

Requirements for standards should influence training, information gathering, evaluation, and research because all of these capabilities should be central to emergency responses. These requirements must be anticipated, and standards should be developed before disasters occur.

Conclusion: A Strategic Approach to Improving Care for People Involved in Emergencies, Major Incidents, and High Consequence Infectious Diseases (HCIDs)

This chapter summarises a model of care to sustain the wellbeing and improve the health of people affected by emergencies of all kinds. The model follows the premises identified in the review by Stevenson and Farmer, and reflects the findings from a number of avenues of evidence and the principles identified in this chapter.

Planning is an important element of the model, as it provides the basis for supporting people through emergencies, incidents, and disease outbreaks. The strategy suggests core actions to support people who are affected. Careful attention is important throughout emergencies. Experience from many sources is that emergencies cause primary stressors and accentuate the impacts of secondary stressors.

Based on the model of care, we propose that the key approaches to be taken into account when planning should include:

- providing services for the people who are directly affected and for the families of people involved in mass incidents
- recognising that social support is a natural and powerful intervention
- establishing the initial support to be delivered for people whose symptoms persist, and assessing those people thought to be at risk of developing a mental health disorder
- providing clear and consistent messages and routes of communication to all key stakeholders regarding access to support and care, including responses to any anticipated incidents or emergencies
- approaches that are evidence based and proportionate, flexible, and timely
- psychosocial care and mental healthcare responses that are provided:
  - as part of a multi-agency response
  - within a clear governance framework
  - to support coordinated delivery of care that manages key interfaces and transitions seamlessly
  - by volunteers and aid agencies, professional practitioners, managers, and staff who are appropriately qualified and have access to training, good leadership, support, and supervision.

We emphasise that a common but erroneous assumption is that everybody involved needs counselling or psychiatric treatment in the immediate aftermath of an incident. Single-session stress debriefing and brief interventions that ask people to re-experience the events that they have survived should not be practised. There are often reports of psychological debriefing being offered to people who have been affected by mass casualty events. Many authors have pointed to how often this approach is used after disasters, despite the evidence that it is unhelpful [21]. In the UK, the National Institute for Health and Care Excellence (NICE) positively advises against offering psychologically focused debriefing for preventing or treating PTSD [22]. However, there are other forms of conversation and support that are appropriate that are not debriefing. Chapters 39, 42, 45, 47, and 48 provide more information.

References

1. Williams R, Bisson JI, Kemp V. Health care planning for community disaster care. In *Textbook of Disaster Psychiatry* 2nd ed. (eds RJ Ursano, CS Fullerton, L Weisaeth, B Raphael): 244–60. Cambridge University Press, 2017.

2. Fullerton CS, Ursano RJ, Weisaeth L, Raphael B. Public health and disaster mental health: preparing, responding and recovering. In *Textbook of Disaster Psychiatry* 2nd ed. (eds RJ Ursano, CS Fullerton, L Weisaeth, B Raphael): 325–39. Cambridge University Press, 2017.

3. McFarlane A, Williams R. Mental health services required after disasters: learning from the lasting effects of disasters. *Depress Res Treat* 2012; 2012: 970194.

4. Inter-Agency Standing Committee. *IASC Guidelines on Mental Health and Psychosocial Support in Emergency Settings: Checklist for Field Use.* Inter-Agency Standing Committee, 2008.

5. Tol WA, van Ommeren M. Evidence-based mental health and psychosocial support in humanitarian settings: gaps and opportunities. *Evid Based Ment Health* 2012; 15: 25–6.

6. Morganstein JC, Herberman Mash HB, Vance MC, Fullerton CS, Ursano RJ. Public mental health interventions following disasters. In *Handbook of PTSD: Science and Practice* 3rd ed. (eds MJ Friedman, PP Schnurr, TM Keane): 570–88. The Guilford Press, 2021.

7. Naldi A, Vallelonga F, Di Liberto A, Cavallo R, Agnesone M, Gonella M, et al. COVID-19 pandemic-related anxiety, distress and burnout: prevalence and associated factors in healthcare workers of North-West Italy. *BJPsych Open* 2021; 7: e27.

8. Cromby J, Harper D, Reavey P. *Psychology, Mental Health and Distress.* Palgrave Macmillan, 2013.

9. Alexander DA. Early mental health interventions after disasters. *Adv Psychiatr Treat* 2005; 11: 12–18.

10. Alexander DA, Klein S. First responders after disasters: a review of stress reactions, at-risk, vulnerability, and resilience factors. *Prehosp Disaster Med* 2009; 24: 87–94.

11. Williams R, Kemp V, Alexander DA. The psychosocial and mental health of people who are affected by conflict, catastrophes, terrorism, adversity and displacement. In *Conflict and Catastrophe Medicine* 3rd ed. (eds J Ryan, A Hopperus Buma, C Beadling, A Mozumder, DM Nott, NM Rich, et al.): 805–49. Springer, 2014.

12. Forbes D, O'Donnell M, Bryant RA. Psychosocial recovery following community disasters: an international collaboration. *Aust N Z J Psychiatry* 2017; 51: 660–62.

13. North Atlantic Treaty Organisation (NATO). *Psychosocial Care for People Affected by Disasters and Major Incidents: A Model for Designing, Delivering and Managing Psychosocial Services for People Involved in Major Incidents, Conflict, Disasters and Terrorism.* NATO, 2009 (www.healthplanning.co.uk/nato).

14. Williams R and Kemp V. Psychosocial and mental health care before, during and after emergencies, disasters and major incidents. In *Health Emergency Preparedness and Response* (eds C Sellwood, A Wapling): 83–98. CABI, 2016.

15. Stevenson D, Farmer P. *Thriving at Work: The Stevenson/Farmer Review of Mental Health and Employers.* Department for Work and Pensions and Department of Health and Social Care, 2017.

16. Williams R, Bisson J, Kemp V. *OP94: Principles for Responding to the Psychosocial and Mental Health Needs of People Affected by Disasters or Major Incidents.* Royal College of Psychiatrists, 2014 (www.apothecaries.org/wp-content/uploads/2019/02/OP94.pdf).

17. Bevan Commission. *Prudent Healthcare: Setting Out the Prudent Principles.* Welsh Government, 2015 (www.prudenthealthcare.org.uk/principles/)

18. Department of Health. *Planning for the Psychosocial and Mental Health Care of People Affected by Major Incidents and Disasters: Interim National Strategic Guidance.* Department of Health, 2009.

19. Misra M, Greenberg N, Hutchinson C, Brain A, Glozier N. Psychological impact upon London ambulance service of the

2005 bombings. *Occup Med* 2009; **59**: 428–33.

20. Drury J. Collective resilience in mass emergencies and disasters: a social identity model. In *The Social Cure: Identity, Health, and Well-Being* (eds J Jetten, C Haslam, SA Haslam): 195–215. Psychology Press, 2012.

21. Brooks SK, Rubin GJ, Greenberg N. Traumatic stress within disaster-exposed occupations: overview of the literature and suggestions for the management of traumatic stress in the workplace. *Br Med Bull* 2019; **129**: 25–34.

22. National Institute for Health and Care Excellence (NICE). *Guideline 116. Post-Traumatic Stress Disorder*. NICE, 2018 (www.nice.org.uk/guidance/ng116).

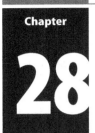

Chapter

28   Facilitating Psychosocial Care for the Public After Major Incidents and During Pandemics

John Stancombe, Richard Williams, and Verity Kemp

Introduction

Chapters 12 and 27 introduce readers to a broad generic approach to caring for people affected by emergencies, incidents, terrorist events, disasters, disease outbreaks, and conflicts (EITDDC). This chapter introduces readers to important concepts and practical aspects of facilitating, managing, and delivering the wellbeing and psychosocial agendas. In Chapter 27 we set out principles for intervening with the psychosocial needs of mass casualties, and briefly explain the model of care that is summarised in Figure 28.1.

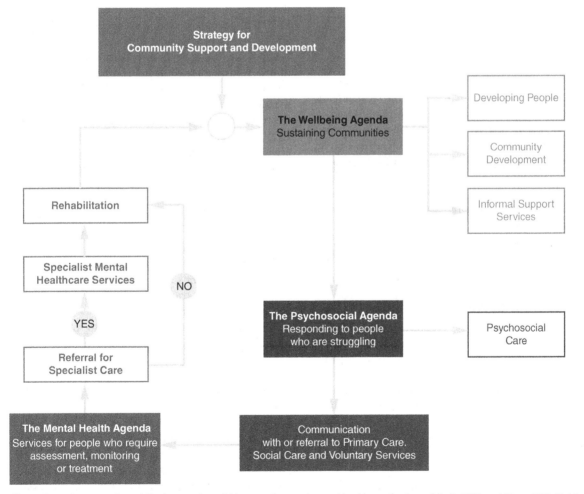

Figure 28.1 An approach to delivering psychosocial interventions and mental healthcare for the public (© R Williams, V Kemp, 2020. All rights reserved).

Table 28.1 Core principles of psychological first aid (PFA) (*Psychological First Aid for Field Workers*. Geneva: World Health Organization, 2011. Reproduced under licence CC BY-NC-SA 3.0 IGO)

a. Provide support through comforting and reflective listening

b. Provide social support for people who are directly affected and for the families and friends who are indirectly affected

c. Reduce the effects of primary stressors (the events or circumstances that caused the problems)

d. Assess people's needs

e. Assist people to feel in control of themselves and their circumstances (i.e., restore their agency)

f. Ensure that adequate welfare, social, and healthcare responses are directed to reducing the effects of secondary stressors

g. Prioritise attention to people who have severe reactions

Although this model was conceived in relation to terrorist incidents before the COVID-19 pandemic began, our experiences during it have confirmed its application to disease outbreaks and many other emergencies, incidents, and disasters. In this chapter we present a brief overview of evidence-informed practice and practice-informed evidence. The recommendations we derive draw on our experiences of what people found helpful and unhelpful after the Manchester Arena bombing in 2017, to highlight practical implications for facilitating more effective delivery of the wellbeing and psychosocial agendas in the future.

Needs for Care and Support After EITDDC

A stratified model of care was initially developed by Richard Williams and his colleagues [1], which brought together work undertaken in Europe [2] with the NATO guidance [3], which was led from the UK and agreed by NATO's Joint Medical Committee. That work led to the development of principles for the Royal College of Psychiatrists [4], a book chapter [5], and a journal article [6]. More recently, NHS England has published guidance based on these principles [7,8].

Core to all of this work is the recommendation that both the wellbeing agenda and the psychosocial agenda should be based on the principles of *psychological first aid (PFA)* (see Table 28.1). The goal is to restore immediate safety and assist people to recover from their experiences [9].

The authors of this chapter recommend that all responders, aid workers, and community leaders should become familiar with the principles. The wellbeing and psychosocial agendas should be organised by community leaders, employers, and social and aid agencies. The role of staff of healthcare services should be to advise on strategic development of wellbeing and psychosocial care services and links with mental healthcare.

The Wellbeing Agenda

Emergencies and major incidents evoke high levels of public concern that can have an enormous impact on the wellbeing and health of people affected. Following EITDDC, people affected can experience widespread and sometimes enduring distress, as well as mental ill health. It can be difficult to predict who will become most seriously affected in the short and longer term, but only a minority of people are likely to develop a mental health disorder that needs assessment and treatment by specialist services [5–8]. Similarly, the COVID-19 pandemic, and the complex system of physical, social, and psychological stressors associated with it, have affected people's wellbeing. However, a minority of people are likely to suffer a mental health disorder [10].

After EITDDC, most people are likely to experience some form or degree of psychosocial distress, and are likely to benefit from informal – but nonetheless important – psychosocial care provided by their families, friends, and wider social networks, or non-mental-health-trained responders from statutory and non-statutory organisations [5].

EITDDC cause major disruption to social life and mental wellbeing. The sheer scale of the COVID-19 pandemic, for example, with its associated complex system of physical, social, and psychological stressors, all of the uncertainties about resolution, and the indirect effects of the resulting economic impacts associated with long-term exposure to loss, stress, and social and economic adversity, have had and are still having impacts on people's wellbeing. This makes awareness of secondary stressors highly relevant. However, in common with EITDDC, although only a minority of people are likely to suffer a mental health disorder, we know that people who are less affluent and who are disadvantaged are at higher risk of more serious consequences [10].

We define wellbeing activities as actions that are intended to bolster recovery environments and ensure that affected people are able to sustain their social connectedness and are provided with social support. Social support is defined as social interactions that provide people with actual assistance, but also embed them in a web of relationships that they perceive to be loving, caring, and readily available in times of need [11].

There are a great many creative activities that have been designed to assist with sustaining wellbeing. It would be inappropriate to attempt to do any more than summarise some of the main principles and a selection of findings from research in this chapter. We review social validation, social connectedness, social support, and the fostering of resilience in terms of their impacts on the wellbeing and psychosocial agendas, and on developing communities.

Social and Professional Validation of People's Experiences Is Important to People Who Are Involved

We draw attention to the importance of social and professional validation of the experiences of people who are involved in emergencies. We draw on findings from our research involving people who experienced the Manchester Arena bombing in 2017 to make the point that validation is an important component of both activities to sustain wellbeing and initiate psychosocial care. Social validation, which is the experience of having one's experiences and/or distress understood and acknowledged by others, emerged as an important social process underpinning our interviewees' experiences of helpful support. However, our interviewees observed that, when they shared their experiences with their partners, close friends, and families, the reactions of the latter moderated the interviewees' attempts at further sharing and their experience of social support. Social invalidation occurs when other people shut down conversations, or are awkward, avoidant, or respond inappropriately [12]. This was a common experience among the interviewees, which inhibited further sharing: 'I just felt like people didn't understand what I was saying, so I kind of stopped talking about it,

because they didn't understand' (Participant 8). Interviewees' experiences of the responses from people at work and in education settings were also mixed. Initially their responses were predominantly positive, and people felt that colleagues provided emotional support and employers readily provided instrumental support in the form of reduced duties or paid leave. However, many said that this support was relatively short-lived, and some thought better-informed practices should be part of human resources and occupational health responses to employees who are affected by untoward events.

People also reported that being told that their experiences are 'normal' can be invalidating. With good intentions, it is likely that people were trying to convey that 'it's okay not to be okay'. However, the message that came through to our interviewees was that their distress was minor, and that it was just part of normal experience. Thus the problem with 'normalising' reactions to major events is that it can be understood as minimising people's experience of distress and delegitimising their need for care.

This is particularly concerning given the growing evidence that invalidating experiences can be more powerful than validating experiences [12–14]. This raises an important issue for messaging but also for availability of services. It suggests that there is a need for more focus on social and authoritative validation in services' responses, and that training people in active listening is very important. It also emphasises the importance of ensuring that the content of information leaflets and online resources is reviewed for content that could be perceived as invalidating.

These findings are consistent with the theoretical work of Andreas Maerker and Andrea Horn [15], who argue that social acknowledgement (defined as survivors' experiences of the reactions of society to their unique state and difficult situation) has an important effect on psychosocial adaptation to the primary stressor after adverse events. The term social here includes not only the person's closest social network (e.g., families, friends) but also significant people (e.g., statutory and voluntary response workers), groups (e.g., in the workplace), and wider society (e.g., impersonal opinions expressed in the media and social media). Social acknowledgement is low if people affected perceive or experience disapproval, misunderstanding, criticism, or rejection. The recent research literature also points to the importance of social acknowledgement in coping and recovery, while simultaneously recognising the multifaceted nature of the concept [15–17]. Our view is that social and authoritative validation can be viewed as specific sources and types of social acknowledgement that are crucial components in sustaining wellbeing and in psychosocial care; this is in line with new experimental research which shows that feeling understood is a fundamental mechanism in the social cure [18].

The Importance of Social Connectedness and Peer Support

The research literature on emergencies and incidents clearly shows that group processes are extremely important sources of coping, adapting, and recovering [19,20]. The effectiveness of this kind of social support turns on people being socially connected with people with whom they share a social identity [21]. These features of social connectedness and embeddedness are important to how people respond after major incidents. The researchers for the Social Influences on Recovery Enquiry (SIRE) (discussed in Chapter 5 and later in this chapter) found abundant evidence to support this premise. Social connection with others who were affected by the Manchester Arena bombing, either in face-to-face groups or via certain personal forms of social media groups, was a key source of support. It was crucial because it provided a forum for unfettered emotional disclosure and a major source of social validation and emotional support. In some cases it opened up access to support or an exchange of information, advice, or practical support. In this sense, it provided people with actual assistance. However, the most important benefit of social connection with others with shared experiences was that it embedded them in a web of relationships that they perceived to be caring and readily available at times of need.

Some interviewees described problems in finding other people with shared experience, and experiencing a feeling of isolation until making this connection. They recommended that facilitating access to groups of survivors should have been available to them earlier. Eventually, many people found such access through attending organised events (e.g., local support groups, family days, workshops). These events not only provided survivors with access to useful information and advice, but also, more importantly, they were a means of making initial connection with others who shared the experience and later

became important long-term sources of support in coping, adapting, and recovering.

These findings are consistent with previous research that demonstrated the usefulness of peer support groups after major incidents and during the COVID-19 pandemic [22–24]. In addition, we show that the benefits of in-person groups also apply to online groups and wider social categories. This in turn means that it is important to consider how peer support groups can themselves be supported. We recommend that people who respond to survivors' psychosocial care and mental healthcare needs after EITDDC should facilitate connectedness between survivors and peer support groups as early as possible.

Fostering Psychosocial Resilience in the Face of Adversity

Psychosocial resilience describes people's ability to cope with stress, and the concept does not imply any lack of impact of events on people's feelings, actions, or performance, but the reverse. It acknowledges that distress followed by recovery is very common if the circumstances are supportive and people can draw on personal and collective sources of psychosocial resilience. Hence bolstering the recovery environment is a key component of both the wellbeing and psychosocial agendas.

Personal psychosocial resilience describes how particular people respond to the challenges that they face. Collective psychosocial resilience describes how groups of people who share a social identity respond to, cope with, and recover from emergencies. This perspective acknowledges that resilience is actively constructed and shaped by cognitive, behavioural, and social processes, such as how an experience of adversity and efforts to cope are perceived, the range and effectiveness of coping strategies, and social processes (e.g., the capacity to cultivate social support and connectedness). A model that draws together personal and collective resilience is offered by Richard Williams and Verity Kemp [25].

Fostering personal and collective psychosocial resilience for all has the potential to buffer the ill effects of untoward events and decrease the risk of negative mental health outcomes. The ongoing challenge is how this can be realised in practice and embodied in recommended actions within emergency guidance, training, and service responses that are likely to facilitate psychosocial resilience [20,21,25].

Community Development

An important contribution to delivering the wellbeing agenda concerns extending the capabilities of working with community leaders to develop local communities and, within them, workplaces and schools, and recreational facilities in the planning stages. The intention is to bring people together so that it is feasible for those who have been affected by adverse events to receive the validation that they seek, and to benefit from social support as well as collective resilience.

The Psychosocial Agenda

As we see in Chapters 5, 12, and 27, and in this chapter, most people who are affected by or involved in EITDDC are likely to experience some degree of psychosocial distress and are likely to benefit from lower-level – but nonetheless important – psychosocial care provided by their families, friends, and wider social networks, or by non-mental-health-trained responders from statutory and non-statutory organisations [6].

Many people who are affected by incidents do not request professional support, or they only come forward months later – for example, after their distress fails to improve, or they develop symptoms of psychiatric disorder [26,27]. In the meantime, they rely on informal social support. We all need to better understand and facilitate this informal support, for two key reasons. First, formal services do not meet everyone's needs, and are not designed to do so. Second, effective informal support is crucial for aiding most people, and it reduces the risk of distress escalating to mental health disorders [28]. Therefore psychosocial care sits between sustaining the wellbeing of people involved in events and recognising the needs of (hopefully) a minority of people for care provided by specialist mental health services.

The boundaries between the wellbeing agenda and the psychosocial agenda are blurred, and the principles underpinning both are similar. However, our research on the Manchester Arena bombing suggests that although informal social support is often protective of people's wellbeing, a more nuanced multidimensional understanding of social support should recognise that inappropriate forms of informal social support are not only unhelpful, but may also potentiate distress and be detrimental to coping and recovery for some people. This has implications for intervention in that it stresses the importance of monitoring the quality of social support and promoting and strengthening the response of immediate and wider social networks that is required. This is one of the features that separates activities to sustain people's wellbeing and psychosocial care.

Validation

Validation is also an important component of psychosocial care. In the research on the impacts of the Manchester bombing, many interviewees reported that eventually receiving validation of their suffering and their entitlement to care, particularly from someone whom they perceived to have special expertise, was a source of great relief and a crucial component of the psychosocial care that they received.

Psychosocial care recognises these matters and should include the capacity to offer authoritative or professional validation. It is defined as recognising and affirming a person's distress and entitlement to care by a person who is perceived to have knowledge or expertise in relation to the psychosocial impact of emergencies, incidents, and disease outbreaks. In our research, we found that it changed how people viewed their distress and eligibility for psychosocial care. In turn, this facilitated their coping and adapting. This highlights the importance of ensuring that processes of validating people's experiences by people whose opinions they respect are available.

Core Principles for Preparing and Supporting People Affected by EITDDC

Table 28.2 summarises a selection of principles on which psychosocial care is based. Each of the activities featured is often cited as an important component or feature of psychosocial care.

The Social Influences on Recovery Enquiry (SIRE)

The Social Influences on Recovery Enquiry (SIRE) explored the experiences and opinions of people who have used the Manchester Resilience Hub. This service was set up to provide a contact point for psychosocial support, mental health advice, and a screening programme to identify people who might require specialist mental health services in the wake of the Manchester Arena bombing in 2017 [12]. SIRE aimed to understand the impact of the bombing on the wellbeing and mental health of people affected,

Table 28.2 Core principles for preparing and supporting people affected by adverse incidents (© R Williams, 2021. All rights reserved)

1. Intervene early to boost the recovery environment by means of general support rather than the use of psychological treatment

2. Base practical interventions on PIES*
   - Proximity
   - Immediacy
   - Expectancy
   - Simplicity of responses

3. Seek out and reduce secondary stressors of significant importance

4. Adopt a selection of interventions that are based on personal psychology
   - Helping to validate people's experiences while being aware that some people do develop a disorder
   - Enabling people by providing social support
   - Providing reflective listening and honest, accurate, and timely information
   - Helping people to restore their agency and perceptions of themselves as effective people
   - Enabling people to seek further help

5. Adopt a selection of interventions that are based on supporting people's membership of families and of social and work groups
   - Social support
   - Peer support
   - Leadership
   - Teambuilding and training in groups that work together
   - Creating and sustaining psychosocial safety in work cultures

* The concept of PIES, developed by the armed forces in the First World War, has been adapted for application to a general population. It provides a practical approach to early intervention for traumatised populations in *proximity* to where people work, with *immediacy* and *expectation* of recovery, and by using *simple* interventions first. Research has shown that military personnel who are managed in accordance with PIES are substantially more likely to remain in the services and to experience good outcomes than are colleagues who are not managed in this way [29].

and their experiences of social support provided by their families, friends, colleagues, and the responding services. It involved in-depth interviews with people, as well as an online survey to:

1. identify what experiences of psychosocial care after the incident helped or hindered people in their coping and recovery
2. learn from participants' experiences how to better deliver and target effective psychosocial care after major incidents in future.

Constraints on Seeking Support are Common

We identified from the research the requirement to overcome the worrying tendency of people to isolate themselves in the short and longer term, and the intrinsic reluctance of people who are distressed to seek help. Mild social withdrawal, which was not associated with reminders of the event or fear of recurrence, was common early on, when it tended to be short-lived. However, some people who were moderately or severely distressed reported early social withdrawal that

became more enduring. In some of these cases, social withdrawal was linked to long-term changes in life-styles, friendships, and membership of social groups. This finding has implications if people's access to the potentially positive effects of social support are limited because social connectedness is a key feature that influences wellbeing and recovery from major incidents. Therefore our view is that an early outreach pro-gramme, which also tracks over time the severity of people's experiences and their behaviour, is required to reduce the risks of people withdrawing from social contacts.

SIRE interviewees received support early on from partners, close friends, and family members. However, many of the interviewees reported reluctance to talk about their experiences, perceiving talking as personal weakness and an unfair burden on others [17–19]. This is consistent with previous studies that have shown that self-appraisal moderates emotional sharing and help seeking from informal sources of support [13,14].

Initial reluctance to seek help from services was also a common theme in the SIRE interviews [10,19]. We found that, as people struggled to make sense of their distress, they were often self-critical of their apparent inability to cope and recover. People who felt that their distress was in some way invalid, or that services were 'prioritising others', were also reluctant to seek help: 'I feel like … I know that I am lucky but then it makes me think like, well, some people did see a lot more and they need it [support] more than I need it, so, like, man up' (Participant 2).

We think reluctance to seek support has implications for intervention. Perhaps, to facilitate a supportive context and promote recovery, it is important that early outreach programmes focus on reducing people's negative self-appraisals that compound their experiences of distress, regulate disclosure and social interaction, and underpin their reluctance to seek help from proximate social networks and official support services.

People Who are Distressed Seek Early and Open Access to Authoritative Sources of Information and Emotional Support

Many research interviewees thought that there could have been more immediate efforts to reach out to people who were affected by the event, so that they did know where to turn if they were seeking validation or care. There was also evidence that some people experienced the Hub's screening algorithm, with its inherent threshold criteria, as a barrier to accessing psychosocial support. Taken together, the interviewees' comments led the researchers to conclude that the public would prefer early access to services and postponement of screening until a little later in the process.

Many interviewees said that knowing that services were available and accessible, if needed, helped to mitigate their distress. In some instances, just having the information about where they could turn if they decided to ask for help gave reassurance. Some interviewees described the importance to them over time of being able to pick up the phone and speak to a practitioner with whom they had already consulted. This was helpful as the need for information, support, and more focused intervention changed over time as a result of the impact of subsequent events (e.g., public inquiries, anniversaries, extended media coverage). Other interviewees thought that regular email contact

from the services provided them with emotional support because it reminded them that their distress had not been forgotten. This finding emphasises the importance of planning, care pathways, and coordinated outreach. It also emphasises the importance of ease of early access to professional validation of people's distress, and access to psychosocial care if their distress persists.

General Practitioners and Primary Care Services Are Seen as Important by People Who Are Distressed

In the early aftermath, many of our interviewees turned to their GPs for assistance. This finding is consistent with the results of other recent research [30]. The interviewees gave a variety of reasons for seeking support from primary care. The most common reason was to seek advice because their levels of distress were affecting their everyday functioning.

To our knowledge, only one previous study has investigated people's experiences of consulting GP services after a terrorist attack [12]. Most of our interviewees thought that their GPs had not been helpful or had provided inappropriate care. Many described encountering limited knowledge of the psychosocial effects of major incidents and appropriate support services, and inappropriate offers of care. The latter included being offered inappropriate self-help leaflets and prescriptions for minor tranquillisers and antidepressants. The interviewees turned to internet searches in these circumstances. A number of parents also stated that they were left disappointed by the care that they were offered in relation to how best to support their children.

Unhelpful experiences of primary care can have adverse consequences. They can reduce further attempts to seek help, and in some cases they can exacerbate distress and affect coping and recovery. We think that this information confirms the vital role of GPs and the importance of briefings for them to expand their background knowledge and build capacity to deliver some components of psychosocial care.

Secondary Stressors are Important Sources of Distress

Research has long identified that the psychosocial effects of adverse events can be influenced by a complex combination of primary and secondary stressors [31]. Indeed, in some studies, people report suffering more from the effects of secondary stressors than from those of primary stressors [32]. Thus the adjective secondary does not mean that a feature is of lesser importance or impact. To date, the lack of conceptual clarity about the nature of secondary stressors has hindered efforts to mitigate their effects through effective, timely interventions [33].

A social model of secondary stressors has recently been published (see Chapter 9). It has ushered in a more coherent and heuristic definition of secondary stressors that includes (a) social factors and people's life circumstances (including the policies, practices, and social, organisational, and financial arrangements) that exist prior to an incident and that affect them during it, and/or (b) societal and organisational responses to an incident or emergency [33]. Utilising this social model in the Manchester research, it was possible to elucidate the common and potent secondary stressors that affected survivors' coping and recovery. Our interviewees described events, policies, and practices that were not inherently based or consequential on the incident itself, but which became sources of substantial stress. The most common stressors were in relation to care services, relationships, work, the media, and wider society.

When distressed people did decide to seek care, some of them did not know how to find the right care or encountered barriers when attempting to access more specialist care. The barriers came in a variety of forms – for example, being turned away due to not meeting services' threshold criteria for care, encountering 'watchful waiting' responses, and the delays caused by long waiting lists. These service responses did not meet our interviewees' preferences for early contact, nor did they provide the validation that so many of them sought. Although there may be scientific reasons for delaying mental healthcare, the responses that people seek go wider than this and include psychosocial care.

Our findings also highlighted the predicaments of many parents in worrying about their children, which also acted as secondary stressors. The difficulties associated with identifying appropriate psychosocial care, combined with the increased burden of caring responsibilities while coping with their own personal distress, were a common experience.

We also emphasise that inappropriate forms of psychosocial care and mental healthcare can compound people's distress. Our finding that some people experienced invalidation by authorities as a secondary stressor is of particular concern: 'one particular place I went to ... she was basically just very dismissive of it all ... she pretty much said "you're not bad enough to treat right now, so we can't do anything for you" ... that actually made me worse, and I didn't want to get any authoritative help after that because ... I clearly can't be helped so what can I do? So, I then turned to alcohol, and I did take drugs' (Participant 13).

Social invalidation by immediate friends and family members acted as an important secondary stressor for some of our survivors [12]. Relationship difficulties that had existed prior to but also had an impact after major incidents also functioned as a secondary stressor: 'That made it [the distress] worse ... she wasn't a mum to me at that point, it was a good 6 months where she was my mum, but she wasn't being a mother ... but at the time, she didn't see what was happening, like I did blame her a lot for a lot of it' (Participant 3).

Unhelpful responses from employers were also substantial stressors. Support in people's workplaces quickly evaporated for some survivors as employers became impatient and their expectations of the survivors returning to pre-event levels of performance increased. In some cases, people were forced to take long-term sick leave or resigned from their jobs because of the stress caused by their perceptions of a lack of understanding and support from employers.

The responses to major incidents from wider social contexts can also function as secondary stressors. In our study, many survivors reported that exposure to news and social media coverage of the event exacerbated their distress. In addition, some participants felt that their psychosocial needs were viewed as less important than the needs of bereaved and physically injured people. This perceived inequity was sometimes a potent stressor: 'I cannot tell you how negative [it] made me feel about myself when Theresa May and everybody was on the news saying, "our thoughts are with the bereaved and the injured people" ... and I'm thinking I shouldn't feel like this because I'm okay, I walked away, why do I feel like this, they've not mentioned us so we should be okay and then it went on, and on, and on and we never got mentioned' (Participant 7).

Public responses to major incidents that are intended to demonstrate social solidarity and provide support can sometimes act as secondary stressors. For example, in Manchester, some survivors reported feeling disconnected from and disturbed by what they perceived as inauthentic displays of public support shown in the city after the event.

In short, these findings indicate that forms of social support as well as aspects of psychosocial care and mental healthcare that were experienced as unhelpful were common and potent stressors that affected survivors' coping and recovery. Importantly, we argue that most of the secondary stressors were socially mediated, and were potentially preventable through more timely and appropriate psychosocial care and intervention.

Practical Aspects of Facilitating Psychosocial Care

The Importance of Inclusive Multi-Agency Planning for Delivering the Wellbeing and Psychosocial Agendas

Together, the experiences summarised here indicate to the authors that it is very important for all of the agencies to come together well before any incident to agree a comprehensive plan with the intention of:

- sustaining the wellbeing of everyone affected (the *wellbeing agenda*)
- identifying and responding to the needs for intervention and support of people who are other than temporarily distressed, but who do not reach the thresholds for further specialist mental health assessment and treatment (the *psychosocial agenda*)
- identifying, assessing, and meeting the needs for treatment of everyone who is identified as potentially having a mental health disorder (the *mental health agenda*).

We conclude from the literature and our work that there is a large group of people who become distressed and do not require specialist mental healthcare, but who do require psychosocial care. Provision for this group of people may not be adequate after many incidents, and consideration should be given to redressing the balance between health protection and promotion and how the wellbeing and psychosocial care agendas can be optimised in practice. These conclusions have several practical implications for planning.

Practical Implications for Planning

1. Actions to Implement the Wellbeing, Psychosocial, and Mental Health Agendas

These actions aim to:

a. orientate the practices of response agencies to support the wellbeing of everyone affected and provide support that promotes natural recovery processes that occur over time for the majority of affected populations

b. respond to people who are struggling by implementing psychosocial care, including facilitating social networks of support among families, peers, and survivors

c. assess people whose needs go beyond these supporting facilities, and create pathways to timely and effective personalised, targeted psychosocial care

d. assess people and create and facilitate access to pathways to timely and effective evidence-based mental healthcare for people with serious mental health needs.

2. A Greater Emphasis on Psychosocial Care in Strategic Planning and Delivery

Planning for and organising psychosocial care merits an important and visible place during every step of planning for responding well to the effects of EITDDC. This relies on collaboration across agencies, organisations, and services in both the planning and delivery phases [22]. This is difficult to achieve with different organisational cultures and expertise coming together without clear leadership and accountability and shared understandings of needs and priorities in terms of what matters to the people affected.

A common language is required. Its bedrock is agreeing and disseminating definitions and common understandings of key concepts – for example, distress, psychosocial resilience, trajectories of recovery, and valuing psychosocial care. It also requires strategic plans for facilitating psychosocial care, with clear aims and purposes, and evidence-informed guidance built into multiagency training and implementation plans. It is also important to be aware of the potential duration of the impacts of incidents on people who are affected. Recovery can take many years. Therefore it is important to consider how support can be maintained in the medium and long term to sustain people.

3. Supporting Wellbeing for Everyone Affected, Including Relatives and Friends of Directly Affected People

Public mental health approaches to prevention rest on universal outreach strategies and surveillance programmes that focus on providing information, opportunities, resources, and encouragement to support coping and recovery processes. This should look to maximise all aspects of people's psychosocial contexts, as well as their own abilities. In practice, making help available in the form of information that may facilitate coping is crucial from the outset. Examples include information about aspects of the event, its effects on people and their families, and what is likely to happen next in terms of what they should do and where to turn if someone needs help. Timely, concise, and accurate information helps to restore a sense of control. Our research has shown that 'screen and treat' approaches can be employed both too early and too late, and, in these circumstances, they can be viewed as unhelpful. Finding out about available psychosocial care can be a challenge for affected people. Moreover, we should not wait for people to bring their problems to us. People do not see themselves as having warranted psychosocial needs, and they may be reluctant to seek help – hence the importance of universal outreach and public mental health interventions.

4. Services That Provide Care According to the Principles of Psychological First Aid (PFA)

It is important to ensure that processes for validation of people's experiences by people whose opinions they respect are available. In practice, this requires active listening to people's needs and concerns, helping them to understand their reactions; the goals are to validate their distress and right to care, and to address any barriers to or restraints on help seeking. It also involves providing a combination of emotional, informational, and practical support in a respectful, accepting manner, linking to resources and services if required, with the aim of facilitating effective coping and recovery. However, this comes with a caveat – even well-intentioned attempts at PFA can have negative impacts. For example, 'normalising' people's distress can invalidate their experiences and exacerbate their distress.

5. Assessing and Monitoring People in Need

Realising the wellbeing and psychosocial agendas require agencies to act together to broaden the scope of surveillance approaches to include monitoring psychosocial distress, other experiences, and their impacts on functioning. Routine mental health screening should be avoided in the early stages because there is little evidence that it confers benefit. Screening measures that identify symptoms of disorders have inherent limitations in specificity and sensitivity, and they can lead to inappropriate, premature pathways to specialist mental healthcare for some people, or overlook the large group of people who may require psychosocial care. Although distress detected through interview and narrative assessments can elucidate the psychosocial context, we should be vigilant for 'red flag' behaviours that may indicate likely chronicity (e.g., social withdrawal, somatic problems, and feelings of shame or guilt), and we should monitor coping and adaptation processes and overall functioning rather than solely assessing the number or severity of symptoms.

We advocate augmenting narrative assessment and regular monitoring to identify people who may need more personalised psychosocial care [12], by in the early stages using a broader range of psychosocial tools that assess wellbeing (e.g., the Warwick-Edinburgh Mental Wellbeing Scales), overall functioning (e.g., the Work and Social Adjustment Scale), and coping abilities (e.g., the Perceived Ability to Cope with Trauma Scale) [34–36]. It is also important to identify the support available within each person's social context, and particularly their closest relationships (e.g., using the Multidimensional Scale of Perceived Social Support) [37], and any hindrances to social support (e.g., using the Social Support Barriers Scale) [13].

6. Attending to the Impact of Secondary Stressors

Although acute exposure to primary stressors may cause distress in the short term, the long-term course of distress is likely to depend on persistent exposure to secondary stressors over time. These are tractable, and recognising them should be included in psychosocial care programmes to mitigate the long-term course of distress and restore functioning. In this regard, the social model of secondary stressors enables a holistic approach to conceptualising and intervening to remedy many of the longer-term and widespread negative psychosocial effects of exposure to EITDDC [33].

7. Strengthening the Contributions of Families, Friends, and Significant Others

People need acknowledgement and emotional and practical support from their close families, friends, colleagues, and acquaintances. However, we cannot assume that this will happen unprompted. Support services should focus on informing, stimulating, and helping to mobilise this support from each person's private/informal support network, be vigilant for 'red flags' (e.g., social withdrawal, reluctance to ask for help, social invalidation), offer simple interventions that facilitate recovery by initiating post-incident conversations with people who feel restricted in talking, and offer social validation to open their access to social support.

Although families can be an important source of support, depending on how family members communicate about their stress their attempts at support can be helpful or harmful. Our research also shows that social invalidation within close relationships can be a strain. Therefore poor-quality informal support can exacerbate distress, affect resilience, and prolong recovery. This more nuanced understanding of received informal social support may explain inconsistencies in studies on received support, which are not controlled for quality [38]. It also suggests that social support may, in certain circumstances in which it is not freely given, require assessment, monitoring, and more focused psychosocial intervention to enable people in distress to make disclosures or seek support. The intention would be to increase relatives' understanding of survivors' experiences and their social validation, and so facilitate intrafamilial communication and support processes.

8. Strengthening the Contribution of Communities: Fostering Collective Support

Activities that bring together people with shared experiences have impacts. The supportive context can be facilitated by enabling survivors to contact other people who have been affected or who have had similar experiences. These contacts can be organised in self-help groups or groups of people with similar experiences. Outreach services can also facilitate workshops and visits to create spaces in which people can talk about their experiences and come together, and these formal group meetings can lead to more informal meetings outside the initial context [39]. Peer support offered by people who have shared experiences provides mutual support and can be a catalyst for social validation, information exchange, and social processes such as local identification.

SIRE and other studies show that collective support can also be effective by using digital technology and virtual internet communities [40,41]. This approach can be exploited during periods of social restrictions and isolation during pandemics. Based on these findings, broader consideration should be given to facilitating informal networks of survivors through physical and virtual meetings [42].

9. Accessible and Scalable Psychosocial Care

There are challenges associated with mobilising sufficient psychosocial care after large-scale events in which affected communities are dispersed over large areas, and during the conditions of pandemics. Ensuring that greater numbers of vulnerable people can access psychosocial care requires more accessible pathways to support [43].

This requires a shift to remote and digital delivery of psychosocial care through, for example, web-based information centres and registration and surveillance programmes, and facilitating access to telehealth resources that provide care and guided self-help. Hence the preparation and response phases of emergency planning and preparedness must include planning and delivery of hybrid service models that integrate specialist and non-specialist agencies, when designing and delivering remote and face-to-face self-directed care and non-specialist and lay supported care using the most efficient and effective empirically supported interventions. There is substantial evidence that lay providers can deliver acceptable and effective care, and there are useful non-specialist provider models that can guide it [44,45].

10. Providing Training and Support for Professionals and Lay Volunteers

Evaluations of almost every disaster emphasise the need for adequate training and developing primary care and other community responders in assessing and delivering psychosocial care [17]. The experiences of survivors of the Manchester Arena bombing support this conclusion. Hence training about the common experiences of distress and the mechanisms of informal social support and how to help to cultivate responsive helpful care should be included in training and support for primary care and community services, as should training in the principles of PFA. Those principles are well suited to the curricula of training for non-specialist frontline workers to prepare them to provide psychosocial care for distressed people, while also ensuring a resilient workforce that can respond effectively to disasters and emergencies [46].

Frontline workers are also likely to benefit from training and support in how to distinguish people who need psychosocial care from those who need mental healthcare, and in how and where people can access focused psychosocial care to avoid prescriptions of inappropriate biomedical treatments and people's premature and inappropriate entry into specialist mental healthcare pathways.

Conclusion

This chapter has built on the general principles that are presented in Chapter 27 to add more detail to delivering the wellbeing and psychosocial agendas that were first identified in Chapter 12. It began with a summary of findings from research on people who agreed to be interviewed 2 years after the Manchester Arena bombing in 2017. Those findings and many papers in the literature provide evidence to support the 10 practical implications for planning and delivering services. They lay the general framework for the contents of substantial numbers of chapters in this book. Elsewhere in Sections 4 and 5, other authors' contributions offer more detail and elaborate the baseline of actions that we have summarised in this chapter. Next this book considers aspects of the mental health agenda in Chapter 29.

References

1. Department of Health. *Planning for the Psychosocial and Mental Health Care of People Affected by Major Incidents and Disasters: Interim National Strategic Guidance*. Department of Health, 2009.

2. Bisson JI, Tavakoly B, Witteveen AB, Ajdukovic D, Jehel L, Johansen VJ, et al. TENTS guidelines: development of post-disaster psychosocial care guidelines through a Delphi process. *Br J Psychiatry* 2010: **196**: 69–74.

3. North Atlantic Treaty Organization (NATO). *Psychosocial Care for People Affected by Disasters and Major Incidents: A Model for Designing, Delivering and Managing Psychosocial Services for People Involved in Major Incidents, Conflict, Disasters and Terrorism*. NATO, 2009.

4. Williams R, Bisson J, Kemp V. *OP94: Principles for Responding to the Psychosocial and Mental Health Needs of People Affected by Disasters or Major Incidents*. The Royal College of Psychiatrists, 2014.

5. Williams R, Bisson JI, Kemp V. Health care planning for community disaster care. In *Textbook of Disaster Psychiatry*, 2nd ed. (eds RJ Ursano, CS Fullerton, L Weisaeth, B Raphael): 244–60. Cambridge University Press, 2017.

6. Williams R, Kemp V. Principles for designing and delivering psychosocial and mental healthcare. *BMJ Mil Health* 2020; **166**: 105–10.

7. NHS England. *Clinical Guidelines for Major Incidents and Mass Casualty Events. Psychosocial Guidelines. Version 2*. National Health Service England, 2020.

8. NHS England and NHS Improvement. *Responding to the Needs of People Affected by Incidents and Emergencies: A Framework for Planning and Delivering Psychosocial and Mental Health Care*. NHS England and NHS Improvement, 2021.

9. World Health Organization, War Trauma Foundation, World Vision International. *Psychological First Aid: Guide for Field Workers*. World Health Organization, 2011.

10. Pierce M, McManus S, Hope H, Hotopf M, Ford T, Hatch SL, et al. Mental health responses to the COVID-19 pandemic: a latent class trajectory analysis using longitudinal UK data. *Lancet Psychiatry* 2021; **8**: 610–19.

11. Kaniasty K, Norris FH. Distinctions that matter: received social support, perceived social support and social embeddedness after disasters. In *Mental Health and Disasters* (eds Y Neria, S Galea, FH Norris): 175–200. Cambridge University Press, 2009.

12. Stancombe J, Williams R, Drury J, Collins H, Lagan L, Barrett A, et al. People's experiences of distress and psychosocial care following a terrorist attack: interviews with survivors of the Manchester Arena bombing in 2017. *BJPsych Open* 2022; **8**: e41.

13. Thoresen S, Jensen TK, Wentzel-Larsen T, Dyb G. Social support barriers and mental health in terrorist attack survivors. *J Affect Disord* 2014; **156**: 187–93.

14. Arnberg FK, Hultman CM, Michel PO, Lundin T. Fifteen years after a ferry disaster: clinical interviews and survivors' self-assessment of their experience. *Eur J Psychotraumatol* 2013; **4**: 20650.

15. Maercker A, Horn AB. A socio-interpersonal perspective on PTSD: the case for environments and interpersonal processes. *Clin Psychol Psychother* 2013; **20**: 465–81.

16. Woodhouse S, Brown R, Ayers S. A social model of posttraumatic stress disorder: interpersonal trauma, attachment, group identification, disclosure, social

acknowledgement, and negative cognitions. *J Theor Soc Psychol* 2018; **2**: 35–48.

17. Jacobs J, Oosterbeek M, Tummers LG, Noordegraaf M, Yzermans CJ, Dückers ML. The organization of post-disaster psychosocial support in the Netherlands: a meta-synthesis. *Eur J Psychotraumatol* 2019; **10**: 1544024.

18. Livingstone AG, Jaman E, Yan M, Adlam A. *They Get Me: Felt Understanding as a Critical Bridge Between Social Identity and Wellbeing*. Society for Personality and Social Psychology (SPSP) Preconference: Happiness and Wellbeing, 9 February 2021 (http://worldmakingthings.org/wp-con-tent/uploads/2022/06/SPSP-happiness-and-wellbeing-preconference-poster.pdf).

19. Haslam C, Jetten J, Cruwys T, Dingle GA, Haslam SA. *The New Psychology of Health: Unlocking the Social Cure*. Routledge, 2018.

20. Williams R, Kemp V, Haslam SA, Bhui KS, Haslam C, Bailey S. *Social Scaffolding: Applying the Lessons of Contemporary Social Science to Health and Healthcare*. Cambridge University Press, 2019.

21. Drury J, Carter H, Cocking C, Ntontis E, Tekin Guven S, Amlôt R. Facilitating collective psychosocial resilience in the public in emergencies: twelve recommendations based on the social identity approach. *Front Public Health* 2019; **7**: 141.

22. Eyre A. The value of peer support groups following disaster: from Aberfan to Manchester. *Bereave Care* 2019; **38**: 115–21.

23. Watkins J. The value of peer support groups following terrorism: reflections following the September 11 and Paris attacks. *Aust J Emerg Manag* 2017; **32**: 35–9.

24. Gregory A, Williamson E. 'I think it just made everything very much more intense': a qualitative secondary analysis exploring the role of friends and family providing support to survivors of domestic abuse during the COVID-19 pandemic. *J Fam Violence* 2022: **37**: 991–1004.

25. Williams R, Kemp V. The nature of resilience: coping with adversity. In *Social Scaffolding: Applying the Lessons of Contemporary Social Science to Health and Healthcare* (eds R Williams, V Kemp, S Haslam, C Haslam, K Bhui, S Bailey): 87–104. Cambridge University Press, 2019.

26. French P, Barrett A, Allsopp K, Williams R, Brewin CR, Hind D, et al. Psychological screening of adults and young people following the Manchester Arena incident. *BJPsych Open* 2019; **5**: e85.

27. Allsopp K, Brewin CR, Barrett A, Williams R, Hind D, Chitsabesan P, et al. Responding to mental health needs after terror attacks. *BMJ* 2019; **366**: l4828.

28. Bonanno GA, Brewin CR, Kaniasty K, Greca AM. Weighing the costs of disaster: consequences, risks, and resilience in individuals, families, and communities. *Psychol Sci Public Interest* 2010; **11**: 1–49.

29. Jones N, Fear NT, Jones M, Wessely S, Greenberg N. Long-term military work outcomes in soldiers who become mental health casualties when deployed on operations. *Psychiatry* 2010; **73**: 352–64.

30. Cyhlarova E, Knapp M, Mays N. Responding to the mental health consequences of the 2015–2016 terrorist attacks in Tunisia, Paris and Brussels: implementation and treatment experiences in the United Kingdom. *J Health Serv Res Policy* 2020; **25**: 172–80.

31. Lock S, Rubin GJ, Murray V, Rogers MB, Amlôt R, Williams R. Secondary stressors and extreme events and disasters: a systematic review of primary research from 2010–2011. *PLoS Curr* 2012; **4**: ecurrents.dis.a9b76fed1b2dd5c5 bfcfc13c87a2f24f.

32. Alfadhli K, Drury J. A typology of secondary stressors among refugees of conflict in the Middle East: the case of Syrian refugees in Jordan. *PLoS Curr* 2018; **10**: ecurrents.dis.4bd3e6437bff47b33 ddb9f73cb72f3d8.

33. Williams R, Ntontis E, Alfadhli K, Drury J, Amlôt R. A social model of secondary stressors in relation to disasters, major incidents and conflict: implications for practice. *Int J Disaster Risk Reduct* 2021; **63**: 102436.

34. Stewart-Brown SL, Platt S, Tennant A, Maheswaran H, Parkinson J, Weich S, et al. The WEMWBS Mental Well-being Scale (WEMWBS): a valid and reliable tool for measuring mental well-being in diverse populations and projects. *J Epidemiol Community Health* 2011; **65**(suppl 2): A38–9.

35. Mundt JC, Marks IM, Shear MK, Greist JM. The Work and Social Adjustment Scale: a simple measure of impairment in functioning. *Br J Psychiatry* 2002; **180**: 461–4.

36. Bonanno GA, Pat-Horenczyk R, Noll J. Coping flexibility and trauma: the Perceived Ability to Cope with Trauma (PACT) scale. *Psychol Trauma* 2011; **3**: 117–29.

37. Zimet GD, Powell SS, Farley GK, Werkman S, Berkoff KA. Psychometric characteristics of the multidimensional scale of perceived social support. *J Pers Assess* 1990; **55**: 610–17.

38. Feeney BC, Collins NL. A new look at social support: a theoretical perspective on thriving through relationships. *Pers Soc Psychol Rev* 2015; **19**: 113–47.

39. Généreux M, Roy M, O'Sullivan T, Maltais D. A salutogenic approach to disaster recovery: the case of the Lac-Mégantic rail disaster. *Int J Environ Res Public Health* 2020; **17**: 1463.

40. Paton D, Irons M. Communication, sense of community, and disaster recovery: a Facebook case study. *Front Commun* 2016; **25**: 4.

41. Drury J, Stancombe J, Williams R, Collins H, Lagan L, Barrett A, et al. The role of informal social support in recovery among survivors of the 2017 Manchester Arena bombing. *BJPsych Open* 2022; **8**: e124.

42. Schildkraut J, Sokolowski ES, Nicoletti J. The survivor network: the role of shared experiences in mass shootings recovery. *Victims Offenders* 2021; **16**; 20–49.

43. Ehrenreich-May J, Halliday ER, Karlovich AR, Gruen RL, Pino AC, Tonarely NA. Brief transdiagnostic intervention for parents with emotional disorder symptoms during the COVID-19 pandemic: a case example. *Cogn Behav Pract* 2021; **28**: 690–700.

44. Barnett ML, Lau AS, Miranda J. Lay health worker involvement in evidence-based treatment delivery: a conceptual model to address disparities in care. *Annu Rev Clin Psychol* 2018; **14**: 185–208.

45. Singla DR, Kohrt BA, Murray LK, Anand A, Chorpita BF, Patel V. Psychological treatments for the world: lessons from low-and middle-income countries. *Annu Rev Clin Psychol* 2017; **13**: 149–81.

46. Wang L, Norman I, Xiao T, Li Y, Li X, Leamy M. Evaluating a Psychological First Aid training intervention (Preparing Me) to support the mental health and well-being of Chinese healthcare workers during healthcare emergencies: protocol for a randomized controlled feasibility trial. *Front Psychiatry* 2022; **12**: 809679.

Chapter

29

Mental Healthcare Required by People Who Are Affected by Major Incidents and Pandemics: Lessons from Research

Jonathan I Bisson

Mental Health Responses to Emergencies, Incidents, Disasters, and Disease Outbreaks

Scoping the Range of Mental Disorders That Survivors Develop

As illustrated in other chapters, experiences of major incidents and pandemics are very personal and are affected by many factors. It is not surprising that mental health responses vary greatly, and it is increasingly well recognised that they encompass a range of different experiences, and that mental symptoms often fluctuate over time [1–3]. The majority of people who are exposed to major incidents and

pandemics will not go on to develop a pathological mental health response, but a minority are likely to do so [4]. Some people will experience symptoms such as anxiety and lowered mood that are self-limiting and should not be viewed as pathological.

Several authors have studied the trajectory of mental health symptoms after traumatic events. For example, Richard Bryant and colleagues undertook a 6-year follow-up study of people admitted to a general hospital for at least 24 hours as a result of physical injury after a traumatic event, and were able to model five distinct trajectories of post-traumatic stress disorder (PTSD) symptoms (see Figure 29.1) [3]. This and other work challenges previously held myths that everyone feels distressed after a traumatic event, and that acute symptoms recover naturally over time

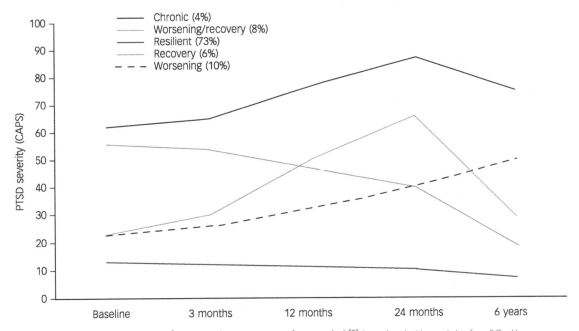

Figure 29.1 Symptom trajectories after traumatic events, over a 6-year period [3] (reproduced with permission from *BJPsych*).

[1,2]. By far the commonest trajectory (seen in almost 75% of this sample) is the so-called 'resilient' trajectory, whereby the people who follow this course never experience distressing mental health symptoms for a sustained period of time. It is very important to note that resilience is affected by context, and that both internal and external factors contribute to it. It is also noteworthy that research evidence consistently suggests that some people will develop long-lasting health and social consequences after traumatic events, and that more in-depth analysis of their experiences and needs should inform future provision of support and care [4].

External factors associated with a more marked and possibly pathological mental health response include greater proximity to the incident and its direct effects [5]. For example, during the COVID-19 pandemic, frontline healthcare workers such as those working in critical care units are likely, on average, to have been exposed to more COVID-19-related traumatic events than the general population. People who have lost a loved one as a result of COVID-19 infection are another group at heightened risk of developing a pathological mental health response as a direct result of the pandemic. For many other people, the stressors associated with the pandemic are likely to be secondary stressors or consequences, such as job loss, financial difficulties, home schooling, inability to socialise, and isolation. Internal factors are likely to be equally important in determining people's mental health responses, and include past mental health problems, family psychiatric difficulties, immediate reaction to stressors, coping style, and perception of social support [6].

This range of external and internal factors is common to many major incidents, especially those that are more complex and more enduring. Given the multiple factors involved in shaping individual people's mental health responses to major incidents and pandemics, and the variation in non-pathological mental health responses to traumatic events, it is not surprising that major incidents and pandemics have been associated with a wide range of pathological responses. PTSD is probably the best known and most widely spoken about reaction to traumatic events, but it is not the only reaction, nor is it the commonest [7,8]. Other common mental disorders encountered after major incidents and pandemics include adjustment disorders, depressive disorders, anxiety disorders, and substance use disorders. Other disorders precipitated more rarely by traumatic events include psychosis, somatic symptom disorders, and obsessive compulsive disorder.

Previous studies have considered mental health responses after a wide range of major incidents. Syntheses of this work have found varying rates of pathological outcomes. PTSD has been the most studied condition, with rates estimated to be 30–40% among direct survivors of disasters, 10–20% among rescue workers, and 5–10% in the general population [9]. More recent systematic reviews have tried to focus on considering the increased likelihood of developing a mental disorder after a natural disaster [10]. This is important work as it takes into account the fact that mental disorder will be present in communities in the absence of major traumatic events. A 1.8-fold increase in incidence of common mental health problems was found after natural disasters [10]. This and other research findings confirm the likely increased prevalence of mental disorders after major incidents, and the importance of this to public and personal health when planning an appropriate response (discussed later in this chapter).

The COVID-19 Pandemic

The COVID-19 pandemic has resulted in a wealth of research on psychological and psychosocial responses to it, and on its mental health consequences, and this is providing a new level of understanding of mental health responses and needs following pandemics.

Despite the fact that much mental health epidemiological research on COVID-19 has been hampered by difficulties in recruiting representative samples of the population as a whole and of specific populations, there are some very good examples of research on representative samples and of longitudinal research involving cohorts of people established before the pandemic.

One of the earliest UK studies reported the results of a survey completed by a representative sample (in terms of age, gender, and ethnicity) of 2,025 adults living in the UK between 23 and 28 March 2020 [11]. In total, 22% scored above standard questionnaire clinical caseness cut-offs for depression, 21% for anxiety, and 16% for PTSD. The authors placed these results, which apparently showed high levels of symptoms of disorder, in perspective by comparing them with the results of other pre-COVID-19 general population surveys (albeit from socioeconomically deprived areas), which found rates of 17% for depressive symptoms, 13% for anxiety symptoms, and 18% for PTSD symptoms. The authors concluded that the immediate impact of COVID-19 appeared to be one of slight elevations in rates of depression and anxiety and a slight reduction in the overall rate of PTSD. The following factors were associated with worse outcomes: younger age, children living at home, estimated personal risk, low income or loss of income as a result of the pandemic, and pre-existing health conditions.

Matthias Pierce and colleagues reported the results of a survey completed by 17,452 adults living in the UK between 23 and 30 April 2020; the participants were members of a study panel that had previously been surveyed in 2018, and were a broadly representative sample of adults in the UK [12]. In 2018, 19% of the participants scored above a questionnaire cut-off for 'mental distress', compared with 27% in 2020, suggesting a small but real increase in pre-COVID-19 levels of mental distress, which was associated with the pandemic. Factors that were associated with increased mental distress were younger age, female gender, and having young children at home.

In 2020, Alex Kwong and colleagues published the results of another study that surveyed a pre-existing cohort (the Avon Longitudinal Study of Parents and Children cohort) during the COVID-19 pandemic [13]. The survey was completed between April and May 2020 by 2,973 adults with a mean age of 28 years. The same people had completed the same questionnaires before the pandemic. Caseness for depression decreased from 24% to 18%, whereas caseness for anxiety increased from 13% to 24%. Overall 'low wellbeing' increased from 8% to 13%. Factors associated with poor outcomes were a history of having been infected with COVID-19, living alone, having no access to a garden, being of younger age, female gender, economic adversity, and pre-existing health conditions.

A high-profile study during the COVID-19 pandemic has been the University College London prospective study following adults within the UK population [14]. A disadvantage of this study, compared with those described above, is that participants were recruited by open advertisement and therefore are not representative of the general population. For example, 76% of the population were female and 70% had a degree or higher qualification. However, the study was large and collected prospective information on symptoms of depression and anxiety through the

pandemic; 36,520 adults were surveyed weekly between March and August 2020. The mean score on the PHQ-9 decreased from 7.4 to 5.8 over this time period, and that on the GAD-7 decreased from 5.9 to 4.1. The mean scores on these widely used measures of symptoms of depression and anxiety were always below thresholds representing likely clinical caseness, emphasising the consistent finding that most people, although affected by the pandemic, had not developed pathological mental health responses to it before August 2020. In fact the results suggest that there was positive adjustment to the situation over time. Factors associated with greater likelihood of experiencing depression and anxiety were female gender, younger age, lower educational attainment, lower income, living alone with children, and a pre-existing mental health condition.

Epidemiological studies from across the world have now been completed and published. Jude Mary Cénat and colleagues undertook a systematic review and meta-analysis of studies that considered symptoms of depression, anxiety, insomnia, PTSD, and psychological distress related to COVID-19 [15]. A total of 55 studies, with 189,159 participants, met their inclusion criteria. The mean prevalence values were 15.97% for depressive symptoms, 15.15% for anxiety symptoms, 23.87% for insomnia symptoms, 21.94% for PTSD symptoms, and 13.29% for psychological distress. The authors concluded that the short-term mental health consequences of COVID-19 were similar across affected countries and across genders. Unfortunately, interpretation of the results is limited by the heterogeneous methods employed by the studies included in the review.

Vulnerable Populations

It is well recognised that closer proximity to traumatic events is associated with increased likelihood of adverse consequences. In the COVID-19 pandemic a major focus has been on frontline healthcare workers, due to the traumatic nature of their work. A number of studies have reported significantly increased rates of clinically significant mental health symptoms among frontline healthcare workers. However, comparison with rates found in studies of the general population is confounded by the probable lack of representativeness of all frontline healthcare workers in the samples studied. For example, Neil Greenberg and colleagues found rates of 40% for possible PTSD,

6% for severe depression, and 11% for severe anxiety among staff working on critical care units [16]. A recent systematic review found 14 studies of health-care workers with rates of significant post-traumatic stress symptoms ranging from 2.1% to 73.4% during the pandemic [17].

Another potentially vulnerable population consists of people with lived experience of mental illness. The National Centre for Mental Health in Wales conducted a survey of members of its pre-existing cohort of people with lived experience of mental illness [18]. The range of self-reported previous diagnoses was broad, with depression and anxiety being most common, and significant numbers of people with other diagnoses, including PTSD, bipolar disorder, schizophrenia, and other psychoses. In total, 2,834 participants took part between June and July 2020; unfortunately, the sample was not representative of all people with lived experience of mental illness. The mean age was 45 years, 78% of the participants were female, and 49% had degree-level education.

The point prevalence was 53% for depression, 42% for anxiety, 67% for poor wellbeing, and 53% for worsened mental health as a result of the pandemic. Around 10% of participants reported an improvement in their mental health during the pandemic. Factors associated with worse outcomes were younger age, difficulty accessing mental health services, low income, income affected by COVID-19, worry about COVID-19, sleeping less than usual, drinking alcohol or taking drugs more than usual, and not feeling socially supported by friends or family. Previous diagnoses most strongly associated with a poor outcome were anxiety, depression, eating disorders, and PTSD.

A follow-up survey, which was completed by around 70% of the original participants between October and November 2020, explored how traumatic people had found the COVID-19 pandemic [19]. In total, 39% reported finding at least one element of the COVID-19 crisis traumatic, which indicates that the majority did not identify their experience as a traumatic one. Respondents were asked to identify the experience that troubled them most, and the vast majority would not have fulfilled the traumatic event criterion for a diagnosis of PTSD, because the event did not cause or threaten serious physical injury, death, or sexual violence [8]. The most commonly reported troubling experience, reported by around 27% of the participants, was 'generalised worry', with 'lockdown and restrictions' being the next most commonly reported troubling experience.

Clear PTSD-qualifying events such as exposure to death accounted for less than 7% of the responses. Other 'most troubling experiences' included exposure to COVID-19, other people not following the rules, the government's response, having to wear face coverings, coverage in the news media, and finances. Just over 13% of all participants reported symptoms sufficient to qualify for a diagnosis of probable PTSD in response to a COVID-19 event, but this decreased to 0.83% when the nature of the traumatic event criterion was included. It is noteworthy that most of the studies of the general population described earlier did not formally consider whether or not people were reporting PTSD symptoms in relation to a qualifying traumatic event.

In addition to the symptoms described previously, the COVID-19 pandemic has raised many questions about its neuropsychiatric impact and possible consequences directly related to the virus itself. There is increasing recognition that an unspecified encephalopathy (delirium) is widely encountered as part of presentations with severe infection [20]. There have also been reports of new-onset psychosis, and of cognitive and behavioural issues that seem to be associated with infection [20]. Longitudinal studies are now underway globally to try to determine the true nature of the neuropsychiatric consequences of COVID-19. Ongoing symptoms after infection with COVID-19 have been labelled *Long COVID*, and comprise a number of physical and psychological symptoms, including fatigue and pain [21]. The exact underlying aetiology of Long COVID is not known, and is probably different in different people. It seems likely that an integrated biopsychosocial approach will be needed to fully understand Long COVID and to help people who suffer from it.

The Evidence Base for Preventing and Treating Mental Health Conditions After Major Incidents and Pandemics

Prevention

The desire to intervene either before or after a traumatic event to prevent people from developing mental health conditions has been a key feature of responses to traumatic events for the last few decades, despite limited evidence on how best to do this. Given the predictable nature of exposure to traumatic events in certain populations (e.g., the armed forces, the emergency services), attempts have been made to engage people in advance interventions that will protect them from later problems. Realistic training has been a mainstay of this, and it is difficult to argue against the face validity of such an approach. It is also difficult to imagine how this could be delivered in a completely realistic way. How can someone be prepared for the death of someone they are working with, or for becoming totally overwhelmed by the numbers of people needing emergency medical attention during a pandemic?

That said, a number of approaches have been tried, including stress inoculation training and attention bias modification training. A recent systematic review concluded that there was insufficient evidence to recommend any pre-incident intervention, although attention bias modification training was noted to show some signs of being beneficial, and further work in this area is clearly warranted [22]. More attention has been paid to universal interventions (prevention delivered to everyone who has been exposed to a traumatic event) and indicated interventions (prevention targeted at certain groups of people). Again the evidence with regard to the efficacy of either approach is disappointing, but there are signals from the research literature that some interventions may be more helpful than others [22].

There has been a lot of interest in a universal intervention commonly referred to as psychological debriefing, in which people who have been exposed to traumatic events are provided with a single session that aims to reduce the risk of mental health sequelae. This was first described as critical incident stress debriefing for groups of ambulance personnel after traumatic events, but was subsequently adapted for use with individual persons, and was termed psychological debriefing. A series of randomised controlled trials and systematic reviews have led to the conclusion that psychological debriefing is ineffective and may cause harm to some people [23]. This has culminated in recommendations that it should not be used, issued by (among others) the National Institute for Health and Care Excellence (NICE) in the UK [24].

More recent systematic reviews of single-session preventative interventions have continued to find an absence of evidence for individual psychological debriefing (PD) [22]. A few studies involving longer-term follow-up have suggested the potential for harm, but meta-analysis of primary endpoints 3–6 months after trauma has revealed a neutral impact [22]. There is still clearly insufficient evidence to recommend

personal PD, and the same is true for group debriefing, although no clear signal of potential harm has been found for this approach. Interestingly, an adapted form of group PD, which included some cohesion training, delivered to army personnel in China dealing with the aftermath of an earthquake, found it to be more effective than standard group PD [25]. It would be premature to recommend any form of debriefing, but this adapted form of group PD seems worthy of further research, and met the criteria for recognition as an intervention with emerging evidence in the latest International Society for Traumatic Stress Studies prevention and treatment guidelines [26].

The best evidence for prevention comes from studies that have identified people with symptoms of PTSD and then provided a more formal trauma-focused intervention, similar to (albeit often briefer than) those interventions provided for treating PTSD [27]. The best evidence is for cognitive behavioural therapy with a trauma focus (CBT-TF), but there is emerging evidence for eye movement desensitisation and reprocessing (EMDR). The evidence for these interventions gets better when it is restricted to individual people, who satisfy the criteria for acute stress disorder in the first month after exposure to a traumatic event, or for PTSD within 3 months after a traumatic event [27]. There is more limited evidence for the preventive value of pharmacological approaches [28]. Hydrocortisone is the only drug for which there is some emerging evidence of prevention of development of PTSD, but the main studies to date have all involved participants who were severely physically unwell, which raises major questions about the generalisability of the findings.

Treatment

There is now good evidence for the efficacy of various treatments for the common disorders encountered after traumatic events. Once a condition has been detected, clinicians are directed to clinical guidelines for evidence-based treatment, such as those produced by NICE in the UK. For depression and generalised anxiety disorder, NICE recommends a stepped approach to treatment that starts with low-intensity psychosocial interventions, including guided self-help programmes for mild presentations with high-intensity psychological approaches, namely cognitive behavioural therapy (CBT) or interpersonal psychotherapy (IPT) for depression, and CBT or applied relaxation for generalised anxiety disorder. Pharmacological interventions are reserved for more severe presentations, and for milder ones that do not respond to low-intensity psychosocial approaches [29,30]. For people who develop alcohol misuse, NICE recommends motivational intervention containing the key elements of motivational interviewing as part of the initial assessment, with harmful drinkers and people with mild dependence being offered a psychological intervention focused on alcohol-related cognitions, behaviour, problems, and social networks [31].

Post-traumatic stress disorder

The evidence base for treating people who have PTSD has expanded significantly in recent years, with the strongest evidence being for trauma-focused psychological interventions, in particular CBT-TF and EMDR [32]. Increased research on specific interventions has allowed more recent guidelines to differentiate between different forms of CBT-TF, resulting in generic CBT-TF, CT-PTSD, cognitive processing therapy (CPT), and Prolonged Exposure being recommended over other types of CBT-TF [26,33]. For less complex presentations of PTSD, eight to twelve 60- to 90-minute sessions are recommended, with some people requiring more therapy, particularly when their presentations are more complex. There is increasing evidence for the efficacy of guided self-help using internet-based CBT-TF programmes for people with mild to moderate forms of PTSD [34]. Such

treatments, which can be delivered entirely remotely, seem particularly relevant to the pandemic context. For PTSD, NICE recommends individual CBT-TF (and EMDR after a non-combat-related trauma), with venlafaxine and selective serotonin reuptake inhibitors being recommended if the person with PTSD has a preference for drug treatment [24].

Service Configuration

A Strategic Model of Care

Optimal service configuration to best deliver the mental healthcare required depends on both resource availability and the nature and magnitude of the major incident or pandemic. Mental health service provision should be one part of a whole system approach, interfacing seamlessly with other elements of the response and contributing to a person-centred pathway. The pathway is most likely to start in the community and involve people from various services and sectors, including first responders, primary healthcare, secondary healthcare (mental and physical), the third sector, and social care. The lack of major advances in recent years means that guidelines published a number of years ago remain relevant [1,35].

A strategic model of care is recommended, as described in Table 29.1 [1]. The absence of strong evidence for specific preventative interventions has led to authors making recommendations, informed by evidence, from a slightly different perspective. For

Table 29.1 Strategic model of care [1]

Purpose	Tasks	Nature
Strategic and operational preparedness	Comprehensive multiagency planning, preparation, training, and rehearsal of the full range of service responses that may be required	Prevention services that are intended to develop the collective psychosocial resilience of communities and which are planned and delivered in advance of disastrous events
Public psychosocial care	Families, peers, and communities provide responses to people's psychosocial needs that are based on the principles of psychological first aid; this component also includes community building	Assessment, interventions, and other responses that are based on the principles of psychological first aid and that are delivered by trained lay people, who are supervised by the staff of the mental healthcare services, and social care practitioners
Personalised psychosocial care and mental healthcare	Access to primary mental healthcare services for surveillance, assessment, and intervention services for people who do not recover from immediate and short-term distress	Access to secondary and tertiary mental healthcare services for people who are thought to have mental disorders that require specialist intervention

example, it has been argued that all actions, interventions, and other service responses should promote a sense of safety, self-efficacy and community efficacy, empowerment, connectedness, calm, and hope [36]. Practical pragmatic support that is provided in an empathic manner and based on the principles of psychological first aid has been recommended as an approach that promotes the factors described by Stevan Hobfoll and colleagues [36]. It is also likely to avoid over-pathologisation and to facilitate detection and referral of people with more significant needs.

Facilitating Detection

It is very important to increase awareness of the possibility of people experiencing problematic mental reactions to major incidents or pandemics; accurate, clear media coverage is an excellent way of doing this. It is also important that the general population knows that experiencing a mental reaction to a traumatic event is expected and should be validated. The experiences of the majority of people are likely to be self-limiting and do not develop into a pathological response; sadly, however, for some people they do, and additional interventions may be required to facilitate resolution. Simple advice delivered through the media, and people across sectors supporting those affected, providing information on what to watch out for and how to seek help if required, are mainstays of facilitating detection.

It has been argued that mass screening of populations should be adopted to facilitate detection. High-profile screen and treat programmes have been set up after some major incidents, such as the London Bombings and the Grenfell Tower fire. Research into the former suggests that it did result in people being detected and treated who would not have come forward otherwise, but the true effectiveness and cost-effectiveness are not known [37]. Anecdotal reports after the Grenfell Tower fire suggested that some people found being asked to complete questionnaires too clinical and transactional. It is important to remember that screening is not without risk, such as raising expectations, not having sufficient staff to cater for demand, the consequences of false-positive findings, and the opportunity costs associated with deploying resources in this way.

The high-quality research that has investigated this, albeit in a military setting, is not supportive of routine screening. A cluster randomised controlled trial of 10,190 UK military personnel found no evidence of increased detection of PTSD, or that personnel received treatment as a result of formal screening after deployment [38]. A longitudinal cohort study of pre-deployment screening of 2,820 UK personnel also failed to demonstrate any benefit [39]. If conventional evidence-based standards were to be applied, there is insufficient evidence to justify screen and treat programmes, but high-quality research is required to explore such approaches further in civilian populations after major incidents and pandemics.

Appropriate Referral and Assessment

It is vital that people know who to consult and that they can easily access an assessment if they are concerned about their mental reaction. In the UK the primary care system is ideally placed to undertake initial screening/triage assessments of people who present to it, and it is important that primary care staff are equipped and have the capacity to undertake this role. Other key members and leaders of local communities also have a major role to play in raising awareness and supporting detection and access to primary care. If a person is assessed as requiring more formal mental health assessment and treatment, this should be arranged by mental health practitioners working in both primary and secondary care settings using a stepped/stratified approach to ensure that affected people are seen by the right person to address their needs. Assessments should be comprehensive and should be undertaken by an appropriately trained person. Questionnaires may assist clinical assessment but should not be relied upon exclusively.

Managing People's Mental Health Conditions

In order to utilise resources optimally, the principles of prudent healthcare should be followed and should aim to direct people to assessment, care, and treatment with the most appropriate person/people [40]. The healthcare system should be configured to deliver simpler forms of treatment at scale in primary healthcare settings, thereby preventing the system from becoming overwhelmed, and ensuring appropriate flows into secondary healthcare for more specialist input. It is very important that clinical assessment, care, and treatment are co-produced, with each person being fully involved and, whenever possible, involving loved ones/carers. A biopsychosocial approach should be taken to ensure that individuals'

Table 29.2 Mental health services required over time [35]

Timeframe	Services required
During the first month	Identification and monitoring of people with high levels of distress, especially if this affects functioning. Formal assessment for health and/or social care services should be made of the needs of people who have psychosocial problems that do not remit given adequate humanitarian aid, welfare services, and social support from their families and communities. Evidence-informed interventions should be available for people with mental disorders
Months 1–3	Identification and monitoring of people with high levels of distress, especially if this affects functioning. Formal assessments should be offered to people who have psychosocial problems that continue or develop 1 month or more after a major incident or disaster. Assessment should take place before any specific intervention is offered, and should consider people's emotional, social, physical, and psychological needs. Evidence-based interventions should be available for people with mental disorders
After 3 months	People who have psychosocial problems that continue or develop 3 months or more after a major incident or disaster should be formally assessed. Assessment should take place before any specific intervention is offered, and should consider people's emotional, social, physical, and psychological needs. Evidence-based interventions should be available for people who have mental disorders. Work and rehabilitation opportunities should be provided to enable those who require them to re-adapt to the routines of everyday life

difficulties are dealt with in a holistic manner. Table 29.2 shows the recommended types of mental health services required over time after traumatic events [35].

Summary

In summary, only a minority of people affected by major incidents and pandemics are likely to develop mental health symptoms of a severity that requires mental healthcare. Those who do develop symptoms are likely to experience a range of different diagnoses depending on the nature of their experiences, the consequences of the event, their environment after the event, and pre-existing factors. The evidence for prevention of mental disorders through formal interventions is very limited, and contrasts with the strong evidence for effective treatments. In order to provide optimal care after major incidents and pandemics, a biopsychosocial framework is appropriate, with mental health service provision being part of a whole system approach. A seamless person-centred mental healthcare pathway for people who are affected is likely to involve first responders, primary care, secondary physical care, the third sector, and social care. The emphasis should be on providing practical pragmatic support in an empathic manner, facilitating detection, appropriate referral, assessment, and management, following the principles of prudent healthcare. Specific considerations, which have service implications, are required for different types of presentation and incident, and for short-, medium-, and long-term impacts.

References

1. Williams R, Bisson J, Kemp V. *OP94: Principles for Responding to People's Psychosocial and Mental Health Needs After Disasters.* Royal College of Psychiatrists, 2014.

2. Bonanno GA. Loss, trauma, and human resilience: have we underestimated the human capacity to thrive after extremely adverse events? *Am Psychol* 2004; 59: 20–28.

3. Bryant RA, Nickerson A, Creamer M, O'Donnell M, Forbes D, Galatzer-Levy I, et al. Trajectory of post-traumatic stress following traumatic injury: 6-year follow-up. *Br J Psychiatry* 2015; 206: 417–23.

4. Stancombe J, Williams R, Drury J, Collins H, Lagan L, Barrett A, et al. People's experiences of distress and psychosocial care following a terrorist attack: interviews with survivors of the Manchester Arena bombing in 2017. *BJPsych Open* 2022; 8: e41.

5. Bryant RA. Post-traumatic stress disorder: a state-of-the-art review of evidence and challenges. *World Psychiatry* 2019; 18: 259–69.

6. Brewin CR, Andrews B, Valentine JD. Meta-analysis of risk factors

for posttraumatic stress disorder in trauma-exposed adults. *J Consult Clin Psychol* 2000; 68: 748–66.

7. World Health Organization. *International Classification of Diseases for Mortality and Morbidity Statistics* 11th revision. World Health Organization, 2018 (https://icd.who.int/browse11/l-m/en).

8. American Psychiatric Association. *Diagnostic and Statistical Manual of Mental Disorders* 5th ed. American Psychiatric Association, 2013.

9. Galea S, Nandi A, Vlahov D. The epidemiology of post-traumatic stress disorder after disasters. *Epidemiol Rev* 2005; 27: 78–91.

10. Beaglehole B, Mulder RT, Frampton CM, Boden JM, Newton-Howes G, Bell CJ. Psychological distress and psychiatric disorder after natural disasters: systematic review and meta-analysis. *Br J Psychiatry* 2018; 213: 716–22.

11. Shevlin M, McBride O, Murphy J, Gibson Miller J, Hartman TK, Levita L, et al. Anxiety, depression, traumatic stress and COVID-19-related anxiety in the UK general population during the COVID-19 pandemic. *BJPsych Open* 2020; 6: e125.

12. Pierce M, Hope H, Ford T, Hatch S, Hotopf M, John A, et al. Mental health before and during the COVID-19 pandemic: a longitudinal probability sample survey of the UK population. *Lancet Psychiatry* 2020; 7: 883–92.

13. Kwong ASF, Pearson RM, Adams MJ, Northstone K, Tilling K, Smith D, et al. Mental health before and during the COVID-19 pandemic in two longitudinal UK population cohorts. *Br J Psychiatry* 2021; 218: 334–43.

14. Fancourt D, Steptoe A, Bu F. Trajectories of anxiety and depressive symptoms during enforced isolation due to COVID-19 in England: a longitudinal observational study. *Lancet Psychiatry* 2021; 8: 141–9.

15. Cénat JM, Blais-Rochette C, Kokou-Kpolou CK, Noorishad P, Mukunzi JN, McIntee S, et al. Prevalence of symptoms of depression, anxiety, insomnia, posttraumatic stress disorder, and psychological distress among populations affected by the COVID-19 pandemic: a systematic review and meta-analysis. *Psychiatry Res* 2021; 295: 113599.

16. Greenberg N, Weston D, Hall C, Caulfield T, Williamson V, Fong K. Mental health of staff working in intensive care during Covid-19. *Occup Med* 2021; 71: 62–7.

17. d'Ettorre G, Ceccarelli G, Santinelli L, Vassalini P, Innocenti GP, Alessandri F, et al. Post-traumatic stress symptoms in healthcare workers dealing with the COVID-19 pandemic: a systematic review. *Int J Environ Res Public Health* 2021; 18: 601.

18. Lewis KJS, Lewis C, Roberts A, Richards NA, Evison C, Pearce H, et al. The effect of the COVID-19 pandemic on mental health in individuals with pre-existing mental illness. *BJPsych Open* 2022; 8: e59.

19. Lewis C, Lewis K, Roberts A, Evison C, Edwards B, John A, et al. COVID-19 related posttraumatic stress disorder in adults with lived experience of psychiatric disorder. *Depress Anxiety* 2022; 39: 564–72.

20. Butler M, Pollak TA, Rooney AG, Michael BD, Nicholson TR. Neuropsychiatric complications of COVID-19. *BMJ* 2020; 371: m3871.

21. Greenhalgh T, Knight M, A'Court C, Buxton M, Husain L. Management of post-acute covid-19 in primary care. *BMJ* 2020; 370: m3026.

22. Bisson JI, Astill Wright L, Jones KA, Lewis C, Phelps AJ, Sijbrandij M, et al. Preventing the onset of post traumatic stress disorder. *Clin Psychol Rev* 2021; 86: 102004.

23. Rose A, Bisson J, Churchill R, Wessely S. Psychological debriefing for preventing post traumatic stress disorder (PTSD). *Cochrane Database Syst Rev* 2002; 2: CD000560.

24. National Institute for Health and Care Excellence. *Post-Traumatic Stress Disorder. NICE Guideline [NG116]*. National Institute for Health and Care Excellence, 2018 (www.nice.org.uk/guidance/ng116).

25. Wu S, Zhu X, Zhang Y, Liang J, Liu X, Yang Y, et al. A new psychological intervention: "512 Psychological Intervention Model" used for military rescuers in Wenchuan Earthquake in China. *Soc Psychiatry Psychiatr Epidemiol* 2012; 47: 1111–19.

26. International Society for Traumatic Stress Studies (ISTSS). *Posttraumatic Stress Disorder Prevention and Treatment Guidelines: Methodology and Recommendations*. ISTSS, 2019 (https://istss.org/getattachment/Treating-Trauma/New-ISTSS-Prevention-and-Treatment-Guidelines/ISTSS_PreventionTreatmentGuidelines_FNL-March-19-2019.pdf.aspx.).

27. Roberts N, Kitchiner N, Kenardy J, Lewis C, Bisson J. Early psychological intervention following recent trauma: a systematic review and meta-analysis. *Eur J Psychotraumatol* 2019; 10: 1695486.

28. Astill Wright L, Sijbrandij M, Sinnerton R, Lewis C, Roberts NP, Bisson JI. Pharmacological prevention and early treatment of post-traumatic stress disorder and acute stress disorder: a systematic review and meta-analysis. *Transl Psychiatry* 2019; 9: 334.

29. National Institute for Health and Care Excellence. *Depression in Adults: Recognition and*

Management. Clinical Guideline [CG90]. National Institute for Health and Care Excellence, 2020 (www.nice.org.uk/guidance/cg90/evidence/full-guideline-pdf-4840934509).

30. National Institute for Health and Care Excellence. *Generalised Anxiety Disorder and Panic Disorder in Adults: Management. Clinical Guideline [CG113].* National Institute for Health and Care Excellence, 2019 (www.nice.org.uk/guidance/cg113).

31. National Institute for Health and Care Excellence. *Alcohol-Use Disorders: Diagnosis, Assessment and Management of Harmful Drinking (High-Risk Drinking) and Alcohol Dependence. Clinical Guideline [CG115].* National Institute for Health and Care Excellence, 2011 (www.nice.org.uk/guidance/cg115).

32. Lewis C, Roberts NP, Andrew M, Starling E, Bisson JI. Psychological therapies for post-traumatic stress disorder in adults: systematic review and meta-analysis. *Eur J Psychotraumatol* 2020; 11: 1729633.

33. Phoenix Australia. *The Australian Guidelines for the Prevention and Treatment of Acute Stress Disorder (ASD), Posttraumatic Stress Disorder (PTSD) and Complex PTSD.* Phoenix Australia, 2020 (www.phoenixaustralia.org/australian-guidelines-for-ptsd/).

34. Bisson JI, Ariti C, Cullen K, Kitchiner N, Lewis C, Roberts NP, et al. Guided, internet based, cognitive behavioural therapy for post-traumatic stress disorder: pragmatic, multicentre, randomised controlled non-inferiority trial (RAPID). *BMJ* 2022; 377: e069405.

35. Bisson JI, Tavakoly B, Witteveen AB, Ajdukovic D, Jehel L, Johansen VJ, et al. TENTS guidelines: development of post-disaster psychosocial care guidelines through a Delphi process. *Br J Psychiatry* 2010; 196: 69–74.

36. Hobfoll SE, Watson P, Bell CC, Bryant RA, Brymer MJ, Friedman MJ, et al. Five essential elements of immediate and mid-term mass trauma intervention: empirical evidence. *Psychiatry* 2007; 70: 283–315.

37. Brewin CR, Fuchkan N, Huntley Z, et al. Outreach and screening following the 2005 London bombings: usage and outcomes. *Psychol Med* 2010; 40: 2049–57.

38. Rona RJ, Burdett H, Khondoker M, Chesnokov M, Green K, Perent D, et al. Post-deployment screening for mental disorders and tailored advice about help-seeking in the UK military: a cluster randomised controlled trial. *Lancet* 2017; 389: 1410–23.

39. Rona RJ, Hooper R, Jones M, Hull L, Browne T, Horn O, et al. Mental health screening in armed forces before the Iraq war and prevention of subsequent psychological morbidity: follow-up study. *BMJ* 2006; 333: 991.

40. Welsh Government. *Prudent Healthcare.* Welsh Government, 2016 (https://gov.wales/prudent-healthcare).

Responding to the Needs of Children, Young People, and Their Families During the COVID-19 Pandemic

Betty Pfefferbaum

Introduction

Chapter 6 introduces readers to the impacts of emergencies, terrorism, and disease on children and their families. Chapter 27 highlights the different mental health needs of certain groups of the population, including children, after disasters. The authors of Chapter 28 describe their research after the Manchester Arena bombing, in which a significant proportion of the people affected were children and their families.

Children constitute an important subset of disaster populations, and they require special attention to protect them from harm and to ensure that they receive the developmentally appropriate services they need [1,2]. Although children have been identified as particularly vulnerable to mass trauma, they also are resilient and respond to social support [3]. This support is central to disaster mental health services. This chapter reviews the current approach to services for children, presents a framework and guiding principles for child disaster mental health response, addresses assessment, examines intervention approaches and the evidence base for intervention, and offers recommendations for future work. The COVID-19 pandemic has presented challenges not adequately contemplated in the existing literature; therefore concerns raised by pandemics are integrated throughout.

A Framework for Response: Guiding Principles and Practical Applications

A framework for addressing children's disaster mental health needs recognises guiding principles that are influenced by a number of overarching considerations regarding services and service delivery, fundamental elements of response, the focus of services and interventions, and the design and structure of service delivery.

Overarching Reflections Related to Services and Service Delivery

General principles in disaster mental health response and practical applications typically consider the importance of the timing of service administration (e.g., disaster phase), the populations being served (e.g., population exposure), and the context (e.g., social resources, cultural issues) in planning and establishing services. Aspects of the setting and providers are also key determinants of the mental health response, and experiences with the COVID-19 pandemic have made it clear that the type of event and event characteristics warrant consideration.

Event

Although epidemics and pandemics are included in the conventional all-hazards approach to disaster management, novel aspects of the COVID-19 pandemic were not previously anticipated in mental health responses to children affected by disasters, which had previously focused primarily on natural and human-made events. Meta-analyses of children's post-traumatic stress reactions and of intervention studies have found similar outcomes across different types of event, but the studies included in these meta-analyses addressed natural and human-made disasters, and did not include studies of biological events or pandemics [4–6]. Furthermore, meta-analyses of interventions have not examined the effect of event characteristics such as magnitude, casualty rates, or duration (e.g., length of conflict) on outcomes from interventions.

The COVID-19 pandemic, with its penetration across entire societies, its soaring morbidity and mortality, and the social, economic, and emotional impact of widely implemented public health measures, has required renewed attention to the effects of disasters and management approaches. For example, restrictive mandates have necessitated attention to reactions not typically assessed in response to disasters (e.g., loneliness), and have dictated modifications in service delivery approaches (e.g., increased use of technology). Moreover, mass trauma reactions and recovery are influenced by the availability and quality of social support, resources, and networks, which may be compromised by physical distancing measures.

Timing

Each disaster phase – preparedness, the acute aftermath, the initial months after the event, and recovery over time – presents distinct challenges, results in diverse needs, and requires appropriate services and resources. As described in this chapter, some services and interventions are designed for specific disaster phases, whereas others are appropriate across multiple phases. An emerging evidence base supports preparedness efforts and interventions for delivery in the early months after the event and throughout recovery.

Children's Characteristics and Population Risk

Children's characteristics (e.g., demographics, pre-existing conditions, previous trauma exposure) influence their disaster outcomes and may be important in the design and use of services and interventions [7]. Except for an important emphasis on developmental appropriateness, these characteristics generally have not been a major consideration in the literature on services and interventions [8]. Population risk, based on children's disaster exposure or experiences (e.g., direct involvement, relationship to victims, community residence, media contact) and reactions (e.g., normative distress, clinically significant symptoms, functional impairment), has been a primary determinant of service and intervention decisions [9].

Context

A variety of social and contextual factors (e.g., population density, cultural and religious beliefs and practices, disaster preparedness and response infrastructures, social support networks, media coverage) have the potential to affect children's mass trauma reactions and their response to services and interventions.

Disasters occur worldwide, but may be especially debilitating in low-resource environments where inadequate infrastructures and disrupted support networks that would foster recovery can impede the response [10].

Service Delivery Settings

Disaster services are administered in various venues, including existing health and mental health, social, and educational systems as well as disaster-specific settings such as shelters [11]. The choice of the setting is determined in part by the characteristics of the event and the damage and disruption generated by it, the experiences of the children receiving the services, the type and goals of the services, the availability of settings and providers, and access [11]. In addition to availability, the choice of provider depends in large part on the exposure and reactions of the children who need services [11]. Directly exposed and/or symptomatic children require the expertise of mental health professionals, whereas trained teachers and paraprofessionals can administer wellness- and/or resilience-focused services and interventions for children whose reactions are not clinically significant [11]. In recent years, access issues and the COVID-19 pandemic have encouraged the use of technological platforms to deliver mental health assistance and interventions.

Because they allow access to large numbers of students in a setting that minimises stigma, schools constitute an ideal setting for delivering services to children [11,12]. The popularity of using schools for this purpose was revealed in a review of studies of child disaster mental health interventions, which found that most interventions were delivered in schools [11]. Teachers and other school personnel have pre-event relationships with children, they understand developmental processes, and they are likely to recognise changes in children's emotions, behaviours, and functioning [11]. Nonetheless, teachers and other school personnel should not be expected to evaluate and manage clinical problems, although they may refer children for these more intense services. Relative to schools, clinical settings may be less accessible and acceptable to families, but these settings are more likely to have the professionals and resources needed to treat children with clinical problems [11]. The COVID-19 pandemic, which resulted in the closure of schools worldwide, virtually eliminated them as a venue for delivering mental health services, and intensified the need for evidence-based decisions regarding the safe opening of schools. Other locations, such as shelters and refugee camps, may be utilised when schools and/or clinical facilities are unavailable – for example, because they have been destroyed by an event [11].

Technological Approaches

In recent years, various obstacles (e.g., access, time, transportation, stigma), along with the popularity of the Internet and other platforms, have stimulated the use of technological approaches to delivering disaster mental health services for children [13]. The COVID-19 pandemic and physical distancing, including the closure of schools and increased concern about the use of in-person health and mental health services, have made it difficult to reach children who are typically served in these venues, and have accelerated the use of technological approaches. An emerging evidence base suggests that telemental health is effective, feasible, and acceptable for use with children, but more research is needed to compare telemental health and in-person care with respect to the quality of care and outcomes [14].

Fundamental Elements That Guide the Mental Health Response

The principles of disaster response acknowledge the importance of community involvement, supportive approaches such as psychological first aid, and communication and information [1]. In a seminal paper documenting distinctive issues related to children, Richard Williams and his colleagues recognise the role and involvement of parents and community programmes in identifying and addressing children's reactions and needs, and they promote the use of developmentally appropriate and practical early interventions for children [8].

Community Involvement in Disaster Management and the Participation of Children

Communities have important roles in disaster management, and should be involved in dialogue and decision making [1,2,15]. This includes eliciting the views and considering the experiences of children, who are not simply passive victims of disasters [1,2,16–18]. Children can serve as resources for preparedness (e.g., hazard and threat identification, drills, family awareness and household readiness), response (e.g., risk communication, evacuation), and recovery (e.g., distribution of resources, peer counselling with potential benefit for children themselves, for families, and for communities) [16–18]. With appropriate adult guidance, involving children provides opportunities to enhance skill development, interpersonal interaction, and self-confidence [16,18]. Although limited in its methodological rigour, the research on children's participation in disaster risk reduction (DRR) programmes suggests that children can contribute to transformational community and community resilience efforts through activities such as risk communication and community mobilisation [19].

Parent and Family Involvement in Children's Services

The principles for providing child disaster services identified by Williams and his colleagues [8] include attention to children's relationships with adults, to parental disaster reactions and needs, and to educating families to recognise and respond to their children's reactions and needs. Family outreach should inform parents about disaster services and, when possible, families should be involved in the assessment of children and in the delivery of interventions [20]. Parents may benefit from interventions aimed at educating them about their own and their children's disaster reactions, and from interventions that address parental reactions and parenting [12]. A meta-analysis of child disaster interventions found that involving parents resulted in better outcomes for children, but interventions that did not involve parents were also effective, which suggests that parental involvement is not essential [21].

Psychosocial Support and Psychological First Aid

Williams and his colleagues promote the use of practical disaster interventions that address concrete needs, encourage children to express their feelings and concerns, offer reassurance, and promote normalisation [8]. Psychological first aid is an evidence-informed set of principles and strategies that can be delivered by clinicians and trained non-clinicians (e.g., paraprofessionals, teachers and school personnel, volunteers). It offers non-intrusive support and timely information about disaster reactions and available resources, assesses basic needs, encourages the measured expression of children's emotional experiences, fosters protection from additional harm, mobilises support, and makes referrals as needed [1,2,20]. Renee Gilbert and colleagues recommend integrating psychological first aid into disaster mental health management in conjunction with assessment, specialised services, and recovery monitoring, and they provide guidelines for evaluation research [22]. Despite a lack of empirical evidence, the literature suggests that psychological first aid is of benefit in the immediate post-event phase [22]. Although generally promoted for use in the early aftermath of a disaster, the principles of psychological first aid find application throughout disaster phases.

Risk Communication and Dissemination of Information

Children need information in order to understand disaster risks and ways to mitigate these risks [16]. Without information, children, like adults, are left to find their own explanations for what is occurring around them, but they can also become overwhelmed by excessive information, especially if it is contradictory. The COVID-19 pandemic witnessed an escalation of fake news, conspiracy theories, and misinformation that contributed to an infodemic in which evolving knowledge and conflicting political, social, and economic interests impeded the delivery of timely, accurate, and trusted information needed to guide public attitudes and health behaviours [23].

In general, children rely on their parents, teachers and other school personnel, and other adults for education and instruction about disasters [16]. Communication should be responsive and interactive, should involve the children themselves, their families, and personnel in schools and other settings where children interact, and should foster interactions among these stakeholders [24].

Issues Related to the Focus of Disaster Services and Interventions

Although children's disaster reactions range from normative distress to a variety of emotional and behavioural reactions, outcome studies have focused largely on post-traumatic stress [4], raising concerns about the extent to which other outcomes are missed [4,15]. Indeed depression and anxiety may be even more pronounced than post-traumatic stress disorder (PTSD) in children who have been exposed to complex emergencies – especially, perhaps, in low-income settings where mental health resources may be particularly limited [25]. Concern about the appropriateness of focusing on trauma and post-traumatic stress in a cross-cultural context reflects an intense debate regarding the application of Western concepts and approaches in non-Western settings, and the importance of cultural and contextual determinants as well as biological reactions in children's mass trauma reactions [26]. Concerns about the appropriateness of a focus on PTSD have been raised in the context of the COVID-19 pandemic as well, because many affected people do not meet the full criteria for the disorder [27,28]. The pandemic also illustrates the importance of considering outcomes not commonly contemplated in disaster work – for example, loneliness in children whose social interactions have been limited over an extended period.

Considerations Relating to the Design and Structure of Services

The design and structure of services and practical applications are guided by principles that recognise the importance of considering mental health issues in general disaster management across service sectors using a multi-layered approach that is organised to address the needs of the various affected populations.

Integration of Disaster Mental Health Services for Children

The importance of integrating disaster mental health services for children extends throughout all disaster phases and across multiple sectors, including those that address government policy as well as those that provide health and public health, social and welfare, education, faith-based, emergency and disaster management, first-responder, law enforcement, media, and other services. The integration of mental health services has the potential to facilitate access, enhance sustainability, and reduce the stigma associated with mental healthcare [29]. Integrated care requires collaboration among mental health programmes, relationships across disciplines and agencies, leadership and coordination, clear delineation of responsibility, consistent terminology, effective communication, agreement about case management, and attention to privacy and other concerns to permit information sharing [15,29].

Of particular importance for children is integration into primary care and into schools where, as discussed earlier, disaster mental health services are commonly provided [11]. The COVID-19 pandemic has highlighted the importance of delivering mental health services in primary care settings where directly and indirectly affected children are more likely to be receiving care. Approaches to integration range from simply co-locating physical and mental health services in the same setting to providing consultation and referral for psychosocial needs, to the use of teams with medical providers and mental health professionals working together to address both physical and emotional issues [30]. Efforts to integrate mental health services into primary care are not new, but it remains unclear how successful these efforts have been with respect to disaster services.

A Multi-Layered Approach to Services

A multi-layered approach is recommended to address the psychosocial needs of various groups in the context of mass trauma [2,15]. This layered approach to services links screening, triage, assessment, and intervention [15] with multiple tiers based on the needs of various populations over time or on the intensity of services [15,29], It includes universal services for the entire population, and targeted services for more affected groups [15,29]. Universal psychosocial public health services and interventions, which are used to foster coping and resilience [9], are intended for all children in the population (e.g., entire schools), regardless of their disaster exposure or reactions, and can be administered without assessment of individual need [9,12,31]. Selective services and interventions are intended to enhance coping in those children who do not manifest clinical outcomes, but who are at heightened biological, psychological, and social risk for developing a mental disorder [31]. These individuals include, for example, children who are directly exposed but who are not distressed or functionally impaired, and those with high levels of post-traumatic stress but no other risk for long-term functional impairment [9]. Indicated services and interventions are intended for children with serious and/or persistent reactions, including those with marked distress, enduring post-traumatic stress and/or other reactions, or other risk factors for adverse outcome [9,31].

Assessment

Assessment is conducted in the early aftermath of an event, and over the course of response and recovery when survivors seek care [15]. It serves to detect children who have serious reactions or mental disorders that require their clinical evaluation and/or treatment [15,32]. As part of the assessment process, those children who have potentially serious reactions should be provided with information and advice and offered follow-up assessment, whereas those with serious reactions should be referred for immediate clinical evaluation and treatment [15].

The problems and needs of affected children can be assessed at both community and personal levels using population surveillance, needs assessment, screening, and individual clinical evaluation. Needs assessment (a cross-sectional determination of disaster effects and needs) and surveillance (monitoring health and behaviour over time) provide assessments at the community level to help plan and direct response activities and to create a baseline from which to detect change over time [32]. Screening is used to identify children with problems and the need for services, and clinical evaluation is used to identify psychopathology [32]. Screening can be administered in sites where children naturally congregate (e.g., schools) to identify those at risk for adverse outcomes from among directly and/or indirectly exposed children or children with unknown exposure [9]. Clinical evaluations are conducted by professionals with children who were directly exposed or whose loved ones were directly exposed, children with pre-existing vulnerabilities, and those determined by screening to be at risk for adverse outcomes [9]. The goal is to identify children with psychopathological reactions who require clinical treatment [32].

Interventions and the Evidence Base for Intervention

Numerous child disaster interventions, based on various approaches and comprising a variety of components, have been developed and evaluated, resulting in an emerging evidence base to support their use for preparedness, in the early post-disaster phase, and across recovery. Clinical treatment is necessary for some children.

Intervention Approaches and Components

Numerous types of interventions and a variety of techniques have been used with children in disaster settings, and many interventions utilise multiple techniques [33]. Cognitive behavioural therapy (CBT) techniques are commonly used, and many interventions include psychoeducation, mostly in conjunction with other techniques [33]. Other interventions include exposure, narrative, relaxation, eye movement desensitisation and reprocessing (EMDR), and mind–body techniques [33]. Many multimodal interventions incorporate components to assist affect regulation, facilitate adaptive coping, build social support [33], and/or address traumatic grief [12]. Little evidence is available on the comparative benefit of the various intervention approaches [12].

Clinical Treatment

Some children, particularly those who are directly exposed or whose loved ones are directly exposed, bereaved children, and children with vulnerability indicators (e.g., pre-existing conditions, prior trauma), may need clinical treatment. Clinical treatment should be based on assessment, foster natural recovery and use familiar supports, enhance coping, address comorbid conditions, and consider the roles and needs of the family [20]. Medication may be necessary in conjunction with other interventions for severe reactions or comorbid conditions [20]. In general, studies have not evaluated mental health treatment such as psychodynamic psychotherapy, family therapy, or psychopharmacological treatment [34].

Preparedness Interventions

Disaster management emphasises preparedness, which is particularly important for children residing in high-risk areas (e.g., locations prone to natural disasters or political violence). Preparedness efforts include a range of activities to educate children about disasters and to improve their own and their family's disaster readiness. Despite methodological limitations, studies suggest that child DRR education interventions increase awareness and knowledge of disasters, enhance preparedness skills and confidence, and reduce negative emotional reactions such as fear

and anxiety [19]. It remains unclear, however, if these interventions facilitate household preparedness or self-protective actions during an event, or if children's gains in disaster preparedness continue into adulthood [35]. Unfortunately, DRR education efforts generally have not involved collaborative efforts within families or communities [19].

Interventions Delivered in the Early Months After the Event

Difficulty establishing services and the priority of providing services rather than focusing on research limit methodologically rigorous intervention research in the early post-event phase. A descriptive review of interventions delivered in the first 3 months after the event revealed generally positive results among studies of a variety of interventions (including CBT, narrative exposure, meditation relaxation, debriefing, EMDR, and innovative approaches such as massage and spiritual hypnosis), and it provided preliminary evidence that interventions implemented in the early months after an event can be effective [36].

The Evidence Base for Intervention and Unresolved Issues

Numerous interventions have been developed and evaluated for use with children who have been exposed to mass trauma. A recent review of publications reporting meta-analyses of randomised controlled trials of child mass trauma interventions using inactive controls revealed a small to medium overall effect of interventions on post-traumatic stress, a non-statistically significant to small overall effect on depression, a non-statistically significant overall effect on anxiety, and a small overall effect on functional impairment [34]. However, the degree to which the results represent meaningful clinical or public health improvement is unclear, especially given that many of the included studies failed to distinguish clinical from non-pathological outcomes [34]. The research also has not determined which component or components of multimodal interventions are responsible for benefit [34], or the extent to which one or more common factors are responsible for adaptive outcomes [33]. Finally, additional research is needed to examine possible moderators of the intervention effect, including, for example, characteristics of the children receiving services (e.g., pre-existing vulnerabilities), of the context (e.g., available resources, preparedness and response infrastructures, culture), of the interventions (e.g., theoretical approach, components, individual or group application, parent involvement, cultural adaptations), and of intervention administration (e.g., timing, setting, providers) [34].

Conclusion

An extensive literature describes the services and interventions used to address the disaster-related needs of children, and key determinants in designing and administering services and interventions. The importance of population risk and context in guiding service delivery decisions has been recognised, but the distinct needs of children with pre-existing conditions, previous trauma exposure, or other vulnerabilities have not been adequately addressed. Although the type of event has not up to now been considered a particularly salient feature in guiding services and interventions, the COVID-19 pandemic has revealed novel challenges associated with pandemics. Thus, the pandemic offers an unparalleled opportunity to give greater prominence to incorporating biological events in the all-hazards approach to disaster management.

Other concerns in the disaster mental health service system include its predominant focus on posttraumatic stress. Additional research on other common outcomes (e.g., depression, anxiety) is warranted, especially in low-resource environments and in the context of pandemics. The literature supports the use of layered mental health services, based on population risk and guided by assessment, but this graduated approach has not been evaluated empirically. The community has an important role in disaster management, and disaster preparedness and educational programmes have demonstrated benefit in fostering children's participation, but attention is needed to expand the involvement of families and communities in these and other intervention efforts. Clearly, although an emerging evidence base suggests that benefit can be derived from a variety of intervention approaches, numerous issues remain unresolved.

References

1. Sphere Association. *Humanitarian Charter and Minimum Standards in Disaster Response*. Sphere Association, 2004 (https://spherestandards.org/humanitarian-standards/).

2. Sphere Association. *The Sphere Handbook: Humanitarian Charter and Minimum Standards in Humanitarian Response* 4th ed. Sphere Association, 2018 (www.spherestandards.org/handbook/).

3. Murray V, Williams R, Johal S. International disaster response. In *Textbook of Disaster Psychiatry* 2nd ed. (eds R Ursano, CS Fullerton, L Weisaeth, B Raphael): 149–61. Cambridge University Press, 2017.

4. Furr JM, Comer JS, Edmunds JM, Kendall PC. Disasters and youth: a meta-analytic examination of posttraumatic stress. *J Consult Clin Psychol* 2010; **78**: 765–80.

5. Pfefferbaum B, Nitiéma P, Newman E. A meta-analysis of intervention effects on depression and/or anxiety in youth exposed to political violence or natural disasters. *Child Youth Care Forum* 2019; **48**: 449–77.

6. Pfefferbaum B, Nitiéma P, Newman E, Patel A. The benefit of interventions to reduce posttraumatic stress in youth exposed to mass trauma: a review and meta-analysis. *Prehosp Disaster Med* 2019; **34**: 540–51.

7. Pfefferbaum B, Jacobs AK, Griffin N, Houston JB. Children's disaster reactions: the influence of exposure and personal characteristics. *Curr Psychiatry Rep* 2015; **17**: 56.

8. Williams R, Alexander DA, Bolsover D, Bakke FK. Children, resilience and disasters: recent evidence that should influence a model of psychosocial care. *Curr Opin Psychiatry* 2008; **21**: 338–44.

9. Pfefferbaum B, North CS. Child disaster mental health services: a review of the system of care, assessment approaches, and evidence base for intervention. *Curr Psychiatry Rep* 2016; **18**: 5.

10. Bonanno GA, Brewin CR, Kaniasty K, La Greca AM. Weighing the costs of disaster: consequences, risks, and resilience in individuals, families, and communities. *Psychol Sci Public Interest* 2010; **11**: 1–49.

11. Pfefferbaum B, Sweeton JL, Newman E, Varma V, Noffsinger MA, Shaw JA, et al. Child disaster mental health interventions, part II: Timing of implementation, delivery settings and providers, and therapeutic approaches. *Disaster Health* 2014; **2**: 58–67.

12. Pfefferbaum B, Newman E, Nitiéma P. Current evidence for selecting disaster interventions for children and adolescents. *Curr Treat Options Psychiatry* 2016; **3**: 192–205.

13. Grolnick WS, Schonfeld DJ, Schreiber M, Cohen J, Cole V, Jaycox L, et al. Improving adjustment and resilience in children following a disaster:

addressing research challenges. *Am Psychol* 2018; **73**: 215–29.

14. Gloff NE, LeNoue SR, Novins DK, Myers K. Telemental health for children and adolescents. *Int Rev Psychiatry* 2015; **27**: 513–24.

15. North Atlantic Treaty Organization (NATO). *Psychosocial Care for People Affected by Disasters and Major Incidents: A Model for Designing, Delivering and Managing Psychosocial Services for People Involved in Major Incidents, Conflict, Disasters and Terrorism.* NATO, 2009 (www.coe.int/t/dg4/majorhazards/ressources/virtuallibrary/materials/Others/NATO_Guidance_Psychosocial_Care_for_People_Affected_by_Disasters_and_Major_Incidents.pdf.).

16. Fothergill A. *Children, Youth, and Disaster.* Oxford Research Encyclopedias, Natural Hazard Science, 2017. Available from: https://doi.org/10.1093/acrefore/9780199389407.013.23

17. Peek L. Children and disasters: understanding vulnerability, developing capacities, and promoting resilience – an introduction. *Child Youth Environ* 2008; **18**: 1–29.

18. Pfefferbaum B, Pfefferbaum RL, Van Horn RL. Involving children in disaster risk reduction: the importance of participation. *Eur J Psychotraumatol* 2018; **9**(suppl 2): 1425577.

19. Amri A, Haynes K, Bird DK, Ronan, K. Bridging the divide between studies on disaster risk reduction education and child-centred disaster risk reduction: a critical review. *Children's Geographies* 2018; **16**: 239–51.

20. Pfefferbaum B, Shaw JA, American Academy of Child and Adolescent Psychiatry Committee on Quality Issues. Practice parameter on disaster preparedness. *J Am Acad Child Adolesc Psychiatry* 2013; **52**: 1224–38.

21. Newman E, Pfefferbaum B, Nirlic N, Tett R, Nelson S, Liles B. Meta-analytic review of psychological interventions for children survivors of natural and man-made disasters. *Curr Psychiatry Rep* 2014; **16**: 462.

22. Gilbert R, Abel MR, Vernberg EM, Jacobs AK. The use of psychological first aid in children exposed to mass trauma. *Curr Psychiatry Rep* 2021; **23**: 53.

23. The Lancet Infectious Diseases. The COVID-19 infodemic. *Lancet Infect Dis* 2020; **20**: 875.

24. Wisner B, Paton D, Alisic E, Eastwood O, Shreve C, Fordham M. Communication with children and families about disaster: reviewing multi-disciplinary literature 2015–2017. *Curr Psychiatry Rep* 2018; **20**: 73.

25. Moss WJ, Ramakrishnan M, Storms D, Siegal AH, Weiss WM, Lejnev I, et al. Child health in complex emergencies. *Bull World Health Organ* 2006; **84**: 58–64.

26. Barenbaum J, Ruchkin V, Schwab-Stone M. The psychosocial aspects of children exposed to war: practice and policy initiatives. *J Child Psychol Psychiatry* 2004; **45**: 41–62.

27. North CS, Suris AM, Pollio DE. A nosological exploration of PTSD and trauma in disaster mental health and implications for the COVID-19 pandemic. *Behav Sci* 2021; **11**: 7.

28. Pfefferbaum B. Posttraumatic stress disorder in children in the context of the COVID-19 pandemic. *J Am Acad Child Adolesc Psychiatry* 2022; **61**: 957–9.

29. Institute of Medicine. *Healthy, Resilient, and Sustainable Communities after Disasters: Strategies, Opportunities, and Planning for Recovery.* National Academies Press, 2015 (www.nap.edu/download/18996).

30. Crowley RA, Kirschner N. The integration of care for mental health, substance abuse, and other behavioral health conditions into primary care: executive summary of an American College of Physicians position paper. *Ann Intern Med* 2015; **163**: 298–9.

31. National Research Council and Institute of Medicine. *Preventing Mental, Emotional, and Behavioral Disorders Among Young People: Progress and Possibilities.* National Academies Press, 2009 (www.nap.edu/download/12480).

32. Pfefferbaum B, Jacobs AK, Houston JB. Children and disasters: a framework for mental health assessment. *J Emerg Manag* 2012; **10**: 349–58.

33. Pfefferbaum B, Sweeton JL, Newman E, Varma V, Nitiéma P, Shaw JA, et al. Child disaster mental health interventions, part I. Techniques, outcomes, and methodological considerations. *Disaster Health* 2014; **2**: 46–57.

34. Pfefferbaum B, Nitiéma P, Newman E. A critical review of effective child mass trauma interventions: what we know and do not know from the evidence. *Behav Sci* 2021; **11**: 25.

35. Johnson VA, Ronan KR, Johnston DM, Peace R. Evaluations of disaster education programs for children: a methodological review. *Int J Disaster Risk Reduct* 2014; **9**: 107–23.

36. Pfefferbaum B, Nitiéma P, Tucker P, Newman E. Early child disaster mental health interventions: a review of the empirical evidence. *Child Youth Care Forum* 2017; **46**: 621–42.

Chapter

31

Social and Educational Impacts of Epidemics and Pandemics

Matthew J Easterbrook, Kathryn J Lester, Alison Lacey, Lewis Doyle, and Vladislav H Grozev

Introduction

The COVID-19 pandemic severely disrupted the educational and social lives of millions of children across the globe. Many governments attempted to curb the spread of the virus by closing schools or allowing them to remain open only for certain students, necessitating a rapid adjustment to remote home learning for schools and families. In the UK, this led to huge variability in the provision of education materials, in children's engagement, and in parents' capacity to support home learning. Although education has been disrupted for millions of children, and recent estimates suggest that school closures were associated with a loss of 0.3–0.9 school years' worth of learning, there are concerns that the brunt of this disruption and its negative consequences are disproportionately experienced by disadvantaged students and families [1]. One consequence of prolonged school closures is therefore likely to be an increase in existing socioeconomic inequalities in educational and socioemotional outcomes [2].

In this chapter, we describe the impacts of the school closures on families' and students' educational and socioemotional development. We draw conclusions from the wider scientific literature, and in particular from three of our own studies. These studies were conducted in the UK between May and July 2020, when British schools were closed to all students except the children of key workers and children identified as vulnerable. The three studies each have different samples and foci, but together offer broad yet deep insights into home learning during the pandemic. The first study is based on an online survey of parents ($n = 3,167$) and teachers ($n = 2,075$) [3]. The second study is based on semi-structured focus group interviews with 20 parents of children with special educational needs and/or disabilities [4]. The third study is based on semi-structured interviews with 21 mothers and their primary-school-aged children [5].

Based on these studies and our reading of the wider literature, we end the chapter by making policy and practice recommendations about how similar events should be navigated in the future to effectively mitigate the potentially devastating impact on children's educational, social, and emotional progress and development. Our data mainly relate to inequality with respect to socioeconomic status (SES), which is the focus of this chapter. Nevertheless, it is important to note that families from ethnic minority and other backgrounds are also likely to have been disproportionately affected by school closures, and should also be prioritised in policies or practices designed to mitigate any impacts of the pandemic [6,7].

Impact: Increasing Inequalities

There are growing concerns about the impact of the school closures on children's academic outcomes, with fears that it may be children from disadvantaged backgrounds who suffer the worst effects. Indeed, early estimates suggest that school closures could increase the social class attainment gap by 36%, with estimates in the range of 11–76% [8]. Emerging evidence endorses these concerns and suggests that COVID-19 caused a lag of 1.6–3 months in students' learning overall, which is thought to be at least 1 month greater for disadvantaged primary school students [9–11]. Other emerging evidence indicates that the pandemic resulted in students from poorer backgrounds and students attending schools in disadvantaged areas learning less and performing worse in assessments than did their peers [12–14].

There are multiple reasons for this growing attainment gap. When learning becomes primarily digital, it further disadvantages low-SES students and exacerbates cultural and environmental differences, particularly when the onus of education is placed on families rather than on schools [2]. We provide evidence related to these mechanisms later in this chapter.

The pandemic also posed a significant challenge to children's social relationships and emotional well-being [15–17]. Recent data show a rise in the prevalence of children's mental health problems compared with 2017, and suggest that children living in a household that was struggling to pay bills and buy food during the pandemic were significantly more likely to experience poor mental health [18]. Families of children with special educational needs and disabilities (SEND) also described particularly adverse impacts of the pandemic and associated social changes on their own and their children's mental health [19].

Parent-report data have also shown fluctuations in children's behavioural, emotional, and attentional difficulties [20]. Greater increases in symptomatology were observed among pre-adolescent children compared with adolescents. This may in part be explained by greater isolation from peers and heightened experiences of family stress, when many parents were trying to balance work commitments with home learning [21,22]. Our own data provide important insights related to the impact of social isolation and parental supervision. Notably, children's behavioural and attentional difficulties were greatest during times of national lockdown, with symptoms decreasing as restrictions eased and schools reopened. However, for children with SEND and those from low-income households, mental health difficulties remained elevated even as restrictions were lifted [20].

Although the emerging evidence justifies concerns that the pandemic is likely to increase educational and mental health inequalities, there is little evidence at present that demonstrates why lower-SES and vulnerable students and families have been disproportionately affected by the pandemic school closures. Therefore, we review the evidence and draw on our own studies to document some of these mechanisms.

Unequal Education

The immediate consequence of the pandemic for education was mass disruption and extreme uncertainty for families and teachers, often resulting in increased stress. As schools closed and learning became remote, the quantity and quality of education that students received varied enormously [23,24]. Some schools had information technology (IT) infrastructure that was sufficient to enable them to rapidly offer their students a rich and interactive remote learning experience. Others did not, and many

prioritised providing pastoral, practical, and extracurricular support for families, such as continuing to provide free school meals and checking on families' welfare, over creating and delivering remote educational resources [25].

Consequently, the disruption that students experienced to their education varied dramatically, particularly in relation to SES [2]. The education of poorer students attending state schools that serve disadvantaged areas may have been severely disrupted for months. Remote education of students from wealthy families who were attending private schools may have increased their learning, because high-quality tuition provided by their school almost from the outset was often complemented by virtual private tuition [26,27].

All three of our own studies revealed stark differences between the educational provision offered by state and independent (fee-paying) schools. The results from the quantitative survey suggested that the majority (89%) of independent schools updated their materials at least once a day, and were much more likely to offer students live interactions with teachers via video streams (85%, compared with 20% of state schools) and a way to interact with peers (82%, compared with 19%). Similarly, parents of children at independent schools were more likely to rate the quality of educational provision as excellent compared with parents of children at state schools (62%, compared with 21%). Teachers in independent schools reported that around 96% of students accessed home learning resources, and around 88% regularly completed the assigned work. The corresponding figures for state schools were 70% and 57%, respectively.

This divide between the state and independent sectors was apparent in the interviews, too, as parents reported feeling frustrated by the speed at which state schools adapted to the new ways of working, and the lack of input that they provided:

> There's such a huge difference between private school education and state school education during lockdown. Not that I would like my child sitting in front of a screen 6 hours a day, but there's a happy medium. They definitely need more input from the schools.
>
> Laurie's mum (Year 6, Study 3)

As well as these stark differences between state and independent schools, engagement with home learning varied according to pupils' characteristics. In the survey, parents reported that, on average, primary school students spent 1–3 hours a day on home learning, whereas secondary school students tended to spend on average 2–4 hours per day. Yet over 25% of primary school children and 15% of secondary school children spent less than 1 hour a day on home learning. Analyses of the survey responses showed that vulnerable children and children from lower-SES households were more likely to spend less time on home learning. From the interviews it was clear that children who were described as self-motivated, self-sufficient, and emotionally resilient were less likely to experience problems accessing the remote curriculum. These findings suggest that closures had a disproportionately negative impact on those students and families who were already struggling.

The Digital Divide and Home Environments

The digital divide refers to SES inequalities in access to technology (e.g., laptops, fast internet speeds). The divide that existed before the pandemic almost certainly means that school closures are likely to have had more of a detrimental impact on lower-SES students, who have less access to the technology that became essential for efficient and effective home learning [27]. Yet the digital divide goes further – pupils from higher-SES backgrounds are more likely to use technology for educational rather than recreational purposes, and to be more confident and motivated with regard to using technology for education. The switch to digital learning therefore disadvantages low-SES students who may be less equipped to navigate the technology needed for learning [2]. However, many schools made efforts to provide educational resources for students who did not have sufficient technology. Over 50% of parents in our studies reported that their child's school supplied alternatives for those students without internet access, but these resources were often delayed or inadequate [24,28].

Lower-SES students are not only more likely to lack IT resources and skills, but also more likely to live in home environments that are not conducive to learning, making home learning more challenging for them [29]. Indeed 45% of parents from lower-SES households who completed the survey indicated that a lack of technology made home learning more challenging for their children, and 35% indicated that an inadequate internet connection was a barrier. Around 60% of parents from lower-SES households indicated that noise was a significant barrier to their children's home learning, and 45% indicated that lack of space

was a problem. This was echoed in the qualitative studies, although the impacts were not exclusive to the most disadvantaged families:

> We had one laptop between all of us. I've lost my job, we're like a comfortable family, but we couldn't afford to buy an extra computer or a printer.
>
> Laurie's mum (Year 6, Study 2)

A particularly concerning finding was that 19% of financially struggling parents (compared with 5% of parents overall) reported that lack of food made home learning more difficult for their child. The data indicate that only around 50% of eligible children received free school meals during the first school closures [30]. Provision of free school meals for students outside of term time, which was spearheaded in a campaign by the UK footballer Marcus Rashford, is likely to have been vitally important in supporting these students and their learning.

Parental Supervision

Family members of lower-SES students are less likely than those of higher-SES children to have the skills, knowledge, and motivation to supervise their children's schoolwork [29]. This is important because parental support and involvement in their children's education are robust positive predictors both of children's attainment and of the effectiveness of home schooling [31–33]. Yet parental involvement also tends to show socioeconomic differences, with more affluent parents tending to be more engaged in their children's education [34,35].

Our survey results showed that availability and confidence to support home schooling differed according to parents' level of education. Overall, parents who had not graduated from university felt less able, motivated, and confident to supervise their children's work, and their children were thus less engaged and spent less time home learning [29]. Parents with bachelor's degrees tended to be more engaged in supervising their children's schoolwork, even if they struggled to find the time to do so [29].

In the interviews, working parents reported finding home schooling particularly stressful because of their limited availability. These parents reported that the competing demands of continued employment and childcare were often unmanageable. Parents with more than one child, or with children with SEND, also reported that home learning was a huge additional pressure that frequently felt overwhelming. This is consistent with recent data which suggest that having a child who struggled with home learning was associated with elevated symptoms of parental mental health difficulties [36]:

> It's constant. They want interaction all the time and it's stressful [trying] to work. Also, you feel this gigantic guilt – pushing your child away and saying, 'I can't be with you just now'.
>
> Peter's mum (Year 4, Study 3)

> It's just me by myself with the five children – it's just me managing on a day-to-day basis and three of them have got additional needs so it's not been easy – it's not been easy at all.
>
> Matthew's mum (Year 6, Study 2)

Lack of parental availability was also associated with poorer wellbeing of children. Children described the experience of having their parents physically present but emotionally unavailable as difficult to manage and associated with increased stress:

> I wish that mum and dad would be more with us because they're usually working. That's one thing I haven't enjoyed.
>
> Peter (Year 4, Study 3)

Social Isolation

For the majority of children, one of the most significant challenges was isolation from their peers during the period of school closures. This reduction in peer interaction is likely to have a negative impact on all children's learning and emotional and social development, and to increase the risk of mental health problems [37,38].

The social and emotional wellbeing of many children deteriorated during the period of school closures, which is consistent with recent data that show an increase in rates of mental health diagnoses and heightened emotional, behavioural, and attentional difficulties during periods of lockdown [18,20].

Almost all of the children who were interviewed reported missing friends, teachers, and the familiar routines of school and extracurricular activities. Feelings of exclusion and distress were felt most acutely by children whose friends were still attending school under key-worker provisions, by only children, and by children with SEND. Some parents believed that this contributed to their children's lack of engagement with home learning:

> She's felt incredibly left out because – all her friends – so, that's probably five or six of her closest friends are all key worker kids and went back.
>
> Zoe's mum (Year 6, Study 3)

He doesn't want to engage [with home learning] as much because I think he feels out of it.

Connor's mum (Year 6, Study 2)

Parents also raised concerns about the longer-term impact of the period of social isolation on their children's ability to make and maintain friendships and develop important social skills, with some parents feeling that their children had regressed in these areas. Prolonged isolation from friends is likely to have made re-establishing friendships upon return to school more difficult, especially for children who struggled with social relationships prior to the pandemic:

> It was very obvious, the first time he met up with people, that they were kind of like a bit, 'Aah! What do we do?'
>
> Theo's mum (Year 5, Study 3)

> She's quite preoccupied with questions like 'What am I into?' She'd make these lists. It's almost like a little mini identity crisis.
>
> Lizzy's mum (Year 3, Study 3)

Parents raised concerns that some children, particularly those with SEND or who had previously found school challenging or anxiety provoking, would find returning to school problematic. These children often experienced the school closures relatively positively, and parents reported that the children's wellbeing often improved due to having fewer stressors and demands:

> He doesn't have to go to school, he doesn't have to go and interact with people, he doesn't have to leave the house. He's having an absolute ball. I've never seen him so happy.
>
> Luke's mum (Year 1, Study 2)

Rates of school attendance following the re-opening of schools were lower for children with additional needs and/or existing mental health difficulties, and for children living in the most deprived areas [39–41]. This finding is problematic because returning to school was associated with improvements in children's mental health [42]. Our analyses of the survey responses also indicated that students from economically disadvantaged families were the least likely to attend school if they were offered the opportunity during the pandemic, potentially compounding the negative emotional and academic impacts of school closures for these students.

Parents were most satisfied with schools that did not just provide home learning materials, but also provided tailored meaningful support and signposting with respect to children's emotional, social, and physical wellbeing, and welcomed communication and collaboration with families. Parents particularly valued consistent and honest pastoral support from schools through frequent phone calls, and educational materials that were engaging, differentiated by ability, and manageable, and which came with clear expectations. These responses helped to alleviate some of the stress that parents felt about home schooling, which was particularly acute if they felt that they could not supervise their children's learning effectively because of lack of time or confidence. This was especially important for families of children with SEND. Parents also felt that a focus on children's social and emotional wellbeing should be a priority when schools reopened, with ample opportunity for children to play and re-establish social relationships:

> It's not just about the work but the connection. Just reminding people that they care about you.
> That's important.
>
> Harry's mum (Year 5, Study 3)

Belonging and Community

Our survey data show that subjective and psychological factors, as well as challenging economic and familial circumstances, play a crucial role in home learning. Parents who believed that educating children was not something for which they should be responsible were more likely to report that home learning was less manageable and more stressful, and that they felt less able and motivated to supervise their children's work [43]. Parents of children at secondary schools who felt that their children did not fit in at school also found home learning more stressful and less manageable.

Furthermore, feelings of belonging, cultural capital, and parents' beliefs that they have a role to play in their children's education were all significantly reduced among parents from lower-SES families – a finding that is often documented in the wider literature [44–46]. This finding was strongly related to children being less motivated, less engaged, and spending less time home learning. Importantly, it was also strongly related to children being less likely to use the resources that the school provided; this explained a remarkably large proportion of the variation in the responses to this question (26% and 45% for primary and secondary students, respectively). This has significant consequences for the

government's catch-up plans, which we elaborate on later in this chapter.

Our brief review of the evidence strongly suggests that shifting the onus of education away from schools and onto families has a greater negative impact on students from lower-SES backgrounds, and will almost inevitably increase socioeconomic inequalities in educational and socioemotional outcomes [2,46].

Longer-Term Impacts

There was variation in the way that schools adapted to the new demands of remote learning as the pandemic progressed. Often adaptation was facilitated by providing training for staff and investing in IT infrastructure. Yet the variations in home learning experiences that were particularly prominent in the early phases of the school closures are likely to lead to increases in inequalities in educational outcomes, thereby compounding existing inequalities.

The increase in inequalities caused by the pandemic is likely to be long-lasting, for several reasons. The pandemic is likely to have ignited a longer-term increase in digital educational provision, which is likely to further disadvantage lower-SES students by morphing the existing digital divide into inequalities in educational outcomes [2]. Our own data are consistent with other research that suggests that providing additional resources aimed at assisting students, especially poorer students, to catch up on their learning losses are likely to be used least by those children who are most in need of this support [47–49]. Worryingly, teachers have been found to have unconscious and unintentional biases that reinforce existing social class inequalities [50,51]. If teachers' reports formed the basis for assessment during the pandemic, as happened in England, lower-SES students might be disadvantaged further.

Although there is understandable concern about the impact of school closures on children's education, the parents in our interview studies felt overwhelmingly that schools should prioritise children's wellbeing and social interaction before addressing academic catch-up. Indeed, the decisions made by some schools to prioritise pastoral support over educational provision were highly valued by parents. By contrast, lack of contact from schools was seen as an important safeguarding concern:

> They [the school] have been signposting, checking in. They've been phoning weekly as well to check that we're

OK and she's alright . . . there's been an awful lot of good going on.

Bella's mum (Year 4, Study 2)

It seems to me that after a month of being in lockdown . . . they don't know who their vulnerable children are anymore.

Ada's mum (Year 5, Study 3)

It will take time for the full impact of school closures – enforced by the pandemic – on children's educational attainment and socioemotional development to become clear, although it seems likely that an entire cohort of children and young people may be disadvantaged, with possible lifelong consequences for children's wellbeing, educational, and occupational outcomes. The loss of learning and the subsequent impact on attainment may lead to an increased risk of chronic underachievement, with consequences throughout their lifespan [52]. Likewise, poor emotional health in childhood is linked to long-term mental and physical health problems and poor academic and occupational outcomes, and emotional health in childhood is the top predictor of adult life satisfaction [53–58]. Of notable concern is research which shows that the mental health of some children, including those with SEND and from more disadvantaged households, has not bounced back as restrictions have eased [21]. If inequalities are not to widen further, it will be especially important that the support needs of these children and their families are met.

Implications for Intervention and Recommendations

Informed by our findings, we make the following recommendations. These should be considered both in planning for future periods of school closures that may necessitate extended periods of home learning, and in any policy or practice that is designed to counteract the detrimental effects of school closures on children's educational attainment and social and emotional wellbeing.

Digital Support

Many schools, especially state schools, initially struggled to respond to the challenge of offering remote digital learning, due to a lack of technological infrastructure and staff expertise. Likewise, many students, particularly those from disadvantaged families, struggled to access and engage with digital educational resources.

As far as possible, education should continue to be face to face, especially for students from lower-SES families, who are more likely to lack the necessary technology to fully engage with remote learning. However, when education must be conducted digitally, schools must ensure that provision is accessible to all by not making it dependent on, for example, availability of high-speed internet or specialist equipment. Schemes that aim to provide students with the necessary IT equipment must be planned and distributed efficiently. Although some schemes were in place during the pandemic, they were often inadequate or were reliant on educational skills that students had not yet developed [59,60]. Successful schemes ensured that all students had access to sufficient IT to learn remotely. Inequalities will increase if students' access to such schemes is limited. Over the longer term, the digital divide must be tackled to avoid similar lockdowns leading to further increases in inequalities in educational outcomes.

If remote digital provisions are necessary, teachers require training and support to feel competent and confident in creating and delivering remote learning. They need to be aware of the available options (e.g., software packages, outsourced content), to identify those resources that are most engaging, and to navigate potential safeguarding problems.

Learning Bubbles

Parents in lower-SES families reported that they often found supervising schoolwork difficult because their home environments were less conducive to learning. A pressing concern among parents was the lack of social interaction for children, which led to feelings of isolation that were harmful to children's socioemotional development and wellbeing.

In order to combat these effects, families of children of similar ages could be placed in learning bubbles, which share supervising responsibilities, pool resources such as laptops, and facilitate group-based social and emotional support. Whenever possible, schools should offer isolated and secure rooms with sufficient internet capacity for bubbles that do not have access to adequate learning environments. Parents need training and support to effectively supervise their children's schoolwork, which teachers could offer to bubbles rather than to individual parents, thereby increasing the efficiency of training. Offering this training before there are any further closures may help both to increase the sense of school community and to enable a rapid response to any future school closures. As far as possible this should be done in person rather than digitally, to avoid any consequences of the digital divide. Bubbles would also help to increase the social and emotional support that families are able to offer each other, and reduce isolation.

Home Learning Curriculum

The delivery and quality of educational resources were strongly related to children's home learning experiences, but varied dramatically across schools. Clear and realistic baseline standards for remote learning provision should be put in place, which give schools appropriate levels of autonomy to deliver a creative curriculum and work responsively to adapt to the specific needs of their students. Baseline expectations for home learning should include regular 'live' contact between children and their teachers, opportunities that encourage play and peer-to-peer interaction, and engaging materials that are differentiated for children of varied abilities and needs.

Balancing Socioemotional Needs, Pastoral Support, and Academic Catch-Up

In the aftermath of the pandemic and any future closures, schools should be given guidance and resources to enable them to focus on children's social interaction, play, physical activity, and mental health. Many children are likely to be anxious about returning to school, and will need support to integrate socially. Play, social interaction, and fostering a sense of belonging will be essential to support these students' wellbeing, socioemotional development, and learning. Fostering a sense of community and belonging, and of caring and support, is likely to be essential to re-engage students with their education. Without these interventions, educational resources and catch-up materials are likely to be less effective.

It is likely that any plans designed to enable children to catch up that involve longer school days, additional teaching, or supplementary resources will be under-utilised by students from families that feel excluded from or unfamiliar with the school system –

precisely those students whose education and socio-emotional wellbeing are likely to be most disrupted by the pandemic. Interventions to mitigate the worst short- and long-term effects of the pandemic on students' education will, in our view, need to first engage the most disadvantaged and alienated students and families with their schools to foster a sense of connection and belonging. Only then are additional resources likely to be utilised and thus be effective. As Harry's mother mentioned in an interview, schools needed to remind people that 'they care about you'.

Schools should consider developing a school closure communication plan that promotes belonging to the school community and continues to foster this sense of community. This should include consistent, regular, and bidirectional communication with families that incorporates pastoral support. The role of schools may have to change in order to re-engage students and families.

Conclusion

Although school closures ordered as a result of the COVID-19 pandemic posed challenges for schools and families across the UK, the impact on disadvantaged children has been particularly severe, exacerbating existing gaps in educational, social, and emotional outcomes. We hope that the results outlined in this chapter will provide insight for schools and policy-makers into the home-learning experiences of families, guide efforts to reduce any educational, social, and emotional impacts on children, and help them to prepare for and minimise the detrimental consequences of any future period of extended school closures.

Acknowledgements

The first study was funded through awards by the European Association of Social Psychology, the University of Sussex's Higher Education Innovation Fund, and the Economic and Social Research Council's Impact Acceleration Account Fast Track Engagement Fund. The second study was funded by a research consultancy payment awarded to A. Lacey from Birmingham City Council. The third study was funded by a grant from the Higher Education Innovation Fund, University of Sussex, to K. Lester. The authors report no conflicts of interest.

References

1. Azevedo JP, Hasan A, Goldemberg D, Iqbal SA, Geven K. *Simulating the Potential Impacts of COVID-19 School Closures on Schooling and Learning Outcomes: A Set of Global Estimates.* Policy Research Working Paper No. 9284. World Bank, 2020.

2. Goudeau S, Sanrey C, Stanczak A, Manstead A, Darnon C. Why lockdown and distance learning during the COVID-19 pandemic are likely to increase the social class achievement gap. *Nat Hum Behav* 2021; 5: 1273–81.

3. Easterbrook MJ, Harris PR, Phalet K, Lisiecka Z, Kosakowska-Berezecka N. *Will COVID-19 Increase Educational Inequalities?* European Association for Social Psychology Rapid Response Funding, 2020.

4. Lacey A. *Family Adjustment During COVID-19 Epidemic: Impact on Children with Special Needs and their Families in Birmingham.* 2020. Available from: https://doi.org/10.31234/osf.io/ex5np.s

5. Lacey A, Banerjee RA, Docklova L, Lester KJ. 'I miss the normalness': mother and child perspectives of well-being and effective remote support from primary schools during COVID-19 school closures. *BMC Psychol* 2023 [manuscript pre-publication].

6. Bayrakdar S, Guveli A. *Inequalities in Home Learning and Schools' Provision of Distance Teaching During School Closure of COVID-19 Lockdown in the UK.* Institute for Social and Economic Research, University of Essex, 2020 (www.econstor.eu/bitstream/10419/227790/1/1703719352.pdf).

7. Dorn E, Hancock B, Sarakatsannis J, Viruleg E. *COVID-19 and Student Learning in the United States: The Hurt Could Last a Lifetime.* McKinsey & Company, 2020.

8. Education Endowment Foundation. *Impact of School Closures on the Attainment Gap: Rapid Evidence Assessment.* Education Endowment Foundation, 2020 (educationendowmentfoundation.org.uk/covid-19-resources/best-evidence-on-impact-of-school-closures-on-the-attainment-gap/).

9. Blainey K, Hannay T. *The Impact of School Closures on Autumn 2020 Attainment.* RS Assessment, 2021 (www.risingstars-uk.com/media/Rising-Stars/Assessment/RS_Assessment_white_paper_2021_impact_of_school_closures_on_autumn_2020_attainment.pdf).

10. Renaissance Learning Education Policy Institute. *Understanding Progress in the 2020/21 Academic Year.* Department for Education, 2021 (https://assets.publishing.service.gov.uk/government/uploads/system/uploads/attachment_data/file/962330/Learning_Loss_Report_1A_-_FINAL.pdf).

11. Rose S, Twist L, Lord P, Rutt S, Badr K, Hope C, et al. *Impact of School Closures and Subsequent Support Strategies on Attainment and Socio-Emotional Wellbeing in Key Stage 1: Interim Paper 1.* Education Endowment Foundation, National Foundation for Educational Research, 2021 (https://educationendowmentfoundation.org.uk/public/files/Publications/Covid-19_Resources/Impact_of_school_closures_KS1_interim_findings_paper_-_Jan_2021.pdf).

12. Domingue B, Hough HJ, Lang D, Yeatman J. *Changing Patterns of Growth in Oral Reading Fluency During the COVID-19 Pandemic.* Policy Analysis for California Education (PACE), 2021 (https://edpolicyinca.org/publications/changing-patterns-growth-oralreading-fluency-during-covid-19-pandemic).

13. Engzell P, Frey A, Verhagen MD. Learning loss due to school closures during the COVID-19 pandemic. *Proc Natl Acad Sci USA* 2021; 118: e2022376118.

14. Maldonado JE, De Witte K. *The Effect of School Closures on Standardized Student Test Outcomes.* KU Leuven, Faculty of Economics and Business, 2020 (https://limo.libis.be/primo-explore/fulldisplay?docid=LIRIAS3189074&context=L&vid=Lirias&search_scope=Lirias&tab=defaulttab&lang=en_US).

15. Cameron L, Tenenbaum HR. Lessons from developmental science to mitigate the effects of the COVID-19 restrictions on social development. *Group Proc Intergroup Relations* 2021; 24: 231–6.

16. Department for Education. *State of the Nation 2020: Children and Young People's Wellbeing.* Department for Education, 2020 (www.gov.uk/government/publications/state-of-the-nation-2020-children-and-young-peoples-wellbeing).

17. Ellis WE, Dumas TM, Forbes LM. Physically isolated but socially connected: psychological adjustment and stress among adolescents during the initial COVID-19 crisis. *Can J Behav Sci* 2020; 52: 177–87.

18. NHS Digital. *Mental Health of Children and Young People in England, 2020: Wave 1 Follow Up to the 2017 Survey.* NHS Digital, 2020 (https://digital.nhs.uk/data-and-information/publications/statistical/mental-health-of-children-and-young-people-in-england/2020-wave-1-follow-up#resources).

19. Asbury K, Fox L, Deniz E, Code A, Toseeb U. How is COVID-19 affecting the mental health of children with special educational

needs and disabilities and their families? *J Autism Dev Disord* 2021; 51: 1772–80.

20. Creswell C, Shum A, Pearcey S, Skripkauskaite S, Patalay P, Waite P. Young people's mental health during the COVID-19 pandemic. *Lancet Child Adolesc Health* 2021; 5: 535–7.

21. Pearcey S, Raw J, Shum A, Waite P, Creswell C. *Report 07: Changes in Parents' Mental Health Symptoms and Stressors from April to December 2020*. Co-SPACE, 2021 (https://cospaceoxford.org/ findings/changes-in-parents-mental-health-symptoms-and-stressors-jan-2021/).

22. Shum A, Skripkauskaite S, Pearcey S, Waite P, Creswell C. *Report 09: Update on Children's and Parents'/Carers' Mental Health. Changes in Parents'/ Carers' Ability to Balance Childcare and Work: March 2020 to February 2021*. Co-SPACE, 2021 (https://cospaceoxford.org/ findings/changes-in-parents-carers-ability-to-balance-childcare-and-work-march-2020-to-february-2021/).

23. Andrew A, Cattan S, Costa Dias M, Farquharson C, Kraftman L, Krutikova S, et al. Inequalities in children's experiences of home learning during the COVID-19 lockdown in England. *Fisc Stud* 2020; 41: 653–83.

24. Cullinane C, Montacute R. *Research Brief: April 2020: COVID-19 and Social Mobility Impact Brief# 1: School Shutdown*. The Sutton Trust, 2020 (www .suttontrust.com/our-research/ covid-19-and-social-mobility-impact-brief/).

25. Julius J, Sims D. *Schools' Responses to COVID-19: Support for Vulnerable Pupils and the Children of Keyworkers*. National Foundation for Educational Research, 2020 (www.nfer.ac.uk/ schools-responses-to-covid-19-support-for-vulnerable-pupils-and-the-children-of-keyworkers/).

26. Borman G. *What Can Be Done to Address Learning Losses due to School Closures?* The Answer Lab, Center on Education Policy, Equity and Governance, 2020 (https://theanswerlab.rossier.usc .edu/wp-content/uploads/2020/ 06/Answer-Lab-COVID-19-Slide-202006-Final-1.pdf).

27. Reimers FM, Schleicher A. *A Framework to Guide an Educational Response to the COVID-19 Pandemic of 2020*. Organisation for Economic Cooperation and Development, 2020 (https://oecd.dam-broadcast .com/pm_7379_126_126988-t63lxosohs.pdf).

28. Children's Commissioner for Wales. *Coronavirus and Me*. Children's Commissioner for Wales, 2021 (www.childcomwales .org.uk/coronavirus-our-work/ coronavirus-and-me-results/).

29. Easterbrook MJ, Doyle L, Grozev VH, Kosakowska-Berezecka N, Harris PR, Phalet K. Socioeconomic and gender inequalities in home learning during the COVID-19 pandemic: examining the roles of the home environment, parent supervision, and educational provisions. *Educ Dev Psychol* 2023; 40: 27–39.

30. Parnham JC, Laverty AA, Majeed A, Vamos EP. Half of children entitled to free school meals did not have access to the scheme during COVID-19 lockdown in the UK. *Public Health* 2020; 187: 161–4.

31. Castro M, Expósito-Casas E, López-Martín E, Lizasoain L, Navarro-Asencio E, Gaviria JL. Parental involvement on student academic achievement: a meta-analysis. *Educ Res Rev* 2015; 14: 33–46.

32. Desforges C, Abouchaar A. *The Impact of Parental Involvement, Parental Support and Family Education on Pupil Achievement and Adjustment: A Literature Review*. Department for Education and Skills, 2003 (https://dera.ioe.ac.uk/6305/).

33. Guterman O, Neuman A. Personality, socio-economic status and education: factors that contribute to the degree of structure in homeschooling. *Soc Psychol Educ* 2018; 21: 75–90.

34. Children's Commissioner for England. *School Attendance Since September: Briefing*. Children's Commissioner for England, 2020 (www.childrenscommissioner.gov .uk/wp-content/uploads/2020/12/ cco-briefing-on-school-attendance-since-september.pdf).

35. Hill NE, Taylor LC. Parental school involvement and children's academic achievement: pragmatics and issues. *Curr Dir Psychol Sci* 2004; 13: 161–4.

36. Davis CR, Grooms J, Ortega A, Rubalcaba JA-A, Vargas E. Distance learning and parental mental health during COVID-19. *Educ Res* 2021; 50: 61–4.

37. Cameron L, Tenenbaum HR. Lessons from developmental science to mitigate the effects of the COVID-19 restrictions on social development. *Group Proc Intergroup Relations* 2021; 24: 231–6.

38. Loades ME, Chatburn E, Higson-Sweeney N, Reynolds S, Shafran R, Brigden A, et al. Rapid systematic review: the impact of social isolation and loneliness on the mental health of children and adolescents in the context of COVID-19. *J Am Acad Child Adolesc Psychiatry* 2020; 59: 1218–39.e3.

39. Children's Commissioner for England. *Stress Among Children in England During the Coronavirus Lockdown*. Children's Commissioner for England, 2020 (www.childrenscommission-r.gov .uk/wp-content/uploads/2020/09/ cco-stress-among-children-in-england-during-the-coronavirus-lockdown.pdf).

40. Department for Education. *Attendance in Education and Early Years Settings During the Coronavirus (COVID-19) Outbreak*. Department for Education, 2020 (https://explore-education-statistics.service.gov.uk/find-statistics/attendance-in-education-and-early-years-settings-during-the-coronavirus-covid-19-outbreak).

41. Sosu E, Klein M. *Socioeconomic Disparities in School Absenteeism After the First Wave of COVID-19 School Closures in Scotland*. University of Strathclyde, 2021.

42. Shum A, Skripkauskaite S, Pearcey S, Waite P, Creswell C. *Report 09: Update on Children's and Parents'/ Carers' Mental Health. Changes in Parents'/Carers' Ability to Balance Childcare and Work: March 2020 to February 2021*. Co-SPACE, 2021 (https://cospaceoxford.org/findings/changes-in-parents-carers-ability-to-balance-childcare-and-work-march-2020-to-february-2021/).

43. Bourdieu P. The forms of capital. In *Handbook of Theory and Research for the Sociology of Education* (ed. J Richardson): 241–58. Greenwood, 1986.

44. Aries E, Seider M. The interactive relationship between class identity and the college experience: the case of lower income students. *Qual Sociol* 2005; 28: 419–43.

45. Bufton S. The lifeworld of the university student: habitus and social class. *J Phenomenol Psychol* 2003; 34: 207–34.

46. Reay D, Crozier G, Clayton J. 'Strangers in paradise'? Working-class students in elite universities. *Sociology* 2009; 43: 1103–21.

47. Andrew A, Cattan S, Costa Dias M, Farquharson C, Kraftman L, Krutikova S, et al. Inequalities in children's experiences of home learning during the COVID-19 lockdown in England. *Fisc Stud* 2020; 41: 653–83.

48. Kim LE, Dundas S, Asbury K. 'I think it's been difficult for the ones that haven't got as many resources in their homes': teacher concerns about the impact of COVID-19 on pupil learning and wellbeing. *Teach Teaching* 2021. Available from: https://doi.org/10.1080/13540602.2021.1982690.

49. Pensiero N, Kelley T, Bokhove C. *Learning Inequalities During the COVID-19 Pandemic: How Families Cope with Home-Schooling*. Southampton Education School, University of Southampton, 2020.

50. Batruch A, Autin F, Butera F. Re-establishing the social-class order: restorative reactions against high-achieving, low-SES pupils. *J Soc Issues* 2017; 73: 42–60.

51. Doyle L, Easterbrook MJ, Harris PR. Roles of socioeconomic status, ethnicity, and teacher beliefs in academic grading. *Br J Educ Psychol* 2022; 93: 91–112.

52. Easterbrook MJ, Kuppens T, Manstead AS. The education effect: higher educational qualifications are robustly associated with beneficial personal and socio-political outcomes. *Soc Indic Res* 2016; 126: 1261–98.

53. Essau CA, Lewinsohn PM, Olaya B, Seeley JR. Anxiety disorders in adolescents and psychosocial outcomes at age 30. *J Affect Disord* 2014; 16: 125–32.

54. Maughan B, Collishaw S. Development and psychopathology: a life course perspective. In *Rutter's Child and Adolescent Psychiatry* (eds A Thapar, DS Pine, JF Leckman, S Scott, MJ Snowling, EA Taylor): 5–16. John Wiley & Sons, 2015.

55. Jaycox LH, Stein BD, Paddock S, Miles JNV, Chandra A, Meredith LS, et al. Impact of teen depression on academic, social, and physical functioning. *Pediatrics* 2009; 124: e596–605.

56. McLeod JD, Kaiser K. Childhood emotional and behavioral problems and educational attainment. *Am Sociol Rev* 2004; 69: 636–58.

57. Knapp M, King D, Healey A, Thomas C. Economic outcomes in adulthood and their associations with antisocial conduct, attention deficit and anxiety problems in childhood. *J Ment Health Policy Econ* 2011; 14: 137–47.

58. Layard R, Clark AE, Cornaglia F, Powdthavee N, Vernoit J. What predicts a successful life? A life-course model of well-being. *Econ J* 2014; 124: F720–38.

59. Parnham JC, Laverty AA, Majeed A, Vamos EP. Half of children entitled to free school meals did not have access to the scheme during COVID-19 lockdown in the UK. *Public Health* 2020; 187: 161–4.

60. Toste JR, Raley SK, Gross Toews S, Shogren KA, Coelho G. 'Eye opening and chaotic': resilience and self-determination of secondary students with disabilities amidst the COVID-19 pandemic. *J Educ Stud Placed Risk* 2021; 26: 157–83.

32 Quarantine, Lockdown, and Isolation in the COVID-19 Pandemic

Samantha K Brooks, Rebecca K Webster, Louise E Smith, Lisa Woodland, and Neil Greenberg

Introduction

The term quarantine has been widely used during the COVID-19 outbreak. Typically, it refers to separation and restriction of movement of people who have not been diagnosed with the infection, but who may have come into contact with others who are infected [1]. This differs from isolation, which is the separation of people who have been diagnosed with a contagious disease. However, the two terms are often used interchangeably, and the COVID-19 pandemic has brought new terms into the public lexicon, such as lockdown (government-enforced restrictions on movement, work, and travel), social distancing (maintaining physical distance from others), and shielding (people at high risk of becoming seriously ill if they were to catch COVID-19 staying at home and minimising their contact with others) [2].

In January 2020, when entire cities in China were effectively placed under mass quarantine, and foreign nationals returning home from China were asked to self-isolate at home or in state-run facilities, it was important to understand the potential psychological impact that quarantine might have [3]. At the time, quarantine and self-isolation had not been the focus of many academic papers. Although previous epidemics and pandemics, including severe acute respiratory syndrome (SARS), swine flu, and Ebola, had involved city-wide quarantine periods for people who had come into contact with infected persons, they were confined to a small number of areas in a small number of countries, and the quarantine periods were relatively short. However, it seemed likely that quarantine might be distressing for those involved, due to the inevitable boredom, separation from loved ones, and loss of freedom, coupled with fear of being infected. We knew from a previous review of distress in healthcare workers involved in the SARS pandemic that staff who were quarantined either at home or at work tended to have poorer psychological outcomes than those who were not quarantined [4]. In addition, reports from previous outbreaks warned of potentially alarming outcomes. For example, an outbreak of SARS in a hospital in Taiwan led to the hospital being cordoned off suddenly and without notice, trapping staff, patients, and visitors inside with no extra food, drink, or medical supplies to sustain them during the quarantine period. This reportedly led to one suicide and one attempted suicide within 4 days of confinement [5].

With an increasing number of countries making plans to quarantine people arriving from China in early 2020, it was apparent that a rapid review was urgently needed to inform policies on how best to apply this quarantine and how to reduce, as far as possible, the negative psychological impacts associated with it. We searched electronic databases for published primary research on the psychological impact of quarantine, in order to better understand what the psychological impact might be, and what factors were associated with this impact. We reviewed 24 studies on previous infectious disease outbreaks that had involved mass quarantines, and our findings are summarised in this chapter.

The Psychological Effects of Quarantine

In total, 23 out of 24 published papers reported negative psychological effects of quarantine. Distress, post-traumatic stress symptoms, frustration, confusion, and anger were common, with a small number of studies further suggesting that these outcomes might be long-lasting. Common mental disorders such as anxiety and depression were reported at significantly higher levels among quarantined people than would be expected in the general population.

Short-Term Impacts

The majority of studies took place soon after the quarantine periods ended, and therefore were only able to discuss the short-term impact on mental health. The immediate psychological responses to quarantine included acute stress [6], anger [7–9], confusion [7,8,10,11], depression [12], distress [13], emotional disturbance [14], emotional exhaustion [9], fear [7,8,11,15–18], grief [17], insomnia [6,15,16,19], irritability [6,19], low mood [19], nervousness [18], numbness [17], and post-traumatic stress symptoms [12,18,20]. A number of studies reported that the loss of usual routine and lack of contact with others led to boredom, frustration, and a sense of isolation [8,10,12,15,16,18,21–24]. Quarantined people also reported fears both about their own health and about infecting others [6,8,12,18,23], often catastrophising any physical symptoms that they happened to experience [15,22].

Studies comparing quarantined and non-quarantined people during a disease outbreak found poorer mental health among people who were quarantined. For example, in 2008 a study of horse owners in Australia who had been quarantined due to an equine influenza outbreak found that 34% of 2,760 quarantined people reported high psychological distress during the outbreak, compared with only 12% in the general Australian population [13]. A study that compared quarantined and non-quarantined parents and children during the SARS and swine flu pandemics found that the incidence of post-traumatic stress symptoms was four times higher in quarantined than in non-quarantined people [20]. In another example, having been quarantined during the SARS pandemic was found to be the strongest predictor of acute stress disorder in hospital staff [6]. Quarantined staff were also significantly more likely to report sleep problems (being exhausted, and having difficulty sleeping), negative emotional effects (feeling detached from others, feeling anxious around febrile patients, and feeling irritable), and negative cognitive effects (poor concentration, and difficulties with decision making), as well as deteriorating work performance.

These short-term psychological effects are perhaps unsurprising – it is easy to see how the loneliness, boredom, and infection fears experienced during quarantine could be potentially traumatic, and it is well established in the literature that potentially traumatic experiences can lead to increases in distress and emotional, cognitive, and behavioural problems in the short term [25]. Typically, these symptoms are likely to resolve on their own within 1 month, so psychological difficulties during the first 4 weeks after quarantine are expected to some extent, and are not necessarily a cause for concern unless they are severe.

Long-Term Impacts

In a study by Hyunsuk Jeong and colleagues, 7.6% of 1,656 quarantined participants reported anxiety symptoms and 16.6% reported feelings of anger during the quarantine period [22]. Four to six months after quarantine, many people appeared to have recovered, with 3.0% reporting ongoing anxiety, and 6.4% reporting still feeling anger. This fits with the existing literature which suggests that people who have experienced a potentially traumatic event will find that their symptoms improve on their own with time. However, several other studies found that levels of psychological distress remained high. For example, in a study by Mutsuko Mihashi and colleagues, 26.2% of 187 participants reported general symptoms of psychological distress 7 to 8 months after quarantine, whereas 39% of the participants in a study by Clete DiGiovanni and colleagues reported feelings of stress several months after quarantine had ended [16,26]. Two studies presented more concerning findings regarding long-term psychological impacts. The first study, involving hospital employees quarantined during the SARS outbreak in China, found that quarantine significantly predicted alcohol dependence and post-traumatic stress symptoms 3 years later [27]. The second study found that being quarantined significantly predicted depression and post-traumatic stress symptoms 3 years after quarantine had ended; this risk was decreased if participants demonstrated altruistic acceptance of risk during the outbreak [28].

Factors Associated with the Psychological Impact of Quarantine

Pre-Quarantine Risk Factors

One study found that negative psychological effects of quarantine were associated with younger age, lower level of education, and having one child [13]. However, another study found no association between psychological outcomes and age, level of education, having one child, marital status, or living with other adults [12]. One study found that having a history of psychiatric illness was associated with experiencing anxiety and anger 4–6 months after the end of the quarantine period [22]. Donna Reynolds and colleagues found that quarantined healthcare workers experienced more severe symptoms of post-traumatic stress disorder (PTSD) and more negative emotions than non-healthcare workers. However, Laura Hawryluck and colleagues found no association between being a healthcare worker and psychological outcomes [12,18].

Risk Factors During Quarantine

Longer duration of quarantine appeared to be associated with poorer mental health [9,12,18]. Although it was not always clear how long was a 'longer duration of quarantine'. Laura Hawryluck and colleagues reported that people quarantined for more than 10 days showed significantly more severe post-traumatic stress symptoms than did those quarantined for less than 10 days [12]. Several studies did not state the duration of their quarantine periods. However, of those that did, 21 days was the longest period.

Having inadequate supplies (e.g., food, water, medical prescriptions, clothing) and accommodation during quarantine was frustrating for people, and continued to be associated with anxiety and anger several months after the end of quarantine [21,22,24]. Supplies from public health authorities were frequently reported to be lacking, participants reported receiving masks and thermometers either late or not at all, and the distribution of food, water, and other items was often delayed or only intermittent, which could be a stressor for people waiting for supplies [8,7,11].

Having inadequate information from public health authorities was also a self-reported stressor. Participants reported a lack of clear information, lack of clear guidelines, and confusion about the purpose of quarantine [7,8,10,11,15,16,23]. Participants in one study believed that their confusion stemmed from lack of coordination between multiple jurisdictions and levels of government, which had led to differences in the style, approach, and content of public health messages [16].

Long-Term Risk Factors

Financial loss resulting from interrupted professional activities due to quarantine appeared to be a risk factor for poor mental health [11,13,22,26]. Perhaps related to this, households with a combined annual income of less than $40,000 (CAD) showed significantly higher levels of PTSD and depression; those with lower incomes were likely to be more affected by the financial impact of quarantine than those with higher incomes [12]. In addition, the financial assistance provided by the government was reported by participants to be inadequate and slow to arrive [8,15].

Another ongoing stressor, which began during quarantine and continued for some time after it, was the stigma associated with quarantine. Although not formally investigated with regard to associations with negative psychological outcomes, participants in many studies reported experiencing negative attitudes from others, including rejection, avoidance, and suspicion [6,8,11,12,15,16,18,23,24,29].

The Psychological Impact of Quarantine for COVID-19

The COVID-19 pandemic has resulted in countries across the globe locking down and quarantining their people for unprecedented lengths of time. In addition to the inevitable boredom, loneliness, and frustration associated with quarantine, many people have also been forced to deal with loss of earnings, loss of social life and hobbies, reduced access to healthcare (including mental healthcare), reduced access to childcare, closure of businesses and schools, job loss or having to adapt to working from home, and inability to travel. It is therefore unsurprising that the mental health impacts of the pandemic are a major concern.

Evidence suggests that a longer duration of quarantine, inadequate or inconsistent information from public health officials and governments, and financial struggles may be stressful and lead to decreased mental health outcomes in people affected by quarantine. This is a concern as the COVID-19 outbreak has, at the time of publication of this book, seen many countries where, during the pandemic, periods of quarantine and lockdown were repeated, governments were criticised for providing insufficient information and imposing constantly changing guidelines without providing a clear rationale, and a great number of people lost their jobs or were unable to work.

Many studies have already been conducted on the psychological impacts of quarantine during the COVID-19 pandemic, and have reported similar results to our rapid review. Mental health outcomes such as anxiety, depression, distress, and suicidal ideation appear to be more prevalent in quarantine-affected people than in those not affected, and they are higher than pre-quarantine levels [30–33]. These mental health impacts are associated with many of the same risk factors that we have previously identified. Lower household income, poor perceived health status, lower perceived control, perceived lack of personal/government support, having older/ageing parents, pre-existing mental or physical health disorders, being a frontline worker, and greater worries about being infected were associated with more negative psychological impacts.

Daisy Fancourt and her colleagues studied the trajectories of anxiety and depression over the 20 weeks after the announcement of lockdown in England, and found similar results to the quarantine data [34]. The highest levels of depression and anxiety occurred in the early stages of the lockdown, and risk factors included female gender, younger age, lower level of education, having pre-existing mental health conditions, and living alone or with children. Interestingly, anxiety and depression levels did decline fairly rapidly, possibly due to people adapting to the circumstances, and to the gradual easing of measures over the 20-week period. However, some of these inequalities in experiences were still evident, with emotionally vulnerable groups, such as people who had pre-existing mental health conditions or those who were living alone, remaining at risk throughout lockdown and its aftermath.

Not only is the psychological impact of quarantine a cause for concern in itself with regard to the mental health and wellbeing of the public, but also the perceived negative impact of restrictions on people's mental health was associated with reduced adherence to lockdown restrictions [35]. This suggests that people's perceptions about the detrimental impact of restrictions on their own mental health may have further negative effects on public health by increasing the spread of the virus. Therefore the benefits of potential interventions to reduce the psychological impact of quarantine are twofold.

Implications for Intervention

When we published our review in early 2020, we recommended minimising the duration of quarantine if possible. However, lifting quarantine too early could lead to a rise in infections and further waves of infection, resulting in longer quarantine restrictions. This was seen throughout the world in 2020. It is important that governments that impose quarantine rules are advised by scientists who have undertaken modelling to estimate how introducing and removing restrictions may affect levels of infection. Although lockdown measures, which allow some

freedom (e.g., leaving home to exercise), are less strict than quarantine, inequalities in mental health have persisted, so it is key to find ways to support vulnerable groups of people in situations in which quarantine or lockdown measures may be needed [34].

People affected by quarantine need increased access to mental health services to manage the increase in psychological problems. These services should include evidence-based psychological interventions to support people in developing and maintaining coping mechanisms, to enhance people's sense of self-control to better manage the adverse effects of quarantine or lockdown [30]. However, pandemic restrictions have resulted in reduced access to mental health services. Psychological first aid workers could help by identifying high-risk groups and by providing information about the quarantine procedure, positive coping strategies, and self-guided interventions (e.g., mindfulness, acceptance-based interventions) [31,36].

A clear rationale for the need for restrictions may also help to reduce the negative psychological impact of quarantine. The public need to be clear about what the COVID-19 risk means, understand why they are being quarantined, and be provided with clear, accurate, and easily accessible information on how best to prevent the spread of infectious diseases. This can be hampered by a lack of coordination between different public health authorities, jurisdictions, and governments. It would be better to have a single knowledgeable spokesperson if possible. Evidence from research on chemical emergencies, for example, suggests that the person or organisation delivering the public health message is as important as the message itself, and that information is perceived as trustworthy if it comes from a spokesperson with a level of authority, who is seen as representative of the people affected [37]. Ideally this person should be involved on the frontlines and be connected to the affected communities [16].

Boredom and isolation contribute to distress. It would be helpful to provide quarantined people with suggestions about reducing boredom. For example, engaging in an existing hobby or taking up new ones may be helpful, particularly if this allows people to feel that they have achieved something or done something useful with their day [36]. Feeling connected to others is also likely to be important. The use of technology to keep in contact with social networks is important; phone calls, video chats, and text messaging may help people to feel connected. Thus social support from community groups may also help to reduce the negative impact of quarantine on psychological health.

Adequate supplies (e.g., food, water, medical supplies) are also imperative, so that people have the capability to quarantine. Studies conducted during the pandemic suggest that financial support is also important. Improved financial support for people who are quarantining may help to ease the distress that quarantine may cause in terms of lost income from not being able to work, and can serve to decrease negative psychological impacts and improve adherence to quarantine measures.

Conclusion

Being quarantined can have a substantial and potentially long-lasting negative psychological impact, and public health officials and governments have a duty of care to ensure that the experience is as tolerable as possible. If quarantine is necessary, restrictions should be designed to minimise psychological distress and reduce the likelihood of longer-term disorders. Helpful actions include ensuring that quarantine lasts for no longer than necessary, providing a timely clear rationale for quarantine and how long it will continue for, providing clear guidelines, advising on meaningful activities to engage in during quarantine, and ensuring that everyone has access to sufficient food, water, medical supplies, and mental health support. Providing clear and accurate information for the public is arguably most important of all, and should be central to all efforts when planning quarantine.

References

1. Centers for Disease Control and Prevention. *Quarantine and Isolation*. Centers for Disease Control and Prevention, 2017 (www.cdc.gov/quarantine/index .html).

2. Manuell M-E, Cukor J. Mother Nature versus human nature: public compliance with evacuation and quarantine. *Disasters* 2011: 35: 417–42.

3. Brooks SK, Webster RK, Smith LE, Woodland L, Wessely S, Greenberg N, et al. The psychological impact of quarantine and how to reduce it: rapid review of the evidence. *Lancet* 2020: 395: 912–20.

4. Brooks SK, Dunn R, Amlôt R, Rubin GJ, Greenberg N. A systematic, thematic review of social and occupational factors associated with psychological outcomes in healthcare employees during an infectious disease outbreak. *J Occup Environ Med* 2018; 60: 248–57.

5. Barbisch D, Koenig KL, Shih F-Y. Is there a case for quarantine? Perspectives from SARS to Ebola. *Disaster Med Public Health Prep* 2015; 9: 547–53.

6. Bai Y, Lin C-C, Lin C-Y, Chen J-Y, Chue C-M, Chou P. Survey of stress reactions among health care workers involved with the SARS outbreak. *Psychiatr Serv* 2004; 55: 1055–7.

7. Caleo G, Duncombe J, Jephcott F, Lokuge K, Mills C, Looijen E, et al. The factors affecting household transmission dynamics and community compliance with Ebola control measures: a mixed-methods study in a rural village in Sierra Leone. *BMC Public Health* 2018; 18: 248.

8. Cava MA, Fay KE, Beanlands HJ, McCay EA, Wignall R. The experience of quarantine for individuals affected by SARS in Toronto. *Public Health Nurs* 2005; 22: 398–406.

9. Marjanovic Z, Greenglass ER, Coffey S. The relevance of psychosocial variables and working conditions in predicting nurses' coping strategies during the SARS crisis: an online questionnaire survey. *Int J Nurs Stud* 2007; 44: 991–8.

10. Braunack-Mayer A, Tooher R, Collins JE, Street JM, Marshall H. Understanding the school community's response to school closures during the H1N1 2009 influenza pandemic. *BMC Public Health* 2013; 13: 344.

11. Pellecchia U, Crestani R, Decroo T, Van den Bergh R, Al-Kourdi Y. Social consequences of Ebola containment measures in Liberia. *PLoS One* 2015; 10: e0143036.

12. Hawryluck L, Gold WL, Robinson S, Pogorski S, Galea S, Styra R. SARS control and psychological effects of quarantine, Toronto, Canada. *Emerg Infect Dis* 2004; 10: 1206–12.

13. Taylor MR, Agho KE, Stevens GJ, Raphael B. Factors influencing psychological distress during a disease epidemic: data from Australia's first outbreak of equine influenza. *BMC Public Health* 2008; 8: 347.

14. Yoon MK, Kim SY, Ko HS, Lee MS. System effectiveness of detection, brief intervention and refer to treatment for the people with post-traumatic emotional distress by MERS: a case report of community-based proactive intervention in South Korea. *Int J Ment Health Syst* 2016; 10: 51.

15. Desclaux A, Badji D, Ndione AG, Sow K. Accepted monitoring or endured quarantine? Ebola contacts' perceptions in Senegal. *Soc Sci Med* 2017; 178: 38–45.

16. DiGiovanni C, Conley J, Chiu D, Zaborski J. Factors influencing compliance with quarantine in

Toronto during the 2003 SARS outbreak. *Biosecur Bioterror* 2004; 2: 265–72.

17. Pan PJD, Chang S-H, Yu Y-Y. A support group for home-quarantined college students exposed to SARS: learning from practice. *J Spec Group Work* 2005; 30: 363–74.

18. Reynolds DL, Garay JR, Deamond SL, Moran MK, Gold W, Styra R. Understanding, compliance and psychological impact of the SARS quarantine experience. *Epidemiol Infect* 2008; 136: 997–1007.

19. Lee S, Chan LY, Chau AM, Kwok KP, Kleinman A. The experience of SARS-related stigma at Amoy Gardens. *Soc Sci Med* 2005; 61: 2038–46.

20. Sprang G, Silman M. Posttraumatic stress disorder in parents and youth after health-related disasters. *Disaster Med Public Health Prep* 2013; 7: 105–10.

21. Blendon RJ, Benson JM, DesRoches CM, Raleigh E, Taylor-Clark K. The public's response to severe acute respiratory syndrome in Toronto and the United States. *Clin Infect Dis* 2004; 38: 925–31.

22. Jeong H, Yim HW, Song Y-J, Ki M, Min J-A, Cho J, et al. Mental health status of people isolated due to Middle East Respiratory Syndrome. *Epidemiol Health* 2016; 38: e2016048.

23. Robertson E, Hershenfield K, Grace SL, Stewart DE. The psychosocial effects of being quarantined following exposure to SARS: a qualitative study of Toronto health care workers. *Can J Psychiatry* 2004; 49: 403–7.

24. Wilken JA, Pordell P, Goode B, Jarteh R, Miller Z, Saygar BG, et al. Knowledge, attitudes, and practices among members of households actively monitored or quarantined to prevent transmission of Ebola virus disease – Margibi County, Liberia: February–March 2015. *Prehosp Disaster Med* 2017; 32: 673–8.

25. Center for Substance Abuse Treatment (US). Understanding the impact of trauma. In *Trauma-Informed Care in Behavioral Health Services*. Substance Abuse and Mental Health Services Administration (US), 2014.

26. Mihashi M, Otsubo Y, Yinjuan X, Nagatomi K, Hoshiko M, Ishitake T. Predictive factors of psychological disorder development during recovery following SARS outbreak. *Health Psychol* 2009; 28: 91–100.

27. Wu P, Liu X, Fang Y, Fan B, Fuller CJ, Guan Z, et al. Alcohol abuse/dependence symptoms among hospital employees exposed to a SARS outbreak. *Alcohol Alcoholism* 2008; 43: 706–12.

28. Liu X, Kakade M, Fuller CJ, Fan B, Fang Y, Kong J, et al. Depression after exposure to stressful events: lessons learned from the severe acute respiratory syndrome epidemic. *Compr Psychiatry* 2012; 53: 15–23.

29. Wester M, Giesecke J. Ebola and healthcare worker stigma. *Scand J Public Health* 2019; 47: 99–104.

30. Burke T, Berry A, Taylor LK, Stafford O, Murphy E, Shevlin M, et al. Increased psychological distress during COVID-19 and quarantine in Ireland: a national survey. *J Clin Med* 2020; 9: 3481.

31. Gan Y, Ma J, Wu J, Chen Y, Zhu H, Hall BJ. Immediate and delayed psychological effects of province-wide lockdown and personal quarantine during the COVID-19 outbreak in China. *Psychol Med* 2022; 52: 1321–32.

32. Lei L, Huang X, Zhang S, Yang J, Yang L, Xu M. Comparison of prevalence and associated factors of anxiety and depression among people affected by versus people unaffected by quarantine during the COVID-19 epidemic in Southwestern China. *Med Sci Monit* 2020; 26: e924609.

33. Xin M, Luo S, She R, Yu Y, Li L, Wang S, et al. Negative cognitive and psychological correlates of mandatory quarantine during the initial COVID-19 outbreak in China. *Am Psychol* 2020; 75: 607–17.

34. Fancourt D, Steptoe A, Bu F. Trajectories of anxiety and depressive symptoms during enforced isolation due to COVID-19 in England: a longitudinal observational study. *Lancet Psychiatry* 2021; 8: 141–9.

35. Smith LE, Amlôt R, Lambert H, Oliver I, Yardley L, Rubin GJ. Factors associated with adherence to self-isolation and lockdown measures in the UK: a cross-sectional survey. *Public Health* 2020; 187: 41–52.

36. Fischer R, Bortolini T, Karl JA, Zilberberg M, Robinson K, Rabelo A, et al. Rapid review and meta-meta-analysis of self-guided interventions to address anxiety, depression, and stress during COVID-19 social distancing. *Front Psychol* 2020; 11: 2795.

37. Carter H, Amlôt R. Mass casualty decontamination guidance and psychosocial aspects of CBRN incident management: a review and synthesis. *PLoS Curr* 2016; 8. Available from: https://doi.org/10.1371/currents.dis.c2d3d652d9d07a2a620ed5429e017ef5

Chapter 33

Reflections on Managing Infectious Diseases in Mental Health Units

Sarah Moslehi, Dominic Aubrey-Jones, Golnar Aref-Adib, and Janet Obeney-Williams

Introduction

On 11 March 2020, when the outbreak of COVID-19 was declared a global pandemic by the World Health Organization (WHO), the senior management at our central London mental health trust designated the acute psychiatric assessment ward as the COVID-19 isolation ward to prevent spread through the other wards. This was necessary due to the challenge for some mentally unwell patients of self-isolating in their rooms, posing a risk to other patients and staff. This chapter describes the challenges faced in providing inpatient mental healthcare during a pandemic.

General Principles That Emerge from the Science

We start with a brief summary of what we knew about COVID-19 and therefore the factors we took into account in our response to the pandemic within our inpatient mental health service.

It is well known that the symptoms and signs of COVID-19 infection may vary from mild to severe illness. One of the reasons why COVID-19 was transmitted so rapidly and caused a pandemic may be attributed to the fact that a high number of infected people remained asymptomatic, and were therefore more likely to transmit the infection to others. One study showed that 59% of COVID-19-positive people did not develop any symptoms [1]. Asymptomatic people with COVID-19 accounted for over 50% of all the viral transmissions. Therefore social distancing and wearing aprons, masks, and gloves were necessary in various settings in order to stop further spread of the virus.

The route of transmission of COVID-19 is via the respiratory tract. Therefore the wearing of masks and maintaining physical distance between people (generally referred to as social distancing) are two of the main methods of reducing the transmission of infectious respiratory particles. However, in a hospital setting, healthcare professionals are in regular contact with people who are known to have or suspected of having COVID-19, and it is often necessary for them to perform procedures within arm's reach of these patients. As a result, it is often not possible to maintain social distancing, which makes the wearing of personal protective equipment (PPE) essential in hospital settings. The wearing of eye protection is believed to provide an additional layer of protection [2].

The Short-, Medium-, and Long-Term Impacts

One of the ways to stop the spread of the virus is to require infected people to self-isolate. Self-isolation can take place on a medical ward, at home, or in a psychiatric ward, depending on the severity of the person's symptoms and other comorbid illnesses (e.g., acute psychiatric relapse). Isolation from other people is likely to have a negative impact on anyone's mental health, but for people who have pre-existing mental health conditions, self-isolation due to the COVID-19 infection may worsen pre-existing mental illness.

It is also possible for some people to develop mental health problems after the pandemic. A study has shown that those who completed a 9-day quarantine were more likely to develop an acute stress disorder compared with a control group. In addition, the quarantined people reported insomnia, anxiety, irritability, poor concentration, and indecisiveness. Those who completed a period of self-isolation after encountering potentially infected people reported experiencing fear, nervousness, sadness, and guilt [3].

Hospital employees who had been self-isolating were also more likely to develop post-traumatic stress symptoms even after a long period of time. As noted in Chapter 32, a study conducted during the equine influenza outbreak in Australia showed that people who had quarantined for several weeks had a 34% risk of developing psychological problems, compared with a 12% risk for the general population [4]. Healthcare professionals who have completed self-isolation may also develop more severe depressive symptoms. In one study, 60% of those who had severe depressive symptoms had quarantined, compared with 15% of those with mild depressive symptoms [5].

Healthcare professionals who had completed a period of quarantine during the SARS outbreak in 2003 showed long-term impacts 3 years afterwards. Alcohol abuse and dependency symptoms were found to be remarkably associated with self-isolation. Compared with the general public, healthcare professionals who had quarantined developed more severe post-traumatic stress symptoms and experienced greater stigma. Other commonly reported adverse outcomes for healthcare professionals included greater feelings of anger, annoyance, fear and frustration, helplessness, loneliness, and unhappiness. They were also more worried about the possibility of infecting others [3].

Pre-isolation factors may also predict the psychological impacts of quarantine. Negative predictive outcomes were linked with female gender, lower educational level qualifications, younger age, and having one child compared with having no children [4]. A medium-term effect of the pandemic on people who had pre-existing psychiatric problems was the experience of feelings of anxiety and anger which developed 3–4 months after the end of quarantine [6].

The duration of quarantine for people who self-isolate due to a confirmed or suspected infection was strongly associated with negative psychological outcomes after 10 days. This indicates that longer than necessary isolation periods result in poorer psychological outcomes [7]. Quarantine, by its very nature, results in reduced contact with others, and many people experience boredom and isolation from society, which results in frustration and distress [8].

There are steps that can be taken to reduce feelings of loneliness and isolation when quarantining during the COVID-19 pandemic. One approach is to use video calls to facilitate staying in touch with loved ones [9]. Video calls can also be used to facilitate professional meetings where multiple agencies are involved in caring for patients.

The Implications for Intervention

SARS-CoV-2 is now understood to be transmitted via the respiratory route [10]. Early in the pandemic,

however, the hypothesis was that SARS-CoV-2 was spread both by droplets and by fomites. The government guidance reflected this, requiring people with symptoms consistent with COVID-19 or a positive test result to isolate at home for 7 days, advice which was later amended to 10 days [11]. Implementing similar principles on psychiatric wards presented unique challenges. First, the transient nature of the population of each ward, because of regular admissions and discharges, provided a setting in which infectious diseases could spread rapidly. Second, mental illness has an impact on patients' ability to isolate. Third, isolation has an impact on patients' mental health – something that people without pre-existing mental illness have struggled with throughout the pandemic [12].

When transforming our ward from a mental health assessment ward to a COVID-19 isolation ward, it was acknowledged by the senior managers of our trust that this setting would not be suitable for all patients with suspected or confirmed COVID-19. They decided that patients who were exhibiting highly agitated and aggressive behaviour, who would normally be best managed on a psychiatric intensive care unit (PICU), would continue to be treated in the appropriate setting. Similarly, patients of advanced age or with significant frailty continued to be treated on a ward for older adults.

In the early days of the repurposing of the ward, polymerase chain reaction (PCR) testing was not available for our patients, so patient transfers were based purely on symptoms known to be consistent with COVID-19 at the time, namely persistent dry cough or fever. Patients were required to isolate in their rooms for 7 days from the onset of symptoms before either being stepped back down to a treatment ward or being discharged home. Later, with increased capacity for laboratories to process nasopharyngeal swabs using PCR, we taught staff on the other wards how to perform nasopharyngeal swabbing. A mass-testing programme across the unit was subsequently rolled out so that any patient in the unit who developed symptoms consistent with COVID-19 could be tested. This allowed them to isolate on their respective wards while the results were pending, and any patients who tested positive were then moved to the most appropriate care setting for them, depending on their mental state and frailty score. It was thus possible to prevent patients who tested negative from being unnecessarily exposed to the virus on our ward.

The wide variation in clinical responses to COVID-19 made it paramount that patients with mild disease should continue to be cared for in a setting more appropriate to their mental health problems, thereby also preventing the local acute trust from becoming overwhelmed [1]. Equally important was the need to identify patients who clinically deteriorated, needing acute hospital care. There were thus a number of simple measures implemented on our ward that enabled patients to continue to be safely cared for on an inpatient psychiatric unit. Increasingly, the frequency of physical observations and utilising the existing daily 'safety huddles' allowed deteriorating patients to be quickly identified and their needs addressed accordingly.

Training from the local respiratory specialist nurse equipped staff to prescribe and administer oxygen via cylinders in emergency scenarios, and via oxygen concentrators for those patients who required small amounts of supplementary oxygen through nasal cannulae, but who otherwise did not require admission to a medical ward. Additional physical health nurses employed by the trust worked with our psychiatric nursing colleagues to ensure that everyone was familiar with the National Early Warning Score 2 (NEWS2) charts [13].

One of the physical health challenges that emerged on the ward was ensuring that patients had adequate intake of oral fluids. The ward layout, consisting of wholly private bedrooms, was not designed with physically ill people in mind. This required purposeful provision of water jugs for each patient regularly throughout the day, and the use of food and fluid charts to monitor their intake. A quality improvement project already in place on the unit that trained nurses in venepuncture and performing electrocardiograms (ECGs) was expanded to support the medical team with these tasks. This facilitated checking the urea and electrolytes of patients who were identified as having poor fluid intake.

As patients were required to isolate in their rooms, the team broke with the tradition of conducting ward rounds in a multidisciplinary team (MDT) room with a junior doctor typing notes at the computer. This was something that patients had previously described as intimidating and too formal. By reviewing patients in their rooms, we helped them to feel more at ease in their interactions with us, and the spread of the virus throughout the unit was minimised. An unexpected benefit of this approach was the valuable information provided about patients' mental states from their attentiveness demonstrated in their care for their surroundings. The success of this new model of ward rounds has changed the way the ward will operate in the future, with more regular and informal ward reviews being conducted at times and places that patients have been empowered to choose for themselves.

Regular input from friends and family members is commonplace in mental health units, and has the benefits of being therapeutic for patients and providing a vital source of collateral information for the staff. Due to the risk of transmission of the virus either to or from visitors to the unit, visiting was suspended when the national lockdown was announced. We used video-calling technology to overcome this challenge and enable valuable therapeutic contact between patients and their loved ones, and also to involve the family in the ward-round process and to keep them updated about the physical and mental progress of their relative [9].

Practical Aspects of Implementing the Principles

In normal times, there is little provision on mental health wards for keeping patients occupied in their rooms, the idea being that part of the therapeutic process involves encouraging their use of communal spaces and interactions with other patients and staff [14]. Therefore one of the challenges of encouraging patients to isolate in their rooms was the lack of provision there. The occupational therapists and activity workers addressed this by developing activity packs comprising materials for artwork and word searches or sudoku puzzles. The trust also prioritised acquiring an iPad for every patient on our ward, and a radio to enable them to listen to music in their room.

Despite being provided with these interventions, some patients struggled to isolate in their rooms. Therefore nursing staff wearing PPE were stationed in the corridors so that they could engage with patients who were struggling to isolate, and direct them back to their rooms if necessary. The trust also developed an involuntary isolation protocol that provided guidance and a legal framework for implementing the Mental Capacity Act 2005. This involved locking the doors to patients' rooms to minimise the risk of spreading COVID-19 to other patients and staff. This was always used as a last-resort intervention, and only for short periods of time. It was reviewed regularly by the medical and nursing staff.

Another challenge unique to encouraging patients to isolate on a psychiatric ward was the influence of their mental states on their ability to isolate. For example, some patients who were psychotic incorporated the pandemic into their delusions, either believing that they had started it and were therefore immune to it, or believing that the staff were part of a conspiracy and had falsified their test results. Being resourceful and providing printed copies of the test results for patients did little to resolve this situation, due to the strength of some patients' delusional beliefs.

As the pandemic was caused by a novel coronavirus, very little was known about the virus itself or the state of disease that it caused. Local and national guidance was updated on a regular basis, and part of the challenge of managing the ward was the need to stay abreast of any developments in the science and in government policy. Relationships fostered with doctors at our local acute hospital over many years proved invaluable in this regard, because they were often among the first to become aware of features of COVID-19 that were not yet widely known, such as the deterioration that patients often experience between days 5 and 10 [15].

Relationships within our own organisation also proved extremely helpful. One of the matrons was redeployed to assist the ward manager in implementing the necessary changes to the structure of the ward. A senior manager also attended our daily safety huddles, and provided a vital channel for escalating any concerns to a senior level on a regular basis. A wartime spirit of 'mucking in' prevailed in the team, further flattening the hierarchy, and resulting in everyone contributing to cleaning the ward when staff absences prevented the usual provision of domestic services staff.

Conclusion

The COVID-19 pandemic has forced a re-evaluation of many aspects of Western civilisation, from a move towards working from home to a renewed appreciation of outdoor spaces. Mental health services have also benefited from the challenges of the pandemic, having been provided with an opportunity to renew the ways in which services are structured. Our in-patient unit in London improved the physical healthcare that we were providing for our patients, rolled out a mass testing programme across the unit, pioneered the use of video-call technology to connect patients with their families, and redesigned the way in which ward reviews are conducted, making them more patient-friendly and empowering. The lessons learned will be invaluable not only for the next pandemic, but also as we explore our 'new normal'.

References

1. Johansson MA, Quandelacy TM, Kada S, Prasad PV, Steele M, Brooks JT, et al. SARS-CoV-2 transmission from people without COVID-19 Symptoms. *JAMA Netw Open* 2021; J4(1): e211383. Erratum in: *JAMA Netw Open* 2021; 4(2):e211383.

2. Public Health England. Guidance COVID-19: investigation and initial clinical management of possible cases. Public Health England, 2020. Available at: https://www.gov.uk/government/publications/wuhan-novel-coronavirus-initial-investigation-of-possible-cases/investigation-and-initial-clinical-management-of-possible-cases-of-wuhan-novel-coronavirus-wn-cov-infection.

3. Chaw L, Koh WC, Jamaludin S, Naing L, Alikhan MF, Wong J. Analysis of SARS-CoV-2 transmission in different settings, Brunei. *Emerg Infect Dis* 2020; 26: 2598–606.

4. Du Z, Xu X, Wu Y, Wang L, Cowling BJ, Meyers LA. Serial interval of COVID-19 among publicly reported confirmed cases. *Emerg Infect Dis* 2020; 26: 1341–3.

5. Lee S, Kim T, Lee E, et al. Clinical course and molecular viral shedding among asymptomatic and symptomatic patients with SARS-CoV-2 infection in a community treatment center in the Republic of Korea. *JAMA Intern Med* 2020; 180: 1447–52.

6. Chu DK, Elie AA, Akl A, Duda S, Solo K, Yaacoub S, et al. Physical distancing, face masks, and eye protection to prevent person-to-person transmission of SARS-CoV-2 and COVID-19: a systematic review and meta-analysis. *J Vasc Surg* 2020; 72: 1500.

7. Taylor MR, Agho KE, Stevens GJ, Raphael B. Factors influencing psychological distress during a disease epidemic: data from Australia's first outbreak of equine influenza. *BMC Public Health*. 2008; 8: 347.

8. Liu X, Kakade M, Fuller CJ, et al. Depression after exposure to stressful events: lessons learned from the severe acute respiratory syndrome epidemic. *Compr Psychiatry* 2012; 53: 15–23.

9. Moslehi S, Aubrey-Jones D, Knowles M, Obeney-Williams J,

Leveson S, Aref-Adib G. Cyberpsychiatry versus COVID-19: using video consultation to improve clinical care in an in-patient psychiatric unit. *BJPsych Int* 2021; 18: E10.

10. Meyerowitz EA, Richterman A, Gandhi RT, Sax PE. Transmission of SARS-CoV-2: a review of viral, host, and environmental factors. *Ann Intern Med* 2021; 174: 69–79.

11. BBC News. Coronavirus: Virus isolation period extended from seven to 10 days. BBC News, 30 July 2020 (www.bbc.co.uk/news/uk-53588709).

12. Fiorillo A, Gorwood P. The consequences of the COVID-19 pandemic on mental health and implications for clinical practice. *Eur Psychiatry* 2020; 63: e32.

13. Brand JW, Morrice DJ, Patteril MV, Mackay JH. National Early Warning Score 2 (NEWS2) to identify inpatient COVID-19 deterioration: the importance of pO_2:FiO_2 ratio. *Clin Med (Lond)*. 2021; 21: e315–16.

14. Gilburt H, Rose D, Slade M. The importance of relationships in mental health care: a qualitative study of service users' experiences of psychiatric hospital admission in the UK. *BMC Health Serv Res* 2008; 8: 92.

15. Parker-Pope T. Why days 5 to 10 are so important when you have coronavirus. *New York Times*, 30 April 2022 (www.nytimes.com/2020/04/30/well/live/coronavirus-days-5-through-10.html).

Chapter

34

Case Study 1: The Omagh Bomb, the Mental Health Response, and the Lessons Learned

Ciaran Mulholland and Michael Duffy

Introduction

On 15 August 1998, 500 pounds of homemade explosives were detonated in a car bomb in the centre of the market town of Omagh, Northern Ireland, causing the deaths of 29 adults and children, along with two unborn twins. Fifteen of the deceased were aged 17 years or younger. A further 400 people were injured, 135 of whom were hospitalised. Many children and young people sustained severe and life-changing physical injuries, including loss of limbs and of soft tissue, scarring, and disfigurement. It was the largest single incident in the Troubles in Northern Ireland, and the scale of the casualties sent shockwaves across the island of Ireland and beyond. The bombing occurred just 6 weeks after the Good Friday Agreement (also known as the Belfast Agreement) had been endorsed in twin referenda in Northern Ireland and the Republic of Ireland. The ensuing widespread hope for a better and more peaceful future magnified the shock and horror caused by the bomb.

By 1998, over 3,700 people in Northern Ireland had died in an estimated 100,000 shooting and bombing incidents over a period of 30 years [1]. One in 12 members of the population had been injured, and 40% had lost a family member or a close friend. It is important to contextualise these figures to the small size of the population, which is just over 1.5 million. For example, the 3,700 deaths in Northern Ireland would be equivalent to 150,000 deaths in the total UK population, or 500,000 deaths in the USA.

Levels of direct participation in the violence were high. Over 50,000 people passed through the ranks of the Royal Ulster Constabulary – the most dangerous armed police force in the world in which to serve at the time. More than 100,000 people served at some point in the Ulster Defence Regiment and its successor, the Royal Irish Regiment (Home Battalions), the largest single regiment in the UK's Army, which was recruited specifically for service within Northern Ireland. The number of people who joined armed paramilitary groups is unknown, but at least 25,000 were imprisoned because of their involvement.

The health and social care professions responded to the impact of the violence on their doorstep with determination and not a little ingenuity and innovation. Several significant organisational and surgical advances resulted and have saved many lives in other conflicts across the globe. The physical impact of violence is all too evident, but the psychosocial impacts can be overlooked. In the context of mass upheavals affecting most of the population, adverse mental health outcomes are to be expected, but there is also ample evidence that the experience of widespread violence often increases social cohesion. Such a 'Blitz effect' was a factor in Northern Ireland's most embattled communities, and acted as a powerful protective factor for many people and families.

Although the generalised population effect may have been ameliorated in this way, it is clearly the case that many of the people who were most directly affected by the violence developed diagnosable and treatable mental health disorders, including post-traumatic stress disorder (PTSD) and prolonged grief disorder (PGD). These conditions were often not adequately treated for obvious and understandable reasons. In the 1970s and 1980s, mental health services remained under-developed, and general practitioners carried the bulk of the workload. Conditions such as PTSD and PGD were not fully understood or lacked diagnostic clarity, and current effective psychological therapies did not exist or were still in their formative stages. One consequence was a reliance on medication in the absence of alternatives. Simplistic conclusions should be avoided, but it is probable that difficulties in accessing psychological therapies resulted in over-prescribing in the past, and this continues up to the present day.

The Community Trauma and Recovery Team

When the Omagh bomb exploded, a systemic approach was in place to address the consequences of physical trauma, but both the immediate and long-term mental health impacts of this mass casualty event required urgent consideration and creation of a bespoke rapid response. Looking back, the success of the mental health response to the Omagh bombing represents a turning point, and the lessons learned have had a lasting impact.

The immediate mobilisation of resources was necessarily focused on surgical care in the local hospital and an airlift of survivors for specialist treatment in hospitals outside the area. Within 48 hours, however, the local health and social care trust had begun the task of developing a comprehensive and integrated mental health response. An experienced team was brought together with the aim of addressing the psychosocial care needs of the hundreds of direct and indirect survivors of the bomb. The ripple effects of the atrocity in a small town (with a population of 26,000) surrounded by a dispersed rural community were immense.

Recognising that existing mental health services were at risk of becoming overwhelmed, the Omagh Community Trauma and Recovery Team (CTRT) was established and remained operational for 3 years. It acted as a central point of access, and provided assessment and therapeutic services. In addition, it provided community and educational initiatives and established links with key community support mechanisms, such as those provided by the clergy, schools, general practitioners, and community and voluntary sector groups.

In total, 2,000 bomb-related contacts were recorded by local general practitioners in the first 3 weeks after the tragedy. During its first year the CTRT received 500 contacts, the majority of them during the initial 4 months. There was a marginal increase in referrals at the time of the first anniversary of the explosion, and over the 3 years in which the CTRT operated there were 622 referrals in total. In addition, in the year after the bombing, local voluntary organisations provided support and counselling services to around 400–500 people. The CTRT was succeeded by the Northern Ireland Centre for Trauma and Transformation (NICTT), which continued its clinical work and research programme while broadening its geographical reach to all of Northern Ireland [2].

Improving Our Understanding of PTSD Through Community Studies

Crucially, the service was evidence based, outcomes focused, and research orientated from the outset. The involvement of international experts Professor David M. Clark and Professor Anke Ehlers of Oxford University not only ensured that the response was based on the best available evidence, but also helped to grow the evidence base through a series of studies that have improved our understanding of PTSD.

We thought it important to explore the varying impacts of the Omagh bombing both to assist in the immediate effort to help survivors, and in order to improve our understanding of the impact of mass casualty events for the future. There were several distinct features of the tragedy that had the potential to contribute to its psychological impacts. First, the number of children who were killed or injured, symbolized by the sight of children's small white coffins, generated severe distress and profound grief. Second, although most of the people who had died during the Troubles were male, the adults who were killed during the Omagh bombing were mostly female, including a pregnant mother of twins. Third, the incident occurred during a period when expectations of violent incidents had diminished greatly. Fourth, people were moved to a perceived place of safety as the two telephone warnings provided inaccurate details of the bomb's location; consequently, the police mistakenly moved people into the area of greatest danger. Fifth, the disaster was caused by human activity, a factor that has been shown to produce higher levels of distress than so-called natural disasters (see Chapters 10 and 12). In addition, there was a widespread assumption that some of the perpetrators came from within the local community. This generated an enduring sense of threat and mistrust that is partially comparable to that experienced after the London tube bombings in 2007, and is in contrast to the perceived external threat associated with the 9/11 attacks in the USA.

Research into Mental Health Disorders Consequent on the Bombing

Four studies examined the impact on adults, adolescents, children, and healthcare staff. The adult study

(n = 3,123; age range 16–92 years) found that six variables linked to a newly developing cognitive model for PTSD accounted for 63% of the variance in PTSD scores – rumination, thought or emotion suppression, nowness of the memory (whether the memory retains a sense of the trauma still being in the present), a muddled memory, negative beliefs about oneself and the symptoms of PTSD, and beliefs about the world being an unsafe place [3,4].

A parallel study, which involved 2,335 adolescents aged 14–18 years, demonstrated that exposure alone is not a precise predictor of risk for developing PTSD. Again the findings emphasised the importance of cognitive factors – what a person is thinking during the event (e.g., the thought 'I am going to die'), negative beliefs about oneself, negative beliefs about PTSD symptoms (e.g., 'I am losing my mind'), rumination, and nowness of the memory [5].

The third study involved 1,945 children aged 8–13 years who were attending 13 schools in the district. An important finding was that comorbid conditions, especially anxiety, had a moderating effect on factors previously reported to predict the emergence of PTSD, such as pre-trauma characteristics (e.g., gender, age) and exposure factors (e.g., whether one was present at the time of the bombing), in predicting probable PTSD [6]. This is an important finding, as when a child presents with high levels of anxiety after a traumatic incident the clinician should screen carefully for PTSD.

The fourth study was a postal survey of 1,064 health service staff [7]. Approximately 50% of them reported professional or personal involvement with the bombing incident. Those who were involved both professionally and personally, particularly those who witnessed the event or those who had experienced previous emotional problems and other psychological traumas, had the highest levels of symptomatology. Although staff with higher levels of symptoms of PTSD were more likely to seek professional help, only a minority did so.

Community Studies Inform Clinical Trials

Two clinical trials were informed by this research, and in both of them therapists were encouraged to target the key PTSD maintenance factors identified in the studies. In the first trial, a consecutive series of 91 patients who had been exposed to the Omagh bombing and had PTSD were recruited to an open trial of trauma-focused

cognitive behaviour therapy (CBT) [8]. There were no major exclusion criteria, and 53% had an additional Axis I disorder. The pre-treatment to post-treatment effect size was 2.47, with a median number of eight sessions. Comorbidity did not predict outcome, nor did lack of social support and status (civilian vs. emergency services personnel). However, continuing physical health problems were associated with poorer outcomes (59% vs. 77% improvement).

The second clinical study, a randomised controlled trial of immediate cognitive therapy versus delayed cognitive therapy, recruited 58 people (60% civilian, 35% police, military, or health service staff, and 5% others) with prolonged and severe PTSD [9]. At the point of randomisation, the mean duration of the current episode of PTSD was 8.9 years (SD = 9.2), with a range of 3 months to 32 years. Subjects demonstrated significant comorbidity (72% had one or more additional Axis I disorders), 19% had been physically injured, and 81% had experienced multiple traumatic events (median 3, range 1–10 events). Despite the complex nature of the presentations of these patients, at 12 weeks the immediate cognitive therapy treatment group scores were significantly lower than the waiting-list group scores on all measures for both completers and the intention-to-treat group ($p < 0.001$). The mean number of sessions was 7.8 (9.2 for completers). The delayed treatment group had similar pre- to post-treatment gains. Factors associated with less improvement were high levels of depressive symptoms and a longer time since the trauma. Factors not associated with improvement were the presence of a comorbid disorder, the presence of enduring trauma-related physical health problems, whether the traumatic event was directly experienced or witnessed, and single versus multiple traumas. One reason for enduring physical health problems not affecting treatment gains was the application of new techniques learned after the open trial, in which there was a negative impact on treatment gains (e.g., using experiments to break the link between chronic pain and the trauma memory).

The evidence accrued in this series of studies helped to inform the further development of the Ehlers and Clark model of PTSD and trauma-focused CBT approaches to treatment, underlining the importance of linking research and clinical practice, including the exploration of themes evident at the population level to identify important target areas for clinicians. Prior to the Omagh studies, the focus of therapy was often on pre-trauma (e.g., gender) and peri-trauma (e.g., type of exposure) factors, whereas these findings suggest that immediate post-trauma factors were more important predictors of which people would go on to develop symptoms of PTSD. The results of the community studies were integrated into clinical practice in the CTRT, with assessment and therapy targeting key risk factors for chronic PTSD, including rumination about the trauma and its consequences, and perceived nowness of traumatic memories. Fewer imaginal exposure sessions, which are often difficult to tolerate, were offered, responses to triggers were understood and modified, and more purposeful use of visits to the site of the trauma was utilised. The result was improved clinical outcomes and more rapid improvement.

An Emerging Concept: Prolonged Grief Disorder

In 1998, approaches to assessing and treating complex or traumatic grief were not well developed. Although most bereaved people recover from the initial intense emotions within weeks or months, some experience difficulties that persist, and they may not seek clinical help despite suffering significant social impairment. Prolonged grief disorder (PGD) was introduced as a diagnostic category in the *International Classification of Diseases 11th Revision (ICD-11)*, published by the World Health Organization, in 2012. It was included as an update to the American Psychiatric Association's *Diagnostic and Statistical Manual of Mental Disorders, Fifth Edition, Text Revision (DSM-5-TR)* in 2020 [10].

In the response to the Omagh bombing, several points quickly became clear in relation to bereavement. First, both primary care and mental health staff were reluctant to pathologise grief, which resulted in a low rate of referral. Second, in the absence of a clear differentiation between PGD and normal grief, when people were referred it was often to non-specialist teams, usually in the voluntary sector, and for generic grief counselling. Emerging evidence at the time, and further research since, have reported little evidence of benefit from this kind of generic grief work [11].

Studying the phenomenology of complex or traumatic grief has provided a rationale for applying the cognitive model of PTSD to the treatment of PGD. We now know that, for people who have PGD, it is important to explore and understand the importance of triggers, appraisals and behaviours (e.g., social withdrawal), and cognitive processes (e.g., rumination, attention) that maintain traumatic grief symptoms and appear to disrupt the integration of the memory of loss with the patient's broader autobiographical memories. Application of the cognitive therapy model for PTSD, with some changes to the protocol, has been reported on elsewhere – for example, by therapists working with people bereaved as a result of the COVID-19 pandemic [12,13].

Organisational and Therapeutic Responses to Trauma: The Lessons Learned

The lessons learned after the Omagh bombing have helped to guide responses to mass casualty events and service developments elsewhere, including providing training, advice, and support. The response to the bombing became a reference point for clinicians and health service managers responding to other large-scale attacks, including the 9/11 attacks in the USA, the Utoya Island mass shooting in Norway, the Manchester Arena bombing and the London Bridge attack in the UK, and, more recently, the war in Ukraine.

We now understand that after large-scale attacks a tailored and phased response is necessary. There is greater awareness that psychosocial responses should be evidence based, and that non-evidence-based interventions, which might cause harm, should be avoided, including non-directive and non-trauma-focused therapies that may facilitate rumination. It is important to differentiate between the need for psychosocial support to assist recovery for people with mild conditions, and the need for psychological and pharmacological treatments for those with diagnosable clinical disorders. Experience of the COVID-19 pandemic reinforces the need for screening to be offered to staff who are exposed to trauma at regular time points, and for trauma-focused CBT (TF-CBT) and/or eye movement desensitisation and reprocessing (EMDR) to be offered at the appropriate time when clinical conditions are emerging, as early treatment leads to better outcomes.

The response to the Omagh bombing has also informed the development of the Improving Access to Psychological Therapies (IAPT) programme in England, which is designed to provide evidence-based psychological therapies at a population level – for example, through the incorporation of session-by-session self-report outcome measures [14].

The Long-Term Impact of the Omagh Bombing in Northern Ireland

The Good Friday (Belfast) Agreement pledged that 'we must never forget those who have died or been injured, and their families'. The tragedy of the Omagh bombing reinforced the impetus for peace and the acknowledged necessity for adequately addressing the long-term consequences of violence. The Stormont House Agreement of 2014 committed government to create a comprehensive, regionalised, and evidence-based trauma network for Northern Ireland. The Regional Trauma Network was created, and today this network involves statutory, community, and voluntary sector organisations in an innovative co-production approach. Its organisational and clinical approaches are directly informed by the experience of Omagh.

The knowledge accumulated also helped to inform the clinical aspects of the implementation of the Troubles Permanent Disablement Payment Scheme [15]. This scheme provides payments to survivors of the Troubles who are physically or psychologically injured, and it was included in the Stormont House Agreement. It opened to applicants in August 2021, and 3,000 people applied during its first year of operation.

We can state with confidence that mental health services in Northern Ireland and worldwide have learned from the response to the Omagh bombing. We know from the Omagh studies that prolonged and severe PTSD, even when accompanied by comorbid conditions, often responds to appropriate evidence-based therapy. Now, decades after the worst years of violence, we can be hopeful of improved outcomes for survivors of conflict in Northern Ireland and elsewhere, even long after the initial traumatic event.

References

1. McKittrick D, Kelters S, Feeney B, Thornton C, McVea D. *Lost Lives: The Stories of the Men, Women and Children Who Died as a Result of the Northern Ireland Troubles.* Mainstream Publishing, 2012.

2. Bolton D. *Conflict, Peace and Mental Health: Addressing the Consequences of Conflict and Trauma in Northern Ireland.* Manchester University Press, 2017.

3. Ehlers A, Clark DM. A cognitive model of posttraumatic stress disorder. *Behav Res Ther* 2000; 38: 319–45.

4. Duffy M, Bolton D, Gillespie K, Ehlers A, Clark DM. A community study of the psychological effects of the Omagh car bomb on adults. *PLoS One* 2013; 8: e76618.

5. Duffy M, McDermott M, Percy A, Ehlers A, Clark DM, Fitzgerald M, et al. The effects of the Omagh bomb on adolescent mental health: a school-based study. *BMC Psychiatry* 2015; 15: 18.

6. McDermott M, Duffy M, Percy A, Fitzgerald M, Cole C. A school based study of psychological disturbance in children following the Omagh bomb. *Child Adolesc Psychiatry Ment Health* 2013; 7: 36.

7. Luce A, Firth-Cozens J, Midgley S, Burges C. After the Omagh bomb: posttraumatic stress disorder in health service staff. *J Trauma Stress* 2002; 15: 27–30.

8. Gillespie K, Duffy M, Hackmann A, Clark DM. Community based cognitive therapy in the treatment of posttraumatic stress disorder following the Omagh bomb. *Behav Res Ther* 2002; 40: 345–57.

9. Duffy M, Gillespie K, Clark DM. Posttraumatic stress disorder in the context of terrorism and other civil conflict in Northern Ireland: randomized controlled trial. *BMJ* 2007; 334: 147–50.

10. Prigerson HG, Boelen PA, Xu J, Smith KV, Maciejewski PK. Validation of the new DSM-5-TR criteria for prolonged grief disorder and the PG-13-Revised (PG-13-R) scale. *World Psychiatry* 2021; 20: 96–106.

11. Litterer DA, Hoyt WT. Effectiveness of grief therapy: a meta-analysis. *J Couns Psychol* 1999; 46: 370–80.

12. Duffy M, Wild J. A cognitive approach to persistent complex bereavement disorder (PCBD). *Cogn Behav Ther* 2017; 10: E16.

13. Duffy M, Wild, J. Living with loss: a cognitive approach to complicated and traumatic grief. *Behav Cogn Psychother* 2023. Available from: https://doi.org/10.1017/S1352465822000674.

14. Clark DM. Realising the mass public benefit of evidence-based psychological therapies: the IAPT program. *Annu Rev Clin Psychol* 2018; 14: 159–83.

15. Mulholland C, Duffy M, McIlwaine R, Coughlan C. *Implementation of Troubles Permanent Disablement Payment Scheme: Rapid Review.* Victims' Payments Board, 2021 (www.victimspaymentsboard.org.uk/sites/victimspayments/files/publications/TPDPS-Literature-Review-final-1.2.pdf).

Case Study 2: A Public Health Survey of People Exposed to the Paris Terror Attacks in November 2015 and Their Consequences

Philippe Pirard and Yvon Motreff

Background

On 13 November 2015, a series of terror attacks took place in Paris. Three bombings occurred near a football stadium in the northern suburbs of Paris, three shootings and one bombing took place in restaurants in central Paris, and there was a mass shooting and hostage-taking at the Bataclan theatre. These attacks left 131 people dead and 643 injured. Several thousand people were highly exposed to events that met the requirements of Criterion A for the definition of post-traumatic stress disorder (PTSD) in the *Diagnostic and Statistical Manual of Mental Disorders, Fifth Edition (DSM-5)* [1].

Hundreds of first responders risked their lives to secure the sites or to provide assistance to the survivors. Affiliated volunteers from the French Red Cross and Protection Civile de Paris were also sent to the various crime scenes [2]. In the days and weeks that followed, the police continued their investigations, and thousands of health personnel continued to care for survivors. After the attacks, Medical and Psychological Emergency Units (CUMP – Cellules d'Urgence Médico-Psychologique) were deployed to provide immediate psychosocial support for affected communities, first in the streets in proximity to the attacks, and later in dedicated information centres set up in the town halls of the districts affected [3]. These centres remained open for 1 month. France's standard healthcare system was responsible for longer-term psychological management. The French Ministry of Health offered free-of-charge consultations with a psychiatrist or a psychologist to people registered as survivors by the Ministry of Justice. People who considered themselves survivors could also contact one of the permanent victim support associations managed by the Ministry of Justice, or one of the several non-governmental victims' associations [4].

Research Objectives

As part of its surveillance and public health policy support missions, Santé Publique France set up the Enquête de Santé Publique post-Attentats du 13 Novembre 2015 (ESPA 13 November survey) in 2016. The aim of this web-based questionnaire survey was to measure the psychotraumatic impact on and the use of care by people who were highly exposed to the attacks of 13 November 2015. This chapter presents two intermediate findings to illustrate the usefulness of the information that this type of survey can provide to guide psychosocial care measures:

- analysis of the prevalence of PTSD and partial PTSD and associated factors among responders
- analysis of the use of mental health support by type of exposure among members of the public.

The data presented here have been published in two different papers, for first responders [2] and members of the public [4], respectively.

Rationale for the Objectives

Terrorist attacks take a heavy psychosocial toll on the lives of people who have endured exposure to these incidents. This is reflected in a high prevalence of mental health disorders (MHD), and specifically PTSD, major depressive disorder, and anxiety-based disorders in the months and even years after the attack. These MHD have negative impacts on people's families, social relationships, and work capacity. It is therefore important to meet the needs of people suffering from MHD in a timely fashion, and to provide appropriate treatment to reduce the intensity and duration of these consequences and their associated social complications.

Some studies recommend providing early and active outreach psychosocial support to meet the needs of populations exposed to terrorist attacks. It is also important to allocate sufficient resources to meet the increased and often long-term demand for mental health support after disasters. Access to mental health support is particularly important for people who have been directly affected by a collective massive attack, as they represent the group that is exposed to the highest risk of psychological sequelae. Yet this access may differ depending on whether an individual person was directly threatened, was a witness to the attack, or learned that a loved one was threatened, injured, or killed.

To date, few studies have focused on both PTSD and partial PTSD in first responders after terror attacks. People exposed to potentially traumatic events can develop symptoms of PTSD without satisfying all of the criteria for a PTSD diagnosis. We call this subsyndromal or partial PTSD. Providing treatment for first responders with partial PTSD is increasingly recommended because partial PTSD can become chronic and may be associated with other psychiatric disorders, functional difficulties, and the need for mental healthcare [5]. As the contexts between the series of attacks differ, and because until now the data have been sparse, there is still a need for more research on risk factors for PTSD and partial PTSD that can be used to develop strategies to reduce the psychosocial burden of terror attacks on first responders.

The Methodology

The Population

The population studied comprised people over 15 years old whose exposure to the attacks on 13 November 2015 met the requirements of Criterion A in the DSM-5 definition of PTSD [6]. This group included people directly threatened (A1), direct witnesses (A2), people who learned of the presence or death of a loved one in the attacks (A3), and first responders (A4) who intervened on the night of 13 November and/or during the following 3 weeks in contexts specifically linked to the terrorist attacks, including health professionals, members of the Paris fire brigade, volunteers from civil protection associations, police officers, and city hall staff.

Recruitment and Data Collection

Information about the ESPA survey was disseminated in the media and using an active approach with key stakeholders including CUMP officers, survivors, and

associations. Furthermore, a study information campaign was complemented by letters delivered to residents living in proximity to the places where the attacks took place [4]. First responders were also solicited by their institutional colleagues, managers, doctors, and psychologists via email, meetings, posters, and videos.

The ESPA is an ongoing longitudinal online survey, and initial data were collected 8–12 months after the attacks using a web-based, self-administered questionnaire. Completed questionnaires and informed consent were provided by 837 first responders and 575 members of the public. The protocol was approved by ethics committees. Data for 663 first responders and 454 members of the public were analysed.

Variables
Mental State

Among first responders, symptoms of PTSD and partial PTSD at the time of the survey were measured using the PTSD Checklist for DSM-5 (PCL-5) [6]. Each PCL-5 item with a rating of 2 ('moderately' or 'higher') was considered to be a PTSD symptom. We then applied the DSM-5 diagnostic rules for PTSD. People considered to be positive for PTSD should show at least one B item (questions 1–5), one C item (questions 6–7), two D items (questions 8–14), and two E items (questions 15–20). Partial PTSD was defined as respondents meeting two or three of Criteria B to E [7].

We wanted to identify respondents from among members of the public for whom engagement with mental health support was essential. Therefore only members of the public who scored as having PTSD with functional impairment were considered. Accordingly, we took into account Criterion G (functional impairment) of the PTSD for DSM-5. PTSD-related functional impairment was defined as answering yes to at least one of the following 'yes/no' questions: Do these symptoms: 1. Make your relationships with your family more difficult? 2. Make it difficult for you to get along with your friends? 3. Make it difficult for you to work well? 4. Cause you problems for your general level of functioning in your everyday life?

Use of Medico-Psychological Care

Members of the public were also asked whether they had received any of the following interventions for psychological problems since the attacks [4]:

- outreach psychosocial support (OPS), whether provided by professional psychologists in the streets immediately after the attacks, or during a visit to one of the ad-hoc information centres, or at a police station, or at a specific occupational medicine support service which was also set up on an emergency basis
- consultation with a mental health specialist (a psychologist or psychiatrist in a hospital, in a unit for the treatment of psychological trauma, or in a Centre Médico-Psychologique, or a private specialist)
- consultation with a GP
- contact with a member of an association for victims (i.e., the Ministry of Justice or a non-governmental organisation).

Regular Psychological Care

Participants were asked whether they had initiated regular psychological care (RPC) since the attacks ('Since the events, have you initiated regular psychological care?'), and on what date [4].

Exposure

Exposure among members of the public was classified according to the following categories: directly threatened (wounded, hit by the blast, targeted by the terrorists, in the indoor or outdoor areas of the restaurants attacked or the Bataclan); direct witness (by sight, hearing, or touch); indirectly exposed (having learned that a loved one was present or had died) [4].

Exposure to the event among first responders was classified into three mutually exclusive categories: (a) having intervened in unsecured crime scenes during the night of 13 November; (b) having intervened in secured crime scenes or scenes distant from the events during the night of 13 November; and (c) having intervened on the day after the 13 November events and/or in the following 3 weeks [2].

Other Variables

Information on gender, age, and educational level was collected.

Mental healthcare history was assessed by asking participants whether they had received any previous mental healthcare (i.e., prior to 13 November 2015) from a psychologist or psychiatrist that lasted for 6 months or more and/or had previously been prescribed antidepressant medication for at least 6 months. They were also asked if they had experienced a difficult life event in 2015 (e.g., divorce, loss of a close relative, serious disease). Each was evaluated on the answers given to yes/no questions.

Participants were asked about their perceived feelings of social isolation using the following question: 'In general, would you say that you feel: very alone, alone, surrounded, or very surrounded?' People who answered 'very alone' or 'alone' were considered to be socially isolated.

Previous exposure to traumatic events was assessed using the following yes/no question: 'Were you confronted with potentially traumatic events during your life in which you felt brutally threatened or that your life was in danger?'

Preparedness to cope with terror attack-related traumatic interventions among first responders [2] was evaluated using four yes/no questions, namely previous training for psychosocial risks, knowing that someone who could help you deal with psychosocial risks and consequences before or after exposure, having been informed about potential psychological risks of such traumatic interventions, and having been trained to provide psychological first aid.

Analyses

Analyses were performed using SAS Enterprise Guide 7.11.

First Responders

The factors associated with PTSD and partial PTSD were computed using a multinomial logistic regression model, giving estimates of odds ratios (OR) and their Wald 95% confidence interval limits. The outcome variables fell into three modalities, namely PTSD, partial PTSD, and neither PTSD nor partial PTSD, with the latter chosen as the reference. Introduction into the multivariate model of the independent variables was based on existing literature or on the significance of the association (gender, first responder category, educational level and exposure to attacks, mental health history, prior traumatic events, training and social support). Intervening during the January 2015 Paris terror attacks and age were also tested.

The Public

The proportions of the different mental health support services used were assessed overall, and according to

Table 35.1 Prevalence of PTSD and partial PTSD by first responder category (*ESPA 13 November* Survey) (*n* = 663)

	PTSD			Partial PTSD		
	n	%	95% CI	*n*	%	95% CI
Firefighters	7	3.4	0.9–5.9	32	15.7	10.7–20.7
Health professionals	10	4.4	1.7–7.0	24	10.4	6.5–14.4
Affiliated volunteers	6	4.5	1.0–8.0	26	19.4	12.7–26.1
Police officers	9	9.5	3.6–15.4	22	23.2	14.7–31.6
Total	32	4.8	3.2–6.5	104	15.7	12.9–18.4

type of exposure (being threatened, witnessing, indirectly exposed) for people with PTSD. Chi-squared tests were used for each mental health support, to test the independence of the distributions between the use or not of the given mental health support, and exposure groups.

PTSD and Partial PTSD Among First Responders and Associated Factors

Results

The overall PTSD and partial PTSD prevalence values in our study sample were 4.8 and 15.7%, respectively, ranging from 3.4% among firefighters to 9.5% among police officers for PTSD, and from 10.4% among health professionals to 23.2% for police officers for partial PTSD (see Table 35.1).

In multivariate analysis, gender was not associated with either full or partial PTSD. Age was not associated either with PTSD or with partial PTSD, and was not retained in the model. Being a police officer was associated with partial PTSD (OR = 2.37; 95% CI = 1.11–5.06) (compared with firefighters). Exposure to an unsecured crime scene was associated with PTSD (OR = 7.26; 95% CI = 1.91–27.54). Having a high-school diploma (compared with a graduate or postgraduate degree) and social isolation were associated with both PTSD and partial PTSD. Not having training on the potential psychological consequences of this type of traumatic intervention (i.e., terror attacks) was associated with PTSD (OR = 4.88; 95% CI = 1.65–14.42). Experiencing a difficult life event in 2015 was associated with partial PTSD (OR = 1.80; 95% CI = 1.07–3.03). Being mobilised for the January 2015 Paris terror attacks but not listing that intervention as a difficult life event in 2015 was negatively associated with partial PTSD (OR = 0.43; 95% CI = 0.23–0.83). Other

associations with having partial PTSD were observed, although they were not significant at a *p*-value threshold of 0.05; in particular, they included exposure to an unsecured crime scene, lack of training, and a history of being prescribed antidepressants.

Discussion

Between 8 months and 1 year after the 13 November 2015 terror attacks in the Paris area, the prevalence of PTSD among firefighters, health professionals, affiliated volunteers, and police officers was 3.4, 4.4, 4.5, and 9.5%, respectively. In comparison, 2 to 3 years after the 9/11 terrorist attacks in the USA in 2001, higher prevalence figures were found for firefighters (12.2%), members of voluntary organisations (7.2%), and emergency medical services, medical, and disaster personnel (17.8%), but lower prevalence values were found for police officers (6.2%) [8]. Lower prevalence figures were found after other recent terror attacks in Europe – for example, the 2004 Madrid terror attacks (1.3% among police officers 5–12 weeks after the attacks) [9] and the 2011 attacks in Oslo and Utøya (0.3% among professional personnel 10 months later) [10]. The prevalence of partial PTSD in the various first responder categories appeared to be higher than was reported in the literature. For instance, it was 15.4% among police officers involved in the 9/11 rescue 3 years later [5], compared with 23.2% in our study sample, and it was 2% among health professional first responders 10 months after the attacks of Utøya [10], compared with 10.4% in our sample.

These differences may be partly explained by differences in the design of the studies, by classification differences in tasks and preparedness between countries for the same first responder category, and by the use of different tools to estimate PTSD symptoms. Differences in exposure between the attacks might also explain variations in prevalence. Furthermore, the preparedness of French institutions after the January 2015 attacks, together with the strong and continued mobilisation of police forces (a state of emergency was declared from November 2015 to October 2017), and other terror attacks in 2016 that targeted, in particular, police officers and military personnel, may all have influenced the prevalence of PTSD.

Just as in our study, most epidemiological studies after terror attacks found that the more people are exposed to the horror of a terror attack, the more likely they are to develop PTSD. This was specifically true for those people who intervened in unsecured crime scenes, those who intervened immediately after an attack [8], and those who intervened directly at the crime scene and who consequently had greater exposure to disturbing stimuli [11]. As with some other studies on PTSD, we found an association between PTSD and social isolation [5]. Whether it constitutes a risk factor for PTSD or is a consequence of PTSD, social isolation should be considered by mental health professionals, particularly for people who have no close family or friends.

As observed in the literature [5], compared with people with the highest levels of education (graduate or postgraduate degree), associations were found with partial and full PTSD for people with a high-school diploma.

In our study, an association was found between PTSD and not having received training on the psychological risks of having to intervene during such traumatic events. Although all of the firefighters had received this kind of training initially, only 60.4% reported having done so. This stark difference stresses the importance of people's perceptions of training.

Compared with respondents who did not intervene in the January 2015 Paris terror attacks, a negative association was found with partial PTSD for those who did intervene but who did not indicate that intervention was difficult in the survey questionnaire. One possible explanation for this is that their experience of intervention both in January and in November 2015 led to their gaining greater experience in dealing with this kind of traumatic event. Another possibility is that they were more resilient by virtue of their experience, their training, or other factors.

We found no association between PTSD or partial PTSD and gender. The results in the literature differ regarding this issue. Female gender was found to be associated with PTSD in some studies [10], whereas other studies found no such association [5].

Use of Mental Health Support Among Members of the Public

Results

With regard to exposure, 35% of the respondents had been directly threatened, 46% were witnesses, and 19% were indirectly exposed (70 people had lost a loved one and 18 people were close to someone who had been injured or directly threatened). In total, 37% of the study sample had probable PTSD.

Overall, 35% of the study sample reported receiving Outreach Psychosocial Support (OPS). With regard to the other types of mental health support, 17% had consulted their GPs, 16% had met a person from an association that provided support for psychological problems, and 39% had consulted a specialist in a structure belonging to the peacetime healthcare system. One-third had initiated RPC. Overall, therefore, 67% of the respondents had used at least one mental health support, and 51% had either consulted a specialist or initiated RPC.

Among people with probable PTSD, the proportions of OPS use were high, and were not significantly different between witnesses, people who were indirectly exposed, and those who were directly threatened (39%, 40%, and 54%, respectively). Witnesses (7% associations, 35% specialist consultations, and 35% RPC) less frequently reported going to an association ($p = 0.004$), consulting a specialist ($p = 0.002$), or initiating RPC ($p = 0.003$) than did those who were indirectly exposed (31%, 43%, and 46%, respectively) and those who were directly threatened (31%, 63%, and 65%, respectively).

Discussion

Comparing the rates of use of mental health support with those measured after other terrorist attacks is difficult. Healthcare systems, survivors' profiles, the amount of time that has elapsed since an attack, the method of interviewing, and the intensity and duration of exposure may all differ between studies and countries. In our study, 67% of the participants had had at least one episode of mental health support since the November 2015 attacks in Paris. More specifically, 51% had either consulted a specialist or started RPC. This is higher than the reported figure of 45% for New York City residents with associated PTSD or severe depression who had received psychological counselling during the first year after the 9/11 attacks [12]. It should also be compared with the figure of 69% for mental health interventions received by people who were directly threatened during the first 6 months after the Oklahoma city bombing on 19 April 1995 [13], and with the 69% of people exposed to the attacks on Utøya Island in 2011 who used a specialised mental health service between 5 and 15 months after the event within the framework of a proactive prevention outreach programme [14].

This relatively high proportion of people with PTSD who received an episode of mental health support may be due to the fact that France ranks high in terms of the availability of GPs and psychiatrists [15], the French healthcare system provides universal coverage, and, in the case of the November 2015 attacks, the French government provided people recognised as survivors with free healthcare services in the form of visits to GPs and specialists. However, we cannot exclude selection bias.

Our study does show that a substantial proportion of people with probable PTSD (35% of those directly threatened, 65% of witnesses, and 54% of those indirectly exposed) did not initiate RPC, and that although recommendations highlight the importance of offering adequate therapy to adults with clinically serious symptoms of PTSD [16], a special effort must be made to promote care for witnesses to attacks, since the proportion of witnesses who reported that they had not used any mental health support was higher compared with people who were directly threatened.

Strengths and Limitations of Web-Based Questionnaire Studies

The number of members of the public who could have been eligible for our survey may be of the order of several thousands. According to the Ministry of Justice, no exhaustive list of survivors exists, and it was not legally possible to obtain a list of them with which to compare our list of participants. Therefore it is not possible to calibrate the sample. Regarding first responders, we estimated that there was a study participation rate of 25% for firefighters and affiliated volunteers. It was not possible to compute the participation rate of police officers or health professionals, but it can be assumed that their participation rates were lower.

The participant selection method certainly introduced selection bias. It is possible that, at the time of the survey, those people who were suffering the most may have felt that it was too difficult to participate.

On the contrary, people who were suffering less might have felt less motivated to participate. As the survey was web based, exposed people who had no internet access were excluded. Accordingly, those people who were most socially disadvantaged were probably under-represented. Furthermore, the methods used to convey information about the survey (i.e., general meetings of victims' associations, letters from certain emergency psychiatrists) probably contributed to the high observed rates of use of mental health support.

As the survey was web based, there was no clinical examination, despite this being the reference diagnostic method. However, we used a validated scale for screening PTSD with good sensitivity and specificity [6]. Moreover, participants' self-reports are prone to recall biases.

Finally, the cross-sectional nature of the study prevented us from assessing whether the observed correlations might be causal. It is therefore not possible to extrapolate our results to the whole population of people who were exposed.

Despite its limitations, our study has strengths. First, stakeholders were involved in the study design, making it more relevant to the issues that they had been facing since the attacks. Second, web-based data collection appears to reduce social desirability bias.

Conclusions

The ESPA 13 November study provides findings that are important for policymaking because it highlights the serious psychological impacts of the November 2015 terrorist attacks in Paris on people who were exposed to the attacks. It also offers a picture of the latter's use of a comprehensive panel of available mental health support interventions, including:

- the beneficial role of associations for survivors and Outreach Psychosocial Support associations in promoting access to RPC in cases of need
- the need for greater efforts to be made to identify and provide care for witnesses to terrorist attacks and for people who had lost loved ones, not just those directly threatened.

Regarding first responders, the ESPA results highlight that special attention should be given to first responders in social isolation, those with low levels of education, and those intervening in unsecured crime scenes. Systematic education and training about the potential mental health consequences of traumatic interventions should be developed for first responders.

In order to improve the representativeness of the samples collected in studies such as the one described in this chapter, it is essential that epidemiologists have access to official lists of survivors to enable medium- to long-term follow-up of people who were exposed to attacks, or to plan for a health registry to be implemented in the case of mass traumatic events [17]. Provided that the ethical rules for protecting and securing personal data are respected, systems to monitor the mental health of exposed people as well as their use of mental health support should be put in place. A second wave of interviews of the ESPA 13 November survey with an open cohort has been launched 5 years after the event. It has been complemented by the collection of retrospective and prospective data on participants' use of healthcare services (i.e., not only mental health support), based on health insurance data records (e.g., visits to private GPs or specialists, prescriptions reimbursed by France's universal healthcare system).

Both data sets should provide us with a more complete perspective on the evolution of mental health support use and general care consumption by members of the public since their exposure to the terrorist attacks.

References

1. Hirsch M, Carli P, Nizard R, Riou B, Baroudjian B, Baubet T, et al. The medical response to multisite terrorist attacks in Paris. *Lancet* 2015; 386: 2535–8.

2. Motreff Y, Baubet T, Pirard P, Rabet G, Petitclerc M, Stene LE, et al. Factors associated with PTSD and partial PTSD among first responders following the Paris terror attacks in November 2015. *J Psychiatr Res* 2019; 121: 143–50.

3. Prieto N, Cheucle E, Faure P, Digard F, Dalphin C, Pachiaudi V, et al. Defusing of victims of the terrorist attacks in Paris. Elements of assessment one-month post-event [article in French]. *Encephale* 2018; 44: 118–21.

4. Pirard P, Baubet T, Motreff Y, Rabet G, Marillier M, Vandentorren S, et al. Use of mental health supports by civilians exposed to the November 2015 terrorist attacks in Paris. *BMC Health Serv Res* 2020; 20: 959.

5. Pietrzak RH, Schechter CB, Bromet EJ, Katz CL, Reissman DB, Ozbay F, et al. The burden of full and subsyndromal posttraumatic stress disorder among police involved in the World Trade Center rescue and recovery effort. *J Psychiatr Res* 2012; 46: 835–42.

6. National Center for PTSD. *The PTSD Checklist for DSM-5 (PCL-5).* US Department of Veterans Affairs, 2013 (www.ptsd.va.gov/professional/assessment/adult-sr/ptsd-checklist.asp).

7. McLaughlin KA, Koenen KC, Friedman MJ, Ruscio AM, Karam EG, Shahly V, et al. Sub-threshold posttraumatic stress disorder in the World Health Organization World Mental Health Surveys. *Biol Psychiatry* 2015; 77: 375–84.

8. Perrin MA, DiGrande L, Wheeler K, Thorpe L, Farfel M, Brackbill R. Differences in PTSD prevalence and associated risk factors among World Trade Center disaster rescue and recovery workers. *Am J Psychiatry* 2007; 164: 1385–94.

9. Gabriel R, Ferrando L, Cortón ES, Mingote C, García-Camba E, Liria AF, et al. Psychopathological consequences after a terrorist attack: an epidemiological study among victims, the general population, and police officers. *Eur Psychiatry* 2007; 22: 339–46.

10. Skogstad L, Heir T, Hauff E, Ekeberg Ø. Post traumatic stress among rescue workers after terror attacks in Norway. *Occup Med* 2016; 66: 528–35.

11. Misra M, Greenberg N, Hutchinson C, Brain A, Glozier N. Psychological impact upon London Ambulance Service of the 2005 bombings. *Occup Med* 2009; 59: 428–33.

12. Boscarino JA, Adams RE, Stuber J, Galea S. Disparities in mental health treatment following the World Trade Center disaster: implications for mental health care and health services research. *J Trauma Stress* 2005; 18: 287–97.

13. North CS, Nixon SJ, Shariat S, Mallonee S, McMillen JC, Spitznagel EL, et al. Psychiatric disorders among survivors of the Oklahoma City bombing. *JAMA* 1999; 282: 755–62.

14. Stene LE, Dyb G. Health service utilization after terrorism: a longitudinal study of survivors of the 2011 Utøya attack in Norway. *BMC Health Serv Res* 2015; 15: 158.

15. Kovess-Masfety V, Alonso J, Brugha TS, Angermeyer MC, Haro JM, Sevilla-Dedieu C, et al. Differences in lifetime use of services for mental health problems in six European countries. *Psychiatr Serv* 2007; 58: 213–20.

16. National Institute for Health and Care Excellence. *Post-Traumatic Stress Disorder. NICE Guideline [NG116].* National Institute for Health and Care Excellence, 2018 (www.nice.org.uk/guidance/ng116).

17. Behbod B, Leonardi G, Motreff Y, Beck CR, Yzermans J, Lebret E, et al. An international comparison of the instigation and design of health registers in the epidemiological response to major environmental health incidents. *J Public Health Manag Pract* 2017; 23: 20–28.

Chapter

36

Case Study 3: Practical Approaches to Delivering Psychosocial and Mental Healthcare for the Public in the UK: Lessons Learned from a Major Incident in Manchester

Alan Barrett, Prathiba Chitsabesan, Paul French, and Chris R Brewin

The Manchester Arena Bombing

This chapter is a case study of the Manchester Arena bombing in the UK in 2017. We focus on practical approaches to delivering psychosocial and mental healthcare for the public and for professional staff, and we consider the generic lessons identified from the experience.

A Chronology of Key Events

The Beginning: Monday 22 May 2017

At 22.31 hours on Monday 22 May 2017, as children and their parents were leaving a pop concert, a suicide bomber detonated an improvised explosive device in one of Europe's busiest events venues – the 21,000 capacity Manchester Arena. In total, 22 members of the public with ages ranging from 8 to 51 years were killed, as was the bomber. Several hundred more were physically injured. Thousands of people were affected psychosocially.

Within the first few hours after the attack, in the absence of mental health featuring within the local emergency preparedness, resilience, and response (EPRR) plan, a mental health response was very quickly created. It mobilised the expertise and experience of local provider mental health trusts, the specialist regional military veterans' service (MVS), and the child and adolescent mental health services (CAMHS) across Greater Manchester. It combined bottom-up expertise with top-down authority within a devolved administration.

The First Days: Key Actions

1. A Humanitarian Assistance Centre was established at a nearby football stadium by the local councils as part of the emergency response plan, supported primarily by British Red Cross volunteers, local social workers, and the police. A casualty bureau, staffed by police, was established.

2. Psychosocial guidance and messaging were developed and circulated to staff of mental health and related services during the first 24 hours after the attack, encouraging these services to follow the principles of psychological first aid [1]. A lead communications manager was assigned to coordinate communication within the wider system.

3. As this was a criminal event, a national victims' charity – Victim Support – established a telephone helpline for the public.

4. Emergency services colleagues contacted the MVS seeking specialist support and information. This led to the MVS being allowed to establish a helpline and a dedicated email address within 72 hours after the attack, which all professionals from the region could access to receive psychosocial support.

5. Psychology clinical leads were invited to attend and contribute to the multi-agency tactical (silver) command meetings. This also enabled subsequent planning for supervision and training requirements of the psychological treatment workforce.

6. Collaboration with responding services present at the tactical command enabled the offer of face-to-face psychological support for staff involved in the response. Grieving families were supported by bereavement nurse specialists at a hotel local to the mortuary, and psychosocial support was provided for them and the hotel staff.

7. An assessment of the capacity required to support the delivery of the psychosocial and mental health response was made.

The First Weeks: Key Actions

1. During the first 2 weeks after the attack, some concert attendees and their families made direct approaches to the mayor's office about the availability of specialist mental health support.

2. Outreach services were established with the purpose of attempting to contact everyone likely to have been affected in order to: acknowledge their involvement in the Incident; assure them that a response was in preparation; offer early screening of any impact; and determine who required a more detailed assessment of any mental health need. People who had attended the concert had come from a wide range of places, including Australia, Thailand, Spain, the Isle of Skye, and Ireland, with the majority from northern England. Understanding where the people involved had come from was important for developing responses that could support those people who were not local to Greater Manchester.

3. A central hub was proposed and established to deliver the full NHS psychosocial response that was thought to be required.

4. Mental health clinicians, including psychologists who specialised in psychological trauma, attended ongoing regional and national multi-agency meetings, enabling them to be briefed, to provide input about appropriate responses and pathways to care, and to assess the capacity and communications that would be required.

Establishing the Greater Manchester Resilience Hub (the Hub)

Representatives from all four mental health NHS trusts in Greater Manchester, strategic clinical network personnel, commissioners, and regional psychological trauma experts agreed that to provide equity of access and reduce variation in local service support, a place was needed to provide a focus for planning and providing psychosocial and mental health services to support people affected by the attack. As Pennine Care NHS Foundation Trust (PCFT) had the greatest number of trauma therapists and CAMHS within the

region, and hosted the regional MVS with expertise in responding to the psychological impact of improvised explosive devices, it was agreed by all providers and commissioners that PCFT should host the all-age psychosocial response to the incident.

Within 7 weeks after the attack, the Manchester Resilience Hub (the Hub) was accommodated, equipped, staffed, and up and running. The MVS had imported its web-based electronic clinical information system, which avoided the firewall restrictions usually created between services. This allowed for adaptations to be made, and offered a higher degree of client confidentiality, suited to survivors of high-profile terrorism. Appropriately skilled and qualified staff were identified and released to work part-time at the Hub.

The Hub provided and continues to provide four pillars of activity, which are described here:

1. Outreach, screening, and, where indicated, assessment and facilitation of access to evidence-based interventions, close to where the clients live. This included commissioning therapy, if not otherwise available. For example, many children and young people experienced difficulty in accessing trauma-focused therapies, due to regional variation in their availability. All children and young people were contacted for a clinical triage in addition to screening, as psychometric measures were considered to be less useful for understanding the needs of children and young people than for adults.

2. Provision of advice, consultation, and guidance for all stakeholders on how best to support the people affected. This included the organising of education conferences, production of resources, training and supervision of staff within other agencies, and offering advice to parents, schools, employers, mental health professionals, and the media.

3. Whole family support included direct telephone and email support for family members of attendees and professional responders, and whole family system assessment and formulation to understand people's needs and views, and plan interventions.

4. Peer support was provided by Hub clinicians facilitating bespoke family events and activities across the north of England and Scotland, to reflect the geographical hot spots of affected

attendees. These events were designed to enable people with similar lived experiences to meet and support each other, while learning how to manage trauma within their families. The Hub provided all clients with details of other peer support offers provided by the voluntary and private sector.

The Principles of the Hub's Approach to Providing a Service

The response to providing psychosocial and mental health services for people who were affected by the bombing was guided by the following principles:

1. Adopting an evidence-informed, values-based approach to psychosocial and mental health interventions after disasters and major incidents. The response was based on the non-diagnostic MVS model, which focused on symptom expression that could be assisted.

2. Understanding that a psychosocial response is not synonymous with a health or clinical response, and therefore needs to be broad, based on an understanding of the capabilities of the voluntary and community organisations in the region.

3. Person-centred care, identifying what the people whom we are seeking to support feel they need, and recognising that what service users want may not be what they need and could cause further harm. There should be an ability to adapt the outreach and active interventions in the future.

4. Ensuring that accepted standards for patient safety, clinical care, and confidentiality of clients are adopted.

5. Looking after the Hub's workforce, including supervision, line management, daily check-in sessions, and encouraging people to develop a personal psychosocial wellbeing plan.

6. Making a whole family offer in recognition that those affected were not limited to the individual people in attendance, and also to enlist the support of family systems around individual people.

7. Enhancing existing services rather than creating new or duplicate services, to enable coordination of existing services and enhanced provision to make pathways smoother for the clients.

8. Using technology to assist with screening the high volumes of people affected.

9. Maintaining a flexible and innovative approach to the services offered.

The Work of the Hub over the First 4 Years

Targeted Outreach, Assessment, and Support after the Manchester Arena Bombing

The work began by supporting and coordinating the psychosocial needs of at least 700 people, whose details had been provided by the police and colleagues working in the acute healthcare services, largely comprising bereaved and seriously injured people, and key witnesses.

Wider Outreach and Screening after the Manchester Arena Bombing

With no prior data-sharing agreements in place, and working within legal constraints for sharing personal data, the Hub requested and received the email addresses of all who had purchased tickets online, approximately 97% of all sales. After careful work by council colleagues to ensure that no one who had been killed in the attack was included on the list, it formed the basis of the next, broader outreach and screening phase, 12 weeks after the attack. The 2005 National Institute for Health and Care Excellence (NICE) guidelines [2,3], current at the time, recommended 12 weeks of watchful waiting that acted as a period of natural recovery before intervention. With permission to use the data only once, everyone on the list was sent a letter that acknowledged their purchase of a ticket, requesting they pass the contents of the letter on to anybody else who they knew had attended or used the tickets, advising them of the Hub support offer and encouraging them, whether or not they were struggling, to participate in an online wellbeing screening programme. This was in addition to other outreach via local media, police, and victim services. Validated self-report measures were utilised as per routine clinical practice, and are described in detail by Paul French and colleagues [4]. Clinicians working in the Hub designed algorithms to enable the web-based system to categorise responses based on clinical risk and symptom expression, which in turn helped the staff to use human resources to triage contacts.

From week 12 after the incident, the mass outreach and screening programme commenced, targeting at least 15,500 people. This resulted in at least 3,790 people seeking psychosocial and mental health support from the Hub over the first 4.5 years.

The first 9 months of screening data indicated that people who responded and were screened earlier (3 months after the incident) tended to be less symptomatic and to show more rapid recovery [4]. More than one-third of adults initially presented with moderate or severe depression and anxiety, and half presented with probable post-traumatic stress disorder (PTSD). Around 25% of children and young people (8–18 years) had clinically significant depression scores, and 83% presented with possible PTSD [5]. In total, 80% of those people who engaged in screening did not live in Greater Manchester. The use of technology helped the Hub to identify and support affected people who lived outside Greater Manchester, including people from other countries. More than ten times as many as the 350 or more people who were physically harmed sought psychosocial support from the Hub. Proactive outreach identified more than 200 people who expressed thoughts of harming themselves and being better off dead for more than half the days of the week, 50% of whom had not planned to seek help for themselves. This alone made the outreach and screening element hugely important, to help to ensure that the death toll did not rise still further.

Facilitating Intervention

With high numbers of people reporting clinically significant levels of need, a large proportion of those who were supported by the Hub received evidence-based treatments, primarily NICE-approved psychological therapies. The existing mainstream commissioned services were used, along with VCSE provision where appropriate, before the Hub used its own limited treatment capacity for complex cases and for people who were otherwise unable to have their needs met. Charitable funding made it possible to commission private therapy for people if it was unavailable but in the best interests of children and young people.

Family Events

The Hub worked on the basis that building relationships with families enabled regular contact and contributed to strengthening support structures. In response to service user feedback, and motivated by the family events held after the Utøya attacks in Norway [6], Hub staff delivered clinically facilitated family events on managing trauma, with voluntary sector staff and police in support. These responses offered a safe environment in which children and adults could meet, validate their experiences, learn more about reactions to single-incident trauma, and improve communication within their families.

Consultation and Advice, including Support for Children, Young People, and Families

Active outreach included working closely with schools and the local health and social care services. The co-location and integration of both adult and child clinicians within the Hub enabled this and facilitated skill sharing across mental health services. The work highlighted varied skills, knowledge, and confidence in the roles that educational establishments have in supporting young people and their parents.

Hub staff have been involved in advising and supporting people after several significant regional, national, and international terrorist and mass casualty incidents since 2017. Learning has also informed mental health guidance from EPRR specialists in NHS England [7].

Site Visits

Based on feedback from people involved in the incident, some people considered that revisiting the scene was important; these visits complemented their trauma-focused therapy. The Hub-facilitated visits took place in person or by using 360-degree video virtual environments created by Salford University's telepresence department.

Training the Workforce in Trauma Therapy

Staff from the Hub and local and national mental health services, including those with experience of working with people after other terrorist bombing attacks, supported specialist training of the local trauma therapy workforce. This training boosted the confidence of the wider workforce.

The Public Inquiry

A public inquiry was established in 2019. The Hub worked in collaboration with it to make it the first trauma-responsive inquiry in the UK. Onsite support was available to everyone involved; families, witnesses, and legal teams were offered bespoke training packages and advice, which were utilised throughout. At the time of publication of this book the public inquiry had only just concluded, so it was not possible to consider more extensive detail about conclusions and processes.

Trusted Relations

Since 2018, the Hub has also held a Home Office contract to embed trauma-informed psychological consultation into complex safeguarding teams across the region. It enables staff of the police, probation, social, third sector, and housing services to better support children and young people at risk of sexual exploitation, county lines gang crime, or relationship abuse.

Healthcare Staff Wellbeing during COVID-19

When COVID-19 reached the UK in early 2020, the Hub, with its experience and expertise in providing large-scale psychosocial support for people, organisations, and systems, was regarded as a regional centre of excellence to be approached to assist in the response by utilising outreach, screening, assessment, advice, consultation, peer support, and referral for and direct delivery of therapy. The work of the Hub in supporting the healthcare workforce during the pandemic, and the subsequent rollout in England of 40 other wellbeing hubs broadly based on the Greater Manchester Resilience Hub model, are described in Chapter 46.

Designing and Delivering a Strategic Psychosocial and Mental Health Response: Lessons Identified from the Manchester Arena Bombing

This section identifies principles that are important for enabling responsible authorities to respond to the impacts of major incidents such as the Manchester Arena bombing. Here we consider the background that is specific to the Manchester locality, the short-, medium-, and long-term impacts experienced, the implications for intervention, and practical aspects of implementing these principles.

Greater Manchester Health and Social Care Partnership is the subject of an arrangement made in 2016 that has devolved responsibility for the money spent on health and social care in the 10 local authorities in Greater Manchester. The partnership approach that was adopted resulted in familiarity with working across geographical, functional, organisational, and political boundaries. Local systems and expertise were trusted and utilised without having to wait for the involvement or approval of national government. This demonstrates that the responsible authorities need to be clear about their jurisdiction, powers, and arrangements for mutual aid, in order to promote a quick, proportionate, and effective psychosocial response.

The response to the Manchester Arena bombing in 2017 was based on established emergency plans that were in place across the NHS, ambulance, fire, and police services, and the 10 local authorities in Greater Manchester. Although NHS colleagues in acute care and ambulance services had routinely planned, practised, and reviewed how to respond to major incidents, staff in NHS mental health services had not been routinely expected to do this. The lesson is that it is advisable to include statutory mental health providers as early as possible in discussions, response plans, and training activities.

In responding to the attack, the mental health and related services adopted a pioneering approach based on their experience of working together and keeping the people affected at the heart of the response. The expertise and experience of the clinical professionals involved were considered to embody good practice, and enabled the acceptance of expert input to the response. This shows how important it is to know who are the local mental health clinical experts, what capacity can be made available to support major incidents, and how the psychosocial and mental health response is to be led.

Being Agile, Adaptable, and Flexible as the Response Develops

New and unexpected developments occur from a range of sources on a regular basis, and can exacerbate psychological distress, so it is important to be able to adapt quickly. Examples from after the Manchester bombing included media intrusion, unsolicited gifts being sent to some affected people and not others, family trips abroad being arranged by travel agencies, and the impacts of perceived inequalities in the distribution of financial gifts. The lesson is that well-meaning but unhelpful offers of help need delicate but robust management.

Communication

From the outset, it was clear that communication was a vital part of the response, taking account of the need for an intergenerational response and of the fact that the people affected had come not only from all over the UK but also from other countries.

The communication strategy had to consider how to provide information that would be helpful to anyone who had been present at the Arena event and anyone who might be affected (e.g., professional staff, volunteers, schools and colleges, concerned members of communities). The language used by all parts of the system, including the police, to convey information to people affected benefited from review by the Hub to ensure that it was trauma-informed, consistent, and accurate. There was also a need to identify unhelpful messages, and effective relationships with local media can be helpful.

Information Sharing

Data-sharing agreements were not in place from the outset. There needs to be an understanding that different agencies have different priorities for protecting confidentiality, and that they have to balance these with their duty to share information.

Utilising Technology Allows Rapid Outreach and High-Volume Screening

Embracing technology is clearly advantageous for efficiency and speed of messaging and screening. However, digital inequalities may be greater for other incidents than was the case for engaging the people who were able to attend this high-ticket-price event. A range of methods of communication (e.g., provision of hard-copy materials, use of signing) need to be considered, and the languages likely to be spoken by the people affected also need to be taken into account.

The Mental Health Workforce

Psychosocial and psychological systems thinking needed to be trauma-informed and trauma-responsive. Clinicians were seconded to the Hub, and this model enabled expertise from the incident to be transferred back into mainstream services. This approach aided access to existing helpful material as well as providing training, support, and supervision of staff and volunteers as well as associated services. Combining staff from child and adolescent, adult, and specialist trauma services made it possible to meet the particular needs of people affected by the Manchester Arena bombing.

Assessing the Effectiveness of What is Being Offered

Information gathering and data capture took place during the early and ongoing stages of the incident and, when combined with user surveys, enabled the establishment of a research team to evaluate screening data, monitor individual people's trajectories of recovery, and gather qualitative data.

Taking Account of Secondary Stressors and Their Impact on the People Involved

Preventive actions were put in place to address the likely impact of secondary stressors (see Chapter 9). They included information about how to access financial advice and other practical financial support for those people whose livelihoods had been affected, and liaison with schools and colleges to advocate for younger victims who struggled with crowds and alarms during breaks, or were unable to concentrate during exams.

Practical Aspects of Implementing the Principles

In Chapter 5, the authors describe the common reactions and trajectories of stress responses across a range of indications and diverse contexts. In this case study, the views of the professional clinical staff who led and were involved in the response are described in terms of the actions taken over time.

John Stancombe and his colleagues sought to understand the experience of distress among people involved in the Manchester Arena bombing by conducting semi-structured interviews with a group of survivors who were not physically injured [8]. They concluded that after many incidents it is likely that provision is inadequate for people who are distressed, because of the ubiquity, duration, and severity of distress. This has implications for policy and service design. They reported the importance of all agencies coming together before any incident has occurred, in order to develop a comprehensive plan, describe interventions that support the wellbeing and psychosocial care of everyone who is involved, and be more aware of the potential duration of effects, particularly for those people who require psychosocial care.

Psychosocial and Mental Health Actions Immediately after and up to 4 Weeks after an Incident

Services and organisations that deliver psychosocial care and mental healthcare should be coordinated through local care pathways and integrated within the wider response and recovery plan and with primary and acute healthcare services. The principle of making evidence-informed and appropriate care available at the right time must be followed at all stages of the clinical pathway.

Primary and community care practitioners have an important role in recognising people who require psychosocial care as well as those people who may be at greater risk of developing mental health problems. They should offer to monitor people at risk and access support for them.

Psychosocial and Mental Health Responses in the Short Term (1–3 Months)

Services should be flexible and use, or expand as necessary, the existing resources available in the health system and local communities. They should collaborate with the voluntary sector and other partner organisations. Everyone affected should continue to be able to access psychosocial care, including those people who do not meet the criteria for referral to specialist mental health services. Institutions should allow everyone confidential access to services. Social media can be used to inform the public about the availability of services.

It may be unclear whether people who continue to be distressed are taking longer to recover because they are affected by secondary stressors, and/or because they have a mental health problem. Early recognition and appropriate referral are particularly important for people who have sustained problems and high levels of stress.

The population affected, and particularly those people at risk of developing mental health problems or who have a history of mental health difficulties, should be monitored and screened to ascertain who needs specialist assessment.

Information about the people affected must continue to be collected, in order to inform any adjustments to the care pathways required, as well as any changes to the assessments and interventions required.

Psychosocial and Mental Health Responses in the Medium Term (3 Months to 1 Year)

It may still be unclear 3 months to 1 year after incidents whether people who continue to be distressed:

- belong to particular groups within the population
- are taking longer to recover
- are experiencing secondary stressors that are maintaining their distress
- have a recognisable mental health problem.

Access to psychosocial care must continue to be available through the first years after the incident, because early recognition and effective responses to their needs are important. In addition, people who may have a recognisable mental health problem require an appropriate referral; this is particularly important for people who have persistent problems and high levels of stress.

As already described in relation to short-term responses, people who are thought to be experiencing secondary stressors should be offered opportunities to explore any suitable non-healthcare interventions that may be required.

Plans for memorials, commemorations, and inquests should be discussed with bereaved people, community leaders, the police, and other partner organisations, and should be culturally sensitive [9].

Research and evaluation should continue to be an integral part of the response to major incidents, and should be set up in the early stages.

Psychosocial and Mental Health Responses in The Long Term (from 1 Year Onward)

People may come forward for help a long time after an incident, and their distress may have remained below the threshold for diagnosis of a mental health problem. Professional practitioners and staff of services often present later than members of the public.

Services should make resources available for at least 5 years after a major incident. The graduated scaling down of psychosocial, monitoring, screening, and mental health services specific to major incidents must be coordinated. In parallel, arrangements should be made to redirect people who are seeking help to services commissioned to provide this as 'business as usual'.

Long-term planning should include assisting people affected by incidents and professionals by informing them how they may react to anniversaries and any further inquests or other legal proceedings.

Conclusions

Psychosocial needs, including mental health impacts, should form part of all emergency preparedness plans. Training and exercising these arrangements should involve the people who are likely to deliver them.

The psychosocial tail following major and mass casualty incidents is often much larger and longer than the immediate and physical effects of the incident, and its impact is likely to vary depending on factors such as pre-incident vulnerabilities, social support available, proximity to the incident, whether people are physically injured or bereaved, and timeliness of access to appropriate interventions. Identification and utilisation of existing expertise within local systems will contribute to a coordinated psychosocial response.

Psychosocial needs are likely to be broad and varied. Therefore coordinated multiagency responses are required to effectively support the people affected. Genuine multiagency collaboration will help to lead to better outcomes for everyone. Clinically informed responses and psychosocially informed systemic work are both possible and desirable.

References

1. World Health Organization. *Psychological First Aid: Guide for Field Workers.* World Health Organization, 2011.

2. National Institute for Health and Care Excellence. *Post-Traumatic Stress Disorder. NICE Guideline [NG116].* National Institute for Health and Care Excellence, 2015. Note to readers: this was the guideline available at the time of the Manchester Arena bombing. It was subsequently superseded by the guideline in reference [3].

3. National Institute for Health and Care Excellence. *Post-Traumatic Stress Disorder. NICE Guideline [NG116].* National Institute for Health and Care Excellence, 2018

(www.nice.org.uk/guidance/ng116).

4. French P, Barrett A, Allsopp K, Williams R, Brewin CR, Hind D, et al. Psychological screening of adults and young people following the Manchester Arena incident. *BJPsych Open* 2019; 5: e85.

5. Allsopp K, Brewin CR, Barrett A, Williams R, Hind D, Chitsabesan P, et al. Responding to mental health needs after terror attacks *BMJ* 2019; 366: l4828.

6. Dyregrov A, Dyregrov K, Straume M, Grønvold Bugge R. Weekend family gatherings for bereaved after the terror killings in Norway in 2011. *Scand Psychol* 2014; 1: e8.

7. NHS England and NHS Improvement. *Responding to the Needs of People Affected by Incidents and Emergencies: A Framework for Planning and Delivering Psychosocial and Mental Health Care.* NHS England and NHS Improvement, 2021.

8. Stancombe J, Williams R, Drury J, Collins H, Lagan L, Barrett A, et al. People's experiences of distress and psychosocial care following a terrorist attack: interviews with survivors of the Manchester Arena bombing in 2017. *BJPsych Open* 2022; 8: e41.

9. Collins H, Allsopp K, Arvanitis K, Chitsabesan P, French P. Psychological impact of spontaneous memorials: a narrative review. *Psychol Trauma* 2022; 14: 1230–36.

The Moral Architecture of Healthcare Systems and Other Organisations

Richard Williams and Verity Kemp

Introduction

This chapter introduces the concept of the moral architecture of healthcare systems and organisations and, by implication, local authority, police, and fire and rescue services. Core to this theme is what helps staff to give of their best, which is related to the support and care that they receive from their employing and deploying organisations, their colleagues, and their families and friends. The chapter also offers descriptions of work undertaken to assess what helps and does not help staff both in a broader context and during the COVID-19 pandemic.

Earlier in the book, Chapter 9 describes, defines, and gives examples of primary and secondary stressors [1]. We know, because healthcare staff have told us, that during the COVID-19 pandemic, secondary stressors affected them to a great degree, and in some circumstances more than primary stressors did. Certainly the concerns raised by staff who seek help very frequently are about secondary stressors, and many of them are about the environments and conditions in which they work [1,2]. Therefore moral architecture includes the arrangements made by employers to reduce to a minimum the secondary stressors that affect their staff. However, it goes further than this because it also includes the supporting arrangements that employers put in place to meet the needs of their staff with a view to helping them to discharge difficult jobs well when they are under pressure. The concept also embraces the vigilance that employers should maintain to prevent pressures from external sources, including performance management, from bringing to bear on staff unnecessary and unintended additional pressures that are not orientated to assisting them to do well.

Arlie Hochschild describes working with people affected by illness and personal problems as 'work done with feelings', and this takes us to the concept of emotional labour [3]. This chapter focuses on the implications of moral architecture for staff in organisations that provide care for people who are unwell. Common experience is that, without the passion, commitment, carefully positioned relationships, and emotional labour of staff, the quality of the care of patients is unlikely to be optimal either routinely or in emergencies [4,5].

In this respect this chapter resonates with Chapter 41, which provides the results of a number of research studies and one qualitative study of interviews given by nurses during the COVID-19 pandemic, which draw attention to the need for health services to be vigilant about sustaining their staff. We think that similar arguments apply in full measure to each of the rescue services that are involved in emergencies, incidents, and disasters. Chapter 41 also provides substantial descriptions by nurses, who were participants in the research, of the many forms that secondary stressors can take.

Thus we begin Section 5 of this book by outlining moral architecture in order to provide a framework for considering the information, experiences, and opinions presented in the eight chapters and four case studies that comprise this section.

Moral Architecture

Our definition of moral architecture refers to the moral and human rights obligations that organisations acquire as employers and through their commitment to delivering high-quality services. Richard Williams and his colleagues and Adrian Neal and colleagues explore this construct in two book chapters [4,5]. In essence their view is that, as well as legal responsibilities to staff, employers have moral responsibilities for them. This concept therefore parallels those of moral distress and moral injury that are covered in more detail in Chapter 39. Thus the moral architecture of organisations includes how well employers discharge implied moral responsibilities, in addition to their legal responsibilities, with a view to protecting and caring for their staff.

In this regard, it is important that responsible authorities recognise the implied psychological contracts between them and the staff whom they employ directly or indirectly, or cause to be employed. These obligations should be reflected in organisations' policies, their design and delivery of services, and their corporate and clinical governance. This means that each healthcare organisation's visions, priorities, structures, activities, leadership, management, and conditions of staff employment should be consistent with its stated roles and espoused values. Usually the ways in which organisations care for their staff test their moral architecture [6].

A survey conducted by NHS Employers in England in 2020 concluded that 'clinicians are working incredibly hard in the most extraordinary circumstances the NHS has ever faced, but without the right safety measures in place, they're still living in fear for their own health and the health of their families. Confidence in the system they work in is low and more must be done to regain that trust' [7]. Thus the advent of COVID-19 brought greatly heightened challenges to healthcare services across the world not only to maintain their ordinary services for the public and continue to meet the support and care needs of their employees, but also to rise to the enormous additional demands in both domains brought by the pandemic. Rapidly we became aware, early in the pandemic that, despite earnest endeavours to do their very best, many services were likely to struggle to meet these demands. This was not only because of their nature and extent during the pandemic, but also because of a substantial legacy of poor relationships with staff prior to the pandemic, which became more apparent as the pandemic progressed in the UK.

Psychological Safety as a Component of Moral Architecture

The concept of psychological safety concerns the degree to which people perceive their work environments as conducive to taking necessary interpersonal risks when working. There is evidence that working environments that are psychologically safe are not only better for the wellbeing and welfare of the staff, but also less likely to result in errors of judgement or mistakes [8]. Leaders and managers should take responsibility for creating working environments that are as psychologically safe as possible, and this therefore includes the need for them to take into account the secondary stressors reported by their staff.

Leaders play important roles in fostering environments that contain their staff's emotions in ways that are realistic and safe, to enhance patient care and prepare staff for new challenges. This requires team leaders to be aware of team members' psychosocial capabilities and training needs and ensure that they receive professional supervision, effective management, and psychosocial support.

Well before the COVID-19 pandemic there were concerns about ensuring the wellbeing and health of healthcare staff. Things have changed for wider society as a consequence of COVID-19 and the measures taken, but healthcare workers and their families have been through very challenging experiences as a result of trying to manage the risks. Past studies have shown that people working in frontline roles, such as firefighters, gain a huge amount of support from their families [9].

Research undertaken before the COVID-19 pandemic among ambulance staff with varying roles has already highlighted the impact of what we would describe as poor moral architecture. Lucy Clark and colleagues undertook a systematic review of the literature on mental health, wellbeing, and support interventions for UK ambulance staff in order to identify evidence gaps [10]. The authors of the review reported that their evidence map provides a context for planning and research into providing for wellbeing of staff after the pandemic.

Kaye Adams and colleagues report on the stress and wellbeing of emergency medical dispatchers who provide remotely crisis intervention for medical emergencies through telehealth support [11]. They have stated that 'organisational membership was negatively affected through perceptions of insufficient positive feedback and the absence of team cohesiveness ... exclusion from ... organisation activated psychological support after traumatic events, promotions, rewards and ceremonies, were all found to contribute to a sense of decreased value by the organisation' [11]. Astrid Coxon and colleagues have studied the experiences of ambulance dispatch personnel, in order to identify key stressors and their impact on staff wellbeing. They found that 'even the most resilient staff stated that at some points they find the pressures of their role, combined with a lack of appropriate support or recovery time, overwhelms any intrinsic motivation for the job' [12]. Susan Clompus and colleagues have researched the subject of staff resilience in their workplaces. Focusing on the experiences of paramedics, they found that 'Participants encountered many situations requiring managerial feedback and guidance, but this was not always forthcoming', and they reported that this may leave staff demoralised [13]. This finding resonates with work by Janice Halpern and colleagues, who conducted a qualitative study of ambulance workers with the aim of characterising critical incidents and eliciting ideas for interventions. They found that the participants valued support from supervisors and peers, and having a 'timeout' period immediately after a critical incident [14]. Research has repeatedly found that peer support, from colleagues, friends, or family members, has been highlighted as a means of dealing with the feelings described as guilt and shame that are experienced by workers, and thereby mitigating the possibility of their developing post-traumatic stress symptoms [15]. Daniel Patterson and colleagues point to the impact of employees' negative experiences in their workplace environments and how this contributes to reduced retention of employees [16]. In their study, Diego Silva and colleagues highlight the importance of what they term moral climate [17]. They report that factors which contribute to a positive moral climate include alignment with the organisation's stated values, transparency about management processes, decisions, and actions, staff engagement in organisational decision making, opportunities to raise and discuss difficult ethical issues without fear of reprisals, public recognition of achievements, respectful relationships among staff, and fair employment practices.

These features of moral climate appear to the authors of this chapter to be similar to our construct of moral architecture. The connection between reducing secondary stressors and moral architecture is striking in the examples that we offer in this chapter, and the link with psychosocial pressures on staff is illustrated in Chapters 38 and 39.

Furthermore, Silva and colleagues emphasise the importance of there being a 'bedside to boardroom' strategy for ethics in healthcare organisations [17]. We agree strongly with this assertion, and Chapter 52 provides a commentary on lessons for public ethics in emergencies that have been derived from the COVID-19 pandemic.

Aspects of Moral Architecture in Events in the USA and the UK

The Long-Term Impacts on Staff of 9/11, and the Implications for Staff Care

Erin Smith and colleagues conducted a qualitative study of the reflections of paramedics and emergency medical technicians on the long-term impacts of their responding to the 9/11 terrorist attacks on 11 September 2001 in New York City [18]. The study contributed to an improved understanding of the long-term impacts on paramedics and emergency medical technicians (EMTs). These impacts were categorised as psychosocial and physical health reflections.

Psychosocial reflections included survivor guilt, ruminating on actions that they had failed to take, and thinking over actions that they had taken and what they might have done differently. A high prevalence of post-traumatic stress disorder (PTSD) was concerning not only on its own account, but also because of the association of PTSD with other mental health disorders, including depression, anxiety, and cognitive impairment (e.g., poor memory, impaired concentration). The ways in which anniversaries were marked created feelings of anxiety and frustration, and participants wanted anniversaries to be marked in more sympathetic and fitting ways.

Physical health reflections included the immense release of toxic dust created by the collapse of the World Trade Center, which caused physical and chemical irritation of the respiratory and gastrointestinal systems of emergency responders as well as people who lived and worked in the Lower Manhattan area. In addition to concerns about respiratory problems, there were growing concerns among paramedics and EMTs about the possibility of developing cancer, and increased rates of cancer were reported.

The conclusion of this research was that paramedics and EMTs continued to suffer the psychosocial, mental health, and physical health consequences of their involvement in the response to 9/11. The effects were ongoing 15 years after the attack, and there are anecdotal reports that this was also the case at the twentieth anniversary in 2021.

The research did reveal responses about which employers could take action to improve their moral architecture, even if they would not have labelled them as such. An example is adapting the ways in which anniversaries are marked to take account of the needs of the people who were responders. Other activities that might have benefited from being adapted to the needs of the responders affected included counselling associated with health research studies. Responders reported often feeling 'rushed and unheard', and the extension of the support and counselling beyond the responders directly involved to include their partners who 'inherited the emotional impact' [18].

The Manchester Arena Bombing in 2017

On 22 May 2017, a suicide bomber detonated an improvised explosive device at the Manchester Arena in the UK. In total, 22 members of the public were killed. Their ages ranged from 8 to 51 years, and the proportion of children and younger people was especially high because of the nature of the concert that they were attending. Several hundred more people were injured physically, thousands were affected psychosocially, and some have been affected by mental health disorders.

Chapters 5 and 28 include findings from the description of the Social Influences on Recovery Enquiry (SIRE) [19,20]. This explored the experiences and opinions of people who used the Manchester Resilience Hub over a period of more than 3 years after the bombing. The potential to improve moral architecture, although it would not be labelled as such, is one outcome of the research. SIRE provided evidence that identified 10 practical implications for planning and delivering services, and we argue that these implications apply as much to the staff whom the services employ, and to volunteers, as they do to the public. They can be summarised as follows:

1. actions to implement the wellbeing, psychosocial, and mental health agendas (see Chapters 12, 27, and 44 for more details)
2. a greater emphasis on psychosocial care in strategic planning and delivery
3. supporting wellbeing for everyone affected, and for their relatives and friends
4. services providing care that is guided by the principles of psychological first aid
5. assessing and monitoring people in need
6. attending to the impact of secondary stressors
7. strengthening recognition of the contributions of families, friends, and significant others
8. strengthening the contribution of communities – fostering collective support
9. ensuring delivery of accessible and scalable psychosocial care
10. providing training and support for professionals and lay volunteers.

Organisational Support during the COVID-19 Pandemic

Research undertaken during the COVID-19 pandemic has demonstrated the importance of organisational support for staff. Neil Greenberg and colleagues suggest that NHS managers should 'prioritize (sic) provision of evidence-based staff support which is likely to . . . improve psychological wellbeing and decrease the likelihood of psychologically unwell staff delivering substandard care' [21]. Catherine Montgomery and colleagues took a sociological perspective to look at the experience of working in intensive care units during the COVID-19 pandemic. Their findings support the importance of considering social and organisational factors that affect staff wellbeing to be an extension of considering individual members of staff [22]. We go further than this, and see team and group activities to develop and improve care for staff as lying at the core of moving towards good moral architecture. A study on the wellbeing, mental health, and work impacts of COVID-19 on first professional responders and frontline workers in Australia highlights many areas that the authors identified as requiring improvement at an organisational level. Communication was highlighted as being important, including the need for improvement of what staff perceived as 'a lack of listening, consultation and trust from their management/leadership team' [23].

In another paper, Greenberg outlines a practical approach for protecting the mental health of healthcare (sic) workers based on contemporary evidence [24]. It takes account of how healthcare workers involved in the COVID-19 response have often been required to work in highly challenging conditions, and are therefore quite possibly at increased risk of manifesting mental health problems. Greenberg points to the probability that healthcare workers have faced morally distressing situations, and the role of managers in supporting them using methods such as Schwartz Rounds. There is an unwritten psychological contract between healthcare staff, their managers, and the public. Staff are more likely to give their all if their employers provide proper support.

Greenberg also asserts that managers of healthcare services have an important role in protecting the mental health of staff [24]. Chapter 47 provides a highly relevant illustration of these points.

Clark and colleagues have developed an evidence map of wellbeing and support interventions for staff of UK ambulance services, and they note that the NHS in the UK was actively engaged in considering the wellbeing and health needs of the workforce before the pandemic [10]. They identified staff working in ambulance services as a priority in the short- and long-term outcomes of the pandemic.

The Impacts of COVID-19 on the Needs of Staff

There is a great deal more that we could say about the impacts of working through the COVID-19 pandemic on the needs of healthcare staff. We summarise the effects here by referring to just two sources.

We know from the NHS Staff Survey for 2019, which was published in February 2020, before the pandemic began, that 40.3% of staff had felt unwell as a result of work-related stress in the previous 12 months. The report on the survey notes that this proportion has been steadily increasing from 36.8% since 2016 [25]. The survey for 2020 shows that the proportion of NHS staff who reported feeling unwell as a result of work-related stress increased by nearly 10% in 2020, as the pandemic took hold [7]. The report for 2020 also found that around one-third of staff (34%) had worked on a COVID-19-specific ward or area at some time, and around half of staff who had done so reported feeling unwell as a result of work-related stress [7]. Taken together, these reports substantiate the evidence that there were problems in caring effectively for staff of the NHS before the COVID-19 pandemic started, which were exacerbated by the experiences of staff during the pandemic. However, the original problems with staff care in overstressed healthcare organisations have yet to be dealt with effectively.

The House of Commons *Health and Social Care Committee Report on Workforce Burnout and Resilience in the NHS and Social Care* was published in June 2021 [26]. It reported on the workforce issues facing staff in the NHS and social care, and took into account the additional impact of COVID-19. It concluded that burnout has a significant impact on and negative consequences for the mental health of individual members of staff, with consequent impacts on colleagues, and on the patients for whom they care.

Conclusion

We started this chapter by defining moral architecture. Providing compassionate, evidence-informed, and values-based care is hard work for healthcare staff. It was hard work before COVID-19, it was even harder during the pandemic, and it has proved harder still since then.

Healthcare organisations should ensure that they support their staff in the best of ways. An explicit approach to ensuring that organisations embrace the concept of moral architecture is required if staff are to be able to continue providing compassionate care.

Elements that indicate that an organisation has good moral architecture include the following:

- compatibility between the training, support, and care of staff offered by an employing organisation and the quality of care that those staff are expected to deliver [4,27]
- compatibility between each organisation's approach to defining and describing its corporate and clinical governance in policy documents and service design and delivery [28]; this is demonstrated by, for example, conditions of employment, the style of leadership, organisational vision and priorities, and structures being aligned with its explicit values and purpose [6]

We propose that organisations can ensure sustenance of compassionate care when they work explicitly towards establishing, developing, and maintaining their responsive moral architectures.

References

1. Williams R, Ntontis E, Alfadhli K, Drury J, Amlôt R. A social model of secondary stressors in relation to disasters, major incidents and conflict: implications for practice. *Int J Disaster Risk Reduct* 2021; 63: 102436.

2. Murray E, Kaufman KR, Williams R. Let us do better: learning lessons for recovery of healthcare professionals during and after COVID-19 *BJPsych Open* 2021; 7: e151.

3. Hochschild AR. *The Managed Heart: Commercialization of Human Feeling*. University of California Press, 1983.

4. Williams R, Kemp V, Neal A. Compassionate care: leading and caring for staff of mental health

services and the moral architecture of healthcare organisations. In *Management for Psychiatrists* (eds Bhugra D, Bell S, Burns S): 377–402. Royal College of Psychiatrists Publication, 2016.

5. Neal A, Kemp V, Williams R. Caring for the carers. In *Social Scaffolding: Applying the Lessons of Contemporary Social Science to Health and Healthcare* (eds Williams R, Kemp V, Haslam SA, et al.): 289–303. Cambridge University Press, 2019.

6. Williams R. A cunning plan: integrating evidence, judgement and passion in mental health strategy. The Inaugural Lecture of Professor Richard Williams, delivered at the University of Glamorgan, November 2000.

7. NHS Employers. *NHS Staff Survey 2020*. NHS Employers, 2021 (www.england.nhs.uk/statistics/2021/03/11/2020-national-nhs-staff-survey/).

8. Bleetman A, Sanusi S, Dale T, Brace S. Human factors and error prevention in emergency medicine. *Emerg Med J* 2012; 29: 389–93.

9. Hill R, Sundin E, Winder B. Work–family enrichment of firefighters: "satellite family members", risk, trauma and family functioning. *Int J Emerg Serv* 2020; 9: 395–407.

10. Clark LV, Fida R, Skinner J, et al. Mental health, well-being and support interventions for UK ambulance services staff: an evidence map, 2000 to 2020. *Br Paramed J* 2021; 5: 25–39.

11. Adams K, Shakespeare-Finch J, Armstrong D. An interpretative phenomenological analysis of stress and well-being in emergency medical dispatchers. *J Loss Trauma* 2015; 20: 430–48.

12. Coxon A, Cropley M, Schofield P, Start K, Horsfield C, Quinn T. 'You're never making just one decision': exploring the lived experiences of ambulance

Emergency Operations Centre personnel. *Emerg Med J* 2016; 33: 645–51.

13. Clompus SR, Albarran JW. Exploring the nature of resilience in paramedic practice: a psycho-social study. *Int Emerg Nurs* 2015; 28: 1–7.

14. Halpern J, Gurevich M, Schwartz B, Brazeau P. What makes an incident critical for ambulance workers? Emotional outcomes and implications for intervention. *Work Stress* 2009; 23: 173–89.

15. Jonsson A, Segesten K. Guilt, shame and need for a container: a study of post-traumatic stress among ambulance personnel. *Accid Emerg Nurs* 2004; 12: 215–23.

16. Patterson P, Probst J, Leith K, Corwin S, Powell P. Recruitment and retention of emergency medical technicians: a qualitative study. *J Allied Health* 2005; 34: 153–62.

17. Silva DS, Gibson JL, Sibbald R, Connolly E, Singer PA. Clinical ethicists' perspectives on organisational ethics in healthcare organisations. *J Med Ethics* 2008; 34: 320–23.

18. Smith EC, Burkle FM. Paramedic and emergency medical technician reflections on the ongoing impact of the 9/11 terrorist attacks. *Prehosp Disaster Med* 2019; 34: 56–61.

19. Stancombe J, Williams R, Drury J, Collins H, Lagan L, Barrett A, et al. People's experiences of distress and psychosocial care following a terrorist attack: interviews with survivors of the Manchester Arena bombing in 2017. *BJPsych Open* 2022; 8: e41.

20. Drury J, Stancombe J, Williams R, Collins H, Lagan L, Barrett A, et al. Survivors' experiences of informal social support in coping and recovering after the 2017 Manchester Arena bombing. *BJPsych Open* 2022; 8: e124.

21. Greenberg N, Weston D, Hall C, Caulfield T, Williamson V, Fong K. Mental health of staff working in intensive care during COVID-19. *Occup Med* 2021; 71: 62–7.

22. Montgomery CM, Humphreys S, McCulloch C, et al. Critical care work during COVID-19: a qualitative study of staff experiences in the UK. *BMJ Open* 2021; 11: e048124.

23. Roberts R, Dwivedi A, Bamberry L, Neher A, Jenkins S, Sutton C, et al. *The Mental Health, Wellbeing and Work Impacts of COVID-19 on First Responders and Frontline Workers in Australia*. Charles Sturt University, 2021.

24. Greenberg N. Mental health of health-care workers in the COVID-19 era. *Nat Rev Nephrol* 2020; 16: 425–6.

25. NHS Employers. *NHS Staff Survey 2019*. NHS Employers, 2020 (www.nhsemployers.org/retention-and-staff-experience/staff-engagement/the-nhs-staff-survey).

26. House of Commons. *Workforce Burnout and Resilience in the NHS and Social Care*. House of Commons, 2021 (https://publications.parliament.uk/pa/cm5802/cmselect/cmhealth/22/2202.htm).

27. Williams R, Fulford KWM. Values-based and evidence-based policy, management and practice in child and adolescent mental health services. *Clin Child Psychol Psychiatry* 2007; 12: 223–42.

28. Warner M, Williams R. The nature of strategy and its application in statutory and non-statutory services. In *Child and Adolescent Mental Health Services: Strategic Approaches to Commissioning and Delivering Child and Adolescent Mental Health Services* (eds Williams R, Kerfoot M): 39–62. Oxford University Press, 2005.

Chapter

38

What Ails Professional Responders, and the Implications for Training and Sustaining Healthcare Practitioners

Jennifer Burgess, Andrew Wood, Suzy Stokes, John Stancombe, and Richard Williams

Introduction

Working in healthcare and the emergency services is recognised to be a rewarding but also highly demanding career choice. Some aspects of these jobs are perceived to be uniquely stressful, such as witnessing injuries, preventing deaths, and being expected to make important decisions under time pressure. As a result, there has been interest from both clinicians and academics in researching the psychosocial effects of working in these environments.

An Orientation to Working in Pre-Hospital Care

There is increasing awareness that working within the field of pre-hospital care can have psychosocial effects on clinicians. This has been brought into sharper focus by the COVID-19 pandemic, which has placed new and increasing demands on our workforce. Clinicians working in pre-hospital care are exposed to stressors, some of which are unique to the pre-hospital environment, whereas others are common across healthcare and workplaces more widely.

Pre-hospital care encompasses a range of clinicians working in diverse environments. In the UK, most practitioners work for NHS ambulance trusts; they include paramedics, call-handlers, and emergency medical technicians. A smaller group of clinicians work in specialist roles – for example, as advanced paramedics with extended skills, within hazardous area response teams (HART), and as doctors and paramedics within specialist teams such as medical emergency response incident teams (MERIT) and helicopter emergency medical services (HEMS).

Healthcare staff who work in pre-hospital environments are exposed to extraordinary events, and may witness suffering, distress, and death with unusually high frequency. Inevitably, some of the impacts are stressful by virtue of the enormity of other people's suffering and their injuries, the responsibilities that staff take on, and the fact that they may have to do demanding and skilful work in hazardous environments. These factors are primary stressors and are inherent in emergencies.

As Chapter 9 shows, secondary stressors are not inherent, but are circumstances, events, or policies that are both directly and indirectly related to work; they may relate to social, organisational, and financial matters. They include perceived job control, autonomy, workload, pay, work–life interface and balance, relationships at work, and the adequacy and effectiveness of employers' responses to primary stressors. They include circumstances that limit people's recovery from stressful events and can sustain adversity. Staff of public organisations have repeatedly commented that secondary stressors affect them to a greater degree than do the primary stressors; importantly, they include factors that are tractable and potentially modifiable by organisations.

Staff working in UK ambulance services are under pressure. Before the COVID-19 pandemic, demand on ambulance services had shown a relentless annual rise of around 5% over the past decade, which has not been matched by equal increases in funding. As a result, staff are being asked to do more with less resources, and have had to adapt to new models of working, such as seeing, treating, and discharging more patients in the community. In part to streamline processes and improve efficiency, there has also been large-scale reorganisation of ambulance services into centralised regional trusts, and within trusts, local community ambulance stations have been consolidated into a smaller number of larger hubs. The effects that these changes have had on the social fabric of these organisations are not well understood. However, it is clear that staff working for ambulance services are feeling the pressure, with some of the highest levels of staff sickness and absenteeism across the entire NHS, and that ambulance trusts are facing chronic difficulties in recruiting and retaining staff. There is alarming evidence that staff working in high-risk professions, such as paramedics, and doctors and nurses working in pre-hospital emergency medicine, have increased rates of stress, distress, burnout, and mental disorders.

Specialist Medical Teams

Some aspects of working within specialist teams such as HEMS and MERIT are thought to be protective for the wellbeing and mental health of clinicians, compared with other areas of pre-hospital care. They include:

- working closely with colleagues in highly developed teams
- working in an open culture, where scrutiny and learning are encouraged
- the many formal and informal opportunities to share and process feelings
- close supervision and support during training
- an ability to influence and effect organisational change.

Frontline healthcare workers in specialist teams, such as HEMS, are directly exposed to extreme and potentially traumatic events with unusual frequency, and they are also exposed to the suffering of the patients for whom they provide care, and of their relatives. These are both types of primary stressors. Primary stressors specific to HEMS include:

- exposure to the risks associated with responding by aircraft or rapid response vehicle
- exposure to on-scene dangers
- frequent, direct exposure to death, to survivors' serious injuries, and to witnesses' suffering
- regular exposure to high-acuity incidents and major incidents.

The matter of exposure as a major risk factor for both people who are directly affected and responders developing mental health problems has been well researched. This is often referred to as the dose effect, whereby 'long-term adverse outcomes are better predicted by the total number rather than the specific nature of environmental risk exposures', which is also described as the cumulative risk model [1].

A Systematic Review of the Literature

Special interest has been paid to first responders and other pre-hospital healthcare professionals, probably due to their role in high-profile incidents or disasters and the perceived demands of the job. Our aim was to conduct a comprehensive review of the literature, in order to evaluate current knowledge of the psychiatric and psychosocial consequences of working in pre-hospital care. In addition, we wanted to identify any factors that could be causative or that could contribute to these impacts.

A systematic review summarises all of the research published on a particular topic by specifying a search strategy and detailed inclusion criteria in advance. The quality of the studies, and therefore the strength of the evidence, is also assessed. This contrasts with other types of review, such as narrative reviews, in which the authors may choose only to discuss research results that support their own view. Our protocol, including our search strategy, was pre-registered on PROSPERO [2]. We searched seven academic databases using keywords, and we hand-searched five relevant journals. We included studies published in English from around the world, with no date limit. This initial search produced 6,365 citations. We removed duplicates, which returned 3,454 abstracts that were screened independently by two members of the team. In total, 359 papers were identified as suitable for further review. Two members of the team independently reviewed the full texts, and 169 papers were found to meet the criteria for inclusion in the review. Some papers reported the results of the same study, and on review 143 separate projects were identified.

Of the 169 papers that met the inclusion criteria, the majority reported quantitative research ($n = 132$), and there were 16 qualitative papers, 9 mixed methods, 11 reviews, and 1 case report. Among the papers that reported quantitative and mixed methods the most common methodology reported was cross-sectional ($n = 130$), with small numbers of cohort ($n = 4$), case-series ($n = 4$), and case–control ($n = 3$) studies. Of the reviews, six were systematic and five were narrative syntheses. The earliest date of publication included was 1988. Figure 38.1 shows that the number of publications per year has increased over the past decade.

Most studies were conducted in Westernised countries (e.g., UK, $n = 22$; Australia, $n = 19$; USA,

$n = 17$; Canada, $n = 13$); however, a small number were conducted in Iran ($n = 6$) and Asia (e.g., India, $n = 2$; China, $n = 1$). It is possible that non-Westernised countries conceptualise the psychosocial impacts of this work in a different way, and therefore were not captured by our search strategy. However, it is likely that this is a particular research interest of countries with extensive healthcare systems and organisations that fund this work. People working in a variety of professional roles participated, the most popular being paramedics (72 samples), EMTs (45 samples), dispatchers (18 samples), nurses (17 samples), and doctors (14 samples).

The Findings

Psychosocial Outcomes

The research team reviewed the quantitative and mixed methods papers and grouped the outcomes into 17 categories (see Table 38.1).

The most studied outcome was occupational functioning (58 papers), which most commonly looked specifically at burnout in professionals, but also included job satisfaction and time off sick. Symptoms of post-traumatic stress (56 papers) and common mental disorders such as anxiety and depression (30 papers about emotional symptoms, and 21 papers on general health and psychopathology) were well researched. However, notably only two papers reported on whether the participants met the criteria for or had been given a diagnosis, and instead the researchers used self-report questionnaires. These types of instruments are usually considered to screen for a particular disorder, and are

over-inclusive compared with clinical diagnosis. Stress, distress, and resilience are important factors that contribute significantly to a healthcare professional's daily experience of their job and their ability to perform it. However, these concepts were not well

Table 38.1 Categories of outcome (an earlier version appears in Williams et al. [3]; amended with the permission of the Faculty of Pre-Hospital Care in the Royal College of Surgeons of Edinburgh).

Quantitative and mixed methods outcomes	Number of papers
Occupational functioning	58
Post-traumatic stress symptoms	56
Emotional symptoms	30
Stress	26
General health and psychopathology	21
Distress	11
Resilience	11
Alcohol and substance use	10
Physical symptoms	9
Quality of life	8
Leaving	6
Wellbeing	6
Relationships	5
Suicide	3
Diagnoses	2
Prescription psychotropics	2
Suicidal ideation	2

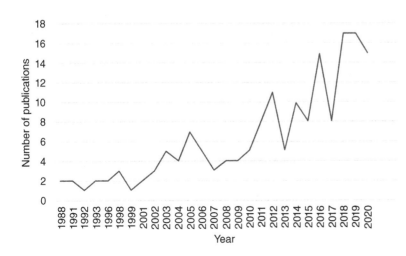

Figure 38.1 Number of publications per year. (Reproduced from Williams et al.[3] with the permission of the Faculty of Pre-Hospital Care in the Royal College of Surgeons of Edinburgh.)

defined empirically. The measurement of stress was especially incoherent – 22 different measures were used, and only two were used more than once. Important outcomes that are likely to have a significant effect on professionals were the least commonly studied – for example, confirmed psychiatric diagnosis and prescription of medication, alcohol and substance use, physical symptoms, suicide, and leaving the profession. Researching these outcomes is likely to be more resource-intensive, and less suited to the cross-sectional questionnaire methodology utilised by most studies. The qualitative research mostly focused on themes of stress and stressors, distress, and resilience, including coping strategies.

Wellbeing, Relationships, and Quality of Life

The question of whether working in pre-hospital care allows health professionals to have healthy and full lives is an important one, yet our review revealed that this was under-researched. The findings were mixed, with samples returning scores that were lower than, similar to, and higher than average on measures of wellbeing and quality of life. However, organisational and social support was associated with greater wellbeing [4,5]. The research on relationships was also limited, and therefore it was not possible to draw conclusions about the effects of working in pre-hospital care on this aspect of professionals' lives.

Stress

Stress as a category of outcome was notable for the inconsistency of agreed definitions and appropriate outcome measures. There is a widely used measure of stress, namely the Perceived Stress Scale [6]. However, this was only reported four times. Comparison of the results from these papers is not possible as they used three different versions of the scale, but all of the papers reported scores lower than or equal to general population norms.

Many papers reported studies for which the authors had written their own questions, or reported the results of validation studies of questionnaires that they had written using a sample of pre-hospital professionals. It is unclear why this category is particularly inconsistent, although there may be a belief that the stressors experienced by pre-hospital healthcare workers are different to those experienced in other occupations, and therefore particular measures were assumed to be required.

Some papers used questionnaires specifically for emergency service professionals, such as the Police Stress Questionnaire and the Emergency Service Personnel Stress Questionnaire. However, ambulance personnel in Devon, UK [7], were asked which work situations caused them stress, and they identified several which could arise in any job, namely inadequate pay, inadequate support from managers, underuse of ability and potential, lack of recognition for good work, inadequate facilities at work, and having to do things that one does not agree with. Only one task – managing injured children – was specific to the emergency services. This suggests a much greater influence of day-to-day organisational and interpersonal stressors than has perhaps been assumed, which has been better highlighted by qualitative work.

Distress and Emotional Symptoms

Our review identified 11 papers that aimed to quantify distress using 6 different measures. Three of these measures have been specifically designed to measure distress, including 2 that are specific to distress related to traumatic events, and the other 3 were originally designed to measure psychological symptoms. Six papers report the results of 5 studies that used the Peritraumatic Distress Inventory, which asks participants to what extent they endorse 13 statements about emotional and physiological distress that they may have experienced in relation to a specific traumatic event [8]. The papers reported a wide range of average scores, with both the lowest mean score (1.39) and the highest mean score (23.15) found in telecommunicators in the USA [9,10], although it is unclear what drives these differences.

Emotional symptoms were most often measured using self-report questionnaires about symptoms of depression and anxiety, such as the Beck Depression Inventory [11] and the Center for Epidemiological Studies – Depression Short Form [12] Several papers report that, on average, pre-hospital professional practitioners were not experiencing symptoms of depression [13,14], although two studies did find higher levels of symptoms in call-handlers [15,9], Several papers also found low average scores on the General Health Questionnaire, a measure of non-psychotic and minor psychiatric symptoms [16].

Occupational Functioning

The Maslach Burnout Inventory (MBI) [17] is the most widely used measure of burnout, and was also the most deployed questionnaire identified by our review (it was reported on 36 times). It is a self-report questionnaire and there are five versions adapted for different populations. Although it was well used, the results were reported in a variety of different ways and the range of scores across papers was large, with some papers identifying lower than average burnout. For example, ambulance driver-rescuers working in Sicily, Italy, scored lower than an Italian normative sample on the Emotional Exhaustion subscale [18]. Other papers reported a high mean score in, for example, a sample of 38 nurses working in mobile emergency medical services in Brazil [19]. Many papers reported a percentage of participants as meeting the criteria for burnout syndrome, although this is no longer recommended due to a lack of diagnostic validity. The fact that the results ranged between 0% and 56% would seem to confirm that this metric is vague and of little use.

Many papers examined associations of other variables with burnout scores, and several factors were repeatedly identified, including having a mental disorder or symptoms, social isolation, personality factors (e.g., neuroticism), experience of aggression from others, and organisational stressors/lack of organisational support. No demographic factor was consistently associated with an increased likelihood of burnout. Burnout was associated with taking sick leave [20]. Two papers found that professionals who work in pre-hospital healthcare in the USA took only a few days of sick leave per year [20,21]. The number of sick days taken by ambulance driver-rescuers in six districts was calculated, and was found to range from an average of 5.3 days to 11.6 days in 1 year [20]. However, in Madrid, Spain, when pre-hospital healthcare workers took an episode of sick leave it lasted for a mean period of 31.48 days (SD = 60.91) [22]. Taken together with the data from the USA, which found that 2.3% ($n = 17$) of EMTs and 4.2% ($n = 56$) of paramedics took more than 10 days of sick leave in a year [10], this suggests that a small number of professionals may be significantly unwell and require extended time off.

Physical Symptoms

The presence of physical symptoms is important, as it predicts important outcomes such as the likelihood of leaving work. However, it has not been extensively studied alongside these psychosocial outcomes.

Average somatisation was found to be low in a large sample of Canadian ambulance service workers [14]; however, over 1 in 10 participants had 'high' levels of somatisation. Around 50% of pre-hospital care workers experience severe fatigue [23–25].

Post-Traumatic Stress Symptoms, Alcohol and Substance Use, and Diagnoses

Symptoms of post-traumatic stress have been a very popular subject of research, with 56 papers reporting on this outcome. The two most commonly used measures were the Impact of Event Scale (IES) [26] and the PTSD Checklist (PCL) [27]. The IES was developed prior to the concept of post-traumatic stress disorder (PTSD). It was designed to measure subjective distress after a specific event by asking about symptoms of intrusion and avoidance. It was revised after the publication of the *Diagnostic and Statistical Manual of Mental Disorders, Third Edition (DSM-III)* in 1980 to include symptoms of physiological hyperarousal [28]. After the publication of DSM-IV, the PCL was developed by the National Center for PTSD within the US Department of Veterans Affairs, based on the diagnostic criteria, and different versions were developed for use in different populations (e.g., the military) [27]. The PTSD Checklist (PCL-5) was updated to reflect the criteria published in DSM-V [29]. Higher scores on both questionnaires indicate more frequent and severe symptoms of PTSD. However, neither instrument can be used to diagnose PTSD.

Using the IES-R, 19–40% of participants were identified as having possible PTSD, although different cut-off scores were used, and 1.1–44.4% using the PCL with a standard cut-off score of more than 31. This is clearly a wide range but also a very high maximum percentage. The lowest PCL percentage was identified in a sample of participants who attended the 2011 terror attacks in Norway [30], and the highest percentage was identified in EMTs and EMCs working in an ambulance service in Ireland [31]. These professionals were also asked about the number of critical incidents they had attended in the last year, and this was found to be higher than in other samples of ambulance personnel. In addition, mean IES scores were found to be similar to those for members of the general population who had experienced traumatic events.

Approximately 1 in 10 professionals who work in pre-hospital care report that alcohol or substance use has become a problem for them [32]. When an average score on a screening instrument such as the Alcohol Use Disorders Identification Test (AUDIT) was calculated [33], overall the sample appeared to be 'low risk' [34]. However, this reporting approach fails to identify the small group for whom alcohol use has become hazardous or dependent.

Very few papers have attempted to identify how many pre-hospital professionals meet the diagnostic criteria for psychiatric disorders, and only one study examined this systematically. A prospective study of 453 paramedics was conducted in the UK [34]. At the start of their training, they were assessed by psychologists using the Structured Clinical Interview for the *Diagnostic and Statistical Manual of Mental Disorders, Fourth Edition (DSM-IV)*, and followed up with repeat assessments over 2 years. In total, 32 participants (8.3%) developed PTSD and 41 participants (10.6%) developed major depression. All except 9 participants no longer met the criteria for diagnosis when assessed again 4 months later.

Qualitative Research Findings

In total, 16 papers were identified, mostly reporting on studies of ambulance personnel in the UK, North America, and Australia. Five key findings were identified.

1. Two papers reported on dispatch personnel or call-handlers [35,36]. They reported that aspects of their work, such as high-volume and emotionally difficult calls, caused them significant distress. This was worsened by a stressful working environment with a lack of resources or support from managers.
2. Ambulance staff who attended incidents reported that certain factors were more likely to increase the distress they felt afterwards – for example, if they had been unable to help or they felt high levels of compassion for the victim or their relatives (e.g., when attending cot deaths and incidents involving children) [37].
3. Resilience and coping were promoted by support and validation from senior staff, families and friends, and the public [38].
4. Organisational factors, such as long hours, inadequate training, and inadequate support from managers, were identified in several papers as significant stressors and aspects of the job that affect recruitment and retention [39]. This was juxtaposed with the knowledge that working in pre-hospital care is a worthwhile and well-respected job.
5. In contrast to the quantitative research, a group of ambulance staff who responded to the 9/11 terrorist attacks in New York reported significant physical and mental health problems that persisted for many years, and half of the sample no longer worked in the emergency medical services [40].

Conclusions

Our review revealed that considerable interest and resources have been directed towards the concern that professional practitioners who work in pre-hospital care may develop burnout and psychiatric disorders in particular, and that they may develop PTSD as a result of attending critical incidents. However, the methods used by most of the studies in our sample were not able to answer these questions, because they used cross-sectional surveys and self-report questionnaires, which are not diagnostic tools. They considerably overestimate the incidence of these problems, as demonstrated by the one high-quality study that conducted clinical interviews and found that only a small percentage of employees met the criteria for PTSD or major depression, and that most resolved over a few months.

However, the high scores on these questionnaires perhaps indicate that pre-hospital professionals often suffer considerable stress and distress. The sources of this stress are not as likely to be, as has often been thought, attending unusual and perhaps high-profile incidents, but are more likely to be related to daily organisational and operational hassles, such as unsupportive managers and a high volume of work to be done despite a lack of resources. Many pre-hospital professionals do experience fatigue and burnout, but despite this continue to attend work, aided by support from their families, friends, and their teams, and in the knowledge that they are doing a well-respected and important job.

Further research endeavours should move away from large questionnaire studies and the topic of post-traumatic stress. Negative experiences such as stress and distress are common, but are poorly defined and under-researched, as are wellbeing and quality of life. Both quantitative and qualitative research highlights how operational and organisational factors have a significant impact on these outcomes, and both clinical and research improvements in these areas could improve the experience of all pre-hospital care providers. In addition, there are small numbers of professionals who develop or have pre-existing psychiatric disorders, which include alcohol and substance use, or who develop severe burnout, or require extended sick leave. It is not clear how these 3 outcomes interact, and it is important that this group of professionals is recognised in order that appropriate support can be provided, and undesirable outcomes averted for the people who work in this crucial area of healthcare.

References

1. Zeanah CH, Sonuga-Barke JS. Editorial: The effects of early trauma and deprivation on human development – from measuring cumulative risk to characterizing specific mechanisms. *J Child Psychol Psychiatry* 2016; 57: 1099–102.

2. Burgess J, Stokes S, Kemp V, Wood A, Batt-Rawdon S, Keith R, et al. *The Psychosocial and Mental Health Impact of Working in Pre-Hospital Medicine: A Systematic Review*. National Institute for Health and Care Research, 2021 (www.crd.york.ac.uk/PROSPERO/display_record.php?RecordID=157165).

3. Williams R, Kemp V, Batt-Rawden S, Bland L, Burgess J, McInerney A, et al. *Valuing Staff, Valuing Patients: The Report on the Psychosocial Care and Mental Health Programme*. Faculty of Pre-Hospital Care, Royal College of Surgeons of Edinburgh, 2022.

4. Petrie K, Gayed A, Bryan BT, Deady M, Madan I, Savic A, et al. The importance of manager support for the mental health and well-being of ambulance personnel. *PloS One* 2018; 13: e0197802.

5. Shakespeare-Finch J, Daley E. Workplace belongingness, distress, and resilience in emergency service workers. *Psychol Trauma* 2017; 9: 32–5.

6. Cohen S, Kamarck T, Mermelstein R. A global measure of perceived stress. *J Health Soc Behav* 1983; 24: 385–96.

7. James AE, Wright PL. Occupational stress in the ambulance service. *Health Manpow Manage* 1991; 17: 4–11.

8. Brunet A, Weiss DS, Metzler TJ, Best SR, Neylan TC, Rogers C, et al. The Peritraumatic Distress Inventory: a proposed measure of PTSD criterion A2. *Am J Psychiatry* 2001; 158: 1480–85.

9. Lilly MM, Allen CE. Psychological inflexibility and psychopathology in 9-1-1 telecommunicators. *J Trauma Stress* 2015; 28: 262–6.

10. Troxell RM. Indirect exposure to the trauma of others: the experiences of 9-1-1 telecommunicators. *Diss Abstr Int Sect B Sci Eng* 2009; 69: 6740.

11. Beck AT, Steer RA, Brown GK. *Beck Depression Inventory*. Psychological Corp., 1996.

12. Andresen EM, Malmgren JA, Carter WB, Patrick DL. Screening for depression in well older adults: evaluation of a short form of the CES-D. *Am J Prev Med* 1994; 10: 77–84.

13. Regehr C, Goldberg G, Hughes J. Exposure to human tragedy, empathy, and trauma in ambulance paramedics. *Am J Orthopsychiatry* 2002; 72: 505–13.

14. Halpern J, Maunder RG, Schwartz B, Gurevich M. Identifying risk of emotional sequelae after critical incidents. *Emerg Med J* 2011; 28: 51–6.

15. Abid SK, Hussain M, Raza M, Naseer R, Durrani M, Ali S, et al. Non emergency calls-depression coupling in call handlers of rescue 1122 Punjab, Pakistan. *Pakistan J Psychol Res* 2019; 34: 43–55.

16. Sanz-Vergel AI, Demerouti E, Mayo M, Moreno-Jimenez B. Work–home interaction and psychological strain: the moderating role of sleep quality. *Appl Psychol* 2011; 60: 210–30.

17. Maslach C, Jackson S. *Maslach Burnout Inventory Manual*. Consulting Psychologists Press, 1986.

18. Ferraro L, La Cascia C, De Santis A, Sideli L, Maniaci G, Orlando IM, et al. A cross-sectional survey on burnout prevalence and profile in the Sicilian population of ambulance driver-rescuers. *Prehosp Disaster Med* 2020; 35: 133–40.

19. França SPdS, De Martino MMF, Aniceto EVdS, Silva LL. Predictors of burnout syndrome in nurses in the prehospital emergency services. *Acta Paul Enferm* 2012; 25: 68–73.

20. Crowe RP, Bower JK, Cash RE, Panchal AR, Rodriguez SA, Olivo-Marston SE. Association of burnout with workforce-reducing factors among EMS professionals. *Prehosp Emerg Care* 2018; 22: 229–36.

21. Marmar CR, Weiss DS, Metzler TJ, Ronfeldt HM, Foreman C. Stress responses of emergency services personnel to the Loma Prieta earthquake Interstate 880 freeway collapse and control traumatic incidents. *J Trauma Stress* 1996; 9: 63–85.

22. Bernaldo-De-Quiros M, Piccini AT, Gomez MM, Cerdeira JC. Psychological consequences of aggression in pre-hospital emergency care: cross sectional survey. *Int J Nurs Stud* 2015; 52: 260–70.

23. Patterson PD, Klapec SE, Weaver MD, Guyette FX, Platt TE,

Buysse DJ. Differences in paramedic fatigue before and after changing from a 24-hour to an 8-hour shift schedule: a case report. *Prehosp Emerg Care* 2016; 20: 132–6.

24. Pyper Z, Paterson JL. Fatigue and mental health in Australian rural and regional ambulance personnel. *Emerg Med Australas* 2016; 28: 62–6.

25. Donnelly EA, Bradford P, Davis M, Hedges C, Socha D, Morassutti P. Fatigue and safety in paramedicine. *CJEM* 2019; 21: 762–5.

26. Horowitz M, Wilner N, Alvarez W. Impact of Event Scale: a measure of subjective stress. *Psychosom Med* 1979; 41: 209–18.

27. Weathers FW, Litz BT, Herman DS, Huska JA, Keane TM, eds. *The PTSD Checklist (PCL): Reliability, Validity, and Diagnostic Utility*. Annual Convention of the International Society for Traumatic Stress Studies, 1993.

28. Weiss D, Marmar C. The Impact of Event Scale-Revised. In *Assessing Psychological Trauma and PTSD* (Wilson J, Keane T, eds): 399–411. Guilford Press, 1997.

29. Weathers FW, Litz BT, Keane TM, Palmieri PA, Marx BP, Schnurr PP. *The PTSD Checklist*

for *DSM-5 (PCL-5)*. National Center for PTSD, 2013.

30. Skogstad L, Fjetland AM, Ekeberg O. Exposure and posttraumatic stress symptoms among first responders working in proximity to the terror sites in Norway on July 22, 2011 – a cross-sectional study. *Scand J Trauma Resusc Emerg Med* 2015; 23: 23.

31. Gallagher S, McGilloway S. Experience of critical incident stress among ambulance service staff and relationship to psychological symptoms. *Int J Emerg Ment Health* 2009; 11: 235–48.

32. Regehr C, Millar D. Situation critical: high demand, low control, and low support in paramedic organizations. *Traumatology* 2007; 13: 49–58.

33. World Health Organization (WHO). *AUDIT: The Alcohol Use Disorders Identification Test: Guidelines for Use in Primary Health Care*. WHO, 2001.

34. Wild J, Smith KV, Thompson E, Béar F, Lommen MJJ, Ehlers A. A prospective study of pre-trauma risk factors for post-traumatic stress disorder and depression. *Psychol Med* 2016; 46: 2571–82.

35. Adams K, Shakespeare-Finch J, Armstrong D. An interpretative phenomenological analysis of

stress and well-being in emergency medical dispatchers. *J Loss Trauma* 2015; 20: 430–48.

36. Coxon A, Cropley M, Schofield P, Start K, Horsfield C, Quinn T. 'You're never making just one decision': exploring the lived experiences of ambulance Emergency Operations Centre personnel. *Emerg Med J* 2016; 33: 645–51.

37. Halpern J, Gurevich M, Schwartz B, Brazeau P. What makes an incident critical for ambulance workers? Emotional outcomes and implications for intervention. *Work Stress* 2009; 23: 173–89.

38. Clompus SR, Albarran JW. Exploring the nature of resilience in paramedic practice: a psycho-social study. *Int Emerg Nurs* 2016; 28: 1–7.

39. Patterson PD, Probst JC, Leith KH, Corwin SJ, Powell MP. Recruitment and retention of emergency medical technicians: a qualitative study. *J Allied Health* 2005; 34: 153–62.

40. Smith EC, Burkle FM. Paramedic and emergency medical technician reflections on the ongoing impact of the 9/11 terrorist attacks. *Prehosp Disaster Med* 2019; 34: 56–61.

Chapter

39

Moral Distress and Moral Injury

Esther Murray and Andrew Wood

Introduction: Self, Other People, and the Moral Dimension of Work

We all have ideas about how we think we will behave in times of crisis, and who we think we will be. Whether we match up to our ideas of ourselves is important in terms of our ability to live with our selves subsequently. In our workplaces we also form ideas, and ideals, about our team and leaders [1,2]. Thus it is important to consider our moral worlds/selves when we think about wellbeing and functioning at work.

Largely due to structural issues such as underfunding, there are substantial tensions between patients' preferences, the ways in which many frontline staff wish to deliver care, and what can be delivered. Staff caught in these tensions are at real risk of becoming distressed, exhausted, and potentially injured. This chapter examines the ways in which thinking about the moral dimension of work might help or hinder our adjustment to these challenging situations in the context of responding to emergencies, whether these are of sudden brief onset or are longer-term and more drawn out.

Most of the work involved in responding to emergencies is based on very specific types of teams, whether outside or inside hospitals. Teams train together to perform complex tasks at speed in high-pressure situations, often using high-fidelity simulation techniques so that many actions become well rehearsed. When a team is familiar with the practice of training to programme a muscle memory so that a set of actions can be followed quickly and safely, it may assume an equivalent ability to programme a set of emotional responses. Certainly in pre-hospital medicine there have been efforts to learn from high-performing sports people in order to avoid phenomena such as 'the yips' – those temporary losses of muscle memory and the ability to make important

decisions that can manifest for no known reason. Some pre-hospital medicine teams use the bucket analogy to address issues of psychological readiness for the task at hand. By sharing the understanding that everyone has a bucket of current life experiences that may be more or less full at any given time, team members can check in with one another using this shorthand. If anyone's bucket is too full, their ability to perform is likely to be impaired. Another frequently used term is bandwidth, which describes the capacity of any member of the team to process information at any given time. When someone's bandwidth is overwhelmed, their situational awareness, focus, and concentration can be lost. Intrusive thoughts and memories can overwhelm available bandwidth.

In most professions in which there is a requirement for expert performance under pressure there is widespread recognition that rehearsal and practice are essential in order to ensure performance. What might be lacking is appropriate consideration of general mental wellbeing before and in the aftermath of a high-pressure event. It may not be sufficient simply to check in with the 'emotional buckets' of the team. Much has been written about learning from error, and the field of pre-hospital medicine draws heavily on findings from aviation and a broad understanding of human factors. It is important to recognise that all factors are necessarily human. Our understanding of how humans interact with machines, workspaces, and equipment is developing and might help to prevent errors in the future. Similarly, an understanding of the effects of pressure to perform might inform training and reduce error. However, we cannot necessarily reduce the emotional or psychological impact of the work itself by this means. Most pre-hospital medicine practitioners tell us that they do not feel so badly about a case if they did everything they could for the patient, in contrast to those events where not enough, or enough of the right thing, was done. Thus the aftermath of a case that is difficult to process is unlikely to be purely related to whether mistakes were made or were perceived as having been made.

This acknowledges the tension between each person's response to an event, their team's response, their organisation's response, and the public response. In this regard, the contents take us back to the scenario described in Chapter 5, where a medical consultant, a medical trainee, and a paramedic reflect on the same event and on each other. All of these perceptions have an effect on each person's ability to process their experiences.

Moral Distress and Moral Injury

The concept of moral distress was outlined by Andrew Jameton in 1984 in his book *Nursing Practice: The Ethical Issues* [3]. It refers to the effects of knowing what should be done for a patient, but also being aware of one's inability to do those things because of situational and organisational constraints such as lack of time, staff, or equipment. Until recently, most of the research on moral distress related to nursing practice, but a recent survey of doctors by the British Medical Association (BMA) reported that the concept of moral distress resonated with their experiences [4]. The concept is of interest in this chapter because it highlights the relationship between organisational issues and personal moral matters. The fact that these issues are becoming more widely and frequently discussed may lead us to think of ways in which we might address them.

The construct of moral injury originated in military populations. More recently it has been extended to healthcare and to healthcare staff [5–7]. The term has been used to describe the psychological sequelae of 'bearing witness to the aftermath of violence and human carnage' [8, p. 700]. It encompasses witnessing human suffering or failing to prevent outcomes that transgress deeply held beliefs, such as the rights of children to be protected by their parents, or the belief that life can and should be preserved by appropriate and timely medical intervention. It also recognises failings in leadership, in situations in which staff are not appropriately resourced, whether in terms of people, space, or equipment. The term was coined by the psychiatrist Jonathan Shay as a result of his years of work in veterans' hospitals in the USA; he said that it stemmed from a betrayal of what is right,

either by the self or by someone in a legitimate position of power, in a high stakes situation [9, p. 182].

It is clear that moral distress and moral injury are closely linked, and there is a suggestion that the difference between them is only one of degree. In their introduction to a journal's special issue on moral injury [10], published in 2019, Brett Litz and Patricia Kerig propose a continuum of moral stressors, which, if they were to occur frequently enough, would result in moral injury. There is an effort in the literature to quantify moral injury, which strays far from Shay's case formulation approach in which he simply tried to explain what he was seeing in his patients. Whatever the intellectual approach, the term is becoming increasingly used in the literature and in interventions. Even before the COVID-19 pandemic, Brandon Griffin and colleagues' integrative review of the term moral injury included 116 articles in its qualitative synthesis alone [7].

Why the Concepts of Moral Injury and Moral Distress Have Been Drawn into the Mainstream

Research on experiences of providing care seems to suggest that work on moral distress was generated from research on the experiences of nurses [11]. However, this began to shift, even before the COVID-19 pandemic, to explore the experiences of moral distress in other staff groups, too [12].

Since the COVID-19 pandemic began, the experience of being unable to provide an appropriate level of care, and the feeling of betraying what is right in a high-stakes situation – either to oneself or to some other person – have become endemic for practitioners at all levels. There is a sharp rise in interest in understanding these concepts as a way of thinking about people's experiences of the pandemic, which I have described as a slow-motion mass casualty event. In her paper on understanding moral injury in COVID-19 [13], Suzanne Shale reminds us that we all build our normative expectations – that is, our beliefs about what people *should* do and our predictions about what they *will* do – over a period of years, and we may not know exactly what these expectations are until they are violated. This is a normal part of our everyday moral lives as citizens. The ways in which handling of the pandemic has violated these expectations have been writ large in official media and social media. As a result, discussions of what was wrong, and what ought to have happened, especially in relation to providing personal protective equipment (PPE) and suitable working conditions for healthcare workers, have become part of the everyday conversation. Thus moral distress and moral injury are no longer the purview of nurses, when they might have been excused as being the experience of those people who delivered more direct patient care and had less control. Instead they have become much more broadly understood as something that could happen to anyone. Indeed, this situation continues as the NHS in the UK, for example, is struggling to recover from the effects of the COVID-19 pandemic.

Definitions: Why 'Moral', and Why 'Injury' and Not 'Distress'?

The suggestion that what is distressing staff is the moral aspect of these restrictions on their work may seem strange, but I argue that placing the problem firmly in the moral sphere will be what enables us to consider remediating it.

To suggest that an issue is moral is to say that it is concerned with the principles of right and wrong behaviour. In most societies there are shared understandings about what constitutes right and wrong behaviour, whether in personal or professional spheres. Certainly we see that people who fall short of the moral standards expected in healthcare are held to account by governing bodies and the law. As well as a shared understanding of right and wrong, we have a personal moral code, which is informed by our life experiences and education. This set of inner values guides our actions, and moral distress helps us to understand the experience of being unable to work in accordance with those values.

The role of values at work forms part of the narrative about work now perhaps more than ever before, and the focus is on personal values, team values, and organisational values. I would imagine that the shift in ways of thinking about values at work is a result of the ways in which we currently understand motivation and performance at work, which are not driven solely by remuneration, but also by a sense of autonomy, belonging, and competence. Research into the occupational psychology of healthcare shows that in order to thrive at work, people need such a sense of autonomy, belonging, and competence, and that this is as true for healthcare workers as for

anyone else [14]. This work is based on social identity theory [15], which postulates that a person's identity is based on the social groups with which they identify. This consideration of work and identity could be useful when thinking about how to tackle the psychosocial aspects of challenging work. Shared values form part of the sense of belonging. In healthcare there is likely to be an assumption about the degree to which values are shared, but the picture may be complicated by the fact that there are many professional groups, and thus subcultures, that do not all share the same values [16]. Since moral injury is defined by one's values having been compromised to such a degree that it is no longer possible to continue as part of a particular group as if nothing has happened, we can see not only that shared values are important, but also that the ability to examine them as a team is paramount for maintaining the health and integrity of the team.

My preference for the term injury over distress, for example, arises from the fact that this chapter focuses on work-based risk, such as a needlestick injury or an injury incurred while loading a patient into an ambulance. Training is in place to prevent workplace injuries like these, but they still happen. The same is true for the psychosocial impact of the work. Where injuries occur at work, the onus is on the employer to mitigate the impact of those injuries, perhaps also changing work-based practice in order to prevent them from happening again. In the case of the psychosocial harms that might occur in the healthcare sphere, some areas are better provided for than others. Psychosocial support in the form of personal support and facilitated debriefing is present as standard in most adult and paediatric intensive care units (ICUs), both for patients and for staff, but not in all areas of healthcare. Debriefing as a regular practice after simulation is also common, though it does not necessarily address concerns that fall into the psychosocial sphere. This is largely because, at the technical level, procedure-based debriefing is initially the safest and most useful type, and a psychological debriefing can take place later, some time after the incident. A widespread culture of taking time to talk regularly and safely would help to mitigate the moral and emotional impacts of the work.

The approach adopted by one helicopter emergency medical service (HEMS) organisation to responding to the needs of its staff, and creating a culture wherein conversations can take place to help to mitigate the effects of moral injury, involves multiple coordinated changes. The aim of these is to effect a change of culture and create a space in which helpful conversations can happen, as summarised here.

- An evidence-based, bespoke wellbeing strategy is introduced. This includes information on best practice, resources, and referral pathways into care, should professional help be required. The strategy is available to all staff, so that they understand what the organisation is able to provide for them.

- All new starters are given an introduction to the psychosocial aspects of working in pre-hospital emergency medicine (PHEM) as part of their induction. The content is guided and supported by mental health professionals, best evidence, and the PHEM curriculum.

- Training is carried out for staff, particularly for those in leadership roles across the organisation, by mental health professionals, on best practice in caring for their staff in the clinical environment.

- A formal Peer Support Network is introduced, which incorporates staff members from across different professional groups within the organisation. The role of peer support is formally recognised, requires training by mental health experts, and is overseen by a local trained mental health practitioner.

- A clinical psychologist is integrated into the team, and is introduced to all new members of staff at the start of their secondment. The psychologist also attends governance meetings when cases are being discussed, and some clinical shifts as an observer. By integrating a mental health expert into the team we hope to diffuse best practice into our culture, and to have someone who is known to the team available for those rare occasions when a crisis hits.

- A focus on mitigating secondary stressors (see Chapter 9) involves a systematic approach to understanding the stressors that most commonly and severely affect staff members, so that they can be mitigated.

Neither moral distress nor moral injury are disorders – they are not the fault or failing of an individual person, but simply ways of conceptualising reactions to exposure to traumatic situations in the course of work. This distinction is important because it offers a non-pathologising perspective on distress. It could also support a shift away from conceptualising psychosocial 'illbeing' as an end point or reason to cease working in the environment.

The Way Forward in Caring for Staff

In Chapter 37, Richard Williams and Verity Kemp suggest that employers have moral as well as legal responsibilities for their staff, and they have called this notion 'moral architecture'. It refers to the moral and human rights obligations that organisations acquire as employers and through their commitment to delivering high-quality services [17].

They argue that it is difficult for healthcare staff to continue to provide compassionate, evidence-informed, and values-based care for their patients if they are not supported by their employers or if there is dissonance between the support, training, and care for staff and the quality of care that they are expected to deliver [18]. This is especially so when employers ask staff to take more than minor risks when discharging their (the employers') responsibilities. These obligations should be reflected in organisations' policies, their design and delivery of services, and their corporate governance [19,20].

Not every difficult experience in a life can be mitigated by preparation. We have a culture in healthcare, and especially in pre-hospital and emergency medicine, which has built on specific types of training in order to make sure that procedures can be carried out safely and with maximum benefit for patients, and this is right and proper. What then becomes problematic is when this same approach is suggested for the mitigation of the experience of moral harms resulting from carrying out the work. Arguably there are potential mitigations, such as proper training, proper provision of equipment, and proper learning from experiences, but the idea that some intervention or selection could prevent moral harms in this arena is a potentially dangerous one. It does not require much imagination to see that screening out people who have a moral compass that might feasibly be disturbed by work with human suffering would affect the experiences of patients under their care. The other suggestion is that training might prevent staff from suffering moral injury, but equally, how could this work? How would we train people not to feel or experience any moral perturbation from their work? And what would be the consequences of this? The problem that arises is not that working in healthcare, and especially in pre-hospital care, is potentially harmful – it is, of course – but that we seek to pathologise and control that harm at the individual level rather than manage it at the group/team level. Such an approach is likely to promote the very experiences that we are seeking to prevent. In a work setting, it is as important to manage the fallout of the work at the team level as it is to manage the preparation for the work.

In 2015, vicarious trauma – that is, being exposed to the trauma suffered by others – was included as one of the potential triggers for developing post-traumatic stress disorder (PTSD) [21]. This was a huge step, as it legitimises the distress suffered by therapists, humanitarian workers, first responders of all kinds, and social workers. We might consider it unfortunate that including these experiences under the umbrella of PTSD, and nowhere else, leaves those who do not develop PTSD with nowhere to go. Embracing perspectives that focus on quite usual, shared human experiences allows workplace cultures to be developed that are able to respond to these experiences through formal peer support. There is no agreed intervention for moral injury or moral distress, despite some proposals to use, for example, acceptance and commitment therapy for its values-based approach. Probably the most useful approach is for each organisation to develop its own support structures based on what works best for its staff. Certainly building on spaces for talking about these experiences will be the beginning of the way forward.

References

1. Steffens N, Haslam S, Kerschreiter R, Schuh S, van Dick R. Leaders enhance group members' work engagement and reduce their burnout by crafting social identity. *Z Personalforsch* 2014; 28: 173–94.

2. Ellemers N, Barreto M. Social identity and self-presentation at work: how attempts to hide a stigmatised identity affect emotional well-being, social inclusion and performance. *Neth J Psychol* 2006; 62: 51–7.

3. Jameton A. *Nursing Practice: The Ethical Issues.* Prentice-Hall, 1984.

4. British Medical Association (BMA). *Moral Distress and Moral Injury: Recognising and Tackling It for UK Doctors.* BMA, 2021 (www.bma.org.uk/media/4209/bma-moral-distress-injury-survey-report-june-2021.pdf).

5. Maslach C, Leiter M. Understanding the burnout experience: recent research and its implications for psychiatry. *World Psychiatry* 2016; 15: 103–11.

6. Murray E, Krahé C, Goodsman D. Are medical students in prehospital care at risk of moral injury? *Emerg Med J* 2018; 35: 590–94.

7. Griffin B, Purcell N, Burkman K, Litz B, Bryan C, Schmitz M, et al. Moral injury: an integrative review. *J Trauma Stress* 2019; 32: 350–62.

8. Litz B, Stein N, Delaney E, Lebowitz L, Nash W, Silva C, et al. Moral injury and moral repair in war veterans: a preliminary model and intervention strategy. *Clin Psychol Rev* 2009; 29: 695–706.

9. Shay J. Moral injury. *Psychoanal Psychol* 2014; 31: 182–91.

10. Litz B, Kerig P. Introduction to the special issue on moral injury: conceptual challenges, methodological issues, and clinical applications. *J Trauma Stress* 2019; 32: 341–9.

11. McCarthy J, Deady R. Moral distress reconsidered. *Nurs Ethics* 2008; 15: 254–62.

12. Whitehead PB, Herbertson RK, Hamric AB, Epstein EG, Fisher JM. Moral distress among healthcare professionals: report of an institution-wide survey. *J Nurs Scholarsh* 2015; 47: 117–25.

13. Shale S. Moral injury and the COVID-19 pandemic: reframing what it is, who it affects and how care leaders can manage it. *BMJ Leader* 2020; 4: 224–7.

14. Kinman G, Teoh K. *Looking after Doctors' Mental Wellbeing during the COVID-19 Pandemic.* BMJ, 2020 (https://blogs.bmj.com/bmj/2020/03/26/looking-after-doctors-mental-wellbeing-during-the-covid-19-pandemic/).

15. Tajfel H, Turner JC. An integrative theory of intergroup conflict. In *The Social Psychology of Intergroup Relations* (eds WG Austin, S Worchel): 33–47. Brooks/Cole, 1979.

16. Morgan P, Ogbonna E. Subcultural dynamics in transformation: a multi-perspective study of healthcare professionals. *Hum Relat* 2008; 61: 39–65.

17. Williams R. A cunning plan: integrating evidence, judgement and passion in mental health strategy. The Inaugural Lecture of Professor Richard Williams, delivered at the University of Glamorgan, November 2000.

18. Williams R, Kemp V, Neal A. Compassionate care: leading and caring for staff of mental health services and the moral architecture of healthcare organisations. In *Management for Psychiatrists* (eds Bhugra D, Bell S, Burns S): 377–402. Royal College of Psychiatrists Publication, 2016.

19. Neal A, Kemp V, Williams R. Caring for the carers. In *Social Scaffolding: Applying the Lessons of Contemporary Social Science to Health and Healthcare* (eds Williams R, Kemp V, Haslam SA, et al.): 289–303. Cambridge University Press, 2019.

20. Warner M, Williams R. The nature of strategy and its application in statutory and non-statutory services. In *Child and Adolescent Mental Health Services: Strategic Approaches to Commissioning and Delivering Child and Adolescent Mental Health Services* (eds Williams R, Kerfoot M): 39–62. Oxford University Press, 2005.

21. American Psychiatric Association. *Diagnostic and Statistical Manual of Mental Disorders* 5th ed. American Psychiatric Association, 2013.

Chapter

40

Consequences for the Mental Health of Families of Responders to Pandemics, Major Incidents, and Emergencies

Rowena Hill

Introduction

This book makes clear the impact on the wellbeing of responders of their responding to, and leading responses to, emergencies, incidents, terrorist events, disasters, disease outbreaks and conflicts (EITDDC), including the UK's management of the COVID-19 pandemic. Responders can be defined as NHS-employed frontline healthcare workers, frontline health or social care workers, local emergency decision-makers, emergency services staff, often referred to as 'Blue Light' responders (e.g., firefighters, police officers, urgent pre-hospital care workers), emergency planners, and community and voluntary sector workers. Chapter 22 makes clear that frequently the first responders come from the public present at an incident, who often intervene before first professional responders arrive at the scene of the event. This chapter does not include the impacts on their families, and it focuses on Category 1 or 2 responders, for whom there is a greater evidence base on which to draw.

The evidence describes a range of impacts on first responders, such as burnout (see Chapter 38), sleep disturbance, moral injury (see Chapter 39), alcohol and substance use, finances and debt, challenges to family relationships and activities, anxiety, depression, and traumatic reactions. Furthermore, there can be occupational stressors that have personal impacts from the organisation within which each responder works. Work pace is one possible source of stress, and we saw that the system and its processes were under huge pressure during the pandemic. This means that health responders were dealing with the demands of both chronic and episodic effects of the pandemic. In other words, sometimes there were periods of acute pressure during the pandemic, in which the pace of work became faster with high workloads. Their timing coincided with high-pressure events such as the waves of transmission or the implementation or relaxing of non-pharmaceutical interventions. These periods were sometimes relatively short in duration, whereas at other times they were not. Other pressures have remained chronic and enduring throughout the management of the pandemic, as they are for other incidents and major emergencies that Category 1 and 2 responders manage.

Common Experiences Among Responders and Their Families

Common expressions of these challenges include responders' mood swings, irritability, unwarranted aggression, unpredictability, and withdrawal from family life. These usual reactions of responders to the abnormal situation of a protracted national emergency also have consequences for the families of the responders. Chapters 4 and 5 recognise this pattern among survivors, responders, and professional responders, and promote the importance of validating rather than normalising these experiences. Professional responders are drawn from many occupations, and researchers have demonstrated the impacts on them and their relationships that arise from responders using emotional numbing or distancing from/avoidance of their families to maintain their wellbeing. This, coupled with the impact of physical separation as a result of the shift system, could be perceived by family members as their responder relatives being physically or emotionally disengaged from family life. Pauline Boss has defined situations like this through non-critical occupation populations as including those people outside of the fire, police, healthcare, military, and pre-hospital urgent care services, as ambiguous loss, when a family member is either physically absent but psychologically present, or physically present but psychologically absent [1]. Psychological absence may occur because responders experience distress and burnout, or as a result of their becoming unwell due to developing depression and/or traumatic reactions. Consequently,

Table 40.1 Threats and resources for families of responders. (Reproduced with permission of the copyright holder, Hill R, 2015 [9], p. 117.)

Threats	Secondary trauma
	Emotional contagion
	Burnout
	Moral injury
	Perceptions of, and coping with, risk
	Perceptions of occupational safety
	Shift work
Resources	Resilience
	Wellbeing
	Psychological mastery
	Family functioning
	Social support

the absence of family members has impacts on the rest of the family.

The effects of living with these impacts, including their effects on family members' own wellbeing, have been documented across all three emergency and essential services [2–5]. The strain from the responders' occupations, and the responders' reactions to that strain, threaten families' resources, structure, and processes [6]. Typically, social support is reported as facilitating an increase in effective coping by responders and their families; it appears to buffer the negative impact of threats [7].

The term family refers to the primary social group of each responder, whose members share biological, social, or experiential commonalities. Families usually have a structure and processes that contribute to family functioning, and which are the systems used by them to adapt, organise, and progress their shared tasks, communications, and activities. There is a need to invest in research in this area to establish the potential problems and outcomes for the wellbeing of responders' families [8]. Table 40.1 lists the potential threats to responders' families, and the potential resources that they have for coping effectively with possible strain.

The literature that considers families of personnel in critical occupations, including the military, the 'Blue Light' services, coastguard, and other essential safety and security occupations, has mostly focused on the prevalence and effectiveness of families providing social support for their responders in response to occupational stress or traumatic stress. There have also been a number of studies across responders' occupations detailing the impacts of shift work on partners' and parents' relationships [10–12].

Understanding the perspectives of families on how the domains of work and families of responders interact, rather than only considering the perspectives of the employees' organisations or the employees, offers the potential to understand the bidirectional relationship of the domains. The relationship between the domains can be positive when it is referred to as family enrichment, and includes the energy, mood, time, psychological resilience, social support, and other resources that responders can gain from their families [13]. The unique opportunities and strains of working as a responder have been shown to affect family members. Consequently, understanding families' perspectives is likely to provide direction to the employing organisations on how they can support their responders and their employees' families, and facilitate a healthy organisation.

Impacts from the COVID-19 Pandemic on Responders and Their Families

More widely across the world, societies saw and continue to live with many changes because of COVID-19 and the measures that have been taken and are being taken to manage the pandemic. However, responders and their families have been through a substantially different experience of the pandemic compared with the public. Past studies have shown that people who work in frontline occupations, such as those in the essential and emergency services, healthcare workers, and people who manage emergencies at the level of local government, receive support from their families. That support can be an effective resource for assisting frontline staff to cope with the strain of the incident. However, people may also require additional support, as Chapter 28 shows.

During the pandemic, and before vaccinations became widely available, many responders were worried about the risk to their families [14–16]. Consequently, they chose to take extra precautions to minimise the risks by, for example, living away from their families, changing certain routines and behaviours, and explaining to their families the system, processes, and safe working practices brought in to protect people from COVID-19. This included working in personal protective equipment (PPE), with the intention of gaining relatives' understanding of the safety processes in place. Responders may have been hesitant to discuss the details and the emotional impact of their work in relation to COVID-19. They might have wanted to protect their families from what they saw or felt, or they might have been obligated by the need to respect other people's confidentiality [17]. Evidence suggests that families can help to alleviate worries by encouraging family members to talk about their jobs and what these entail. Not all responders were attending a place of work throughout the pandemic.

The literature is still lacking in evidence that has adopted a family perspective sufficient to enable an understanding of the impacts and benefits for their families of home working by responders, whether or not working from home is recommended. Identifying positive family coping with spillover from the work domain of energy, mood, and time, for example, is likely to enable learning and policy development to inform the management of any future major incidents, including adverse or extreme weather events, to implement home working policies.

There have been social and emotional impacts from the changes to work patterns that have necessarily been created by the pandemic, including changes to shift patterns, to the nature and pace of jobs, to social perceptions of workers' roles, and to working practices, as well as the challenges of addressing the backlog of business-as-usual activities across the wider public services. These changes to working practices were commonly in place for at least the first 6 months of the pandemic within the UK. This is a long time for responders to undertake different roles and activities compared with their substantive permanent roles. Given the evidence in the literature that demonstrates the strain that unclear or varying role definitions have on people, it could be inferred that experiencing this in the context of a large-scale global pandemic could cause significant strain for the people affected. This includes firefighters and police aiding ambulance services and working in community hubs, police understanding their commitments in enforcing the Coronavirus Act 2020, broad sweeping changes to ways of working in public services, reallocation of healthcare staff to COVID-19 temporary roles, secondments across local governments, and working to ensure that the local responses were enacted and monitored.

Empirical Evidence from Responders in the First Year of the COVID-19 Pandemic in the UK

During the first year of the COVID-19 pandemic, empirical data were collected from across the UK at three time points, namely March, June, and September 2020. The participants were local strategic leaders from the emergency response agencies, including local authorities, emergency and essential services, NHS England (NHSE), Public Health England (PHE), now known as the UK Health Security Agency (UKHSA), local resilience structures such as Local Resilience Forums, and representatives from governmental departments. Data collection focused on creating discussion on what was going well, what was not going well, and what support was needed, as well as personal reflections [18–21].

Within these data, responders clearly highlighted the impact on their families of their work during the pandemic. This included their understanding and perception of risk to themselves and their families of contracting COVID-19. One participant described it as a 'massive, emotionally challenging area for front-line staff'. This is because responders reported that they were making some very difficult personal decisions about the risk to themselves and their families. They confronted their own mortality, and participants described their practical steps to ensure that their affairs were in order should they contract and die of COVID-19. Responders described it as their duty to their families to ensure that this was completed.

Respondents also reported the personal costs to their families of physical exhaustion, and the cost of emotional exhaustion. In addition, they described missing the physical contact and proximity of their families and friends, and their perceptions of the reductions in their support. They described the emotional harm caused by seeing the large numbers of COVID-19-related deaths, and how this had consequences for their ability to be present with and connected to their families.

This situation became more complicated over time, and as their own families contracted COVID-19. Their accounts describe the additional challenge of their own families being ill or dying from the very virus they were trying to manage in their work life. This affected the relationships between their family members and themselves, as they were unable to step away from managing the pandemic. It had become the sole focus of their work, and then also became the main focus within their homes, too. This made the virus even more omnipresent for responders and their families than it was for the wider public; they felt that their lives had become saturated by the pandemic (see Chapter 54). All of these experiences should be set against the context of the virus and its consequences causing one of the most disruptive and intrusive experiences in living memory.

In their responses, the responders discussed the risks to themselves of the immense pressures placed on them as a result of the limited number of people trained and their ability to take on certain roles. In addition, the need to work intensely and at a fast pace came at a cost not only to their own physical and mental health but also to the wellbeing of their families. Some responders described the nature, magnitude, and the length of time working under such pressure. These direct experiences caused them to suffer, and also to sacrifice time with their families. In the discussions, some responders also offered their opinions that their marriages could not sustain for much longer the circumstances posed by their responses to the pandemic and being in such adverse roles for so long. Another impact on families was that because responders were 'living in a constant state of on-call', their children now reacted negatively to the ringtone of their phone. The pandemic has presented a unique set of challenges due to the protracted and ubiquitous nature of the emergency, and it is still doing so.

Selin Tekin and colleagues studied the experiences and views of and mental health impacts on frontline healthcare workers and families in the UK during the pandemic. They identified the experiences and needs of family members of healthcare workers as having been largely absent from the literature. They support the need for further research to explore their experiences more fully [22].

Empirical Evidence About Other EITDDC

Other studies have looked at incidents that are more discrete, shorter in time scale, or specific to certain geographical or societal impacts. They identify the impacts of these more circumscribed EITDDCs on responders' families. For example, research into events such as hurricanes and flooding suggests that, when an incident occurs in the responders' home community, they and their families become survivors

of the event [23–26]. Consequently, the resources of their families are affected, through reduced capacity of social support networks in the local geography, the reduced safety of their homes and livelihoods, and their reduced energy for supporting responders.

Prior to the COVID-19 pandemic, evidence from research conducted with family members of firefighters [2] showed that:

- families and relatives have a strong need for their sacrifices to be recognised
- relatives and families avoid engaging with the perceived occupational risk of their family members, instead trusting their training, their equipment, and their firefighting colleagues
- being a relative or family of a firefighter provides a shared identity and support network
- families often try to undertake ongoing assessments of their relatives or family members to calibrate the health and wellbeing of their firefighters.

When these findings are contextualised in the literature relating to the research on family impacts from the roles of other responders, the impacts are found to have four principal domains in common. Figure 40.1 focuses on staff of the NHS to illustrate the impact on families of the responder's occupation. There are four principal domains – living with distress, shared sacrifices, the responders' 'families' at work, and perceptions of risk.

Figure 40.1 suggests that families are actively engaged in managing the impacts that result from their responders' occupations. They seek ways to actively support their responders in processing events and coping (living with distress), they seek support for themselves and others to legitimise their experiences (family at work), they manage their perception of risk and safety (risk perception), and they recognise the burden from a lot of the sacrifice that the responders' occupations cause to family life (sacrifices).

A second source of recent data collected throughout the COVID-19 pandemic also echoes these findings regarding a career of impacts from being a responder. Niamh McNamara and colleagues undertook a programme of research to explore the challenges faced by firefighters transitioning into retirement [27]. This research was scheduled to take place in 2020, and it therefore continued, taking account of the context of the pandemic. One strong theme that emerged from this research was the notion

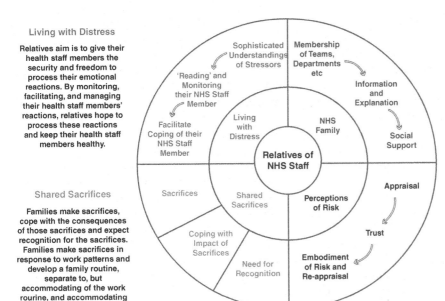

Living with Distress

Relatives aim is to give their health staff members the security and freedom to process their emotional reactions. By monitoring, facilitating, and managing their health staff members' reactions, relatives hope to process these reactions and keep their health staff members healthy.

Shared Sacrifices

Families make sacrifices, cope with the consequences of those sacrifices and expect recognition for the sacrifices. Families make sacrifices in response to work patterns and develop a family routine, separate to, but accommodating of the work rourine, and accommodating the health staff member when available.

The NHS Family

The 'work family' (or NHS family) is a wider collective group that includes NHS colleagues, NHS spouses and children. The main function of this 'family' is to provide both a social support network and friendships among healthcare staff and their families. Relatives are enabled to speak of both emotional and practical difficulties and share experiences of coping, establishing common feelings and also common understanding of the health staff members' roles.

Perceptions of Risk

Relatives are aware of the perceived dangers of their health staff members' occupation. They trust that training procedures, equipment, experience of their health staff members, and their work colleagues will protect them. This enables families to manage the percived level of risk.

Figure 40.1 The impacts on families of their relationships with NHS staff. (© R Hill, R Williams, V Kemp, 2020. All rights reserved.)

that families were prioritised by responders in retirement because their families had sacrificed so much while the responders were in their occupations. This theme arose from a number of programmes of study of other responders and occupational groups. Disruption to family life, inability to attend all key social events or celebrations due to the shift work, and the emotional burden of being a responder meant that although families absorbed these strains, doing so was not without cost. When transitioning into retirement, responders were clear that their families were to become one of the highest-priority social groups in which to invest. These findings echo the retirement literature for other responders and critical occupation groups [8].

Practical Conclusions and Solutions

The personal impacts on responders and the impacts on their families must be considered in relation to their context, culture, and group dynamics if effective practical solutions are to be developed to support emergency responders. Conservation of resource theory can be used as a framework for achieving this (see Chapter 54).

Conservation of resource theory was initially developed by Stevan Hobfoll [28]. Hobfoll argued that resources used to protect a person from a stressor

could be studied in isolation, but that unless all resources that could be used to cope are considered, coping could not be fully researched. Although originally developed as a theory to explain stress, its potential to explain adaptation, that is, the opportunity for a person to alter their future behaviour to facilitate coping, or to build their resilience against future threats, was soon recognised. Hobfoll's theory focused on situating coping resources within a pool and acknowledging the context, rather than simply studying individuals. Conservation of resource theory also acknowledges the ability of people to gain, preserve, and build resources in preparation for any potential threat. This assumes that people attempt to gain, preserve, and build resources within different structural tiers [29]. Structures at personal, family, group, community, and cultural levels are different resources available to any one person (see Chapter 54 for further explanation), and sustaining access to these wide-ranging resources motivates people to protect them. The loss of resources, or access to them, is what jeopardises people's wellbeing. Resources are defined as things within the environment of a person or group that they can draw upon to manage stress and increase their resilience against negative emotions and cognitions. This includes universally valued resources such as health, peace, self-preservation, wellbeing, family, and a positive sense of self [30].

The resources are not isolated from each other, but are referred to as 'pools' at the personal level and 'reservoirs' at the group level. The tiers of people within the dynamic mean that these resources are collective and flow between the tiers. Hobfoll suggests that the resources, and conservation of resource theory, integrate 'the individual-nested in family-nested in tribe' [31, p. 338]. He goes on to define these terms, but for the purposes of this chapter the person is the responder, the family is the immediate family of the responder, and the tribe is the employer of the responder.

The theory advocates that resources do not appear, and should not be tested, in isolation from one another, but that they appear in clusters, which usually present together. Major resources, such as the personal characteristic of self-esteem, are synonymous with associated resources such as optimism. This clustering phenomenon is termed 'resource caravans' by Hobfoll, who explains that these caravans are so named because they travel with groups and individual people throughout their lifespans [32]. Caravan passageways are conditions that nurture, support, and enrich the resources of groups or individual people, or, in the negative context, conditions that impoverish and frustrate these resources. Whereas passageways define the developmental lifespan quality of a person's resource caravan, pathways are structures within which resources are supplied, protected, shared, fostered, and pooled.

For an employer of responders, there is a social responsibility to develop policies that facilitate an engaging resource ecology [32]. These are organisations and structures that actively encourage 'pooling' of resources for the employees, departments, or groups to access when needed in order to meet the employing organisation's needs and goals. Suggesting that the wellbeing of their employees is (in part) facilitated by their relatives means that responding organisations have an additional interest in the relatives of their responders as they offer effective resources that enable their employees to manage stress and increase resilience against negative emotions and cognitions [33].

Recommendations

- It has been clearly established that the work of emergency responders has impacts on their family members. Families can be seen as contributing to their relatives' employers due to the role they occupy in diffusing for their relatives, and buffering health issues, thereby promoting employees' capacities. The social support that relatives provide is an essential part of increasing and maintaining resilience, reducing stress, and maintaining occupational effectiveness. As part of their delivery of initial training, organisations that employ responders should develop and deliver messages for the families of their trainees, to educate and prepare them for the impacts associated with the work of emergency responders with the explicit aim of minimising those effects. The armed forces and some emergency services in different cultures already include this as part of the initial training stages. The messages are nuanced as the responders progress and their roles change with career progression. This allows for self-management of families through their preparation and legitimisation of the impacts, if and when these occur.

- Evidenced-based support mechanisms for responders should become a key area of focus, building on the widely reported lessons from the COVID-19 pandemic as the nature of strain on people in these occupations has changed, particularly in relation to system health and moral injury. The support for these people has suffered over the years of austerity following the financial crash as the public purse strings were tightened. The same is happening again after the public expenditure on the pandemic response, but this should not be allowed to persist for the staff and their families who have sacrificed so much for society. The support offered to responders by their employers needs to be prioritised, facilitated through appropriate funding from the public purse, with conditions that the funds be spent on evidence-based support structures with appropriate, quality-assured, and accredited processes overseen by appropriate governance structures, and with built-in evaluations to monitor their effectiveness.

- Messages that are acceptable for key workers to share with their families (if they are comfortable doing so) should be embedded in training and practice. Some key workers were hesitant about discussing with their families the details and emotional impact of their work. This was due to their motivation to protect their families from the reality of their work, or concerns that their families might not respond constructively. Advice given to key workers should include how to structure the conversation with family members, what responding constructively might look like, how to initiate discussions about the experiences that they have in their work as responders, and how to facilitate social support for their families.

- The development of reliable credible resources to support families should be completed, and these resources should be made available to families if they need them. Information about the resources could be stored on a known website to allow families to seek reassurance, guidance, and knowledge to enable their own management of their particular situations. Attendance at major incidents could trigger a reminder of these resources for responders, and in turn for their families, to ensure awareness of support as responders progress through their careers.
- The literature suggests that as responders and their families start to gain resources from these

initial activities, they will want to seek out more, in order to harvest more resources for future use. Therefore ensuring the longevity of these solutions is an important aspect of achieving a successful support ecology. They should be actively looked after and facilitated, and responses should not be initiated for a short time before moving the resource elsewhere. The sustainability and continuation of any support for families and responders should have a sustainability plan going forward for at least the next 15 years.

Conclusion

By facilitating a resource-rich caravan for responders' families, employers are investing in the human capital of their organisations as well as the psychosocial health of their staff. Policy development should continue to follow the evidence base that should follow the experiences of the global pandemic to produce leading practice in supporting responders' wellbeing.

References

1. Boss P. Ambiguous loss research, theory, and practice: reflections after 9/11. *J Marriage Fam* 2004; 66: 551–66.

2. Hill R, Sundin E, Winder B. Work–family enrichment of firefighters: 'satellite family members', risk, trauma and family functioning. *Int J Emerg Serv* 2020; 9: 395–407.

3. Davidson AC, Berah E, Moss S. The relationship between the adjustment of Australian police officers and their partners. *Psychiatry Psychol Law* 2006; 13: 41–8.

4. Regehr C. Bringing the trauma home: spouses of paramedics. *J Loss Trauma* 2005; 10: 97–114.

5. Hill R, Pickford R, Abdelmalak E, Afolayan S, Brittain M, Nadeem L, et al. *Mapping the Health and Wellbeing Across the Firefighting Career and Assessing the Current Demands*. Nottingham Trent University, 2023.

6. Hobfoll SE, Spielberger CD. Family stress: integrating theory

and measurement. *J Fam Psychol* 1992; 6: 99.

7. Schumm JA, Vranceanu AM, Hobfoll SE. The ties that bind: resource caravans and losses among traumatized families. In *Handbook of Stress, Trauma, and the Family* (ed. DR Catherall): 33–50. Routledge, 2014.

8. Sharp ML, Harrison V, Solomon N, Fear N, King H, Pike G. *Assessing the Mental Health and Wellbeing of the Emergency Responder Community in the UK*. King's College London, 2020.

9. Hill R. Occupational related consequences for relatives of firefighters. PhD Thesis, Nottingham Trent University, 2015.

10. Mikkelsen A, Burke RJ. Work–family concerns of Norwegian police officers: antecedents and consequences. *Int J Stress Manag* 2004; 11: 429.

11. He N, Zhao J, Archbold CA. Gender and police stress: the convergent and divergent impact of work environment, work–

family conflict, and stress coping mechanisms of female and male police officers. *Policing* 2002; 25: 687–708.

12. Schumm WR, Bell DB, Resnick G. Recent research on family factors and readiness: implications for military leaders. *Psychol Rep* 2001; 89: 153–65.

13. Greenhaus JH, Powell GN. When work and family are allies: a theory of work–family enrichment. *Acad Manag Rev* 2006; 31: 72–92.

14. Cabarkapa S, Nadjidai SE, Murgier J, Ng CH. The psychological impact of COVID-19 and other viral epidemics on frontline healthcare workers and ways to address it: a rapid systematic review. *Brain Behav Immun Health* 2020; 8: 100144.

15. Shaukat N, Ali DM, Razzak J. Physical and mental health impacts of COVID-19 on healthcare workers: a scoping review. *Int J Emerg Med* 2020; 13: 1–8.

16. Ann SM, Gaughan AA, Macewan SR, Gregory ME, Rush LJ, Volney J, et al. Pandemic experience of first responders: fear, frustration, and stress. *Int J Environ Res Public Health* 2022; **19**: 4693.

17. Løvseth LT, Aasland OG. Confidentiality as a barrier to social support: a cross-sectional study of Norwegian emergency and human service workers. *Int J Stress Manag* 2020; **17**: 214.

18. Hill R, Stewart S, Potter A, Pickford R, Smith K. *Managing the First 230 Days*. C19 National Foresight Group, 2020.

19. Hill R, Guest D, Pickford R, Hopkinson A, Daszkiewicz T, Whitton S, et al. *Covid-19 Pandemic: Second Interim Operational Review*. C19 National Foresight Group, 2020.

20. Hill R, Guest D, Pickford R, Hopkinson A, Daszkiewicz T, Whitton S, et al. *Covid-19 Pandemic: Third Interim Operational Review*. C19 National Foresight Group, 2020.

21. Hill R, Guest D, Hopkinson A, Towler A, Pickford R. *Covid-19 Pandemic: First Interim Operational Review*. C19 National Foresight Group, 2020.

22. Tekin S, Glover N, Greene T, Lamb D, Murphy D, Billings J. Experiences and views of frontline healthcare workers' family members in the UK during the COVID-19 pandemic: a qualitative study. Eur J Psychotraumatol 2022; **13**: 2057166.

23. Jenkins SR. Coping and social support among emergency dispatchers: Hurricane Andrew. *J Soc Behav Pers* 1997; **12**: 201–16.

24. O'Toole M, Mulhall C, Eppich W. Breaking down barriers to help-seeking: preparing first responders' families for psychological first aid. *Eur J Psychotraumatol* 2022; **13**: 2065430.

25. Casas JB, Benuto LT. Work-related traumatic stress spillover in first responder families: a systematic review of the literature. *Psychol Trauma* 2022; **14**: 209–17.

26. Porter KL, Henriksen RC. The phenomenological experience of first responder spouses. *Fam J* 2016; **24**: 44–51.

27. McNamara N, Muhlemann N, Stevenson C, Haslam C, Hill R, Steffens N, et al. Understanding the transition to retirement for firefighters: a social identity approach. *Nottingham: The Firefighters Charity*. Available from: https://irep.ntu.ac.uk/id/eprint/49070

28. Hobfoll SE. Conservation of resources: a new attempt at conceptualizing stress. *Am Psychol* 1989; **44**: 513.

29. Halbesleben JR, Neveu JP, Paustian-Underdahl SC, Westman M. Getting to the "COR": understanding the role of resources in conservation of resources theory. *J Manag* 2014; **40**: 1334–64.

30. Hobfoll SE. Conservation of resources and disaster in cultural context: the caravans and passageways for resources. *Psychiatry* 2012; **75**: 227–32.

31. Hobfoll SE. The influence of culture, community, and the nested-self in the stress process: advancing conservation of resources theory. *Appl Psychol* 2001; **50**: 337–421.

32. Hobfoll SE. Conservation of resource caravans and engaged settings. *J Occup Organ Psychol* 2011; **84**: 116–22.

33. Brunsden V, Hill R, Maguire K. Managing stress in the fire and rescue service: a UK informed global perspective. *Int Fire Service J Leader Manag* 2014; **7**: 27–39.

41

Lessons for Structure, Workforce Planning, and Responding to Emergencies from Nurses in the COVID-19 Pandemic

Jill Maben and Anna Conolly

Background

Nurses, like other healthcare professionals, have been lauded and applauded during the COVID-19 pandemic and called heroes [1]. Indeed, the pandemic has not only shone a spotlight on the importance and complexity of their work in delivering care to the sickest patients [2], but has also shone a very welcome spotlight on the need to look after nurses' psychosocial wellbeing.

In the UK's National Health Service (NHS) hospital, community, and primary care settings there are around 350,000 nurses and midwives directly employed by NHS organisations, constituting one-third of the total workforce [3]. Nurses remain one of the most trusted professions [4], but not always the most valued.

Nursing has never been seen as a 'safety-critical industry' [5], yet nurses spend the most time with patients, notice and act on signs of deterioration, and provide life-saving interventions every day that go largely unnoticed. Changes to the skills mix in nursing and the delegation of what many consider essential nursing skills to others have undermined the importance of patients' assessment and moved registered nurses away from patients and from much of this so-called 'invisible' safety-critical work [5]. As Alison Leary has stated, 'In other safety-critical industries the benefit of expertise is when that expertise is close to risk' (i.e., patients) [5, p. 3761]. In nursing, a response to the workforce supply issues has been to develop a new care role, a second-level nurse, the nursing associate role, to 'act as a bridge between the registered and non-registered workforce' [16, p. 38]. Thus frontline hands-on care is something for less skilled workers to do, and the skilled experienced registered nurses are removed from the bedside to be managers of care delivery, with non-registered workers undertaking task-based care.

Leary has argued cogently that a narrow focus on care delivery as a series of tasks to be completed, rather than delivering person-centred care, together with the reductionist, efficiency-based approaches to the workforce crisis, underestimates workload in complex, high-risk nursing work [7]. Managerial discourses of efficiency overwhelm nurses' knowledge of patients as whole people, and task-based work is unsatisfying for nurses, compromising their ideals and values, resulting in reported burnout and many nurses leaving the profession [8].

Furthermore, there is a whole host of legacy issues that have resulted in the nursing workforce not being optimally prepared for the COVID-19 pandemic, and nurses being put under extreme pressure. Decades of little or no workforce planning [5,7,9], underfunding of the health service workforce, and significant staffing shortages have led to significant structural challenges [6,10]. In 2019, there were already 46,000 nursing vacancies across the NHS, with considerable difficulty in recruiting and retaining staff. A King's Fund report published in 2019 predicted a shortfall of 108,000 full-time-equivalent registered nurses within the next 10 years if current trends continued [11]. Even before the pandemic, pressure in the health and care system was taking its toll on staff and was not sustainable. Staff were described as 'running on empty' and as the 'shock absorbers in a system lacking [the] resources to meet rising demands' [10].

A decade ago, nursing workforce experts James Buchan and Ian Seccombe identified periods of boom and bust in nurse workforce planning, particularly in relation to student nurses, with overseas recruitment used to fill gaps [5,9]. This cycle has continued. The arrival of Brexit, the COVID-19 pandemic, and removal of the nursing bursary have resulted in a perfect storm for the profession. An already depleted workforce was asked to step up to face the challenge of an unprecedented global pandemic.

Over time, there has also been a reduction in previous systems that supported nursing practice, helped to manage infection control issues, and helped nurses to live relatively well on fairly low salaries. For example, in the not too distant past, hospitals provided cheap accommodation, free car parking, and access to a uniform laundry. Few nurses have access to subsidised accommodation today, even in central London or other expensive cities. Nurses are expected to launder their own uniforms even in a pandemic, which requires fatigued nurses to shower, disrobe, and wash uniforms at the end of an exhausting shift before leaving work, or to disrobe before entering their homes to protect their relatives. Car parking charges, although suspended during the pandemic, were subsequently re-introduced, leaving staff feeling undervalued and frustrated. It continues to be difficult to recruit and retain registered nurses in expensive parts of the country. The average annual basic pay for doctors is double that of nurses. Yet nurses' access to funded time or fees for continuing professional development (CPD), which is required for re-registration, are scarce, are often not ring-fenced, and remain poor compared with the access and funding received by most doctors [12].

Any health service needs healthy, motivated staff to provide high-quality patient care, yet the workforce challenges and legacy issues outlined in this chapter combine with an ever increasing workload to take their toll on staff [6,10]. Specific challenges relating to the pandemic have also been identified. The risks to healthcare workers' health from contracting COVID-19 have been high during the pandemic, with England and Wales experiencing the highest rate in the world of deaths of healthcare workers from COVID-19, particularly workers from Black and ethnic-minority groups [13]. There have been calls for COVID-19 to be classified as an occupational disease, but little action has been taken [14], and there have also been calls for the outdated UK guidance on personal protective equipment (PPE) in workplaces to be rectified [15].

The start of 2020 saw poor access to PPE in the face of the pandemic, with widespread reports of inadequate access to PPE across the world and specifically in the UK [13]. This was particularly the case for social care workers and some nurses, – for example, community and mental health nurses, who reported wearing black bin liners and other inadequate equipment. The toll on nurses' mental health has been

significant. A survey of nurses in 2020 found that almost a third of nurses who responded reported traumatic stress symptoms 3 months after the first pandemic peak. A lack of confidence in infection prevention and control training was associated with increased symptoms of post-traumatic stress disorder (PTSD) at all three time points [16].

In terms of supporting the mental health of staff through the pandemic, there were several rapid syntheses of the literature on interventions and activities to support the psychosocial wellbeing of staff during the extreme challenges of the pandemic, many of which were found to be useful [e.g., 17,18].

Although there is a wealth of evidence to support the importance of psychosocial wellbeing at work for emergencies, such as localised epidemics and global pandemics, most evidence-based interventions for healthcare staff focus on individual people, with the responsibility to remain well, by looking after their own mental health and wellbeing, resting firmly with individual nurses. There are few team-based or organisation-wide interventions to support wellbeing at work, notable exceptions being Schwartz Rounds, Balint groups, and group supervision [e.g., 19]. Much has been written about the notion of 'resilient' nurses, and how the responsibility to be 'resilient' is left for each to manage and maintain [20,21]. This can let organisations off the hook [22], and can make nurses feel that if they are not coping they are not 'resilient enough', despite facing the most challenging work conditions (extremely ill patients, high demand, low staffing, and a poor skill mix). There is now something of a backlash against resilience-based training interventions targeted at individuals, with many arguing that the structural aspects of work need to improve considerably to support people's resilience, and that it is not an individual's sole responsibility to be resilient and bounce back.

In a recent review we examined the service architecture (structural features of work), comparing how work is organised across four professions (nurses, midwives, paramedics, and doctors) in order to identify the resulting impacts on wellbeing in these professions [23]. We note that nursing and midwifery are female-dominated, with gender pay gaps, often extra caring responsibilities, and a preponderance of lower-paid roles. Professions other than medicine had ageing workforces, yet turnover and retention were problematic across all professions. All professions reported high job stress, with sickness absence rates for nurses, midwives, and paramedics 3 times higher than those for doctors, and presenteeism nearly double [23].

What has been shown to help healthcare staff is peer support, and more formal one-to-one talking therapy support may be needed by some staff in due course. Peer support provides opportunities for staff to connect with each other and share experiences, talk to each other, and be heard by peers who understand what the job entails (Chapter 48 provides more information). An analysis of 179 studies of interventions for doctors found that those that emphasise relationships and belonging, such as creating a people-focused working culture, were more likely to promote wellbeing. It was concluded that multilevel interventions to tackle mental ill health are most likely to be successful [24]. Yet, as we have suggested, many interventions (e.g., mindfulness training, resilience building, mentoring) are frequently geared towards improving the coping mechanisms of individual people [25]. At an organisational level, some interventions improve practice, such as increased uptake of psychosocial support through Schwartz Rounds and Balint groups [26]. A synthesis of evidence in 2018 found that reflective spaces such as Schwartz Rounds (but also Balint groups, restorative supervision, after-action reviews, etc.) provide positive benefits for individuals through, for example, increased self-awareness, job satisfaction, or overall wellbeing, and most provided some evidence of positive benefits to 'others', such as colleagues and patients [19].

We now turn our attention to the specifics of the COVID-19 pandemic and the experiences of nurses in the UK by drawing on data from our qualitative longitudinal study of the impact of COVID on nurses (the ICON study).

How the COVID-19 Pandemic Affected Nurses' Psychological Wellbeing in the UK

Since the World Health Organization (WHO) declared a pandemic on 11 March 2020, there has been much research examining the effects of working during COVID-19 on different sectors of the nursing and healthcare workforce (e.g., [18,27,28]). Although most of this research has been cross-sectional, it has raised concerns about the emotional impact of working during the pandemic. We explored the detailed narratives of nurses' experiences of COVID-19 in the ICON qualitative study, by conducting up to four interviews longitudinally with two cohorts of nurses ($n = 50$) across the trajectory of the pandemic. The participants were from a wide range of working environments, and we asked them about the possible impacts of working during the pandemic on their psychosocial and emotional wellbeing.

The interviews were undertaken using a narrative method, with participants invited to tell interviewers about their experiences. Topic guide prompts were only used when required [29]. We used NVivo12 to organise the data, and developed inductive codes and subsequent themes across the data. We wrote summaries or pen portraits of participants' interviews, which reduced fragmentation of the data and aided our narrative analysis [30]. The themes identified are outlined in Tables 41.1 and 41.2 (to which we come later), and we present our data here through two exemplar case studies because they represent the majority of the themes in our data and illuminate the challenges and support encountered by nurses in the UK. The two cases are particular nurses' experiences (we use the pseudonyms Annabel and Gaby), and we use quotes from their narratives. They worked in very different environments, and their jobs required different levels of experience and support; this reveals similarities and differences both between and within the themes. The first case study describes the experiences of Annabel, a nurse who worked in an intensive care unit (ICU) before COVID-19, and who continued to do so during the first and second waves of the pandemic. The second case study shares the experiences of Gaby as a nurse who was redeployed to a community hospital. In this context, being redeployed means being assigned to work in a new setting or area (usually COVID-19 wards or ICUs during the pandemic), away from one's usual role. Although there were some positive aspects of working during the pandemic, such as the sense of camaraderie and pulling together, Annabel and Gaby – like most nurses in our sample – recounted their experiences of working in the pandemic as mostly negative, and both of them were deeply affected by their experiences.

Annabel: An ICU Nurse

COVID-19 brought about a change in patient cohorts for the majority of our interviewees, with many

Table 41.1 Analytic themes and their presence in Annabel and Gaby's narratives

Overarching theme	Sub-theme	Annabel	Gaby
Moral distress due to care delivery	Work left undone		✓
	Increased patient acuity and death	✓	✓
	Contagion fears	✓	
Systemic challenges	Insufficient training, staff, and specialist environments	✓	✓
	PPE shortages	✓	✓
	Limited opportunity to speak up	✓	✓
Emotional exhaustion	Survival mode	✓	
	Burnout and PTSD symptoms	✓	✓
	Intention to leave	✓	✓
Support accessed	The importance of collegial support	✓	✓
	Avoidance of support provided by the NHS	✓	✓

nurses unused to seeing so many critically ill patients with limited clinical options and high mortality rates. We use the term deathscapes to conceptualise nurses' working environments that are characterised by high rates of mortality, and we use this concept to describe the environments during the COVID-19 peaks in the UK [22]. Most of the nurses whom we spoke to reflected on the impact of increased inpatient mortality on their psychosocial wellbeing, as Annabel did:

I switched from [thinking] … I'll be fine … to all of a sudden thinking, no, this is awful … I was sat on the nurses' station next to three other people having this conversation with family members and it was like [the same conversation] over and over again and they'd die and next, next, literally … quickly turn the bed around, next. It felt like a conveyer belt. It felt surreal. …

Then … I had three weeks off work because I was really unwell [with COVID-19] I think it hit me when I was rock bottom … emotionally and physically.

Annabel's description of her ICU as an almost factory-like conveyer belt of death powerfully conveys the sheer volume of patients who were dying, and the sense of powerlessness that healthcare professionals experienced during this time as their actions had very few positive impacts on patients' health in the first wave of the pandemic. Throughout her interview, Annabel emphasised the differences between her normal working practices and those she experienced during the UK's COVID-19 waves. For example, before COVID-19, deaths were well managed with relatives prepared and present. However, excluding family members during COVID-19, in order to keep them safe and prevent spread of the disease, placed more emotional responsibility on nurses to provide support for patients at the end-of-life stage, and meant that deaths were rarely as well managed as practitioners would have preferred. Annabel's ICU extended into other hospital wards where the only barrier between one patient and the next was a curtain. Thus, due to the make-do nature of the space she was working in, Annabel found that:

I don't feel like we could uphold patients' privacy and dignity as well because the curtains, as you know, don't hide the sound, but we didn't have side rooms to put patients in. We just had to give end of life care as best we could in the bays surrounded by possibly other awake [patients]. … So it was traumatising for the other patients. … It wasn't personalised, we couldn't be sat with the family surrounding them and be anticipatory.

The lack of appropriate resources, such as whether there were single rooms, or equipment such as ventilators or PPE, was mentioned by all of the nurses who participated in the study. Although Annabel was only in her second year as a registered nurse and ICU nurse, she also became responsible for supervising nurses and healthcare assistants who had been redeployed to help in the crisis. Due to the increased numbers of patients that she was caring for, Annabel also found supervising nurses challenging:

All of a sudden, there are four patients in a bay. I'm used to nursing one-to-one. These are the sickest patients … they were on filters, they were on dialyses, they were on heart medication, they were on all sorts and [there were] four of them and these nurses were turning to me and saying, 'Annabel, what do I do for this?' I'm thinking I don't know … I've only been here 18 months.

Previous research has shown that training deficits can undermine nurses' ability to feel able to enact positive change and improve outcomes for patients. These feelings can lead to a lack of engagement, reduced job satisfaction, and depersonalisation [31].

Nurses' work environments during the COVID-19 pandemic involved negotiating stressors that were both psychological and physical in nature, such as wearing PPE. Annabel recounted a shift in stressors as a result of limited PPE supplies:

> Well, I didn't go to the toilet I remember for two days because we had a gown shortage . . . you couldn't have a drink. If you got your lunch break you were lucky [as a result I became unwell]. I didn't go to the toilet because I was so worried that I'd use all the PPE.

The toll taken by working in this manner was both emotional and physical, resulting in Annabel becoming physically unwell. Additionally, a fear of contamination and infecting loved ones caused many nurses to experience extensions to their working days as they stayed on site after their shifts to shower and decontaminate:

> I'd finish my shift at half seven, but I never left until about quarter past eight because I'd be handing over four patients . . . and then I'd go and wait in the queue for a shower and then at 9 o'clock I'd be home and then I'd be going for another shower and then I'd go to bed and then I'd do it all again the next day. I tried not to think about it really at the time . . . what I was doing.

The relentlessness of Annabel's working days are striking, but she, like many other nurses, continued to work throughout the pandemic. Annabel's stoicism is common among nurses in the NHS [32], and the majority of the nurses in our study reported that stoicism was intertwined with their professional identity. A notable feature that the majority of our interviewees shared was the feeling that they could not discuss their experiences of nursing during the pandemic with family members and non-nursing friends:

> I tried not to talk to my family because I just couldn't cope with hearing their worries, [it] was not helpful because I thought I've just got to get through this, I've just got to do it.

Like many of the study participants, Annabel did not use any of the Apps or other wellbeing resources that the NHS or hospitals provided. She cited the stigma within the NHS associated with healthcare professionals not being able to cope with their jobs as a possible reason why she chose to avoid professional help, as well as the need to keep going, and therefore not having the time to take the lid off her emotions at that stage. She reflected that she had worked too much during this period, and she wished that she 'hadn't been allowed to do so much overtime'.

We found that the vast majority of the participants in our study valued their own support groups in which they shared their experiences with colleagues who had 'been through the same thing'. Similarly, Annabel did confide in a colleague about some aspects of her experiences. They shared voice notes of their experiences, having witnessed similar events, which they could talk about and support one another.

However, Annabel's interview for the ICON study was the first time she had spoken at length to anyone about her experiences of and feelings about COVID-19. This was not at all uncommon. Rather like war narratives, nurses kept their traumatic experiences buried deep. The process of taking part in our study, and having a compassionate stranger listen carefully to their stories, was described by the vast majority of nurses as cathartic and therapeutic [33]. Processing her experiences in the research interview allowed Annabel to acknowledge, for the first time, that she had left her ICU post because she needed to get away and find a different environment in which to work. She no longer felt able to continue to provide care for very sick patients during further waves of COVID-19. She stated that she was now ready to access some talking therapies, citing sleep disturbances and anxiety as indicators that she might have some traumatic stress to process. Again, this was not at all uncommon.

Annabel's narrative highlights the fact that extra stressors created by the COVID-19 pandemic were felt by nurses who were accustomed to working in high-stress and end-of-life environments, such as ICUs. For those nurses who were redeployed from community settings into environments with large numbers of intensely sick COVID-19 patients, the stressors experienced were even further amplified, as is illustrated by Gaby's case.

Gaby: A Redeployed Community Nurse

Although many public health nurses continued their work in the community during the COVID-19 pandemic in the UK, some were redeployed to other areas within the NHS. Gaby was working as a health visitor prior to the pandemic, a position that gave her autonomy and job satisfaction. At the onset of the pandemic in the UK, and like other nurses in the study who possessed a strong sense of moral duty towards both patients and colleagues, Gaby volunteered to be redeployed, and moved into a very different clinical setting, a community hospital.

Due to inadequate testing of COVID-19-positive patients referred by local hospitals to the community hospitals, the virus spread quickly in the latter. The patients who were admitted during the first COVID-19 wave were experiencing severe levels of respiratory illness, and thus presenting an entirely new type of patient for the permanent staff who worked there. As a member of redeployed staff, Gaby spoke of the Matron's relief ('Thank God you're here') when she first arrived. Gaby found the work in this community hospital to be some of the hardest in her long career, as it was so psychologically and physically demanding:

> You're answering bells, so you haven't got the time to clean everything thoroughly ... you're just running all the time. You are leaving people on the toilet ... or you are not answering a bell, or somebody needs to be made more comfortable on their bed. Nothing is what you're used to doing. So, you're starting to build up this guilt.

Gaby believed that the treatment her patients received during her redeployment was greatly at odds with her nursing values, which normally involved her going the extra mile and delivering compassionate care. Therefore the guilt or distress that Gaby described regarding the treatment that her patients received was moral in nature (moral distress) because she was constrained from providing the quality of care that she felt she should be providing [34]. Gaby was highly critical of the care that the patients in this unit received, due to the understaffing and the lack of choices about their care that patients and their relatives were given. Gaby's criticisms focused mostly on systemic failures, such as the lack of PPE, the unsuitability of the rehabilitation hospital for providing appropriate infection control measures, and colleagues who were struggling with COVID-19-related decisions that included assigning patients to end-of-life care pathways, due to either fears of contagion or inexperience and being out of their depth:

> A doctor there put a lady on an end-of-life pathway and I said to him, 'Why?' And he didn't really know. I was going off shift and I said to the nurse I was handing over to, 'Please get her daughter in, because I have no clue as to why this decision has been made, but she needs to see

her daughter'. . . . They got her daughter to come ... I think her daughter seeing her saved her life, but she wasn't [an end-of-life patient]. It seemed that anyone that showed any sign of deterioration [was put on an end-of-life pathway].

Like many other nurses in our study, Gaby did attempt to speak up and raise concerns with managers and doctors, yet organisational deafness was prevalent during the COVID-19 pandemic. Concerns were were frequently not acted upon, as the voices of those who tried to speak out against poor decision making and unsafe working conditions were silenced [35].

Similarly to other nurses in the study, Gaby's feelings of psychological insecurity in her new role were characterised by personal risk calculations. She referred to a risky situation in which a colleague had found herself:

> One of my [redeployed] colleagues who did a night shift on her own had somebody who had a fall and didn't know what the protocol was, and it's huge isn't it? And it's that kind of risk taking as well. . . . You're in a new environment, long shifts, you've got a long drive, trying to make sure that you're upskilling – there was a pressure to upskill every day.

On top of the other stressors, Gaby described how the pressure to upskill and take on extra duties was a risk she was not prepared to accept. This resonated with many of the redeployed nurses to whom we spoke in our study. After several months of redeployment, Gaby herself caught COVID-19 and became quite unwell. She attributed her contraction of COVID-19 to the poor infection control measures at the community hospital. She reflected some months later on what she had been through:

> I think that I was definitely having signs of trauma ... because I would go home and I really couldn't, you know there's still people now, and I think about their names every day, even now, and I think about them, and it just makes me so sad ... I think everybody there, we wanted to just look after people, and you feel that you've not looked after them [very well].

Gaby described a sense of being haunted. She was, and still is, unable to forget her interactions with some of her patients, or to remove or emotionally disentangle them from her (un)conscious mind. This sense of a 'haunted mind' is not uncommon within caring environments, particularly in spaces of care that generate difficult emotions or moral or ethical dilemmas [35]. Drawing on Emma Rowland's work [36, p. 33], we argue that, as was the case for many of the nurses in our study, the collision between Gaby's private and public emotional worlds threatened her ability to create emotional distance between herself and her patients.

For Gaby, like Annabel, the effect on her wellbeing was great and she referred to her 'signs of trauma'. Repeated exposure to traumatic and distressing events without sufficient psychosocial preparation or support has been found to have a cumulative effect on nurses' mental health, making them vulnerable to PTSD [31]. People who have PTSD often become haunted by and re-live the traumatic event through nightmares and flashbacks, and they may experience feelings of isolation, irritability, and guilt; these symptoms were experienced by both Annabel and Gaby.

In her later interviews, Gaby anticipated a public inquiry into the healthcare that patients received during the COVID-19 pandemic, and expressed her desire for the relatives of patients who had died to ask difficult questions to reveal how substantially care in the NHS was altered and what could be done to prevent such deficits in compassionate care during future pandemics. During her third interview, Gaby announced that she had reduced her working hours significantly and was about to retire. Like many other participants who planned to leave the NHS in the aftermath of COVID-19, Gaby described the immediate positive impact that this had on her wellbeing.

In summary, we have used two cases studies to illuminate the intense and unique stressors that the COVID-19 pandemic presented to nurses in the UK, and the effects they had on nurses' psychosocial wellbeing. These stressors were experienced by nurses who worked in a variety of different settings, including both those who were redeployed and those who were not.

Although some mental health impacts may be short-term responses to the crisis, others have the potential to cause long-term effects across groups of healthcare staff. Some of the recommended strategies that were offered were useful. For example, our participants recognised the psychosocial benefit that they gained from sharing their experiences with colleagues who had 'been through the same thing' and understood what they had experienced. Nurses who worked in supportive teams found this support face to face, whereas others gained support virtually through WhatsApp or Facebook groups. We also advocate that peer support should be provided at a structural level in spaces and environments provided by managers, to ensure that no workers are left out. Our

data support the statement by the British Academy that 'there is an urgent need to restore nurse well-being and develop a national COVID nursing workforce recovery strategy focusing on valuing the nursing workforce and nurse retention' [37, p. 15]. We call for more considered systemic support to be generated and consistently provided for nurses and other healthcare workers to ensure the future of professional practice and the security of society. The avoidance of a mass exodus from nursing, and of any further worsening of recent shortages in the UK and global nursing workforce, depend on putting the right support in place now. It is to this subject that we turn next.

Insights from the COVID-19 Pandemic for the Future Management of Psychological Wellbeing in Nursing and Other Healthcare Staff during Health Emergencies

It is imperative that healthcare professionals feel that their needs are being met and that they are safe in their work environments [38], particularly during emergencies. Thus, in a crisis, staff need their immediate basic physiological and safety needs to be met as per Maslow's hierarchy of needs, published in 1943 (see Figure 41.1). Only when these basic needs are met, and the threat recedes, can they begin to access psychosocial support to meet their wider needs. In Table 41.2 we present data from the ICON qualitative study, noting that the staff in our study required very different kinds of support at different times.

Using our adapted version of Maslow's hierarchy of needs [38], which places organisational responsibility at the core, we have explored the key issues and strategies that the ICON study participants reported. We have used Maslow's hierarchy to indicate the type of need and/or strategy to which participants were referring, and the extent to which it was or was not helpful. As indicated in Table 41.2, the needs and requirements to which our participants referred were intersected by notions of temporality, with different strategies required at different times, across the trajectory of the pandemic.

Notably, many of the ICON study participants did not access interventions (e.g., mindfulness Apps, 'wobble rooms', online 'Zoom' wellbeing sessions,

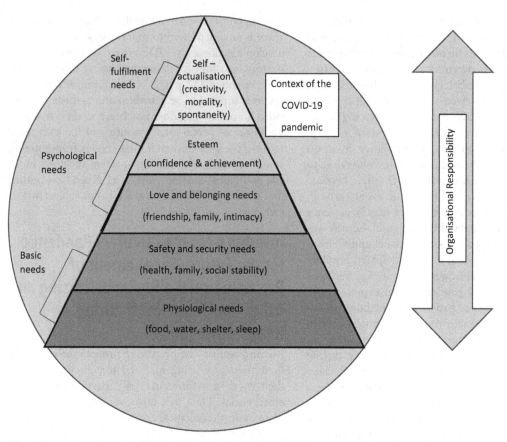

Figure 41.1 Adapted version of Maslow's hierarchy of needs, published in 1943.

counselling, psychology sessions) due to time con-straints and not wishing to access resources outside shift hours, or because of physical barriers such as sessions not being set up at the site where staff were working. Our participants needed to meet their basic needs for safety and physiological needs first. Inadequate staffing levels were a major factor that inhibited implementing informal and formal interventions. Psychological first aid recognises this matter.

Managerial interventions were also highlighted by participants as frequently lacking, with many nurses stating that they felt unvalued by their managers, and that they would not be able to discuss their emotions with the managers. Talking about mental health at work is still felt to be a stigmatising experience, with many staff suggesting that some line managers would not have the necessary tools or knowledge to do this well. The ICON participants spoke of their need to confide in people who were not necessarily trained

psychologists, with many preferring to talk to work colleagues. Many of the ICON participants (including Annabel) reported that taking part in the study was cathartic [33]. As interviewers, we were aware of the need to be good listeners and to provide psychological first aid through the medium of active listening [33].

We call for more work to be done at a national level to address stigma within the healthcare services, along with the notions of nurses as stoical, and con-ceptualisations of resilience as a valued individual trait rather than an organisational responsibility [21]. We argue that it is imperative, for the long-term psychosocial and physical safety of staff in healthcare services and of people using those services, to prioritise higher staffing levels along with specified funding in order to build actions to sustain wellbeing into the weekly routine of all healthcare staff. Much of our learning can be applied to all staff in healthcare organisations. Returning to the structural and legacy issues that we outlined at the beginning of this

Table 41.2 Specific strategies that support nurses (or not) over time. (Note that these strategies are categorised according to the levels of Maslow's hierarchy of needs; see Figure 41.1.)

	Helpful	Not helpful
Early days		
Physiological needs	Ensuring time in which to take breaks and be able to consume drinks/food and use toilet	Limiting breaks, or no access to a safe break space
	Access to (free) food provided	Not ensuring equity of access to free food for all frontline NHS workers, whether redeployed, in hospitals, or in community settings
	Free parking and access to parking spaces on site	
Safety and security needs	Training required prior to redeployment in skills and possible traumatic incidents which may be encountered	Mindfulness Apps
	Adequate supplies of equipment needed (e.g., PPE)	'Wobble' rooms
	Creating a compassionate listening culture with 'someone to talk to' (e.g., team member, colleague, psychologist) in every unit/healthcare setting	One-to-one sessions with a psychologist offered via line-manager as gatekeepers
	Calming strategies (e.g., quiet time during shift to access wellbeing resources)	Online wellbeing resources offered for nurses to engage with during their home time (wellbeing needs to be embedded into their shift time)
	Greater consideration of nurses' working shifts and hours	
Love and belonging needs	Buddy system to ensure skills/training competency and for checking in on mental health and wellbeing	Extremely condensed training or no support from colleagues in redeployed setting
	Creating time and space for co-workers to talk to each other during shifts	Not ensuring adequate recovery time through monitoring or limiting the numbers of extra shifts nurses could do (too much overtime)
		Limiting interaction with other nurses (e.g., due to COVID restrictions in staff-room spaces)
Esteem	Managers need to give nurses choices about redeployment	
	Professional supervision sessions to be offered to all nurses with space allocated/created on shift for attendance	
Six months		
Physiological needs	Perks such as free parking/access to parking to continue	
Safety and security needs	Informal anonymous individual counselling opportunities at work	Counselling offered via the organization, with line-managers as gatekeepers
	Free gym membership	
Love and belonging needs	Improved organisational communication	Organisational communication through social media channels
Esteem	Requirement for leadership culture to be compassionate	

Table 41.2 (*cont.*)

	Helpful	Not helpful
	Psychologists available in staff rooms at break times, offering opportunities to listen and talk ad hoc	Leadership/management culture that encourages presenteeism (e.g., praising people for not taking time off after a stressful event)
One year plus		
Safety and security needs	Compulsory group psychology/debriefing sessions	
	Free gym membership	
	More frequent team meetings where voicing of issues/concerns is encouraged/normalised with traceable pathways of action after concerns have been raised	
	Managers undertaking regular clinical shifts to increase visibility among the team and increase their awareness of contemporary clinical needs and issues	
	Greater awareness of individuals' skills, and offering training to complement their expertise	
	Organisation-wide reconsideration of nurses' working shifts and hours to support rest and psychological wellbeing	
Love and belonging needs	Creating more satisfactory spaces in which staff can take breaks and communicate with each other	COVID-19 restrictions in small staff rooms preventing staff from talking to each other
	Working to make teams more supportive, and getting to know each other (e.g., away days)	
Esteem	Individualised meaningful 'thank you' tokens/messages for frontline COVID-19 healthcare workers	Tokenistic messages of thanks or symbols (e.g., badges proving that people had worked at the frontline during COVID-19)
	Recognising nurses' skills with fair pay increases	
Self-actualisation	Treating nurses as individual people (e.g., recognising each nurse's needs and achievements)	

chapter, and to conclude, Table 41.3 provides examples of structural, organisational, and team learning from the COVID-19 pandemic, identifying the conditions that allow nurses and other healthcare staff to flourish and remain psychologically well in emergencies such as the COVID-19 pandemic.

Conclusions and Summary

Nurses have provided the most care, 24 hours a day, 7 days a week, for patients during the COVID-19 pandemic, and they continue to do so. Despite best efforts, the workforce was neither well prepared nor well supported, with legacy issues (e.g., poor workforce planning, staff shortages) and unsafe working conditions (e.g., inadequate training, limited PPE, insufficient staffing) making care provision during the pandemic even more difficult and perilous. The nurses in our study continued to put patients' needs first, often to the detriment of their own health, and we have outlined valuable lessons in the form of structural, organisational, and team learning to support psychosocial wellness in emergencies and disease outbreaks such as the COVID-19 pandemic.

Table 41.3 Structural, organisational, and team learning from the COVID-19 pandemic for supporting the psychosocial wellness of practitioners involved in emergencies

Structural learning

- Recognise nursing and healthcare work generally for the safety-critical work that it is
- Recognise the importance of personalised and holistic care, and avoid fragmenting care into tasks that are delegated to others
- Ensure that long-term workforce planning focuses not only on the supply side of planning but also on retention of valuable staff
- Ensure that there are adequate staff to meet current demand and to account for known changes and likely losses of staff (e.g., due to retirement):
  - Invest in healthcare to provide adequate human resources to enable staff to do their jobs well and avoid burnout and moral distress
  - Identify and ameliorate the impacts of national policy that affect emigration and migration of previous healthcare workforces globally and nationally
  - Invest in the pipeline (supply) through financial support to educate healthcare staff for the future, but also focus on the retention issues ('leaky bucket')
- Recognise and ameliorate inequalities in pay and reward by, for example, prioritising access to CPD for nurses as well as others, and reducing risk (e.g., among ethnic-minority staff during COVID-19)
- Move swiftly to support the workforce with adequate PPE and vaccinations, and consider classifying disease outbreaks (e.g., COVID-19) as an occupational disease

Organisational and team learning

- Ensure easy or easier access to psychosocial wellbeing interventions (on site) as needed
- Consider investing in administrative support for hard-pressed care staff/staff concierge to reduce the administrative burden and improve support for staff
- Invest in training for the whole workforce in psychological first aid and how to support staff in crisis/poor psychological health
- Reframe psychosocial wellbeing as an organisational and team responsibility, rather than being solely the responsibility of individual people
- Consider redeployment rotations where possible in emergencies, in order to reduce the burden on individuals and teams
- Help staff to feel valued (e.g., by giving positive feedback, or by being generous with time off for staff who have been redeployed or gone out of their way to help, before they return to their previous work)
- Ensure equity and parity of staff, and reduce hierarchies (e.g., a nurse may have been on the waiting list for a car parking permit for years, yet a new consultant receives a permit immediately)
- Consider providing education and training for all staff in the importance of psychological safety, allowing staff to speak up about concerns without fear or detriment [39]
- Validate poor psychological health of healthcare staff due to the challenges of work – it is OK not to be OK – and reduce stigma (see Chapters 5, 27 and 28)
- Improve and invest in pandemic readiness (including adequate supplies of PPE, and PPE that fits)
- Consider communicating more about the safety levels of different types of PPE; reassure staff that the safest and most up-to-date PPE would be bought, not the cheapest
- Invest in suitable environments in which staff can relax and spend time with each other while on breaks, so that they can begin to process their work and decompress

References

1. Conolly A, Maben J, Abrams R, Rowland E, Harris R, Kelly D, et al. 'Fallen angels': shifting discourses of nursing over the trajectory of the COVID-19 pandemic. Submitted to Human Relations.

2. Jones-Berry S. COVID-19: Boris Johnson's nurses say praise helps raise profession's profile. *Nursing Standard*, 23 April 2020.

3. Nuffield Trust. *What Kind of Staff Make Up the NHS Workforce.* Nuffield Trust, 2021 (www.nuffieldtrust.org.uk/resource/the-nhs-workforce-in-numbers#1-what-kinds-of-staff-make-up-the-nhs-workforce).

4. IPSOS. *Trust in Professions.* IPSOS, 2021 (www.ipsos.com/sites/default/files/ct/news/documents/2021-12/trust-in-professions-veracity-index-2021-ipsos-mori_0.pdf).

5. Leary A. Safety and service: reframing the purpose of nursing to decision-makers. *J Clin Nurs* 2017; 26: 3761–3.

6. Health Education England. *Raising the Bar Shape of Caring: A Review of the Future Education and Training of Registered Nurses and Care Assistants.* Health Education England, 2015.

7. Leary A. The healthcare workforce should be shaped by outcomes, rather than outputs. *BMJ Opinion* 2019 (https://blogs.bmj.com/bmj/2019/05/31/alison-leary-the-healthcare-workforce-should-be-shaped-by-outcomes-rather-than-outputs/).

8. Maben J. The art of caring: invisible and subordinated? A response to Juliet Corbin: 'Is caring a lost art in nursing?' *Int J Nurs Stud* 2008; 45: 335–8.

9. Buchan J. Seccombe I. Using scenarios to assess the future supply of NHS nursing staff in England. *Hum Resour Health* 2012; 10: 16.

10. Ham C. UK Government's autumn statement: no relief for NHS and social care in England. *BMJ* 2016; 355: i6382.

11. Beech J, Bottery S, Charlesworth A, Evans H, Gershlick B, Hemmings N, et al. *Closing the Gap: Key Areas for Action on the Health and Care Workforce.* Nuffield Trust, The Health Foundation, and the King's Fund, 2019.

12. Mlambo M, Silén C, McGrath C. Lifelong learning and nurses' continuing professional development, a metasynthesis of the literature. *BMC Nurs* 2021; **20**: 62.

13. Amnesty International. *Exposed, Silenced, Attacked: Failures to Protect Health and Essential Workers during the Pandemic.* Amnesty International, 2020 (www.amnesty.org/en/wp-content/uploads/2021/05/POL4025722020ENGLISH.pdf).

14. Leary A. Why does healthcare reject the precautionary principle? *BMJ Opinion* 2021 (https://blogs.bmj.com/bmj/2021/03/12/alison-leary-why-does-healthcare-reject-the-precautionary-principle/).

15. Gould D, Purssell E. *RCN Independent Review of Guidelines for the Prevention and Control of Covid-19 in Health Care Settings in the United Kingdom.* Royal College of Nursing, 2021 (www.rcn.org.uk/professional-development/publications/rcn-independent-review-control-of-covid-19-in-health-care-settings-uk-pub-009-627).

16. Couper K, Murrells T, Sanders Anderson J, Blake H, Kelly D, Kent B, et al. The impact of COVID-19 on the wellbeing of the UK nursing and midwifery workforce during the first pandemic wave: a longitudinal survey study. *Int J Nurs Stud* 2022; 127: 104155.

17. Williams R, Murray E, Neal A, Kemp V. *Top Ten Messages for Supporting Healthcare Staff during the COVID-19 Pandemic.* Royal College of Psychiatrists, 2020 (https://tinyurl.com/wm7e3pn).

18. Ustun G, COVID-19 pandemic and mental health of nurses: impact on international health security. In *Contemporary Developments and Perspectives in International Health Security,* 2021 (dx.doi.org/10.5772/intechopen.96084).

19. Taylor C, Xyrichis A, Leamy MC, Reynolds E. Maben J. Can Schwartz Center Rounds support healthcare staff with emotional challenges at work, and how do they compare with other interventions aimed at providing similar support? A systematic review and scoping reviews. *BMJ Open* 2018; **8**: e024254.

20. Traynor M. *Critical Resilience for Nurses.* Routledge, 2017.

21. Conolly A, Abrams R, Rowland E, Harris R, Kelly D. Kent B, et al. 'What is the matter with me?' or a 'badge of honor': nurses' constructions of resilience during COVID-19. *Glob Qual Nurs Res* 2022; 9: 23333936221094862.

22. Maben J, Bridges J. COVID-19: supporting nurses' psychological and mental health. *J Clin Nurs* 2020; 29: 2742–50.

23. Taylor C, Mattick K, Carrieri D, Cox A, Maben J. 'The WOW factors': comparing workforce organisation and wellbeing for doctors, nurses, midwives and paramedics in England. *Br Med Bull* 2022; 141: 60–79.

24. Carrieri D, Pearson M, Mattick K, Papoutsi C, Briscoe S, Wong G, et al. Interventions to minimise doctors' mental ill-health and its impacts on the workforce and patient care: the Care Under Pressure realist review. *Health Serv Deliv Res* 2020; 8: 19.

25. Cheshire A, Ridge D, Hughes J, Peters D, Panagioti M, Simon C, et al. Influences on GP coping and

resilience: a qualitative study in primary care. *Br J Gen Pract* 2017; 67: ve428–36.

26. Maben J, Taylor C, Dawson J, Leamy M, McCarthy I, Reynolds E, et al. A realist informed mixed-methods evaluation of Schwartz Center Rounds® in England. *Health Serv Deliv Res* 2018; 6: 37.

27. Montgomery C, Humphreys S, McCulloch C, Doherty A, Sturdy S, Pattison N. Critical care work during COVID-19: a qualitative study of staff experiences in the UK. *BMJ Open* 2021; 11: e048124.

28. Greenberg N, Weston D, Hall C, Caulfield T, Williamson C, Fong K. Mental health of staff working in intensive care during COVID-19. *Occup Med* 2021; 71: 62–7.

29. Riessman C. *Narrative Analysis.* Sage, 1993.

30. Hollway W, Jefferson T. *Doing Qualitative Research Differently.* Sage, 2013.

31. Kinman G, Teoh K, Harriss A. *The Mental Health and Wellbeing of Nurses and Midwives in the United Kingdom.* Society of Occupational Medicine, 2020.

32. Kirk K, Cohen L, Edgley A, Timmons S. 'I don't have any emotions': an ethnography of emotional labour and feeling rules in the emergency department. *J Adv Nurs* 2021; 77: 1956–67.

33. Conolly A, Maben J, Abrams R, Rowland E, Harris R, Kelly D, et al. Researching distressing topics ethically: reflections on interviewing nurses during the COVID-19 pandemic. *Int J Soc Res Methodol* 2022.

34. Morley G, Bradbury-Jones C, Ives J. 'What is 'moral distress' in nursing? A feminist empirical bioethics study. *Nurs Ethics* 2020; 27: 1297–314.

35. Jones A, Kelly D. Deafening silence? Time to reconsider whether organisations are silent or deaf when things go wrong. *BMJ Qual Saf* 2014; 23: 709–13.

36. Rowland E, Emotional geographies of care work in the NHS. PhD thesis, Department of Geography, Royal Holloway, University of London, 2014.

37. British Academy. *The COVID Decade: Addressing the Long-Term Societal Impacts of COVID-19.* British Academy, 2021.

38. Maslow AA. Theory of human motivation. *Psychol Rev* 1943; 50: 370–96.

39. Edmondson A. Psychological safety and learning behavior in work teams. *Adm Sci Q* 1999; 44: 350–83.

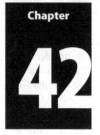

Chapter

42

Intelligent Kindness Under Stress: Working with Intensive Care Unit (ICU) Staff During The Pandemic

Penelope Campling

Introduction

Over the course of my career I have become increasingly interested in the culture of healthcare, how we create the conditions for good practice, how we do the best for our patients, and how we get the best out of our colleagues, our teams, and our organisations. At the heart of my thinking is the concept of intelligent kindness [1].

During the pandemic I have been working as a psychotherapist with intensive care unit (ICU) clinicians, trying to support individual people and groups as they struggle with a situation and pressures that are pushing them to their limits. In this chapter I make observations drawn from this work, and I link them to the concept of intelligent kindness. Although my direct experience is of the situation in one city in the UK, what I have read, and heard, suggests that it is by no means an exception.

The concept of kindness often gets reduced to a sentimental fuzzy niceness – an optional extra in the great enterprise of healthcare. However, the kindness I am talking about is informed by intelligence and motivated by a sense of kinship that drives us to cooperate with, look out for, and do better for each

other. It is integral to good practice, to efficiency, and to outcome. I have used a virtuous circle, which is illustrated in Figure 42.1, to model these links. All of the individual steps in the virtuous circle make a difference, affecting the health and wellbeing not just of patients, but also of staff and of the system as a whole [2]. If we get them right, the work and the culture will thrive; if we neglect them, the enterprise will suffer, the job will start to feel toxic, and the environment will be hostile.

A Healthy Culture

I had not worked with clinicians in ICUs previously, and from the beginning I was impressed by their attitude to the work, their dedication, and their conscientiousness. So many of them told me how much they loved their job – or used to love their job before COVID-19 hit. Most of them felt supported by their immediate teams and talked appreciatively about their colleagues, not just from their own profession but with an empathy for the pressures on the other health professionals they were working alongside. They seemed to understand the importance of investing time in building and nurturing relationships, recognising

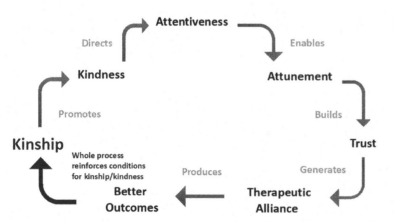

Figure 42.1 The virtuous circle.[2] (Reproduced with permission from Cambridge University Press.)

that the patients' prognoses were significantly improved if their families were actively engaged in the enterprise. Team-building rituals, such as buddy schemes, taking coffee breaks together, and tea and toast at the end of a night shift, were prioritised. The consultants worked closely as a team, doing handover ward rounds together so that they could share their intelligence, and ensuring they were not left on their own with a difficult decision to make. Many of the nurses saw the ICU as an environment in which they could 'do the job properly', enjoying the sense of gratification that comes from focusing on just one patient and giving them their full attention.

This positive team culture stood them in good stead during the first stage of the pandemic. I was enormously impressed by their capacity to step up, take the initiative, and think creatively. Because they see some of the most critically ill patients in the hospital, they were used to managing high levels of anxiety and tension, and were well able to switch in and out of a 'command and control' type of organisation when necessary. Crucially, however, they seemed to balance this with a strong sense of camaraderie, chirpy banter, and care for each other. They were grounded in a sense of kinship, and in turn displayed mutual attentiveness, attunement, and trust, building the therapeutic alliances that lead to better outcomes and wellbeing for all. In short, they seemed to embody the sort of healthy culture I try to capture in the virtuous circle in Figure 42.1. They were used to a relatively high number of their patients dying, but were comforted by knowing that they had done everything possible to treat them, and when death was inevitable they took pride in the humanity of their 'end-of-life' care. By all accounts they seemed to learn and adapt extremely fast to the unpredictable nature of a new disease, and to have an admirable capacity to problem solve 'on the hoof'.

My work with groups and individual clinicians at the end of the first wave of the pandemic found teams worn out and sensibly anxious about what the future would bring. They were able to reflect upon the impact of the pandemic, aware of the cost to themselves. Generally speaking, however, they were proud of how they had managed. Some were struggling more than others, but there was a sense of a crisis managed well and, on balance, a sense of post-traumatic growth rather than post-traumatic trauma.

Sadly, this was not the end, and there was of course no recovery time. At least two new variants were to emerge in the UK in the next year, both of them more infectious and more deadly than the initial one. I drafted this chapter in August 2021, after another gruelling 12 months and with no end in sight. Now, at the time of publication of this book, 3 years later, it is very clear just how much the culture has been challenged by the realities of COVID-19.

Working as a psychotherapist with a multidisciplinary group of people at various levels of seniority, I became aware of my role as some sort of witness as events unfolded. In the rest of this chapter, I use these observations and reflect on the steps of the virtuous circle in order to draw a picture of how the healthy culture that I first encountered on ICUs was, and continues to be, threatened. The virtuous circle is of course only a model – there are many ways in which it could have been depicted. Nevertheless, it can be a helpful way into exploring the complexity of a culture.

Kindness Motivated by a Sense of Kinship

At the heart of the virtuous circle is the idea that kindness is driven by a sense of kinship – the profound sense that we are all part of one human family, and that we will treat the patient in front of us, and our colleagues, with the same care as we would treat our close families and friends. Because the virtuous circle is concerned with exploring and nurturing the conditions for kindness, the system as a whole is an important focus, and is seen as intertwined with what happens between a patient and a clinician. I find it helpful to imagine that I am switching between different lenses – a bifocal approach – centring on the relationship between clinician and patient, but always mindful of how this is affected by the culture of healthcare in the organisation and beyond.

During the first wave of the pandemic, most patients either arrived on the ICU already intubated or were intubated soon after arrival. Thus most patients were unable to speak. Therefore it was difficult to get to know them. Most of them were admitted to hospital already very ill and unaccompanied by a family member. The details that help us to see the person within the patient were often absent. A number of staff members whom I saw were troubled that they could not remember any of the patients' names. It is unusual to be dealing with just one illness, and staff were aware that they had developed a sort of resigned and rather impersonal attitude to the patients – just another COVID-19 case – with resonances of an industrial production line. Despite all of this, personal characteristics often broke through staff defences. One doctor was haunted by a young man who died and who had children exactly the same age as his own. A nurse broke down in tears because she had been unable to save a previously healthy 70-year-old who reminded her of her father, and many others were aware that the patients could so easily have been their own parents. ICU staff are used to patients dying, but it is unusual in this day and age for people who were fit and well a week or two earlier to become ill so quickly and deteriorate so rapidly.

During the first wave, families were not allowed to visit. This meant that many patients died a frightening and lonely death. Staff were only too aware of this. Although they understood the need for infection control, it went against everything they held important and caused them significant moral distress. Everything possible was done to help patients' families to feel connected to the patients, with staff organising final goodbyes using iPads or relaying last words on the phone. Many of the clinicians to whom I spoke were haunted by these scenes of grief-stricken intimacy in such desperate circumstances. Some of the nurses spent their off-duty time using needles and thread to make pairs of hearts out of scraps of material, giving one heart to the relatives and placing the other by the patient – a touching recognition of the need to connect with one's nearest and dearest, even if this can only be done symbolically. Perhaps most importantly, staff determined that no one should go through the experience alone, and they tried to stand in for family members, particularly when it was clear that patients were dying, and end-of-life care had been commenced.

The process of communicating with the families was often described in harrowing terms. Staff were having to break bad news to people to whom they had never previously spoken, and whom they had never seen face to face, while aware, particularly during the first year of the pandemic, that many of these family members were also socially isolated, with no one around them to give them comfort. These clinicians are experienced, skilled communicators of bad news, but the starkness of these circumstances left many of them disturbed.

During the second year of the pandemic, visiting rules became less restrictive, but contact between patients and their families was still compromised by the need to prevent spread of infection, with family visits kept short and family members required to wear full personal protective equipment (PPE). Likewise, communication between staff and the families of their patients remained restricted and difficult, and very far from the ongoing, carefully facilitated communication that was the pre-pandemic ideal.

What I was hearing from so many people was a horribly compromised struggle to preserve and hold on to kinship and kindness, with touching successes and painful limitations.

Attentiveness and Attunement

A sense of kindness drives us to do the best for the other person, helps us to hold that person in mind, and directs our attention, picking up on the small things that can make all the difference to an otherwise traumatic experience. A patient who is receiving thoughtful attention is likely to experience a sense of attunement, a confidence that their needs are understood, and a consequent reduction in anxiety. In what ways has this dynamic been affected by COVID-19?

The first issue was PPE. Protective clothing was hugely important in protecting staff from infection, but no-one liked wearing it. It is horribly hot, uncomfortable and restricts movement. Visors, masks and hoods affect vision and hearing, and it is difficult to make oneself heard. As well as feeling isolated and depersonalised, clinicians worried that their clinical astuteness was compromised by their diminished vision and hearing, let alone the feeling of clumsiness that comes from dripping with sweat and wearing three layers of plastic gloves. They were also aware of how they must appear to the patient and how difficult it was to communicate their humanity from behind these layers of 'armour'.

ICUs across the country adapted to the increased pressure on their services by opening more beds, often expanding into operating theatre space. Finding more room was difficult enough, but the real shortage was in skilled staffing. Staff from across the hospitals were redeployed to ICU at the start of the pandemic but it is such a highly technical area that many found it overwhelmingly frightening or struggled with the skills required. It was also difficult for the specialist ICU nurses who found themselves caring for many more patients than they were used to as well as helping the staff who had been redeployed. Their attention was spread thinly.

Although the numbers of COVID-19 patients in ICUs remained high, there was soon pressure to try to maintain normal services as well as address the backlog of major heart and cancer operations that had been so long postponed. This required high numbers of staff and put enormous pressure on the unit. Redeployed staff had returned to their normal services. It seemed as if ICUs had been left to manage an extremely difficult situation with ever diminishing resources. Some staff, particularly nurses, moved on, retired early, or resigned. Others were on sick leave, many of them with mental health problems. Almost unbelievably, the payment to nurses for overtime across the Trust was reduced and the number of medical training posts in anaesthetics was cut. The fact that these overstretched clinicians couldn't give individual patients the attention they would ideally have liked to give them continued to take its toll.

At a team level, it is more difficult to attend to each other when beds are spread out geographically as they were during surges in the numbers of COVID-19 cases. Some nurses felt trapped and forgotten, looking after patients in rooms some distance away from the main hub of activity. Although WhatsApp groups and other forms of social media were useful forums for keeping in touch at the start of the pandemic, more recently they have been experienced by many as persecutory, with frequent desperate calls for staff to volunteer to cover extra shifts. Even at their best, they do not compensate for the lack of informal face-to-face communication between work colleagues.

As any management student knows, the culture of the coffee room or its equivalent in an organisation is significant. Informal conversation nurtures team cohesiveness, mutual awareness, and support, and can stimulate the emergence of creative ideas. This culture has been severely curtailed. Informal space was the first to be used for extra beds. Nurses found that their breaks were shortened, with the need for 'donning and doffing' their PPE eating into the time, and it was almost impossible to timetable a break to coincide with a colleague. Comforting, relaxing rituals such as tea and toast at the end of a shift, or indeed a visit to the pub to chat over the day, were not possible. Of course, many senior staff were very attentive and worked all hours to try to keep their staff safe and maintain morale, but it was noticeable how many junior staff felt isolated and alone with their struggle, cut off from their peer group and excluded from clinical discussions.

At the level of the organisation, the lack of attention received by the ICUs has been much commented upon. Perhaps this was done better in other places, but there was no perception that the top level of management understood what their key frontline teams were up against, or that they had them in mind even during the first wave of the pandemic. PPE was the obvious example – especially in the early days, it was left to senior staff in the units to step up and do what they could to protect their teams.

At a wider level, some government communications were also far from helpful. Again the issue of PPE is the obvious example, with the Secretary of State both denying that there was a problem and exaggerating what was being done to remedy it. This was widely perceived as reflecting a lack of appropriate concern for and attention to the safety of healthcare staff.

It is important to remember just how afraid staff were of dying, particularly at the start of the pandemic before vaccination was possible. Two clinicians referred themselves independently to my service in January 2020 because they were frightened by what they were observing in China and Italy. They were scared both by what they saw looming on the horizon – it was not even designated a pandemic at that time – and by the lack of appropriate fear and consequent lack of concern shown by those people who should have been playing a major part in protecting us, namely the government, and top managers in their organisations.

Despite the high number of healthcare staff who died from COVID-19, I found that people talked less about the fear of their own death (although they seemed relieved when I asked about this) than about the fear of infecting other people, particularly close family members – anxiety that was at the front of their minds. It was heartbreaking, particularly at the start of the pandemic when PPE was so hard to obtain, to hear the lengths to which people were going to scrub themselves clean, and the elaborate rituals that they followed when they got home (no contact until they had stripped off, put their clothes in the washing machine, showered, and disinfected their car, their keys, and their mobile phone). Many slept apart from their partner, and some of them distanced themselves from their families, staying for months in cheap hotels, or in a caravan on the driveway.

When we are at our most vulnerable and facing something frightening, it is important to feel that this is understood and appreciated, particularly when it is for the collective good and when significant risk is involved. It should not be beyond people in power to convey such understanding in words and deeds. Some governments managed this better than others. In the UK, the government was not seen as appropriately attentive or in tune with the experiences of the people who were dealing with the brunt of the pandemic. Most of the staff whom I saw were angry at the way the government exploited the UK grass-roots ritual of clapping healthcare workers on a Thursday evening. They felt that the rhetoric of kindness and kinship – for example, 'all being in it together' – was betrayed by the lack of proper attention, and did not match the government's actions.

It was a story, then, of exhausting and often troubled efforts to maintain attentiveness and attunement in almost impossible conditions, accompanied by a sense that the clinicians themselves received little of either.

Trust and the Therapeutic Alliance

A good therapeutic alliance means that the patient and their family have a basic trust in the clinician/clinical team and believe that they have their best interests at heart. Kindness, attentiveness, and attunement to their needs promote such a trusting relationship, but, as we have seen, these characteristics of care have been made much harder to sustain under COVID-19. It is difficult to win the trust of someone when you are wearing PPE, with most of your face hidden by a mask, hood, and visor. ICU is always a noisy, high-tech, frightening environment for patients, but never more so than during the pandemic, with patients dying around them and staff looking more like characters in a science-fiction movie than regular doctors and nurses. In normal times it is the calm attentiveness of the staff that soothes patients' fear. Although clinicians have learned to express themselves by exaggerating their 'eye language', and have become adept at making themselves heard through mask and visor, it is not surprising that many patients were and are fearful and mistrustful.

More widely, the issue of trust and the therapeutic alliance that it nurtures seems to have become particularly complicated during the pandemic, with mistrust being whipped up in subgroups of the population, sometimes leading to groups of protestors outside hospitals claiming that COVID-19 is 'just a conspiracy'. When I wrote this chapter, the majority of patients admitted to ICUs in the UK were those who had chosen not to be vaccinated. Some of these patients just never got round to it and regretted their inaction, whereas others were ardent anti-vaxxers with a deep mistrust of doctors even before they set foot in the unit.

This is a difficult dynamic for clinicians to manage on a personal level. It is common for members of staff to seek my help after a hostile complaint or accusation from a grief-stricken relative. Such mistrust aggressively expressed can test an exhausted clinician to their limits. It is not uncommon for their tired psychological coping mechanisms to fail them, and for these clinicians to feel suddenly overwhelmed by the personal cost of the work and to decompensate dramatically. During the worst few months at the start of 2021, staff were battling a deep sense of helplessness in relation to the number of patients who were dying despite all their efforts. Being misunderstood and attacked verbally – or sometimes even physically – often seemed to be the trigger that pushed them over the edge. One doctor, whom I had been seeing regularly, eventually went off sick in response to social media reporting a speech at a rally of anti-vaxxers asking for a 'Nuremberg-type trial' for all doctors and nurses involved in the pandemic. Many people more generally were struggling with their feelings about a family member or friend who had taken up an extreme contrary view about the pandemic, but it is particularly hard for clinicians who have put themselves at risk working on the frontline and seen the ravaging effects of the virus – the untimely and horrible deaths – up close.

Trust, and a good therapeutic alliance, work in everyone's favour. Patients' anxiety is reduced, thereby increasing their fortitude and even enhancing their capacity to heal [3,4]. Anxiety in the clinical team may also be minimised, with staff members feeling less self-protective and defensive, more open to the experiences of their patients, more attentive, and more kind. In some cases this positive dynamic may even alter the outcome. It certainly improves and sustains the team culture, its members' optimism and wellbeing, and their capacity for cooperation and mutual support. It is not difficult to see how a surplus of mistrust can work in the opposite direction.

Final Thoughts

Many ICU staff continue to suffer from mental health problems, a few directly attributable to their experience during the pandemic, but more often due to ongoing stresses that got a lot worse during this time. Some of them will be helped by psychosocial support to take stock of their experience at work and process some of the feelings involved. However, therapy is of minimal help when exhaustion is profound and ongoing pressures are as bad or worse than ever.

Putting committed effort into making the wider system and culture as healthy as possible is vital. This means helping team leaders and other senior staff to deal with their anxieties, frustrations, risks, and lack of resources. However, most importantly, it means helping them to keep a focus on sustaining healthy relationships between the people who are doing the work. Leaders need to notice and understand what is happening to the teams in their organisations, and help to develop a repertoire of ways to support their wellbeing. It is really very simple – if we want clinicians to be kind and caring and to give of their best, they need to feel that they are being treated kindly by their employing organisation and the wider healthcare system. This is the focus of Chapter 37 at the beginning of this Section, in which the reciprocity between the quality of patients' care and that of the staff is termed moral architecture. This relationship is always critical, but never more so than in a pandemic.

References

1. Heath I. Kindness in healthcare: what goes around. *BMJ* 2012; 344: e1171.

2. Ballatt J, Campling P, Maloney C. *Intelligent Kindness: Rehabilitating the Welfare State* 2nd ed. Cambridge University Press, 2020.

3. Weinman J, Ebrecht M, Scott S, et al. Enhanced wound healing after emotional disclosure intervention. *Br J Health Psychol* 2008; 13: 95–102.

4. Cole-King A, Harding KG. Psychological factors and delayed healing in chronic wounds. *Psychosom Med* 2001; 63: 216–20.

Chapter

43

The Role of Occupational Health Services and Responding to Staff Who Have Long COVID

Clare Rayner

Introduction

This chapter gives an overview of what occupational health services can do for workers and employers, what we mean by occupational health, and how occupational health services can help in the event of a pandemic or disaster. I use Long COVID as an example of how health services might be organised and delivered at scale to meet a new health need.

What Is Occupational Health and What Do Occupational Health Services Do?

When people use the term occupational health they usually mean the occupational health service or department within a community's health services. In simple terms, occupational health services protect the health of workers. Typically, practitioners of this specialty do not prescribe or encroach on the role of healthcare practitioners who are treating the same people as their patients. I use the term worker as the currently accepted term for *any* person who works, because there are many models of employment (e.g., employed, self-employed, contractor, zero-hours contractor).

It is fair to say that many people do not know what occupational health is and does. I have found that people are more aware of it if they have worked in private sector organisations, such as large commercial employers or high-risk industries. This is not to say that the public sector has no occupational health provision – it does, and this is often extensive. Occupational health and occupational medicine are little-known specialties among healthcare staff, largely because many of them have little or no exposure to the specialty during their training. Occupational health services are typically located in or close to workplaces, with confidential records held separately from any other health service records. The armed forces in the UK make substantial investments in this

specialism, because sustaining fighting power means keeping their workforce as well as possible.

Occupational health is a complex discipline, dealing primarily with:

1. the effect of work on people's health (prevention and management of occupational diseases or occupationally aggravated diseases)
2. the effect of health on work (how people's health problems affect their ability to work, 'fitness to work' assessments, protecting vulnerable workers, and rehabilitation)
3. hazard and risk management in work environments; this should involve strategic direction at senior management level, involvement in writing policies, and project management.

There can be overlap between occupational health and public health – for example, the joint investigation by public and occupational health specialists into the source of a cluster of cases of lead poisoning in the children of lead workers [1]. In some countries, occupational health sits as a subspecialty of public health. Emergencies, incidents, disasters, and disease outbreaks (EITDDC) definitely afford opportunities for this kind of joint working. Figure 43.1 summarises the foci of occupational and public health services.

Occupational health professionals (nurses, doctors, and vocational rehabilitation therapists) are trained to assess psychological and physical health problems. They also advise on workplace adjustments to enable safe working within legal and ethical frameworks. These practitioners must balance the needs of workers, employers, and public safety, and be able to justify their advice to many stakeholders. They assess and understand workplaces and the complex interaction between people's health and their work.

My interest in occupational medicine stemmed from an early interest in public health. It seemed to me that it was more effective to prevent health problems than to treat complications, and that prevention

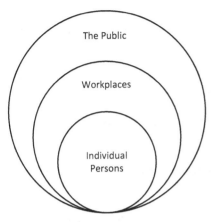

Figure 43.1 The foci of concern of occupational and public health services.

saved suffering, complications, and money. I was impressed by the detective work of Dr Snow, which led to the discovery that a communal water pump was the source of the 1854 cholera outbreak in London.

What Are Workplaces?

Occupational health professionals have an extraordinarily wide remit, essentially because tasks, workplaces, and the potential hazards are so varied. Today, a workplace can range from one's home to a factory, an office, a public building, a hospital, a remote mining facility, or military operations at 50 degrees Celsius.

First and foremost, we aim to prevent occupational disease. Occupational diseases, toxic exposures, and accidents can be disfiguring or life limiting (think of the effects of asbestos or aniline dyes). The same agent may cause one disease or death in high dose and another in low, repeated dose (e.g., pesticide poisoning). As occupational diseases are inherently preventable, it is important to prevent exposure to known hazards.

We have come a long way. Great leaps in social development, such as the Renaissance in Europe and the Industrial Revolution in Britain, led to new diseases. Bernardino Ramazzini, a physician in Padua, advised, 'When you come to a patient's house, I may venture to add one more question: what occupation does he follow?' Hans Christian Andersen based his story 'The Little Match Girl' on the plight of young female workers in London who went on strike because their exposure to phosphorus, used in the manufacture of matches, eroded their skin and

jawbones. They died of 'phossy jaw', which is a bacterial bone infection. Their strike action led to phosphorus being replaced by a less toxic substance. Mad hatter's disease was a neuropsychiatric disorder caused by exposure to the mercury that was used to stiffen top hats. Today, the most common occupational disorders are psychosocial [2].

Our principles of practice are prevention, prevention, prevention, and prevention – anticipation of a problem after exposure, early detection and early treatment, and risk assessment and management, using the hierarchy of controls [3]. These principles apply in the context of psychosocial hazards and in disasters and pandemics.

Hazard Management

There are four types of workplace hazard – chemical, biological, physical, and psychological. A hazard is 'something with the potential to cause harm', and risk is 'the likelihood of that harm occurring' under the circumstances of the work being done. Where a significant risk remains after endeavours to reduce it, legislation requires actions to prevent workers from being exposed to it. Occupational health professionals have a duty to advise both employers and workers, and to protect the public. The more complicated the work environment, the more comprehensive the occupational health service needs to be. Thus, for a high-hazard, high-risk environment, it should be led by a consultant occupational physician advising on strategy and policy at senior management level.

Pre-Emptive Activity in Incidents and Disasters

The key aspects of managing an EITDDC are anticipation, prevention, planning, and managing potential risks. People responsible for planning a response to an EITDDC should not forget to involve occupational health specialists and occupational hygienists (the scientific and technical experts on assessing and measuring hazardous exposures, and the controls needed).

In major incidents involving explosions, fire, or leakage (e.g., Bhopal in 1984, Piper Alpha in 1988, the World Trade Center in 2001, Fukushima in 2011), hitherto unknown combinations of hazardous substances may occur, with unknown effects on health. There are differences in the way that major incidents and pandemics begin. Often a major incident appears to begin with a single catastrophic event (although in most human-made disasters there is likely to have been a series of unnoticed contributory events), whereas in an infectious disease outbreak, such as COVID-19, the beginning may be less obvious. In both types of event the risk assessments need to be updated as the situation evolves.

In the uncontrolled initial environment that characterises incidents and disasters, the environment must be 'secured' immediately to prevent further injuries or deaths. Only then should an employer send in their rescue teams, otherwise there is a risk of creating a second cohort of potential victims. Because it may not be possible to implement effective structural controls, professional first responders (fire and rescue, ambulance, police, and health staff) must be provided with suitable personal protective equipment. Other measures include administrative controls (e.g., rotas, rest periods, maximum exposure times) and information and education for workers and the public.

The escape of hazardous materials from a workplace might lead to serious injury or death, and occupational health services should establish, in advance if possible, treatment pathways with response services and hospital emergency departments. Examples include escape of hydrogen fluoride, a chemical used in oil extraction and refining, which can erode skin and bone, or a potential escape of chlorine gas.

Psychosocial Hazards and Risk

Hazards to mental health at work can be grouped into aspects of work design that are associated with poor health, low productivity, and increased rates of accidents and sickness absence. These aspects are demand, control, support, relationships, roles, and change, known colloquially as 'the six domains of stress' [4]. A range of psychosocial problems may result, including distress and traumatic stress responses. In the event of a major incident, people who are on-site at the time and professional first responders from the emergency services may be faced with horrific, stressful, or life-threatening situations.

During the COVID-19 pandemic, health staff have been faced with wave after wave of poorly controlled community infection, and staff burnout has been a serious concern. As with physical hazards, everyone should be alert to delayed or prolonged psychosocial effects. It behoves all governments to take every control measure that is reasonably possible (ventilation, administrative measures, protective equipment, and appropriate psychosocial support) to reduce the risk of repeated infections in the population and ease the severe pressure on healthcare staff.

Supporting Staff During a Disaster or Pandemic

A range of psychosocial interventions can be made available for staff, which address the short-, medium-, and long-term effects of their work experiences. When setting up appropriate support and treatment services for staff, occupational health service practitioners should seek advice from specialist colleagues in the mental health services. The employers of all staff who may be exposed to an EITDDC should have a disaster plan that includes a coordinated psychosocial response to the disaster as per national guidance, and should anticipate the risk of continued exposure to trauma-inducing environments [5,6]. The disaster plan should explain how immediate practical help, information and support (including psychosocial care and peer support), and access to specialist mental health, evidence-based assessment, and treatment services are to be provided. Effective trauma-focused cognitive behaviour therapy (TF-CBT) interventions that are used to prevent and treat post-traumatic stress disorder (PTSD) include cognitive processing therapy, cognitive therapy for PTSD, narrative exposure therapy, and prolonged exposure therapy. Debriefing as an intervention is not recommended, as it has been shown to be ineffective, and in some cases may worsen outcomes.

Ambulance personnel and police have told me that apart from their colleagues, no one can imagine the sights they have seen as professional first responders on scene, and they find it difficult to express them to people who have not experienced them. In these and other trauma situations, peer support can be helpful. Emergency planners should also be aware that it is common for the first responders to be members of the public, who often intervene before the professional first responders arrive. These people also require support and psychosocial and mental healthcare. Chapter 22 in this book provides more information about the potentially important roles of members of the public, including bystanders, and Chapter 48 in this Section discusses peer support.

It is important to watch out for the 'second ring', which consists of those people who have been indirectly exposed to traumatic circumstances. They may be near to the situation, but not frontline, and incidents may affect the relatives of frontline workers and bystanders. Complex feelings may arise for which they also need support.

We must remember that some workers undertake safety-critical duties in which there is a risk to self or others, and they may need a period of 'time out' or temporary alternative duties before they are sufficiently recovered to be able to revert to normal duties.

Prolonged Illness with COVID-19 and Responding to Staff

The COVID-19 pandemic presents health services with the twin challenges of managing acute COVID-19 and Long COVID. Although COVID-19 was initially thought to be a respiratory illness, the underlying problem is damage to and inflammation of the lining of blood vessels, which results in endotheliitis [7,8]. As blood vessels supply every part of the body, there are multiple symptoms, and neural tissue is especially vulnerable. Consequences include blood clots and an increased risk of cardiovascular events in the year after infection, even in young people [9,10].

Risk factors for infection include immunocompromise, vascular disorders, diabetes, and being in one of a range of occupations (e.g., health and social care, education, bus or taxi drivers, working in poorly ventilated spaces such as poultry slaughterhouses) [11]. People who work in the health, social care, and education sectors are also more likely to develop Long COVID.

Long COVID (also known as post-COVID syndrome, post-COVID sequelae, or long-haul recovery) is COVID-19 with the same pathological processes occurring as in the early stage – that is, persistent infection, blood clots, and immune dysfunction [12]. The diagnostic criteria include symptoms lasting for 12 weeks or longer, for which specific health problems have been excluded.

The fact that millions of people, including key workers, are affected by sequelae of long duration and by the impact on their day-to-day activities suggests that some reconfiguration of health services is going to be necessary. The UK Defence Medical Services led with recommendations in April 2020, and developed a programme of treatment and rehabilitation that results in 90% of people returning to work within 3 months [13].

This integrated model of care incorporates initial rest and avoidance of triggering activities, followed if necessary by investigations for organ damage, and then by tailored physical rehabilitation.

We know from other health conditions that early intervention leads to earlier recovery – the 'stitch in time saves nine' approach. There is evidence in COVID-19 that the onset of immune-driven complications occurs after around 3 months, so it appears to be important to prevent this from happening [14].

Early Health Interventions in Long COVID

Early health interventions in Long COVID include:

1. public health messaging advising sufferers to rest during the first stage, and to avoid sports while they are experiencing cardiac and respiratory symptoms
2. early symptomatic treatment to counteract the damaging inflammatory response; there are compelling reasons for advising this, including evidence from previous pandemics [15]
3. standardised baseline screening for common or red flag issues if troublesome symptoms persist beyond 4 weeks [16]; this should include taking a full history, face-to-face examinations, and specialist referrals (commonly to cardiology, respiratory medicine, and neurology) where indicated
4. rehabilitation services, aimed at improving or maintaining function, directed towards physical, psychological, cognitive, speech, and language impairments, and also making available social and financial advice.

Resource Implications

All of the considerations discussed in the previous section have implications for delivering health services. Baseline screening could be undertaken in a 'one-stop shop' setting, ideally medically led. Even if healthcare resources are limited, advice on early rest and the need for pacing can be provided. Complications such as perimyocarditis can be diagnosed on the basis of clinical history, as was standard practice until recent years, and patients should be managed clinically initially. Research is already defining some of the microvascular pathology. No healthcare system is likely to sustain such expensive investigations for everybody affected, but this research could be translated into pragmatic techniques for prevention, as well as informing treatments.

Cascade learning should be designed and enacted to inform delivery of services. Experienced figures in the medical field have pointed out that great leaps in understanding have occurred in the aftermath of disasters, and I believe we are already seeing this with COVID-19.

It is important to co-produce solutions with people who are affected, as they know their limitations, symptoms, priorities, and preferences. They also know their communities, and can be well-informed advocates for their own recovery and care.

Return to Work: What Works

My final word goes to the many workers who have experienced prolonged illness with COVID-19, especially those who may have contracted the infection through workplace exposure, and have also faced delays in recognition and treatment of their symptoms. This situation has caused huge distress.

In many health conditions, early intervention leads to early recovery and early return to work [17]. Work itself is beneficial to recovery, and should be viewed as an important health goal and outcome [18]. People who have been ill with COVID-19 for more than 2 years are likely to need intensive support. Occupational health professionals focus on managing the impact of symptoms on people's functioning and their jobs, rather than on specific diagnoses. We are used to implementing health surveillance and rehabilitation programmes, and this sets an important precedent for adjusting services to meet the needs of people who have Long COVID.

The most effective workplace adjustments for Long COVID are [19]:

1. a prolonged, phased return to work
2. an individualised return-to-work plan [20].

A 'standard' 4-week phased return to work by people with Long COVID often leads to relapse. Occupational health professionals have found it best to start with minimal hours and duties, which are very slowly increased over a period of months in order to achieve a sustained return to work.

The return-to-work plan is the crucial element of helping people with health problems to achieve a timely return. There should be regular managerial review and readjustment of the plan to reflect the relapsing–remitting nature of the condition. This should be a collaborative process, focusing on what *can* be done, not on what cannot, and identifying obstacles to return to work and actions that will overcome those obstacles.

There are two cautions with regard to people with Long COVID returning to work. First, strenuous physical activity is contraindicated in the presence of uninvestigated chest pain, because there is a risk of exercise-induced sudden cardiac death in people who have acute myocarditis, or oxygen desaturation at rest or exertion [21]. Thus cardiorespiratory clearance is required before any strenuous activity is undertaken [19]. Physical exertion should be adapted if people have autonomic dysfunction or other symptom exacerbation. Second, cognitive dysfunction is common and may affect safety-critical tasks. An updated risk assessment should be made under work conditions.

I acknowledge the challenge of the COVID years for occupational health services and practitioners who have had to adapt a small workforce to address the needs of a severe, disabling illness that has affected many workers.

When this chapter was written in 2022, there were 2 million people, mainly of working age, reporting Long COVID, out of a total workforce of approximately 31 million in the UK. Faced with this situation, employers should take pragmatic approaches to working practice and focus on core business functions. I hope that one outcome of the pandemic will be some increased flexibility, including more people being able to work from home, and that we relinquish outdated practices.

Conclusion

There is no economy without health, and there is 'no health without mental health'.

References

1. Kar-Purkayastha I, Balasegaram S, Sen D, et al. Lead: ongoing public and occupational health issues in vulnerable populations: a case study. *J Public Health (Oxf)* 2012; 34: 176–82.

2. Health and Safety Executive. *Work-Related Ill Health and Occupational Disease in Great Britain*. Health and Safety Executive, 2021 (www.hse.gov.uk/statistics/causdis/).

3. Health and Safety Executive. *Hierarchy of Controls, Leadership*

and *Worker Involvement Toolkit.* Health and Safety Executive, 2021 (www.hse.gov.uk/construction/lwit/assets/downloads/hierarchy-risk-controls.pdf).

4. Health and Safety Executive. *What Are the Management Standards?* Health and Safety Executive, 2022 (www.hse.gov.uk/stress/standards/).

5. NHS England and NHS Improvement. *Responding to the Needs of People Affected by Incidents and Emergencies: Guidance for Planning, Delivering, and Evaluating Psychosocial and Mental Healthcare.* NHS England and NHS Improvement, 2021.

6. National Institute for Health and Care Excellence. *Post-Traumatic Stress Disorder. NICE Guideline [NG116].* National Institute for Health and Care Excellence, 2018 (www.nice.org.uk/guidance/ng116).

7. Fogarty H, Townsend L, Morrin H, Ahmad A, Comerford C, Karampini E, et al. Persistent endotheliopathy in the pathogenesis of long COVID syndrome. *J Thromb Haemost* 2021; 19: 2546–53.

8. Bonaventura A, Vecchié A, Dagna L, Martinod K, Dixon DL, Van Tassell BW, et al. Endothelial dysfunction and immunothrombosis as key pathogenic mechanisms in COVID-19. *Nat Rev Immunol* 2021 21: 319–29.

9. Kell DB, Laubscher GJ, Pretorius E. A central role for amyloid fibrin microclots in long COVID/PASC: origins and therapeutic implications. *Biochem J* 2022; 479: 537–59.

10. Raman B, Bluemke DA, Lüscher TF, Neubauer S. Long COVID: post-acute sequelae of COVID-19 with a cardiovascular focus. *Eur Heart J* 2022; 43: 1157–72.

11. Verbeeck J, Vandersmissen G, Peeters J, Klamer S, Hancart S, Lernout T, et al. Confirmed COVID-19 cases per economic activity during autumn wave in Belgium. *Int J Environ Res Public Health* 2021; 18: 12489.

12. Couzin-Frankel J. What causes Long Covid? Here are the three leading theories. *Science* 2022; 376: 1261–5.

13. Barker-Davies RM, O'Sullivan O, Senaratne KPP, Baker P, Cranley M, Dharm-Datta S, et al. The Stanford Hall consensus statement for post-COVID-19 rehabilitation. *Br J Sports Med* 2020; 54: 949–59.

14. Nalbandian A, Sehgal K, Gupta A, Madhavan MV, McGroder C, Stevens JS, et al. Post-acute COVID-19 syndrome. *Nat Med* 2021; 27: 601–15.

15. Fedson DS. COVID-19, host response treatment, and the need for political leadership. *J Public Health Policy* 2021; 42: 6–14.

16. Master H, Chaudhry A, Gall N, Newson L, Glynne S, Glynne P. *Draw On Expert Opinion to Optimise Care for Long COVID.* Medscape UK, 2022 (www.guidelinesinpractice.co.uk/infection/draw-on-expert-opinion-to-optimise-care-for-long-covid/456989.article).

17. Waddell G, Burton AK, Kendall NAS. *Vocational Rehabilitation: What Works, for Whom, and When?* The Stationery Office, 2008.

18. Council for Work and Health. *2019 Healthcare Professionals' Consensus Statement for Action: Statement for Health and Work.* Council for Work and Health, 2019 (www.councilforworkandhealth.org.uk/wp-content/uploads/2019/05/Health-and-Work-Consensus-Statement.pdf).

19. Rayner C, Campbell R. Long COVID implications for the workplace. *Occup Med (Lond)* 2021; 71: 121–3.

20. Burton K, Bartys S. The smart return-to-work plan: Part 1: The concepts. *Occup Health Work* 2022; 19: 22–6.

21. Lampejo T, Durkin SM, Bhatt N, Guttmann O. Acute myocarditis: aetiology, diagnosis and management. *Clin Med* 2021; 21: e505–10.

Chapter

44

A Framework for Designing, Developing, and Delivering Psychosocial and Mental Healthcare

Richard Williams and Nick Ambler

Introduction

In 2017 a series of terrorist attacks in Manchester and London, and the Grenfell Tower fire, raised concerns about the psychosocial and mental health impacts on survivors to very high levels. In parallel, the importance of caring effectively for staff of healthcare services before, during, and after mass casualty events has been increasing since the 9/11 terrorist attacks in the USA. That event has had a huge and persisting toll on professional first responders. Indeed the twentieth anniversary of the event in September 2021 refocused awareness on the impacts on the persisting physical and mental health and the late presentations of so many responders of all kinds [1]. This resonates with our contemporary concerns about health and social care staff who have responded to patients' needs over a long period of time, since the SARS-CoV-2 pandemic began in 2020.

The COVID-19 pandemic has driven home just how dependent patients are on the continuing good health of those people who provide their healthcare. Yet staff of healthcare services have been poor at looking after themselves, in utter contrast to their delivery of exceptional care for their patients. For too long, matters pertaining to mental health have been seen as reflecting conditions to be diagnosed and managed by mental health professionals, and stigma, although slowly diminishing, has remained prominent. However, the truth is that managing the mental health of healthcare staff is both simple and complex, and is a matter that should fall first to the teams in which they work, second to occupational health and primary care services, and third, but least often, to specialist mental health services. Each of these echelons of care is important, and they are all interdependent. Staff may develop experiences that are indicators of mental disorders, and in these circumstances they should be referred rapidly and without delay to mental health practitioners. However, although routes to specialist

mental healthcare should be negotiated routinely and well rehearsed in all organisations, there is much that employing organisations could and should do to help the majority of their staff to cope, adapt, and learn from their experiences routinely as well as in emergencies. Our model of care brings these matters together in a logical strategic sequence.

In this chapter we pull together learning from this book relating to caring for staff of health and social care organisations. However, we begin by presenting the reflections of a clinical psychologist attached to an intensive care unit (ICU), and then develop the model of care and unpack its important constituents in the remainder of this chapter. We can clearly see ways in which an influential member of staff has wrestled with constructing a non-pathologising and popular approach to supporting staff working in that ICU.

A Postcard from an ICU Psychologist

As I write, in autumn 2022, there have been almost 2 years of exceptional pressures in ICUs. Again we are experiencing an easing off from the brutal effects of COVID-19. One thing I have learned is not to imagine that we have reached the end. There have been too many false dawns. I sense that the hardest part is yet to come, recuperating the psychosocial wellbeing of our staff, just to get back to where we were pre-pandemic. What have we learned about this so far?

I am a clinical psychologist attached to a 48-bed ICU. My role includes staff support, particularly for the 240-strong nursing team. This became a priority 3 years before the pandemic, when the staff turnover was over 30%, much the same as in other ICUs in the National Health Service (NHS). That takes a toll on stability and morale in a team, and on the budget (training, recruitment, and agency cover). We had formed a workgroup to tackle this, avoiding talk of burnout and focusing on the positives, following core principles from the Institute for Healthcare Improvement's *Joy in Work*. We conducted one-to-one interviews within the nursing team, structured around the theme 'What matters to you', in order to bolster the sense of meaning, purpose, and satisfaction about ICU work. I led the interview training, but the one-to-one interviews were strictly between nurse colleagues. Many of them were recorded, and qualitative analysis revealed half a dozen recurring themes. It emerged that what mattered most was teamwork, and experiences of having made a difference under stress.

Next, small group discussions about 'the stones in our shoes' identified hassles in everyday work experience, discussed the potential solutions, and then tried them. This built a sense of agency, as within-team discussions collectively achieved improvements. Gradually, over a period of 2 years, morale seemed to be rising, and it did not feel like a coincidence when monthly staff turnover decreased to its best ever level – no vacancies, and a recruitment waiting list. Then COVID-19 began.

We had forewarning and so we reorganised to make ready, including psychosocial support preparations. We ran presentations about managing intense work stress, prompting greater attention to self-care. We set up a dedicated self-referral psychology service.

Looking back, I think that there were missteps. Our efforts were appreciated, but it soon became clear that sharing knowledge about the effects of intense work stress did not alter what people did to cope. Very few used the self-referral service. Previous studies revealed that frontline workers tend not to use psychological services during major incidents. Media reports of a high prevalence of post-traumatic stress disorder (PTSD) among frontline staff, based on cross-sectional surveys, were alarmist and misleading. The timing, nature, and prevalence of the disorder were misjudged. This is not to deny that some people have been profoundly affected, but I think that PTSD is about persistent symptoms after a stressor has ended, not while it is ongoing. We have been dealing with prolonged high-intensity work, the threat of becoming overwhelmed, the accumulation of distressing experiences, and, above all, exhaustion, the psychology of which is different. If you gather a group of people, set them tasks, and then crank up the pressure, one by one they will falter until none are left. This is fine for a TV game show, but not for healthcare. The terms resilience and burnout are divisive, focusing inwardly on individuals when the real issue is external. Addressing

the extraordinary demands that are being placed on a team is more important than personal variations in the capacity to keep going.

From the build-up onwards, through each wave, all non-essential activities were cancelled. There simply wasn't time for them. Keeping the ICU running was the only game in town. Between the waves there was some space. It was then that we resumed our pre-COVID methods, organising one-to-one interviews about the impact of such high-intensity working and how to help. Recordings (which averaged 12 minutes) were analysed for themes, and this revealed much about teamwork, physical conditions, support, and emotional challenges (both negative and positive). Exhaustion was a universal theme. Most people felt a strong sense of achievement and of 'loving' their ICU team. A number described memories of highly stressful events that they could not shake off. Many felt that they had reached their mental, emotional, and physical limits. However, we also learned that these brief interviews between nurse colleagues, who had previously been too busy to stop and talk in this way, had a powerful intrinsic value ('thank you for asking'). Hearing each other's recent experiences, both good and bad, provided an outlet. A high-functioning team makes time for informal mutual support, but circumstances had obstructed that process. Perhaps we had found a means of restoring it.

We introduced peer support training, to provide knowledge, skills, and confidence to enable nurses on the ICU to take the initiative with delivering psychosocial support for each other. Although it had been conceived for critical incidents, we decided to adopt a proactive approach, consisting of a one-to-one 'check-in chat' between each nurse and a peer supporter, as a routine supportive process. These chats are conversational rather than problem focused, but they explore any issues that emerge. We had learned how quickly ICU nurses cut to the chase when talking to a colleague. After all, they know each other and will both have experienced being in the thick of it. The check-in chat could lead to a handover to the ICU psychologist (myself) if appropriate, for booked one-hour discussions, which were supportive but still informal in nature. Surprisingly, this option caught on, overcoming the barrier for accepting help. Many people had reduced their hours and were looking elsewhere, for self-preservation – getting out before burnout kicked in. There was plenty to discuss.

Under intense pressure, there is a mindset in the ICU to 'crack on', but there is not a 'don't ask, don't tell' attitude of emotional reserve. Instead the uptake of support seems to be a matter of timing and who is providing the support. When the ICU is extremely stretched, setting up a counselling clinic simply does not work. Afterwards, the impulse to arrange psychological debriefing meetings may be strong, but research evidence suggests that it is ill-advised. Recuperation is not achieved through single events or an extra day off. It requires a prolonged strategy, a flexible pluralistic model, better terminology, and heuristics through which to adapt the approach to each new situation.

The numbers of cases of COVID-19 are falling, but pressures remain high. During the pandemic the ICU has been a very different work experience. Large numbers of staff are thinking about leaving. For some this is a natural step, but to lose those for whom ICU work is in their blood seems tragic. Becoming an ICU nurse implies a degree of personal calling. Not everyone wants to walk a mile in those shoes, nor can they, but some are really good at it. Right now we need to find the best ways to help them to reconnect with the joy in this vocation.

Nick Ambler, October 2022

This postcard illustrates some very important learning points. It is critical to respond to staff as the capable people they are, despite their doubts, fatigue, and fears, and not to see them as patients unless that is really necessary. It is important to remain aware that, despite notable reductions in recent years, stigma still abounds. Looking through Nick's postcard, we find comments that suggest that the following observations, constructs, approaches, and interventions are highly important when responding to colleagues' preferences and needs:

- Recognise the importance of co-production in getting responses right. This means that the people for whom responses are intended should be fully engaged in their design and delivery [2–5], otherwise, and all too often, there is a tendency for responses to inadequately reflect the needs of colleagues as they see them.
- Social support is very powerful.
- We should be aware of the trajectories of how support is mobilised in the face of emergencies and incidents and then deteriorates as time passes [6].
- Membership of teams is very important. The shared social identities that come from team

membership provide the motive force behind social support, and that is why people prefer the support of their families and those colleagues whom they trust. Having a shared social identity also separates teams from workgroups that do not necessarily experience this sharing.

- We must realise how important it is to focus on helping colleagues to restore their sense of agency. Both personal and team efficacy are important to team members.
- People need time to reflect on intense experiences.
- Staff should have a person or place to which they can go for immediate support.
- We should all be aware of the power of secondary stressors (see Chapter 9) [7].

A Model of Care to Meet the Needs of Staff of Healthcare Organisations

The model of care that we set out here harks back to Section 1 of this book, and the model of care for communities that we presented in Chapter 12. Chapters 27, 28, and 29, in Section 4 of the book, develop the contents of that approach for the public. In the present chapter, however, we develop that approach into a model of care for healthcare staff. It is based not only on the generic model but also on colleagues' experiences and opinions, as presented in other chapters in Section 5. Generally, the pandemic has rendered staff of healthcare organisations more sensitive about their health but also more open to talking about their mental health needs in relation to both work and home. We see this illustrated in Chapters 4 and 5. Nick Ambler identifies and discusses some of the sensitivity that should be afforded to staff. Our colleagues did not get this quite right initially, but changes in how support was offered during the pandemic have resulted in much greater impacts. We must learn from this.

Our model, summarised in Figure 44.1, builds on the work reported by Dennis Stevenson and Paul Farmer, which one of us (RW) has translated into the wellbeing, psychosocial, and mental health agendas [1,3,8]. Thus we include many of the matters that we have learned about from staff during past emergencies and incidents, as well as lessons from caring for staff through the pandemic, and we offer a framework through which to take in the wisdom presented in this book.

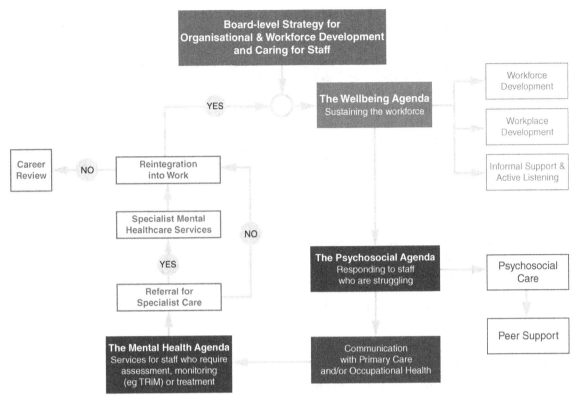

Figure 44.1 A model of care. (© R Williams, V Kemp, 2021, all rights reserved.)

We have observed in previous work a powerful tendency within organisations to read models such as these as describing structures and procedures. Therefore, we point out that this model is intended to be neither structural nor linear. It is intended to be strategic, and to emphasise a functional approach to caring for and supporting staff. It shows how those functions are linked, but care may proceed in both directions through this model, and people may be fast-tracked to mental healthcare if that is warranted, or, often, they may cycle between the wellbeing and psychosocial agendas.

Delivering the Wellbeing, Psychosocial, and Mental Health Agendas

As in the postcard presented earlier, this chapter focuses mainly on the wellbeing and psychosocial agendas. That is not intended to in any way diminish the vital importance of meeting the mental health agenda, but it reflects the focus of this book on a wide readership and the actions that non-mental health practitioners and managers can contribute. Here we present further ideas about how the wellbeing and psychosocial agendas might be developed. Much of this material was developed by us and a team of specialists for the Faculty of Pre-Hospital Care at the Royal College of Surgeons of Edinburgh [9]. We reproduce and develop here some of that material, albeit in generalised form, and we are grateful to the Faculty for allowing us to do so.

Training for Professional and General Managers

The first matter that we consider important is that general and professional managers at all levels should be offered training. A paper published in *Lancet Psychiatry* reviews the impact of a well-constructed randomised controlled trial of a 4-hour training programme for commanders of firefighters in Australia, which aimed to increase their confidence in speaking with staff about wellbeing and mental health [10]. The research showed that this intervention led to a significant reduction in work-related sickness leave and a return of £10 for every pound invested.

After the earthquake sequence in Canterbury, New Zealand in 2010–2011, the impact of measures to enhance employees' wellbeing was monitored [11]. That study suggested that attention needs to be paid to longer-term recovery of staff. Targeting employees' wellbeing and psychosocial needs is a low-cost strategy that can ensure positive functioning through a lengthy recovery period. It benefits both the organisation and individual members of staff [11]. This research recommends that managers should:

- validate employees' and managers' efforts and flexibility during a crisis
- give more autonomy to local managers
- use flexible performance management by giving local managers discretion to enhance performance and create a learning culture for a variety of reasons, including the evidence that better psychological safety tends to reduce mistakes [12]
- focus on the wellbeing and psychosocial care of employees.

The Wellbeing Agenda

The term wellbeing is used in this book to refer to the need of every member of staff for sources of support to ensure that they are able to continue to develop, enjoy the stimulation of their work, and flourish. Every member of staff, for example, requires effective leadership and to be a member of a cohesive team that is supporting and nurturing.

The wellbeing agenda focuses on the importance of supporting staff who are thriving to continue to do so. It recognises the pivotal role of team leaders and managers, as well as those people with responsibility for organisational policy, in developing teams by focusing on:

- addressing people's physical healthcare needs
- continuing to develop leadership
- strengthening teams, team membership, and teams' cohesion
- offering Schwarz Rounds, modified to suit the settings in which staff work
- ensuring preparedness, training, and support for staff so that they are always able to look out for each other
- ensuring that every member of staff has a 'buddy' to whom they can turn for support
- ensuring that every member of staff has a person or place to which they can go to receive support in a timely way

- ensuring that staff have space and time for reflection and recovery
- seeking and addressing organisational and workplace factors that affect people's physical, social, and work capacities
- reducing secondary stressors
- continuing to work on reducing stigma.

In order to maintain the wellbeing of those people who are coping well with the demands of their work, organisations should support their employees to deal with a range of challenges, such as:

- sleep and shift work
- transition from one role to another (e.g., from trainee to consultant), and re-deployment of staff to non-familiar roles, and across the working lifespan
- life transitions (e.g., parenthood, the menopause, bereavement)
- physical health, especially back pain
- drug and alcohol use
- bullying
- mental health, especially awareness of how to protect one's mental health.

People's relationships can either support or undermine their resilience. Their abilities to form and maintain relationships with others at home and at work, as well as with strangers at times of greatest need, and to accept support are key strengths. These social relationships are powerful influences on how people cope with adversity, ill health, and emergencies. People who show good outcomes tend to perceive that they are are entitled to, and do receive, support because of their membership of their team.

Every person and every organisation involved in planning for and responding to incidents and emergencies should understand how people may react to emergencies and incidents. They must also understand the factors that affect how well people cope, including the importance of relationships, social support, leadership, and care.

Twelve Pivotal Approaches to Sustaining the Wellbeing of Staff

The approaches to the wellbeing agenda that we have identified thus far can be summarised under the 12 pivotal approaches listed here.

1. Provide clear messages about the priorities of work and care for staff within organisations.
2. Ensure that every employee has a person or place to which they can go for immediate support, and

ensure that staff have space and time for reflection – for example, a buddy system among colleagues.

3. Ensure that work is based upon effective teams, and that team cohesion is supported by employees training together as well as working together.

4. Ensure that leaders are effective and supportive, because these approaches enable people to develop team cohesion.

5. Intervene early with staff who are distressed. This requires bolstering the working environment, and listening rather than therapy or counselling.

6. Learn and use active listening and hearing skills.

7. Seek out and remedy secondary stressors, before they affect staff if possible.

8. Ensure that employees are offered opportunities for integration with their peers, because social support is key.

9. Remember that colleagues' sense of personal efficacy and agency is important in their recovery.

10. Be clear about who will and who will not benefit from a 'medical' approach (a minority of people may develop diagnosable mental health disorders for which they require specialised mental healthcare, but most do not).

11. Support staff in the face of negative public perceptions.

12. Get the workplace culture right. The actions and policies in this list are all critical to creating environments at work that are conducive to staff giving of their best. This means that policies and actions for supporting staff must be separate from those for staff discipline and performance management.

The Nature of Social Support

Social support is based on people perceiving that they have good social networks that offer them support. It promotes people's wellbeing and recovery in many settings [13]. Social support consists of social interactions that provide people with actual assistance that also embed them in a web of relationships that they perceive to be caring and readily available in times of need [14,15]. It includes emotional, informational, and operational components.

The Psychosocial Agenda

Psychosocial Care

From time to time, members of staff may struggle at work and/or at home. They may well recover with support from their families and colleagues. Some people who are struggling, including those who are distressed for longer periods, may benefit from interventions based on the principles of psychological first aid (PFA) that are not medical in nature, and which do not seek to pathologise their needs and methods of meeting them. Social support is critical to meeting the needs of people in these circumstances. Some members of staff may find that being able to call on colleagues for peer support is extremely helpful. This approach is named psychosocial care because many of the factors that cause concern lie in the social and psychological areas rather than reflecting medical needs. It is based on taking a non-pathologising, non-medical approach to meeting the needs of staff who are struggling. The approach taken here is founded on the lessons learned from Section 3 of this book.

The number of people affected by emergencies, incidents, disasters, and disease outbreaks (EITDDC) may be very substantial despite the fact that the majority of distressed people are unlikely to develop a mental disorder. Intervening early can reduce the risk of their developing disorders later. Psychosocial care emphasises responding to the needs of staff by focusing on:

- strengthening the contributions of teams and enabling members to actively listen to, hear, and support each other
- developing peer support [16]
- providing mental health training for professional and general managers [10]
- setting workplace cultures to recognise and augment post-traumatic growth – that is, positive psychological changes experienced because of adversity and other challenges that give rise to higher levels of functioning
- working according to the principles of PFA to provide psychosocial care with the intention of [17,18]:
  - reducing the risks of morbidity
  - reducing absence through sickness
  - reducing the risks of presenteeism
  - promoting personal growth and learning.

In practice the principles of PFA require leaders, managers, and practitioners to:

- adopt a practical approach to early intervention based on the acronym **PIES**
- seek out and remedy secondary stressors

- consider establishing peer support programmes because they bring staff in departments and teams together and may prevent the development of more serious problems
- develop care pathways that link the wellbeing, psychosocial, and mental health aspects of the organisation's workforce plans into the clinical and governance roles in pre-hospital care.

The **PIES** approach describes a practical approach to early intervention, and two rigorous studies show that its adoption reduces the risk of people developing mental health diagnoses later [19,20]. It calls for psychosocial care interventions to be offered in **P**roximity to where staff work, with **I**mmediacy, in **E**xpectancy of good outcomes, and using **S**implicity of interventions.

However, organisations are advised to avoid routine screening because there is little evidence that it conveys benefit inside organisations.

Psychological First Aid

One approach that is an important component of psychosocial care is PFA. The principles of PFA are identified as being central to psychosocial interventions for the public and staff during and in the immediate aftermath of incidents and emergencies. PFA is not a single intervention or treatment and, as originally described, its basic objectives are to:

- establish a human, compassionate, and non-intrusive connection with affected people
- enhance people's immediate and continuing safety
- provide physical and emotional comfort and calm for overwhelmed people
- establish people's immediate needs
- offer practical assistance and information
- connect survivors with social support networks
- support adaptive coping
- clarify the availability of services, and signpost survivors to sources of help, assessment, and further intervention.

Furthermore, PFA recognises the importance of the matters that we list here.

- Attending to basic needs (safety, security, food, sanitation, shelter, interventions for acute medical problems, etc.) is the first and highest priority.
- People affected by EITDDC need rapid, effective action followed by sustained service responses that may require medium- and long-term mobilisation of resources.

- Organisations and services should understand people's preferences for informally provided support, but also their needs for responsive formal services.
- The emphasis of psychosocial universal care (discussed later in this chapter) should be on empowering affected people and communities at work and at home, and restoring their agency.
- The public should be actively engaged in delivering responses to the psychosocial needs of communities and individual people after disasters and major incidents.
- The public must be trusted with accurate information that is provided regularly by credible people, because the public should be regarded as part of the response and not solely as part of the problem (see Chapter 22).
- Formal services should be made available that offer psychosocial care interventions for people whose needs are not met informally by their families and colleagues.

Peer Support

Peer support is an intervention that involves a supportive relationship between people who have experiences in common. It is rooted in the knowledge that 'hope is the starting point from which a journey of recovery must begin' [21]. Peer supporters can inspire hope and demonstrate the possibility of recovery. They are valued for their authenticity because they can relate to the challenge. They draw from their experiential knowledge – the happenings, emotions, and insights of their experiences – as they listen to and interact with peers who seek their help. More information on peer support can be found in Chapter 48 and in the documents prepared for the Faculty of Pre-Hospital Care at the Royal College of Surgeons of Edinburgh [9,16].

Universal, Selective, and Indicated Psychosocial Interventions

Psychosocial interventions are categorised as universal, selective, or indicated.

- *Universal psychosocial interventions* are intended to offer primary prevention. They should be started as soon as possible, within hours of each incident's impact, and should continue to be available for months afterwards (i.e., into the recovery phase). Universal psychosocial interventions should be readily available to staff of the emergency services. They should also:

- be family- and community-orientated
- be based on the principles of PFA
- address people's practical needs and their relief from distress, and aim to build community coping and support.

- *Selective psychosocial interventions* should be offered as public mental health interventions for groups of people who are identified as being at higher risk of developing mental disorders. People should be assisted to identify and resolve, if possible, any persisting secondary stressors that may be maintaining their distress and dysfunction.

- *Indicated psychosocial interventions* should be offered to people who, after an initial personal screening of their experiences and needs, are found to have persisting distress that is accompanied by dysfunction, or whose assessments suggest that they have symptoms of a mental disorder that do not meet the criteria for diagnosis.

Universal and selective psychosocial interventions may be offered without or before assessment of people's personal needs.

Currently, the evidence for many popular psychosocial interventions is regarded as thin, although it is improving in strength as research findings become available. However, more techniques need to be developed and evaluated. Nonetheless, universal and selective interventions, based on the principles of PFA, are unlikely to cause harm. The guidance on PFA also draws attention to the evidence for the positive impacts of social integration and social support on people's health. In addition, as Section 3 in this book shows, there is a lot of evidence to support the positive impacts of the social cure approaches.

This situation becomes more challenging when designing and delivering indicated psychosocial interventions. Internationally, the SOLAR programme has recently published evidence for the effectiveness of a focused indicated intervention for adults whose needs fall short of requiring treatment for mental disorders [22]. Similar testing and validation work is in hand to develop an indicated programme for children and young people.

The Role of Occupational Health Services

Occupational health is a specialist clinical service that aims to provide benefits for staff and organisations by contributing to the productivity of organisations through investing in the health and wellbeing of their workforces. Chapter 43 describes succinctly the roles of occupational health. In 2019, NHS Employers in the UK produced a guide to ensure that NHS organisations are clear about what they should expect from their occupational health service and how to ensure that the service works to enable staff to deliver safe, effective, and efficient patient care [23]. It commented that, where NHS organisations prioritise staff health and wellbeing, performance is enhanced, patient care is improved, staff retention is higher, and sickness absence is lower. There is also evidence that access to good occupational health support improves staff engagement and can contribute to cultural change.

Additional standards relating to their ability to deliver six 'core' services is required of occupational health services that deliver care for the NHS. This consists of [23]:

- prevention – preventing ill health caused or exacerbated by work
- timely intervention – early treatment of the main causes of absence in the NHS
- rehabilitation – a process to help staff to stay in or return to work after illness
- health assessments for work – supporting organisations to manage attendance and retirement
- promotion of health and wellbeing – using the workplace to promote improved health and wellbeing
- teaching and training – promoting the health and wellbeing approach among all staff, and ensuring the availability of future occupational health staff.

The Mental Health Agenda
Mental Healthcare

Some staff may have more persistent needs, and a moderate number may have needs that go beyond psychosocial care. The approach taken in this book recognises that some people may require skilled mental health assessments by general practitioners, occupational health teams, or psychiatric services. They may need to be assessed for mental health disorders by staff of a specialist mental health service. The mental health agenda focuses on responding to the needs of staff whose symptoms indicate that they may require specialist mental healthcare by:

- ensuring access to occupational healthcare to enable staff in need to receive assessments of their needs
- creating service-level agreements with specialist mental health providers to ensure ease of access for certain staff to timely and reliable mental healthcare.

Key Ways of Responding Immediately to Staff Who Become Distressed at Work

It is important to recognise that stress and distress are common reactions and are not usually harbingers of pathology. That is probably because working in small teams over long (12-hour) shifts provides opportunities for natural conversations and peer support. It is important to develop a culture wherein people feel valued and safe, and can form relationships with their colleagues. This also emphasises an important principle of having psychosocially informed conversations embedded within organisations' cultures.

Validation and Invalidation of People's Experiences

As we have seen in Chapter 28, people who are affected by EITDDC regard social and professional acknowledgement of their experiences as key to their recovery. This process is called validation, and it involves recognition or affirmation of a person's distress (see Chapter 5). Often colleagues and family members are those most important sources of validation. Authoritative validation is that aspect of validation and establishing entitlement to care offered by a person who is perceived to have specialist knowledge or expertise in relation to the psychosocial impacts of EITDDCs. It emphasises the importance of ensuring that opportunities are created for other people, whose opinions are respected, to recognise and acknowledge their experiences. Authoritative validation confers positive connotations on a person's distress and their wish to seek support. It challenges negative self-evaluations (i.e., people seeing their distress or seeking help as a sign of weakness or inadequacy).

Research shows that it is all too easy to invalidate people's experiences by using words such as 'normal'. That word may be interpreted as the listener not being interested. Supervising staff and colleagues should develop ways of listening to each other and reflecting that minimise the risks of invalidation.

Listening ... and Hearing

Not being listened to makes people feel undervalued. In contrast, active listening – that is, making a conscious and practised effort not only to hear the words that another person is saying but also, more importantly, to try to understand the complete message that is being sent – is core to helping to support the health and wellbeing of colleagues. It is suggested that:

- 85% of what we know, we learn from listening
- 45% of our time is spent listening
- a person recalls 50% of what they have just heard, and only 20% of it is remembered long term.

We can improve our listening skills with practice.

Leadership

Managers and team leaders have a core role in addressing the impacts of stress on the workforce of their organisations. In the first instance, managers and team leaders should be mindful of their own needs. They need access to sources of care and support in order to be able to manage the stress of their own roles. Their responsibilities for other people should be acknowledged.

Managers and leaders can champion the approach to wellbeing in their organisations and help to embed it into the culture. This involves creating a culture of safety within organisations but also creating a focus on valuing staff communicating their feelings (it is OK to speak up, to admit one's fears, weaknesses, mistakes, and uncertainty and to express emotion). Both should be components of psychological safety and governance practices. It is important that leaders are familiar with key concepts relating to psychosocial care of their staff, and that they can shape the culture of teams and environments that are psychosocially informed and safe. People should also lead by example, and it is important for leaders to share examples of mistakes that they have made and to be open about their weaknesses. This is powerful modelling that encourages other people to behave in open ways that support wellbeing. Furthermore, it is important that leaders address issues as they arise, and focus on clinical excellence.

Enabling Staff to Access Support

Staff may find it difficult to consider seeking support. We suggest that managers and leaders and their organisations have a responsibility to ensure that staff can access support when they are concerned about their own wellbeing or that of colleagues. Access to wellbeing services is aided by:

- a clear description of the services being offered, with entry points being well defined and signposted, and a description of the people at whom each element of the service is aimed
- a clear statement that confidentiality will be respected for people accessing services, and that such access will not affect their professional jobs
- every effort being made to facilitate access to services by, for example, allowing time to use services and facilitating IT access.

The key to most mass casualty triumphs is in planning – having a plan, preparing an organisation to be able to deliver elements of the plan, and then empowering staff to follow that plan when a crisis occurs. This is never truer than when responding to the wellbeing, psychosocial, and mental health needs of staff who are involved in all kinds of emergencies. Work to plan and design services should be done well in advance of any incident if the benefits are to be realised during and in the aftermath of a significant event.

Avoiding Re-Traumatisation

Some organisations have governance processes in which cases are scrutinised in a systematic way. These case reviews often involve a technical debriefing and discussion of cases in detail, and the experience is often valued highly as conveying learning. However, there is also the potential for this type of reflection to create situations in which clinicians might be expected to recount the events of an incident and to re-live difficult or distressing events in front of peers, colleagues, and supervisors. There is evidence that 'emotional debriefing' of this nature has the potential to cause harm, and that it should be avoided. Therefore it is important to understand and select cases for open peer review in cognisant and sensitive ways that take into account the mental health risks of re-traumatisation.

Conclusion

This chapter takes the lessons from across this book to create a model of care for staff of healthcare and other organisations involved in responding to EITDDC through which the wellbeing, psychosocial, and mental health agendas can be delivered. At the very least, this model provides a framework for planning, decision making, and review to ensure that the essential elements of a coherent approach to meeting the mental health needs of staff are all present. Chapters 45, 47, and 48 provide illustrative information.

References

1. Smith EC, Burkle FM. Paramedic and emergency medical technician reflections on the ongoing impact of the 9/11 terrorist attacks. *Prehosp Disaster Med* 2019; 34: 56–61.

2. Murray E, Kaufman KR, Williams R. Let us do better: learning lessons for recovery of healthcare professionals during and after COVID-19. *BJPsych Open* 2021; 7: e151.

3. Williams R, Murray E, Neal A, Kemp V. *The Top Ten Messages for Supporting Healthcare Staff during the COVID-19 Pandemic.* Royal College of Psychiatrists, 2020 (top-ten-messages-williams-et-al.pdf).

4. Fancourt D, Bhui K, Chatterjee H, Crawford P, Crossick G, DeNora T, et al. Social, cultural and community engagement and mental health: cross-disciplinary, co-produced research agenda. *BJPsych Open* 2021; 7: e3.

5. San Juan NV, Aceituno D, Djellouli N, Sumray K, Regenold N, Syverson A, et al. Mental health and well-being of healthcare workers during the COVID-19 pandemic in the UK: contrasting guidelines with experiences in practice. *BJPsych Open* 2020; 7: e15.

6. Kaniasty K, Norris FH. Distinctions that matter: received social support, perceived social support and social embeddedness after disasters. In *Mental Health and Disasters* (eds Y Neria, S Galea, FH Norris): 175–200. Cambridge University Press, 2009.

7. Williams R, Ntontis E, Alfadhli K, Drury J, Amlôt R. A social model of secondary stressors in relation to disasters, major incidents and conflict: implications for practice. *Int J Disaster Risk Reduct* 2021; 63: 102436.

8. Stevenson D, Farmer P. *Thriving at Work: The Independent Review of Mental Health and Employers.* HM Government, 2017.

9. Williams R, Kemp V, Batt-Rawden S, Bland L, Burgess J, Murray E, et al. *Valuing Staff, Valuing Patients: The Report on the Psychosocial and Mental Health Programme.* Faculty of Pre-Hospital Care, Royal College of Surgeons of Edinburgh, 2022.

10. Milligan-Saville JS, Tan L, Gayed A, Barnes C, Dobson M, Bryant RA, et al. Workplace mental

health training for managers and its effect on sick leave in employees: a cluster randomised controlled trial. *Lancet Psychiatry* 2017; 4: 850–58.

11. Malinen S, Hatton T, Naswall K, Kuntz J. Strategies to enhance employee well-being and organisational performance in a postcrisis environment: a case study. Available from: https://doi .org/10.1111/1468-5973.12227.

12. Bleetman, A, Sanusi, S, Dale, T, et al. Human factors and error prevention in emergency medicine. *Emerg Med J* 2012; 29: 389–93.

13. Hill R, Sundin E, Winder B. Work–family enrichment of firefighters: 'satellite family members', risk, trauma and family functioning. *Int J Emerg Serv* 2020; 9: 395–407.

14. Kaniasty K, Norris FH. Longitudinal linkages between perceived social support and posttraumatic stress symptoms: sequential roles of social causation and social selection. *J Trauma Stress* 2008; 21: 274–81.

15. McFarlane AC, Williams R. Mental health services required after disasters: learning from the lasting effects of disasters. *Depress Res Treat* 2012; 2012: 970194.

16. Williams R, Kemp V, Stokes S, Lockey D. *Peer Support: An Introductory or Briefing Document*. Faculty of Pre-Hospital Care, Royal College of Surgeons of Edinburgh, 2020 (fphc.rcsed.ac.uk/media/2841/ peer-support.pdf).

17. Williams R, Bisson J, Kemp V. Health care planning for community disaster care. In Textbook of Disaster Psychiatry (eds R Ursano, C Fullerton, L Weisaeth, B Raphael): 244–60. Cambridge University Press, 2017.

18. World Health Organization. *Psychological First Aid: Guide for Field Workers*. World Health Organization, 2011.

19. McDuff DR, Johnson JL. Classification and characteristics of Army stress casualties during Operation Desert Storm. *Hosp Community Psychiatry* 1992; 43: 812–15.

20. Solomon Z, Shklar R, Mikulincer M. Frontline treatment of combat stress reaction: a 20-year longitudinal evaluation study. *Am J Psychiatry* 2005; 162: 2309–14.

21. Mental Health Commission of Canada. *Toward Recovery and Well-Being: A Framework for a Mental Health Strategy for Canada*. Mental Health Commission of Canada, 2009.

22. O'Donnell ML, Lau A, Fredrickson J, Gibson K, Bryant R, Bisson J, et al. An open label pilot study of a brief psychosocial intervention for disaster and trauma survivors. *Front Psychiatry* 2020; 11: 483.

23. NHS Employers. *Your Occupational Health Service: Guidance*. NHS Employers, 2019 (www.nhsemployers.org/system/ files/media/Your-occupational-health%20service-October-2019_0 .pdf).

Chapter

45

Case Study 1: Caring for Teams – An Organisation-Wide Approach to Wellbeing, Psychosocial Care, and Mental Healthcare

Verity Kemp, Sarah Robbins, Christine Howard, Gary Strong, Mark Thomas, and Richard Williams

Introduction

This case study builds on the contents of Chapters 12, 27, 28, 29, 37, and 44 to illustrate approaches to promoting wellbeing and initiating psychosocial care to support the mental health of the staff of public sector services in the UK. It focuses on staff who work in emergencies, including those in the fire and rescue, police, ambulance, and search and rescue services, often referred to in the UK as the Blue Light services. This case study uses information provided in Chapters 37 and 44 to identify what can be done to assist the work of employing organisations to promote the mental health of all employees – that is, senior, middle, junior, general, and professional managers and their staff. It describes important concepts in both the planning and delivery of interventions.

This case study picks out themes from Chapter 44 to show how they are being implemented in the UK. It draws on work undertaken by the authors for MindEd, a project supported by Health Education England. (The material produced for that project, including an online learning tool – with content design led by RW and VK, who own the copyright for this – can be found at https://www.minded.org.uk/Component/Details/712211) Two of the authors (RW and VK) have led the Psychosocial Care and Mental Health Programme for the Faculty of Pre-Hospital Care at the Royal College of Surgeons of Edinburgh (the report on it is available at fphc.rcsed.ac.uk/media/3140/valuing-staff-valuing-patients.pdf). This chapter summarises material in the programme's report [1], as well as material in the MindEd Blue Light project's resources. The authors are grateful to the Faculty for allowing us to develop here some of the contents of that report.

Working in one of the emergency services tends to be regarded as being inherently stressful. Working with people who are unwell or in crisis means doing a job that is rich in social meaning, and it requires emotional labour from employees [2]. We also know that people who choose helping as a career tend to believe more in the kind of work that they do than in the level of pay that they receive. However, this can create the circumstances in which people experience moral distress. This kind of work often requires intense interactions with other people, and the pace and content mean that it can interfere with the way that staff members would ideally want to carry out their work.

The Stevenson/Farmer Review

In earlier chapters, this book references *Thriving at Work*, the report of the Stevenson/Farmer review [3]. We draw on its content again here. It is a review of mental health and employers and it is concerned with all organisations, showing that the human cost of poor mental health is huge through impacts on the lives of employees and people around them at work and at home. We know that there can be higher rates of mental health problems and suicide for employees in certain work settings. The report recommends that employers foster employees' good mental health by attending to three challenges that were illustrated in Chapters 28 and 44 [2,3].

The authors of this chapter have developed that approach to identify the three agendas that it generates [4].

- The wellbeing agenda is concerned with assisting employees to thrive at work. Wellbeing is about feeling good and functioning well, and is influenced by each person's experience of life, including their work and relationships at home.

- The psychosocial agenda is concerned with supporting staff who are struggling or who are distressed. Psychosocial care describes interventions for people who are distressed or struggling, or who have symptoms of mental health problems that do not meet the criteria for a diagnosis, whether or not they also experience social or work dysfunction.

- The Mental Health Agenda is concerned with enabling people whose needs appear to go beyond struggling, and may indicate that they are developing a mental disorder, to access timely mental healthcare, to recover, and to return to work.

The Problems Faced by Staff

The findings of a poll conducted in 2016 by Mind, the mental health charity in England and Wales, were that one in four emergency service workers had considered ending their life, and 41% had been prescribed medication to deal with work-related problems [5]. Mind's follow-up survey in 2019 found that only 34% of staff rated their current mental health as being good or very good. In total, 21% of staff of all emergency services stated that their mental health was poor or very poor, compared with 14% in 2015 [5]. Thus, even before the COVID-19 pandemic, there were indications that matters were getting worse, and it appears entirely likely that the mental health problems of many staff deteriorated during the pandemic [6].

Before the COVID-19 pandemic occurred, reports from a number of organisations (e.g., the NHS Staff Survey, Police Care UK) emphasised the need to consider and maintain the health and wellbeing of the workforce [7,8].

The General Medical Council has highlighted workplace stress as affecting doctors' health and having an impact on patient safety and medical staff retention [9]. The NHS Staff Survey reported that 40.3% of staff were feeling unwell because of work-related stress in the previous 12 months [7]. The British Medical Association (BMA) has found that doctors experience moral distress (see also Chapter 39) when there is no growth in support to match the increasing numbers of patients seen and the complexity of their needs [10].

The *House of Commons Health and Social Care Committee Report on Workforce Burnout and Resilience in the NHS and Social Care* was published in June 2021 [11]. It reported on the workforce issues facing staff in the NHS and social care, and took into account the additional impact of COVID-19.

It concluded that burnout has a significant impact and negative consequences for the mental health of members of staff, with consequent impacts on colleagues and the patients they care for. It recommended that the NHS should provide additional support for its staff, which will require removing barriers to seeking help and embedding a culture in which staff are explicitly given permission and time away from work to seek help when it is needed.

Public Sector Policies and Plans

General Programmes

The MIND Blue Light Programme provides mental health support for emergency services staff and volunteers across England and Wales. Each service has also continued to develop its own programmes to support the health and wellbeing of staff.

The NHS

The NHS People Plan

The NHS People Plan for 2020 provided a clear commitment to protecting the health and wellbeing of NHS staff as well as creating compassionate and inclusive environments wherein staff can thrive [12]. Its proposals for improving the health and wellbeing of NHS staff included providing a designated wellbeing guardian in each organisation, safe spaces for staff to rest and recuperate, access to psychological support and treatment, and physically healthy workplaces.

Ambulance and Other Healthcare Services

The Association of Ambulance Chief Executives (AACE) and the College of Paramedics (CoP) have each developed material to support the health and wellbeing of ambulance service employees, volunteers, and their families [13–15]. There are support services offered by The Ambulance Service Charity (TASC) [16]. NHS England and Improvement and the Samaritans published a brief guide online in 2020 [17].

The BMA's charter proposes that employers develop a supportive structure based on a culture that supports mental health and wellbeing, a wellbeing strategy, embedding health and wellbeing into line management, accessible support services, creating safe and healthy workplaces, actively fostering peer support, and supporting staff during sickness leave and on return to work [10].

A *Lancet Psychiatry* paper has reviewed the impact of a 4-hour training programme for commanders of firefighters in Australia, and showed that a 4-hour mental health training programme for managers led to a significant reduction in work-related sickness leave and a return on investment of £9.98 for every pound spent on the training [18].

The Police Services

The National Police Chiefs' Council (NPCC) launched a National Police Wellbeing Service – Oscar Kilo – through the College of Policing [19]. Each force commits to its own wellbeing initiatives, using primarily peer support groups and Trauma Risk Management (TRiM) as adapted for civilian services, including the NHS. For example, the Derbyshire Constabulary works closely with Mind and with charities such as PTSD999.org, and is looking at online wellbeing seminars [20].

Fire and Rescue Services

The National Fire Chiefs Council (NFCC) has signed Public Health England's Concordat for Better Mental Health [21]. This consensus statement describes the shared commitment of the sector to work through local and national action to prevent mental health problems and promote good mental health. This commitment is reflected in priorities for the fire and rescue workforce.

Each fire and rescue service has developed its own approaches to deliver against the priority [22]. Fire and rescue services also have support mechanisms for staff following their exposure at traumatic incidents.

Practical Approaches

Achieving improvements in care for the staff of statutory sector organisations requires employers to pay attention to their organisations' cultures, and the matters described in this section of this chapter, in order to achieve the objectives. Chapter 44 includes a description of 12 key approaches, known as the Golden Approaches to Sustaining Wellbeing of Staff, that are imperatives for all organisations in any approach to caring for the wellbeing, psychosocial, and mental health needs of their staff.

Primary and Secondary Stressors

In the context of disasters and emergencies, it is essential to differentiate between primary and secondary stressors [3,23,24].

Primary stressors are the sources of worry, anxiety, and stress that stem directly from the events and consequential tasks that the staff of services face at work (e.g., death, dying, violence). As Chapter 39 shows, moral distress and moral injury are primary stressors of particular current concern that have increased substantially during the pandemic [4].

Secondary stressors are: 1. social factors and people's life circumstances (including the policies, practices, and social, organisational, and financial arrangements) that exist prior to and impact people during an incident, and/or 2. societal and organisational responses to an incident or emergency [24]. They include the adequacy and effectiveness of employers' responses to events, and their expectations of employees' performance, the career aspirations of staff, and concerns of staff about their training, the conditions in which they work and live, and their work–life balance. We recognise, for example, that accountability processes, although essential to learning and to professional and organisational development, should be managed carefully because otherwise they may become stress inducing [2,25].

Staff of public organisations repeatedly comment that secondary stressors affect them to a greater degree than do primary stressors. The COVID-19 pandemic has resulted in much greater appreciation of the frequency and disproportionately deleterious impacts of secondary stressors. Thus the situations described by various organisations also demonstrate the impact of secondary stressors as the healthcare and Blue Light services began their responses to the primary stressors posed by the COVID-19 pandemic.

Employers should identify and tackle primary and secondary stressors in day-to-day work, and should create a plan to increase efforts to sustain their staff when they are preparing for, facing, and recovering from challenging circumstances and crises. The evidence suggests that it is important to create a mixed approach based on a variety of methods when implementing the advice offered in this chapter. This requires employers to put in place actions to work on the three agendas that were summarised earlier in the chapter. We now summarise the actions that should be considered.

A Strategic Approach to Delivering the Objectives: A Model of Care

In Chapters 12, 27, and 28 we describe a framework to improve the health and wellbeing of the public, and in

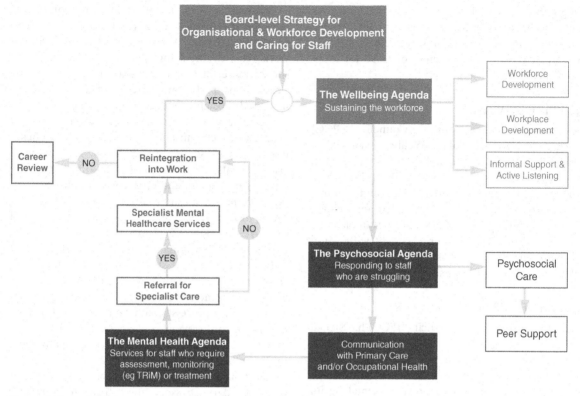

Figure 45.1 A model of care. (© R Williams, V Kemp, 2021, all rights reserved.)

Chapter 44 we develop that framework for people who work in the healthcare, rescue, and Blue Light services. The framework follows the categories identified in the Stevenson/Farmer review and consists of a set of core principles and a model of care. Figure 45.1 is reproduced from Chapter 44; it offers a model for caring for people at work. However, it is important to reiterate here what we stated in Chapter 44. This model is intended to be neither structural nor linear. It is intended to be strategic, and to emphasise a functional approach to caring for and supporting staff. It shows how those functions are linked, but care may proceed in both directions through this model, and people may be fast-tracked to mental healthcare if that is warranted, or often they may cycle between the wellbeing and psychosocial agendas.

Core Principles

It is important for services to implement core principles in caring for and supporting their staff, and to act on the three agendas derived from the report of the Stevenson/Farmer review in supporting and caring for staff. The model of care underpins these intentions.

The principles on which it sits are based on the principles of psychological first aid [26], and include:

1. agreeing and disseminating definitions in frequent use to ensure common understanding
2. orientating services to staff members and their families in the cultures in which they live, relate, and work
3. translating lessons from evidence and experience into plans and frameworks for delivering on the wellbeing, psychosocial care, and mental health agendas
4. integrating plans for the wellbeing, psychosocial care, and mental health agendas into all policies
5. ensuring that communications are effective, because they are fundamental to sustaining the integrity of services and reassuring staff
6. emphasising social connectedness and social support in creating comprehensive programmes
7. working to agreed minimum standards that take account of the range of circumstances that might be encountered.

This is a summary of a selection of principles that are covered more substantially in Chapter 27 [27].

The Wellbeing Agenda

The wellbeing agenda focuses on the importance of supporting staff who are thriving by recognising and actively supporting team leaders' pivotal roles in developing staff and their workplaces, and in developing teams, teamworking, and team cohesion, by:

- addressing people's physical healthcare needs
- continuing to develop leadership
- strengthening teams, team membership, and teams' cohesion
- ensuring preparedness, training, and support for staff so that they are always able to look out for each other
- ensuring that staff have space and time for reflection and recovery
- seeking and addressing organisational and workplace factors that affect people's physical, social, and work capacities
- reducing secondary stressors
- continuing to work on reducing stigma.

Examples of responses to meeting the wellbeing needs of people at work are provided by AACE, NPCC, and the NFCC, which have published material to support their staff that also provides signposting to specialist services. Examples include:

- Oscar Kilo – the source of information about the National Police Wellbeing Service [19]
- Five Ways to Wellbeing (Derbyshire Mind for Derbyshire Police) [20]
- health and wellbeing support for ambulance service employees, volunteers, and their families (AACE, CoP, and TASC) [13–17]
- psychological first aid programmes (various organisations and services) [26].

The Psychosocial Agenda

The number of people affected by emergencies, incidents, disasters, and disease outbreaks (EITDDC) may be very substantial despite the fact that the majority of distressed people are unlikely to develop a mental disorder. Intervening early can reduce the risk of their developing disorders later. Psychosocial care emphasises responding to the needs of staff by focusing on:

- strengthening the contributions of teams and enabling members to actively listen to and support each other
- developing peer support [28]

- providing mental health training for professional and general managers, particularly in the skills required to enable staff to discuss any problems that they have [18]
- ensuring that workplaces recognise and augment opportunities for post-traumatic growth (PTG) – that is, positive psychological changes experienced because of adversity and other challenges that give rise to higher levels of functioning
- working according to the principles of psychological first aid to provide psychosocial care with the intention of:
  - reducing the risks of morbidity
  - reducing absence through sickness
  - reducing the risks of presenteeism
  - promoting personal growth and learning [26,27].

Practical interventions are best provided using the **PIES** approach, which reduces the risk of people developing mental health diagnoses later. It calls for interventions to be offered in Proximity to where staff work, with Immediacy, in Expectancy of good outcomes, using Simplicity of interventions [29,30]. However, we emphasise that it is important to avoid routine screening because there is little evidence that it conveys benefit inside organisations.

The Mental Health Agenda

The mental health agenda focuses on responding effectively to staff whose needs may indicate that they appear to require specialist mental health assessment and/or care by:

- ensuring access to occupational health services (see Chapter 43) to enable staff in need to receive assessments of their needs
- creating service-level agreements with agencies that ensure ease of access for certain staff for timely and reliable specialist mental healthcare.

Sustaining Staff in Challenging Circumstances and Crises

Core Approaches

Planning is important for sustaining staff of all sectors through an upsurge in activity caused by the occurrence of an emergency, a major incident, or an outbreak of serious illness. The advantage of the three agendas identified here is that they apply both to unusual circumstances and to 'business as usual'. Thus this chapter identifies the core actions for these situations. Careful attention to the wellbeing and mental health of staff is important throughout emergencies. Experience from the COVID-19 pandemic is that emergencies cause unusual primary stressors and accentuate the impacts of secondary stressors. Chapter 44 presents ideas about how the wellbeing and psychosocial agendas might be developed.

A paper for managers reported a longitudinal study of work to enhance employees' wellbeing after the earthquake sequence of 2010–2011 in Canterbury, New Zealand, which suggested that attending to longer-term recovery of staff is necessary to ensure positive organisational functioning. Targeting employees' wellbeing is a low-cost strategy that can ensure positive functioning throughout a lengthy recovery period [25]. The paper recommended that managers should focus on:

- validating employees' and managers' efforts and flexibility during a crisis
- giving more autonomy to local managers
- flexible performance management by giving local discretion to managers to manage performance and create a learning culture, because increased psychological safety may reduce mistakes [3]
- the wellbeing and psychosocial care of employees.

Preparation as Crises Begin

Supporting teams to prepare for what is to come means providing anticipatory briefings and critical information that should enable people to feel in a better place to understand what is likely to happen and how they might respond. An example of a psychosocial briefing is provided by Richard Williams and his colleagues [31]. Preparation means:

- providing information about the feelings that people are likely to have in preparation for potential distress that they may experience
- reducing anticipatory anxiety by sharing what may happen
- being honest and open about what is happening, and why, helps to reduce the risk of moral injury and moral distress
- enhancing knowledge of, and support from, managers

- focusing on leadership, teamwork, and team cohesion – this is critical
- preparing a range of interventions for people who become distressed, including ensuring ease of access to them.

Conclusions: An Agenda for Developing Staff Care in the Public Sector

This case study presents an overview of the stress that affects staff who work in the emergency and healthcare services. Managers at all levels have two major tasks when tackling the impacts on the workforce of their organisations. First, they should be mindful of their own needs, because there is common experience that responsibilities for other people may bring additional stress; managers also need sources of care and support. The approach taken in this chapter is as applicable to them as it is to any other member of the workforce. Second, managers have important opportunities to influence the cultures of their organisations and to embed an approach to all three agendas into the framework of their organisations to the benefit of the whole workforce.

The authors agree that, although there are differences in the roles, responsibilities, and cultures of the police, fire and rescue, search and rescue, and health services, and their staff may experience stress differently, there is also common ground in the ways in which stress affects everyone. Recognising primary and secondary stressors is common to all organisations, which should be aware that although primary stressors are very powerful, the secondary stressors are very common, may have more impact than do the primary stressors, but many are tractable if they are recognised and there is careful planning.

This chapter supports the single stepped approach proposed in Chapter 44 with the intention of embedding the wellbeing agenda for all employees, psychosocial care for employees who are struggling, and agreed pathways for people who appear to need specialist mental healthcare. We draw attention to the potential for people to grow, post traumatic growth (PTG), that can be augmented by attending to the three agendas. Richard Tedeschi has identified education, emotional regulation, disclosure, narrative development, and services as routes to increasing the likelihood of PTG [32].

References

1. Williams R, Kemp V, Batt-Rawden S, Bland L, Burgess J, McInerney A, et al. *Valuing Staff, Valuing Patients: The Report on the Psychosocial and Mental Health Programme.* Faculty of Pre-Hospital Care, Royal College of Surgeons of Edinburgh, 2022.

2. Williams R, Kemp V. Caring for healthcare practitioners. *BJPsych Advances* 2019; 26: 116–28.

3. Stevenson D, Farmer P. *Thriving at Work: The Stevenson/Farmer Review of Mental Health and Employers.* Department for Work and Pensions and Department of Health and Social Care, 2017.

4. Murray E, Kaufman KR, Williams R. Let us do better: learning lessons for recovery of healthcare professionals during and after COVID-19. *BJPsych Open* 2021; 7: e151.

5. Mind. *Blue Light Programme Research Summary 2016–18.* Mind, 2018 (www.mind.org.uk/media-a/4861/blue-light-programme-research-summary_2016-to-18_online.pdf).

6. Williams R, Kaufman KR. Narrative review of the COVID-19, healthcare and healthcarers thematic series. *BJPsych Open* 2022; 8: e34.

7. NHS Employers. *NHS Staff Survey 2019.* NHS Employers, 2020 (www.nhsemployers.org/articles/nhs-staff-survey-2020).

8. Police Care UK. *Policing: The Job and the Life Survey.* Police Care UK, 2018.

9. General Medical Council. *The State of Medical Education and Practice in the UK.* General Medical Council, 2018.

10. British Medical Association. *Caring for the Mental Health of the Medical Workforce.* British Medical Association, 2019.

11. House of Commons Health and Social Care Committee. *Workforce Burnout and Resilience in the NHS and Social Care: Second Report of Session 2021–22.* House of Commons, 2021.

12. NHS England. *We are the NHS: People Plan for 2020/21 – Action for Us All.* NHS England, 2020 (www.england.nhs.uk/publication/we-are-the-nhs-people-plan-for-2020-21-action-for-us-all).

13. Association of Chief Ambulance Officers. *Supporting Ambulance Staff on Mental Health and Wellbeing.* Association of Chief Ambulance Officers, 2019 (https://aace.org.uk/mentalhealthandwellbeing/).

14. College of Paramedics. *Paramedic Mental Health and Wellbeing.* College of Paramedics, 2023 (https://collegeofparamedics.co.uk/COP/Member_/Paramedic_Mental_Health_and_Wellbeing.aspx).

15. College of Paramedics. *Guidance for Managers on Psychosocial Support and Mental Wellbeing of Ambulance Personnel in a Pandemic.* College of Paramedics, 2020 (collegeofparamedics.co.uk/COP/News/Covid-19/Guidance_for_managers_psychosocial_support_and_mental_wellbeing_of_ambulance_personnel_in_a_pandemic.aspx).

16. The Ambulance Staff Charity (TASC). *Mental Health Support.* TASC, 2020 (www.theasc.org.uk/services-we-offer/mental-health/).

17. NHS Leadership Academy. *Supporting Others in Difficult Times: A Samaritan's Guide to Helpful Conversations.* NHS Leadership Academy, 2020 (https://people.nhs.uk/guides/supporting-others-in-difficult-times/).

18. Milligan-Saville JS, Tan L, Gayed A, Barnes C, Dobson M, Bryant RA, et al. Workplace mental health training for managers and its effect on sick leave in employees: a cluster randomised controlled trial. *Lancet Psychiatry* 2017; 4: 850-85.

19. National Police Wellbeing Service. *Oscar Kilo.* National Police Wellbeing Service, 2023 (www.oscarkilo.org.uk/).

20. Derbyshire County Council. *Five Ways to Wellbeing.* Derbyshire County Council, 2023 (www.derbyshire.gov.uk/social-health/health-and-wellbeing/mental-health-and-wellbeing/five-ways-to-wellbeing/five-ways-to-wellbeing.aspx).

21. Office for Health Improvement & Disparities. *Prevention Concordat for Better Mental Health.* Office for Health Improvement & Disparities, 2023 (www.gov.uk/government/publications/prevention-concordat-for-better-mental-health-consensus-statement/prevention-concordat-for-better-mental-health).

22. Mind. *Mental Health in the Emergency Services: Our 2019 Survey Results – Fire Service.* Mind, 2019 (www.mind.org.uk/media-a/4848/2019-survey-fire-service-summary.pdf).

23. Lock S, Rubin GJ, Murray V, Rogers MB, Amlôt R, Williams R. Secondary stressors and extreme events and disasters: a systematic review of primary research from 2010–2011. *PLoS Curr* 2012; 4: ecurrents.dis.a9b76fed1b2dd5c5bfcfc13c87a2f24f.

24. Williams R, Ntontis E, Alfadhli K, Drury J, Amlôt R. A social model of secondary stressors in relation to disasters, major incidents and conflict: implications for practice. *Int J Disaster Risk Reduct* 2021; 63: 102436.

25. Malinen S, Hatton T, Naswall K, Kuntz J. Strategies to enhance employee well-being and organisational performance in a postcrisis environment: a case study. *J Contingencies Crisis Manag* 2019; 27: 79–86.

26. NHS England. *Psychological First Aid Training for Staff and*

Volunteers. NHS England, 2020 (www.nhsemployers.org/news/ 2020/06/free-psychological-first-aid-in-emergencies-training-for-frontline-staff-and-volunteers).

27. Williams R, Bisson JI, Kemp V. Designing, planning and delivering psychosocial and mental health care for communities affected by disasters. In *Textbook of Disaster Psychiatry*, 2nd ed (eds R. Ursano, CS Fullerton, L Weisaeth, B Raphael): 244–60. Cambridge University Press, 2017.

28. Williams R, Kemp V, Stokes S, Lockey D. *Peer Support*. Royal College of Surgeons of Edinburgh, 2020 (https://fphc.rcsed.ac.uk/ media/2841/peer-support.pdf).

29. McDuff DR, Johnson JL. Classification and characteristics of Army stress casualties during Operation Desert Storm. *Hosp Community Psychiatry* 1992; 43: 812–15.

30. Solomon Z, Shklar R, Mikulincer M. Frontline treatment of combat stress reaction: a 20-year longitudinal evaluation study. *Am J Psychiatry* 2005; 162: 2309–14.

31. Williams R, Murray E, Neal A, Kemp V. *The Top Ten Messages for Supporting Healthcare Staff during the COVID-19 Pandemic*. Royal College of Psychiatrists, 2020 (top-ten-messages-williams-et-al.pdf).

32. Tedeschi RG. Growth after trauma. *Harvard Business Review*, July–August 2020 (https://hbr .org/2020/07/growth-after-trauma).

46

Case Study 2: The Impacts of COVID-19 on Healthcare Staff – Lessons from a Selection of Interventions Put in Place During the Pandemic

Kate Allsopp, Sonya Wallbank, and Richard Williams

Introduction

The first lockdown in the UK started in March 2020 [1]. Subsequently, UK restrictions eased, before there were two more waves in autumn 2020 through to 2021, and another two lockdowns. Early in 2021, the UK government began a huge rollout of vaccines [2]. When we drafted this chapter in 2022, confirmed daily cases of COVID-19 were rising again rapidly due to the highly transmissible Omicron variants, with additional fears for the winter ahead around the combined impacts of influenza and COVID-19. Since then rates have declined, but rates of COVID-19 in the UK and around the world still remain higher than many members of the public realise, and healthcare staff have been under massive pressure for more than 3 years with services across the UK affected during 2022 and 2023 by high rates of staff sickness absences and difficult industrial relationships. As we update the chapter in July 2023, the preceding 7 days in England have seen 1,912 people testing positive with 147 deaths with COVID-19 shown on the death certificates and 760 people admitted to hospital.

This chapter outlines the impact of the COVID-19 pandemic on healthcare staff in the UK. The UK's healthcare is delivered predominantly by the National Health Services (NHS). Therefore this chapter draws on key strategies and support for NHS staff in particular. It should also be noted that there are four distinct national health services, one in each of the four countries that comprise the UK; these are described collectively as the NHS hereafter.

The Approach in the NHS

Pre-Existing Challenges

Before the COVID-19 pandemic began, the NHS workforce was under significant pressure. Staff shortages were evidenced in England with 100,000 vacancies across NHS trusts, that is, an average of 1 in 11 posts being vacant overall and 1 in 8 nursing posts [3]. Staff shortages were evidenced by an average of 1 in 12 unfilled medical posts and 1 in 8 unfilled nursing posts [3]. Sickness absence in the NHS was approximately 2.3% higher than in other industries, and around 1 in 11 staff were leaving the NHS every year [4].

> The workforce crisis was the biggest issue facing the health and care system before the emergence of COVID-19. NHS hospitals, mental health services and community providers were operating with more than 100,000 full-time vacancies and staff were working under strain with high levels of sickness absence and work-related stress [5].

The UK sickness absence rate remained relatively flat between 2010 and 2018, standing at 2.0% in 2018 [6,7]. NHS staff sickness rates rose from 3.8% in April 2018 to 4.1% in April 2019. This was the highest level at that time of year in more than a decade, and represented more than 1.4 million full-time equivalent days lost in that month alone [6]. Consequently, the workforce was overstretched, and gaps were plugged by temporary agency staff, leading to a negative impact on staff wellbeing [8], and over 38% of staff in the NHS in England were reported to be suffering from work-related stress [9].

A review observed a significant and widespread work-related emotional impact on staff [10]. The year before the pandemic began, the King's Fund reported that [11]:

- 25% of secondary care nurses and midwives in England were considering leaving their organisations due to stress
- 24% of students had dropped out of undergraduate nursing courses because they were unable to cope

- 34–51% of UK nurses and midwives reported being unwell due to work stress each year
- 40% of nurses and midwives experienced bullying, harassment, and abuse in 2018–2019
- over 50% of nurses and midwives had gone into work despite not feeling well enough to perform their duties.

Work Content and Career Choices

People who choose helping as a career tend to believe more in the kind of work that they do than in the pay they receive. However, staff being too busy to do their work to their satisfaction creates incongruence between the ideal of the work and the reality, and can create personal conflict and moral distress [12]. The members of this workforce are less likely to need to be asked to work above and beyond their roles, and they identify with the role of helper rather than with being helped themselves. Consequently, presenteeism is significant, and people are often very unwell before they agree to take any significant time off. The subsequent negative impact on the health and wellbeing of staff is well documented, and is a significant risk factor for negative long-term outcomes [13]. The need to draw attention to implicit overworking and a tendency to avoid seeking help was key to informing the strategy adopted by NHS England during the pandemic.

The Response of the NHS in England

We set out the paragraphs in this section to indicate the broad approach that appeared to us to be taken by the NHS in England.

Prepare

Initially, managers and frontline teams were faced with the need for urgent and increased preparatory activity. Clinical services not deemed urgent or time critical were put on hold, leaving some staff seeing themselves as underused. Others were confined to their homes by their health history requiring them to shield from higher risks of becoming infected; this rendered some unable to undertake meaningful tasks.

Supporting teams – that is, staff designated either formally or informally to support their colleagues in providing urgent pandemic responses – needed to help to keep staff informed about what was going to happen and to acquire and develop a range of interventions to help staff to cope (see Chapter 47 for a

description of these principles in action). They can be summarised as follows.

1. *Validation.* Validating people's feelings and experiences, and preparing them for potential distress by offering self-help and highlighting the importance of distraction, coping, and resilience strategies (e.g., talking to colleagues, sleep, hydration, exercise, healthy diet), was especially important during the preparatory phase when hospitals were not all uniformly operating in active stages and at capacity.

2. *Reducing anticipatory anxiety.* It was important to share information about what changed workplaces may look and feel like, in order to address anticipatory anxiety during the waiting and preparatory stages. The plan was to reduce the element of surprise and to support staff returning to services (e.g., from retirement) to be prepared for the changed situation.

3. *Preparing people for learning new skills.* This involved supporting people to upskill quickly and still feel safe within their boundaries by providing policies and guidance about decision making and team working in the new way required by the new infectious disease.

4. *Enhancing managers' knowledge and support.* Being honest and open about what is happening and why is an essential ethic that encouraged people to feel safe within their changing workplaces. It included ensuring that leaders were visible, and that people had confidence in the decisions being made and in the leader who was making them.

5. *Reducing the risk of moral distress and moral injury.* Understanding potentially morally distressing and injurious experiences and having strategies to prepare for them have been shown to be effective in reducing their impact. The strategy of the NHS appeared to be that the focus for staff needed to be on understanding the complex decisions required of them, but accompanied by their being enabled to take the time and space afterwards to reflect on them. Chapter 39 in this book covers this topic in more detail.

6. *Leadership and teamwork.* The NHS decided that fostering team cohesion was critical. This implied focusing on how teams function in a crisis, ensuring that team members can rely on each other, and noticing whether any members of a

team need help or additional support. The natural leaders for this work might not be the most senior or the usual team leaders, and the principle adopted was enabling the right people to lead in the crisis.

Through the Peak of the First Wave (March to August 2020)

During the 'active' stage of the crisis, the impact on staff varied depending on:

- their roles and proximity to areas with higher levels of infection
- whether they were part of direct care delivery
- their work in a support function
- whether they were at home either working or shielding.

The NHS People team responsible for the work anticipated that a range of reactions, including stress, grief, loss, and complex bereavement, would be normal for the type of events to which staff were exposed. Esther Murray and colleagues provide a commentary on the psychosocial experiences of staff from their perspectives [14]. Anxiety, depression, post-traumatic stress disorder (PTSD), and other serious mental health conditions were predicted to affect a smaller proportion of staff. As a result, an offer of comprehensive support was designed to focus on line managers and team responses as well as local and national support for staff who became distressed or developed other needs for psychosocial care. Alongside this was an offer of assessment and treatment for people who developed serious mental disorders. This accords with the approach outlined in Chapters 27, 28, and 29. Responses to the increased demand for occupational health services and other local support were also planned, with return-to-work strategies enabling short-term redeployment elsewhere and ensuring that staff had time to recover.

A review summarises findings from more than 148 papers regarding the impacts on the mental health of staff who were affected by COVID-19 and their work in the pandemic [15]. Another review summarises the findings from 22 studies from 14 countries published by one journal [16]. Many of these papers report cross-sectional analyses of data collected from convenience samples by self-reported surveys conducted at single time points. Although they provide snapshots of the impacts, and generally show high levels of symptoms of anxiety, depression, and PTSD, they do not allow conclusions to be drawn about diagnosis or causality.

The Psychosocial Impacts of the COVID-19 Pandemic on Healthcare Staff

Mental Health

A national survey of 4,378 NHS clinical and non-clinical staff has demonstrated that groups particularly affected by self-reported symptoms of depression, anxiety, and post-traumatic stress included people identifying as women, people of younger age, and nurses [17]. Staff reporting greater exposure to morally injurious experiences were more likely to report clinically significant symptoms of depression, PTSD, and alcohol use. In addition, other research shows that people who reported histories of problems with their mental health prior to the pandemic were more at risk [17].

Evidence that has been accumulating from major incidents and terror attacks (e.g., the 9/11 terrorist attacks in the USA in 2001, the shootings and bombings in Paris in 2015, the terrorist attacks in London in 2005 and 2017, and the Manchester Arena bombing in 2017) indicates that professional responders may take several years to present with problems to mental health services for assessment and treatment, if at all. Regrettably, this tends to follow a common pattern of prolonged significant deterioration, often associated with increased use of alcohol, breakdown of relationships, and difficulties staying in employment. The impacts of responding to the pandemic are yet to be fully seen, and we know from responses to other large-scale incidents that we are likely to be seeing the real needs of staff unfold over the next 2 to 7 years or more [18,19].

Burnout

Alongside the risk of moral distress and moral injury, one of the chief concerns for healthcare staff has been burnout. Occupational factors that have significant associations with burnout include, in particular, redeployment and working in a role specifically related to COVID-19 patients [20–22]. Concerns about personal protective equipment (PPE) were also a key predictor, whereas reduced ability to rest and recover during breaks has been associated with a clinically significant increase in work-related burnout regardless of job role [20,22]. Other contributory challenges reported by staff included lack of control over changes in work roles, rotas, and locations, poor communication from managers, feeling under-supported, and pressure at work (that may be embedded in the culture) to skip or reduce breaks [20].

Younger age and pre-existing difficulties have been found to be important factors contributing to burnout [22]. Those people who experienced burnout were more likely to have medical conditions associated with higher risk from COVID-19, such as diabetes and chronic obstructive pulmonary disease (COPD), and were almost four times more likely to have had depression previously [22]. With these findings in mind, a number of agencies, Royal Colleges, and professional groups provided advice for healthcare staff and their managers, and we cite one example [23].

Redeployment

Redeployment within healthcare roles is frequently cited in studies of the psychosocial impact of COVID-19 (e.g., [21]). In particular, forced redeployment [24], redeployment to intensive care units (ICUs) [25], and redeployment with training that was perceived as inadequate [25] all contributed negatively. Survey findings from 90 UK surgical trainees redeployed to ICUs showed that, although nearly all participants felt that their experience in the ICU would benefit their future careers, over half also felt that the redeployment had had a negative effect on their mental health [26]. However, a survey of 161 junior doctors found that almost 40% felt that the pandemic had had a negative impact on their careers [27]. In particular they reported that the pandemic had adversely affected their opportunities to complete training requirements, resulting in the need to extend their training.

A number of important challenges associated with redeployment have been highlighted [28]. The changing NHS workforce necessitates delivery of appropriate, timely training, and strategies must be adaptable to manage variable numbers of patients, such as those who need care in an ICU. Clear and consistent communication in a rapidly changing environment can be challenging, particularly when it is exacerbated by wearing PPE. Furthermore, demands outside clinical practice, such as caring responsibilities and the availability of leisure activities, have additional impacts [28].

Staff From Black, Asian, and Minority Ethnic Communities

Ethan Shone has estimated that over 850 members of health and social care staff died with COVID-19 between March and December 2020 [29]. Preliminary analysis of 119 deaths of healthcare workers up to 22 April 2020 found that people from Black, Asian, or minority ethnic communities accounted for 63% of these deaths, despite people from the same backgrounds representing just 21% of NHS staff nationally [30]. Of those who died, 64% of nursing and support staff and 95% of medical staff were from Black, Asian, and minority ethnic backgrounds, compared with 20% and 44%, respectively, of NHS staff in the same occupational groups nationally.

Under pressure to explain the disparity across ethnic groups, Public Health England (now the UK Health Security Agency) examined the impact of COVID-19 on Black, Asian, and minority ethnic groups [31]. The report found that existing social and economic inequalities may in part explain the disproportionate impact on these communities, and include racism, discrimination, and stigma. The impact of the virus replicated, and in some cases worsened, existing health inequalities, such as an increased prevalence of obesity, diabetes, and asthma. Higher occupational risk has been reported, including the likelihood of working in frontline roles, as well as racism and poor experiences of healthcare, leading to people being less likely to seek care when they need it, or less likely to voice concerns (e.g., about inadequate PPE). The answers are likely to be multifactorial, but there is now widespread acknowledgement that healthcare workers from Black, Asian, and minority ethnic groups were at higher risk of COVID-19-related death. As the vaccination programme began in 2021, the priority group consisted of people at highest risk, including a stream dedicated to increasing uptake from communities that were hesitant about receiving the vaccine [32].

Studies have shown that ethnicity is also a significant factor in the mental health impacts of COVID-19, which is again linked with pre-existing mental health inequalities and compounds physical risk [33–36]. Regarding the UK's population, it has been suggested that deterioration in mental health from pre- to mid-pandemic may have involved an interaction between ethnicity and gender, whereby men who identified with minority ethnic groups experienced a greater increase in distress compared with men who identified as white. Men who identified as Bangladeshi, Indian, or Pakistani experienced the greatest deterioration in mental health. Women's mental health deteriorated regardless of ethnic group, and at a similar rate to that in men from minority ethnic groups [37]. At the time of publication of this book, there have been few studies examining the specific impact of COVID-19 on NHS staff from Black, Asian, or other minority ethnic communities. However, preliminary findings from the one research study that has been conducted suggest that NHS clinical staff from these groups report significantly more symptoms of post-traumatic stress than do colleagues who identify as white [17]. Qualitative research has highlighted the emotional burden of structural workplace inequalities, racial injustice, and cultural insensitivity experienced by staff from minority ethnic communities during the pandemic [38].

Intervening to Support and Care for Staff

Help Seeking and Outreach

Reluctance to seek psychosocial care and mental healthcare is common among healthcare providers in general. A survey of GPs and psychiatrists showed that barriers to help seeking included fear of letting colleagues down (73.1%), fear of letting patients down (51.9%), and concerns about confidentiality (53.4%) [39]. Likewise, a rapid review of help seeking by healthcare staff during the pandemic found that healthcare workers reported low interest in seeking professional help; instead, many staff relied more on social support and social contact [40].

An exploration of physicians' attitudes towards burnout has described a ubiquitous but mythical professional culture of 'invincibility' among doctors, whereby staff feel that they are expected to be 'superhuman' [41, p. 10]. Furthermore, the post-disaster literature suggests that staff may take time to come forward for support, if they come forward at all, after having traumatic or distressing experiences while engaging in their professional duties [42]. For example, research conducted with paramedics and ambulance personnel 15 years after the 9/11 terrorist attacks in the USA found that despite 80% of participants being diagnosed with PTSD after the attacks, only 50% had sought support [43]. Reservations reported by participants included fear of being seen as weak, unfit to work, or unable to cope, and not wanting to worry loved ones [43]. Therefore active outreach and engagement with health and social care staff communities is a core part of the service model of the staff mental health and wellbeing hubs that were created in England over a period of 2 years (2021–2023).

Team-Based Support

Few papers published when this chapter was drafted in 2022 address the impact of the pandemic on staff teams, or the effectiveness of team-based interventions. Since then, the research literature has been expanding. However, the early literature suggests that the traditional focus of personal psychological interventions to reduce distress and mental health symptoms may be at odds with the organisational challenges that represent important factors that contribute to staff distress [40]. One study found that frontline NHS staff placed greater emphasis on systemic issues at work, such as understaffing, adequate breaks, access to PPE, and community support, than did staff support guidelines, many of which focused predominantly on avoiding psychiatric impacts [44]. Furthermore, research conducted before the pandemic found that doctors resisted and even resented individual wellbeing-focused interventions in the absence of systemic changes such as addressing organisational pressure and staff shortages [41].

Therefore continuing systemic issues may explain the greater appetite for and uptake of team-based support. NHS England set up a network of staff mental health and wellbeing hubs in direct response to the pandemic, which required a flexible approach that was responsive to the needs of the health and social care system. In response to demand from the NHS, the hubs began to integrate team-based consultation and support into their core service provision. Team-focused work may include consultation with managers, teams of managers, or entire teams, to help to identify support needs and resolve issues and challenges, as well as workshops, training, or bespoke sessions to support staff teams in developing skills and approaches to manage these challenges. The Lancashire and South Cumbria Resilience Hub also provides workplace trauma support using a 'train-the-trainers' approach to cascade training throughout teams about, for example, trauma-informed responses to workplace incidents. Other supportive interventions include facilitated peer support sessions, team resilience, and reflection sessions.

The Staff Mental Health and Wellbeing Hubs

The resilience hub approach is an innovative service model that was originally developed after the Manchester Arena bombing in 2017. It aimed not only to respond to the mental health needs of young people, adults, and emergency response workers affected by the bombing, but also to ensure that expertise in mental health screening and trauma management could be sustained and repurposed for responding to future crises. Therefore, when the pandemic began, the expertise and infrastructure were already available locally in Greater Manchester to provide large-scale support and mental health screening. The Hub was adapted in Greater Manchester to support NHS, social care, and emergency service key workers throughout the COVID-19 pandemic. This model was replicated across England and there were 40 staff mental health and wellbeing hubs, funded by NHS England until funding for most was withdrawn in 2023[45].

The hubs vary at a local level, but their shared purpose was to support the mental health and wellbeing of health and social care staff affected by the COVID-19 pandemic [46]. For example, the Greater Manchester Resilience Hub model predominantly utilises the 'screen-and-refer' approach that was used after the Manchester Arena bombing, in which key workers initially complete online mental health screening measures, before receiving supportive telephone or email follow-up by the Hub's clinicians, in which a referral may be made to other mental health services, such as Improving Access to Psychological Therapy (IAPT) services, for formal psychological interventions if these are deemed clinically necessary. By contrast, at the Lancashire and South Cumbria Psychological Resilience Hub, following screening and assessment, high- or low-intensity psychosocial interventions were typically provided directly by the Hub team, to enable timely access to services for staff who would not otherwise be given priority.

During the initial set-up of the first hubs in 2020, the focus had been largely on the mental health screening and support of individual staff members. However, consistent with the help-seeking literature described in the previous section, in the first hubs to be set up, two things became clear. First, individual uptake of support was considerably lower than anticipated, and second, requests from managers and teams for team-based support were growing.

Challenges for the Future

In this closing part of the chapter, we draw together some of the lessons learned, by 2022, from the COVID-19 pandemic.

Lessons from Science and Recommendations for Science and Future Research

At the time of publication of this book we are clear that the COVID-19 pandemic has had a range of impacts on the mental health of the public and of the staff of health and care services. There have been huge numbers of research studies and very many publications. Yet documenting and quantifying the impacts remains a challenge. In part this reflects the imprecision of terminology and its diffuse employment, but it also reflects the methodologies used thus far, and this results in difficulties in comparing the findings from different studies. A critique of the methods used has been presented by Richard Williams and Kenneth Kaufman [16].

We note that much of the evidence regarding endeavours to quantify the personal mental health impacts of the first 2 years of the COVID-19 pandemic is based on self-report survey data, using standardised mental health questionnaires that are intended to assist clinicians in screening populations of people for the presence of mental health disorders. A selection of these papers has been published thematically; they show high rates of symptoms of depression, anxiety, and post-traumatic stress [16]. However, by the end of 2021, few of the publications reported findings from clinical interviews. This raises two challenges. First, how are we to interpret the meaning of frequencies of symptoms of conditions that lie at the serious end of a potential list of mental health impacts derived from self-reports on questionnaires? Clinical interviews of the same people often yield lower levels of diagnoses. The second challenge is how we construe the conditions suffered by people who report symptoms but who fail to reach the thresholds for presumptive diagnoses.

Two of us (KA and RW) have been involved in researching the mental health impacts of the Manchester Arena bombing in May 2017; similar challenges appear in that work. Therefore we used a combination of qualitative and quantitative methods to study the people affected and the sorts of experiences that our participants reported as describing their distress [47] (see Chapter 28). Often, in other accounts, research participants' distress after emergencies is reported as being short term in nature. However, what struck us forcibly was just how many people continued to be distressed, but remained subthreshold on screening, 2 to 3 years later. We were also struck by the following:

- the ubiquity of distress as described colloquially by people who are affected by emergencies
- the impact of secondary stressors
- the effects of shared social identity on people's recovery
- the importance to survivors of validation of their experiences, and of informal social support provided by their families and by people who had experienced the same event [47,48].

At the time of publication of this book there is insufficient longitudinal evidence to allow direct comparison of the levels of distress, burnout, other psychosocial needs, and mental health disorders among NHS staff before and during the pandemic. We need better descriptions of the breadth of the short-, medium-, and long-term impacts.

Chapter 9 on secondary stressors describes how many members of the public and the staff of healthcare services were working in suboptimal conditions before the pandemic started. We make similar points in this chapter; it is important to note the pre-existing, pre-pandemic levels of burnout, and of sickness due to mental health difficulties, within this workforce. It is also clear that many secondary stressors began before the pandemic and attained more serious implications during it, whereas others arose as a consequence of problems stemming from the response (e.g., problems with PPE) [49].

We call for more research, but with carefully constructed samples that are representative of the population of people at risk, and including interviews with members of the sample. We should prioritise longitudinal studies based on mixed methods and probability sampling. We should also devise better methods for examining distress and the impact of untoward events on people's functioning, both at work and socially.

The pandemic has shown just how important are social relationships at work [15,16,40]. Functional teams are very protective of staff, so we recommend that important topics for research should include the impact of untoward events on teams and the empirical evaluation of team-based interventions.

The Implications of What We Have Learned for Interventions to Support Members of Staff

There is a range of matters about which we need to develop further understanding. We summarise them here.

- Staff retention. More than 900 staff lost their lives through the pandemic. What will this mean for how many staff members elect to stay in the health services?
- It is important that all staff are able to trust the systems in which they work (matters such as lack of adequate PPE, value, safety, and pay have all been revealed to be important by the pandemic).
- We need to determine how we can identify and intervene to help people who manifest longer-term mental health problems including those staff who delay seeking help.
- It is important that managers offer regular health and wellbeing discussions to ascertain the support needs of their staff. Support for mental health and wellbeing should be embedded within organisations, encourage staff to seek support early, and begin to change the culture regarding help seeking among this population.
- All members of staff should be given appropriate opportunities to process their experiences and reduce the natural distress that this work evokes (e.g., restorative supervision [50]). This resonates with the paper by Murray et al. [14].
- We should understand how people are supported outside work by exploring what we can do to ensure that staff have support networks, especially if their families are unavailable.
- We should ensure that staff have regular periods of time off, because they are less likely to want to spend time away from their workplaces during crises.

- We should provide staff with accurate and authoritative information.
- We should ensure that healthcare teams have training and up-to-date information on the mental health consequences of their exposure to emergencies, major incidents, and high-consequence infectious diseases.
- Occupational health teams should develop and test practical ways of looking after staff, enabling them not only to return to work but also, importantly, to remain employed.

Practical Aspects of Implementing the Lessons from Science and Experience

Supporting Teams and Systemic Changes

An important topic is creating approaches through systemic changes to support staff who work together, with a view to them becoming teams rather than groups.

- *We should create integrated approaches to supporting staff in the future.* We should adopt an approach that recognises pre-existing and other secondary stressors as well as those relating to the primary event.
- *We should recognise that resilience lies in teams.* Teams that function well enhance the ability of their members to manage distress arising from work.
- *We should understand the importance of the relationships of staff with their supervisors and managers.* Strong and positive relationships with managers facilitate access of their staff to specific

intervention techniques to assist people in dealing with distress.

- *We should recognise that equipping staff with the skills to engage in safe conversations with colleagues is empowering.* These conversations provide a supportive presence before, during, and after incidents, and enable staff to develop relationships with mental health staff and a supportive culture and infrastructure within workplaces in the build-up phase before events begin [51].
- *Training to prepare employees helps them to cope with the psychosocial impacts of their work.* This includes encouraging supportive relationships in workplaces, and developing listening skills and empathy, but it is important that programmes are based on co-production [52].

Concluding Comments

This survey of the impacts of COVID-19 on healthcare staff in the UK covers briefly what we do and do not know. It is clear that we are reporting at an early stage in terms of knowing the numbers of staff who have developed mental disorders, although the effects on them of working for an extended period of years in circumstances that are unprecedented in the history of the NHS are plain. The stress, strain, and continuing fatigue have been almost palpable.

We are privileged to have learned so much from so many selfless people, and we have tried to distil here a sense of learning points for the future.

References

1. Wahlquist C, Rawlinson K, Campbell L, Gayle D, Perraudin F, Davidson H. Italy Covid-19 death toll rises to 21 as UK confirms 20th case – as it happened. World news, *The Guardian*, 1 July 2020.

2. Sample, I. NHS aims to give 35m flu jabs amid warnings of up to 60,000 deaths. *The Guardian*, 8 October 2021.

3. The Health Foundation, King's Fund, and Nuffield Trust. *The Health Care Workforce in England: Make or Break? Joint Briefing.* King's Fund, 2018 (www .kingsfund.org.uk/sites/default/

files/2018-11/The%20health%20care%20workforce%20in%20England.pdf).

4. Royal College of Nursing. *10 Unsustainable Pressures on the Health and Care System in England.* Royal College of Nursing, 2021.

5. The King's Fund. *The Road to Renewal: Five Priorities for Health and Care.* The King's Fund, 2021 (www.kingsfund.org.uk/publications/covid-19-road-renewal-health-and-care).

6. The King's Fund. *NHS Sickness Absence.* The King's Fund, 2019.

7. Office for National Statistics. *Sickness Absence in the UK Labour Market.* Office for National Statistics, 2018.

8. Sizmur S, Raleigh V. *The Risks to Care Quality and Staff Wellbeing of an NHS System under Pressure.* The King's Fund, 2018.

9. NHS England. *NHS England Publishes Latest NHS Staff Survey Results.* NHS England, 2018.

10. Williams R, Kemp V. Caring for healthcare practitioners. *BJPsych Advances* 2020; 26: 116–28.

11. The King's Fund. *NHS Sickness Absence.* The King's Fund, 2019.

12. Wallbank S. *The Restorative Resilience Model of Supervision: An Organisational Training Manual for Building Resilience to Workplace Stress in Health and Social Care Professionals.* Pavilion Publishing and Media Limited, 2016.

13. Manthorpe J, Iliffe S, Gillen P, Moriarty J, Mallett, J, Schroder H, et al. Clapping for carers in the Covid-19 crisis: carers' reflections in a UK survey. *Health Soc Care Community* 2022; 30: 1442–9.

14. Murray E, Kaufman KR, Williams R. Let us do better: learning lessons for recovery of healthcare professionals during and after COVID-19. *BJPsych Open* 2021; 7: e151.

15. Ntontis E, Luzynska K, Williams R. *The Impact of COVID-19 on the Psychosocial and Mental Health Needs of NHS and Social Care Staff: Final Report on Literature Published Between 2021 and 2022.* The Open University, 2022.

16. Williams R, Kaufman KR. Narrative review of the COVID-19, healthcare and healthcarers thematic series. *BJPsych Open* 2022; 8: e34.

17. Lamb D, Gnanapragasam S, Greenberg N, Bhundia R, Carr E, Hotopf M, et al. Psychosocial impact of the COVID-19 pandemic on 4378 UK healthcare workers and ancillary staff: initial baseline data from a cohort study collected during the first wave of the pandemic. *Occup Environ Med* 2021; 78: 801–8.

18. Lowell A, Suarez-Jimenez B, Helpman L, Zhu X, Durosky A, Hilburn A, et al. 9/11-related PTSD among highly exposed populations: a systematic review 15 years after the attack. *Psychol Med* 2018; 48: 537–53.

19. Chau SWH, Wong OWH, Ramakrishnan R, et al. History for some or lesson for all? A systematic review and meta-analysis on the immediate and

long-term mental health impact of the 2002–2003 Severe Acute Respiratory Syndrome (SARS) outbreak. *BMC Public Health* 2021; 21: 670.

20. Gemine R, Davies GR, Tarrant S, Davies RM, James M, Lewis K. Factors associated with work-related burnout in NHS staff during COVID-19: a cross-sectional mixed methods study. *BMJ Open* 2021; 11: e042591.

21. Denning M, Goh ET, Tan B, Kanneganti A, Almonte M, Scott A, et al. Determinants of burnout and other aspects of psychological well-being in healthcare workers during the Covid-19 pandemic: a multinational cross-sectional study. *PLoS One* 2021; 16: e0238666.

22. Ferry AV, Wereski R, Strachan FE, Mills NL. Predictors of UK healthcare worker burnout during the COVID-19 pandemic. *QJM* 2021; 114: 374–80.

23. Williams R, Murray E, Neal A, Kemp V. *Top Ten Messages for Supporting Healthcare Staff during the COVID-19 Pandemic.* Royal College of Psychiatrists, 2020.

24. Kisely S, Warren N, McMahon L, Dalais C, Henry I, Siskind D. Occurrence, prevention, and management of the psychological effects of emerging virus outbreaks on healthcare workers: rapid review and meta-analysis. *BMJ* 2020; 369: m1642.

25. Khajuria A, Tomaszewski W, Liu Z, Chen J-H, Mehdian R, Fleming S, et al. Workplace factors associated with mental health of healthcare workers during the COVID-19 pandemic: an international cross-sectional study. *BMC Health Serv Res* 2021; 21: 262.

26. Payne A, Rahman R, Bullingham R, Vamadeva S, Alfa-Wali M. Redeployment of surgical trainees to intensive care during the COVID-19 pandemic: evaluation of the impact on training and

wellbeing. *J Surg Educ* 2021; 78: 813–19.

27. Salem J, Hawkins L, Sundaram A, Gates J, Suleman S, Mistry M, et al. COVID-19 and the impact on doctor wellbeing and training. *Physician* 2021; 6: 1–8.

28. Juan NVS, Camilleri M, Jeans JP, Monkhouse A, Chisnall G, Vindrola-Padros C. Training and redeployment of healthcare workers to intensive care units (ICUs) during the COVID-19 pandemic: a systematic review. *BMJ Open* 2022; 12: e050038.

29. Shone E. More than 850 health and social care workers have died of Covid in England and Wales since the pandemic began. *The Scotsman*, 27 January 2021 (www.scotsman.com/health/coronavirus/more-than-850-health-and-social-care-workers-have-died-of-covid-in-england-and-wales-since-the-pandemic-began-3114202).

30. Cook T, Kursumovic E, Lennane S. Exclusive: deaths of NHS staff from covid-19 analysed. *Health Service Journal*, 22 April 2020 (www.hsj.co.uk/exclusive-deaths-of-nhs-staff-from-covid-19-analysed/7027471.article).

31. Public Health England. *Beyond the Data: Understanding the Impact of COVID-19 on BAME Groups.* Public Health England, 2020.

32. Iyengar KP, Vaishya R, Jain VK, Ish P. BAME community hesitancy in the UK for COVID-19 vaccine: suggested solutions. *Postgrad Med J* 2022; 98: e134–5.

33. Bhui K, Stansfeld S, Hull S, Priebe S, Mole F, Feder G. Ethnic variations in pathways to and use of specialist mental health services in the UK: systematic review. *Br J Psychiatry* 2003; 182: 105–16.

34. Barnett P, Mackay E, Matthews H, Gate R, Greenwood H, Ariyo K, et al. Ethnic variations in compulsory detention under the Mental Health Act: a systematic

review and meta-analysis of international data. *Lancet Psychiatry* 2019; 6: 305–17.

35. Grey T, Sewell H, Shapiro G, Ashraf F. Mental health inequalities facing UK minority ethnic populations. *J Psychol Issues Organ Cult* 2013; 3(suppl 1): 146–57.

36. Smith K, Bhui K, Cipriani A. COVID-19, mental health and ethnic minorities. *Evid Based Ment Health* 2020; 23: 89–90.

37. Proto E, Quintana-Domeque C. COVID-19 and mental health deterioration by ethnicity and gender in the UK. *PLoS One* 2021; 16: e0244419.

38. Jesuthasan J, Powell RA, Burmester V, Nicholls, D. 'We weren't checked in on, nobody spoke to us': an exploratory qualitative analysis of two focus groups on the concerns of ethnic minority NHS staff during COVID-19. *BMJ Open* 2021; 11: e053396.

39. Adams EFM, Lee AJ, Pritchard CW, White RJE. What stops us from healing the healers: a survey of help-seeking behaviour, stigmatisation and depression within the medical profession. *Int J Soc Psychiatry* 2010; 56: 359–70.

40. Muller AE, Hafstad EV, Himmels JPW, Smedslund G, Flottorp S, Stensland SØ, et al. The mental health impact of the covid-19 pandemic on healthcare workers, and interventions to help them: a rapid systematic review.

Psychiatry Res 2020; 293: 113441.

41. LaDonna KA, Cowley L, Touchie C, LeBlanc VR, Spilg EG. Wrestling with the invincibility myth: exploring physicians' resistance to wellness and resilience-building interventions. *Acad Med* 2022; 97: 436–43.

42. Bentz L, Vandentorren S, Fabre R, Bride J, Pirard P, Doulet N, et al. Mental health impact among hospital staff in the aftermath of the Nice 2016 terror attack: the ECHOS de Nice study. *BMC Public Health* 2021; 21: 1372.

43. Smith EC, Burkle FM. Paramedic and emergency medical technician reflections on the ongoing impact of the 9/11 terrorist attacks. *Prehosp Disaster Med* 2019; 34: 56–61.

44. Vera San Juan N, Aceituno D, Djellouli N, Sumray K, Regenold N, Syversen A, et al. Mental health and well-being of healthcare workers during the COVID-19 pandemic in the UK: contrasting guidelines with experiences in practice. *BJPsych Open* 2020; 7: e15.

45. NHS England. *NHS Expands Mental Health Support for Staff after Toughest Year in Health Service History*. NHS England, 2021 (www.england.nhs.uk/2021/02/nhs-expands-mental-health-support-for-staff-after-toughest-year-in-health-service-history/).

46. Rimmer A. Staff wellbeing: NHS England expands support with 40 hubs. *BMJ* 2021; 372: n559.

47. Stancombe J. Williams R, Drury J, Collins H, Lagan L, Barrett A, et al. People's experiences of distress and psychosocial care following a terrorist attack: interviews with survivors of the Manchester Arena bombing in 2017. *BJPsych Open* 2022; 8: e41.

48. Drury J, Stancombe J, Williams R, Collins H, Lagan L, Barrett A, et al. Survivors' experiences of informal social support in coping and recovering after the 2017 Manchester Arena bombing. *BJPsych Open* 2022; 8: e124.

49. Williams R, Ntontis E, Alfadhli K, Drury J, Amlôt R. A social model of secondary stressors in relation to disasters, major incidents, and conflict: implications for practice. *Int J Disaster Risk Reduct* 2021; 63: 102436.

50. Wallbank S. Recognising stressors and using restorative supervision to support a healthier maternity workforce: a retrospective, cross-sectional, questionnaire survey. *Evid Based Midwifery* 2013; 11: 4–9

51. Smith E, Walker T, Burkle FM. Lessons in post-disaster self-care from 9/11 paramedics and emergency medical technicians. *Prehosp Disaster Med* 2019; 34: 335–9.

52. Brooks S, Das S. Mental health and psychosocial aspects of COVID-19 in India: the challenges and responses. *J Health Manag* 2020; 22: 197–205.

Chapter

47

Case Study 3: Lessons from Delivering Support for Staff Working at the Nightingale COVID-19 Hospital in London

Derek K Tracy and Neil Greenberg

Introduction

In the spring of 2020, like much of the rest of the world, the UK faced the first wave of the COVID-19 pandemic, with data from earlier-hit countries showing that the existing healthcare system risked becoming completely overwhelmed. In particular, the bed supply in acute hospital and critical care units (CCUs)/intensive care units (ICUs) appeared to be inadequate, with modelling predicting that London alone faced a shortage of 4,000 CCU beds. The governmental response prioritised the Nightingale temporary hospital concept, with seven planned COVID-19 field hospitals. The London Nightingale was the first built and largest of them, and the only one to accept critically ill patients. Built within the ExCeL exhibition centre in East London, it was designed to take up to 4,000 fully intubated patients, necessitating a predicted 16,000 clinical staff, and many more ancillary staff, to run it 24 hours a day. Surrounding hotels were requisitioned as accommodation for staff, and, supported by the military, it was ready to open, at far below maximum capacity, within a matter of weeks. The first wave of the pandemic was a substantial challenge for the healthcare system, but it did not overwhelm existing capacity in the manner that had been feared, and local hospitals were able to absorb most of the demand. Ultimately, the London Nightingale was mothballed after a couple of months or so of operation, treating in total just 55 ventilated Londoners, with clinical outcomes comparable to those of the surrounding NHS trusts.

It was anticipated that the Nightingale would draw its staff from a wide range of London's healthcare workers, initially on a volunteer basis. There were discussions about how it might prove necessary to rota staff in from London hospitals and primary care practices, but this was not required. Nevertheless, the staff had a wide range of professional backgrounds and experience levels, and included some newly qualified doctors and nurses whose final-year graduation had been fast-tracked because of the pandemic. The enormous temporary hospital, which still looked like an exhibition centre, was a novel, alien, and potentially overwhelming environment for staff. COVID-19 was new to everyone, and most staff did not have intensivist training or experience of working with ventilated patients or with patients who had such high mortality rates. The volunteers were enthusiastic and keen, but inevitably faced many stressors at a time when they were also experiencing the same lack of support and resources that was being endured by the rest of the population in the era of lockdown, social distancing, and closure of public recreation facilities.

Given the scale of the task, support for staff wellbeing and mental health was deemed a priority. A bespoke Nightingale mental health team (NMHT) and support plan were created to deliver support in an evidence-based manner. This included drawing on the large body of research on mental health outcomes from other disasters and pandemics, including the experiences of the armed forces. This chapter provides an overview of the support plan, its background and supporting scientific rationale, and the practical experience of its implementation [1]. It utilised core preventative medicine principles – that is, *primary prevention*, which aims to stop the initial onset of any difficulties, *secondary prevention*, which focuses on people with possible emerging mental health disorders, and *tertiary prevention*, which involves managing staff who have developed disorders.

Primary Prevention

There are reliable data to support the view that effective practical and psychological preparation mitigates against frontline healthcare workers developing work stress-based and trauma-based problems [2]. In this regard, the London Nightingale faced particular challenges, including some unknowable aspects of a huge hospital that was still under construction, a viral pandemic that had never been previously encountered, with rapidly evolving national and local guidelines, and a very wide range of staff, most of whom were operating well outside their professional and perhaps also personal comfort zones and experiences. All of the staff would be placed in new teams with unfamiliar colleagues, in a new site, with new managers, and a lack of external resources in a society that was increasingly shutting down. Inevitably, this situation would lead many or most to question their competencies and abilities, and, as a direct consequence, to risk moral injury – a condition in which extreme emotional reactions occur when a person's moral code is strongly challenged. Primary prevention requires frankness and honesty about likely physical and emotional hazards, which is a real challenge when these matters are not necessarily clear.

Despite this, we could nevertheless be upfront with volunteer healthcare workers at the Nightingale about what we did and did not know in this testing venture, and the likely difficulties that we would all face. We included a new joiners' letter at induction that did not sugar-coat the probably traumatic and morally challenging work that staff would undertake. Staff were advised that patients were likely to die despite their best efforts, and were reminded that the difficult environment was going to be novel to almost everyone. They were advised to reflect on their personal suitability for the role and the work, in the light of any personal risks or additional stresses that they might face. The concept of moral injury was openly introduced, and it was noted how volunteers might face clashes with their own moral or ethical code during a pandemic [3]. However, staff were also congratulated on volunteering, advised that most people would not develop mental health problems, and informed that post-traumatic growth was among the more commonly expected sequelae. In addition, they were likely to form new friendships and develop new learning during their time at the Nightingale.

A 'psychological PPE (personal protective equipment)' programme was established that delivered brief non-technical information to enable staff to consider coping strategies for better managing their wellbeing and mental health during their time at the Nightingale. This was also another opportunity to reflect upon their personal suitability for the role. Direct examples were provided, such as concerns about living with someone who was particularly

vulnerable to the effects of infection with SARS-CoV-2, or adverse past experiences of working clinically with very unwell patients. Notably, this was not a form of pre-screening using psychometric testing or evaluation. Research has clearly demonstrated that such an approach is typically inaccurate at predicting people's subsequent performance, and moreover can inadvertently discriminate by inappropriately excluding staff who would be perfectly competent to undertake roles such as those required of our volunteers [4].

What the evidence does show with regard to primary prevention is that staff cohesion is positively associated with good mental health, and that this can be fostered organisationally and developed. Many of the data come from the armed forces and show the importance of both horizontal (colleagues) and vertical (managers/leaders) relationships [5]. Indeed the resilience of an organisation has been shown to rely more on the strength of these social bonds than on the strengths of individual members of staff.

Operationally, staff cohesion took several forms at the London Nightingale. At a horizontal level, a practical initial step was a buddy system that paired members of staff from any professional group, so that they could look out for each other and actively check in on each other's wellbeing across a given shift. At a vertical level, there is good evidence that so-called 'psychologically savvy' supervisors can have a crucial role in supporting the wellbeing of their staff and teams [6]. Work from the armed forces has demonstrated that, even in the most arduous environments, so long as there is the right leadership ethos, team members can avoid developing mental health problems, and indeed function well and thrive. The NMHT worked in a bespoke manner with managers and shift leaders to discuss this, and the qualities, skills, and attributes of good supervisors. These include effective and regular communication, avoiding open criticism of others, looking out for others' safety, and not trying to look good at the expense of the team. Training was provided in active listening, which research data have demonstrated is an effective method of growing supervisors' confidence in talking with their teams about mental health. High-quality research on firefighters in Australia has linked this skill to reduced sickness absence [7]. The Nightingale mental health plan emphasised the importance of post-shift reviews, both for the paired buddies and for shift-supervisor-led discussions. Staff were encouraged to share their experiences (emotional as well as practical/clinical ones) and to look out for colleagues who appeared to be distressed, encouraging them to speak to a peer support worker, as described in the next section.

Secondary Prevention

Even with optimal primary preventative measures, it was clear that some staff would develop work-based mental health problems. They were anticipated to primarily involve depressive and anxiety disorders, adjustment disorders, substance misuse, and post-traumatic stress disorder (PTSD). The UK's National Institute for Health and Care Excellence (NICE) guidance on PTSD recommends, in the first instance, active monitoring of people who have been exposed to traumatic events [8]. This is because, in most cases, early symptoms are likely to resolve and therefore do not require intervention. However, where they do not resolve, appropriate assessment, support, and treatment are necessary.

At the London Nightingale, a small cadre of 'welfare walkers' was engaged with 'walking the floor' to actively watch for any distressed staff, particularly during shift breaks and handovers. They had unique easily identifiable lanyards, about which all staff had been informed on induction, and staff were aware that they could directly approach the welfare walkers at any point. Regular signposted drop-in sessions at coffee-break stations were arranged and advertised. The underpinning principle, following a peer support model [9], was one of supporting the busy managers and shift coordinators, who would be at the disadvantage of lacking established relationships with their teams. The approach involved low-key chats and catch-ups, to encourage engagement. Interventions could range from helping staff to access food and refreshments, or to recharge their mobile phones, to talking through how difficult a person's day might have been. Throughout, the welfare walkers were supported by and had access to the full multidisciplinary NMHT.

There were some initial requests from the Nightingale's (non-mental health) senior managers for us to allocate mental health professionals who would be directly embedded within the CCU wards. Although this appeared to be potentially sensible, it risks introducing a psychological debriefing or post-incident counselling approach, which evidence has shown is at best ineffective, and in fact can actually be harmful [10], For this reason it is discouraged by NICE. This should not be confused with a manager- or leader-led operational review or debriefing, which is a key part of good leadership practice. The difference is that the latter process explores the causes of specific outcomes, and how these can be used to improve performance.

A related potential input, which again perhaps seems sensible but that lacks evidence and should not be instigated, is post-exposure psychological health screening. The well-intentioned principle of this is an attempt to rapidly identify staff with emerging mental health difficulties via questionnaires. The problem is that, even setting aside its snapshot cross-sectional nature, it has been shown that concerns about reputation, confidentiality, and what employers might do with such data limit the honesty and accuracy of replies. Even more egregious are anxieties that employers might feel falsely assured that they are doing something and providing effective support and cover for their staff, when people who are struggling are not being picked up. Consistent with this, data from UK military personnel have confirmed the ineffectiveness of such screening [11].

More broadly, research confirms that most people with mental health problems do not seek or receive help for their difficulties. UK figures show that this might include an astonishing 70% of people with PTSD. Stigma related to mental illness is, sadly, endemic across all walks of life, from the public, through the armed forces, to healthcare professionals [12]. Mindful of this, the NMHT, working with the hospital's communications department, devised a campaign strategy and advertising about mental health and available resources. Staff were reminded to look after themselves and to look out for their colleagues, and were given accurate up-to-date contact details for a range of different local and national resources and supports using emailed newsletters, print and electronic posters and videos, business cards, and white boards. The endeavour was visibly supported by the hospital's senior managers, including the chief operating officer and medical director. A key message was that 'it's OK not to be OK'.

A forward liaison or forward psychiatry model was delivered by the psychiatrists and mental health nurses who comprised the NMHT. This meant that they too would walk the floor with a 'nip-it-in-the-bud' model of engaging with staff and shift managers, rather than waiting to be approached. No booking or referral systems were needed – staff would be seen whenever they asked or dropped in. Good visibility, destigmatising access, and low barriers to being seen rapidly were key. Assessments aimed to find ways to return staff to work, even if this necessitated some change of role, function, or hours – for example, shifting from a bedside position to the role of supporting other staff donning and doffing their PPE.

The principles underpinning this model of returning distressed staff to work are sometimes referred to as **PIES** – Proximity, Immediacy, Expectancy, and Simplicity. Proximity involves keeping staff as close as possible to their original roles, even if with temporarily altered duties, rather than sending them home or signing them off work. Immediacy involves rapid assessment and support to try to prevent unnecessary further deterioration. Expectancy is a philosophically positive outlook that most people should be able to continue to work, and involves reminding staff of the great jobs they had been doing despite the pressures, and reassuring them that all necessary support is available as required. Finally, simplicity of solutions encourages the use of straightforward options, such as recommending a good night's sleep, speaking to a loved one, and so forth. Not only has the PIES model been shown to work in minimising immediate distress and maximising functioning, but the data show that it helps to improve longer-term wellbeing and self-esteem, and the avoidance of labelling oneself as someone who cannot handle pressure [13].

Tertiary Prevention

The nature of the London Nightingale, which was solely a CCU, meant that there were limitations to the type and number of redeployment options for staff who might be struggling. If this was not possible, staff might be deemed unable to continue to work there and potentially be returned to their original clinical team or signed off as unfit to work. The NHMT liaised closely with the onsite occupational health department, which was located in an office next door. There was also the facility to refer staff on for any further intervention or treatment that might be required (e.g., trauma-focused cognitive behavioural therapy for PTSD).

Conclusions

Fortunately, the London Nightingale was never needed at anything close to its operational capacity, and it was closed in 2021. Therefore the effectiveness of its mental health plan was never fully tested, although it operationalised and ran an evidence-based tiered model of care for staff for the full duration.

We believe this plan provides a blueprint that is transferable to other sites, units, and healthcare services outwith large-scale CCUs [14], and which might be modified locally to support the mental health of staff. Healthcare leaders have a particular responsibility to ensure that their workforce is adequately supported and the mental health of their staff is a suitably high priority [15], and the lessons learned should endure after the pandemic [16]. The core principles are to encourage the development of a psychologically savvy workforce and managers, to provide clear accurate advice and guidance, and to adopt a 'nip-it-in-the-bud' approach to support. It is important to avoid medicalising normal distress, to focus on supporting relationships across teams and with managers, and to encourage working where this is possible.

References

1. Tracy DK, Tarn M, Eldridge R, Cooke J, Calder JDF, Greenberg N. What should be done to support the mental health of healthcare staff treating COVID-19 patients? *Br J Psychiatry* 2020; 217: 537–9.

2. Mulligan K, Jones N, Woodhead C, Davies M, Wessely S, Greenberg N. Mental health of UK military personnel while on deployment in Iraq. *Br J Psychiatry* 2010; 197: 405–10.

3. Greenberg N, Docherty M, Gnanapragasam S, Wessely S. Managing mental health challenges faced by healthcare workers during COVID-19 pandemic. *BMJ* 2020; 368: m1211.

4. Opie E, Brooks S, Greenberg N, Rubin GJ. The usefulness of pre-employment and pre-deployment psychological screening for disaster relief workers: a systematic review. *BMC Psychiatry* 2020; 20: 211.

5. Jones N, Campion B, Keeling M, Greenberg N. Cohesion, leadership, mental health stigmatisation and perceived barriers to care in UK military personnel. *J Ment Health* 2018; 27: 10–18.

6. Jones N, Seddon R, Fear NT, McAllister P, Wessely S, Greenberg N. Leadership, cohesion, morale, and the mental health of UK Armed Forces in Afghanistan. *Psychiatry* 2012; 75: 49–59.

7. Milligan-Saville JS, Tan L, Gayed A, Barnes C, Madan I, Dobson M, et al. Workplace mental health training for managers and its effect on sick leave in employees: a cluster randomised controlled trial. *Lancet Psychiatry* 2017; 4: 850–58.

8. National Institute for Health and Care Excellence. *Post-Traumatic Stress Disorder. NICE Guideline [NG116]*. National Institute for Health and Care Excellence, 2018 (www.nice.org.uk/guidance/ng116).

9. Greenberg N, Langston V, Jones N. Trauma risk management (TRiM) in the UK Armed Forces.

J R Army Med Corps 2008; 154: 124–7.

10. Greenberg N, Brooks S, Dunn R. Latest developments in post-traumatic stress disorder: diagnosis and treatment. *Br Med Bull* 2015; 114: 147–55.

11. Rona RJ, Burdett H, Khondoker M, Chesnokov M, Green K, Pernet D, et al. Post-deployment screening for mental disorders and tailored advice about help-seeking in the UK military: a cluster randomised controlled trial. *Lancet* 2017; 389: 1410–23.

12. Woodhead C, Rona RJ, Iversen A, MacManus D, Hotopf M, Dean K, et al. Mental health and health service use among post-national service veterans: results from the 2007 Adult Psychiatric Morbidity Survey of England. *Psychol Med* 2011; 41: 363–72.

13. Solomon Z, Shklar R, Mikulincer M. Frontline treatment of combat stress reaction: a 20-year longitudinal evaluation study. *Am J Psychiatry* 2005; 162: 2309–14.

14. Patel RK, Sweeney MD, Baker CSR, Greenberg N, Piper SE, Shergill SS, et al. If not now, when? Enhancing cardiologists' psychological well-being as a COVID-19 gain. Heart 2021; heartjnl-2020-318852.

15. Greenberg N, Tracy DK. What healthcare leaders need to do to protect the psychological well-being of frontline staff in the COVID-19 pandemic. *BMJ Leader* 2020; 4: 101–2.

16. Greenberg N, Brooks SK, Wessely S, Tracy DK. How might the NHS protect the mental health of health-care workers after the COVID-19 crisis? *Lancet Psychiatry* 2020; 7: 733–4.

Chapter

48

Case Study 4: Delivering Peer Support

Morwenna Maddock, Verity Kemp, and Richard Williams

Introduction

This chapter draws together information about the concept of peer support. We define this as a supportive relationship between people who have experiences in common. We explore some of the background matters relating to its principles, the skills that practitioners require, and matters relating to practice. We also provide advice based on implementing peer support in a critical care unit (CCU). The aim of this chapter is to illustrate a general approach rather than provide a detailed plan.

Peer support is one intervention within a wider comprehensive approach to assisting staff in coping with the stress that arises from their work. This approach is recommended in Chapters 41 and 44. In the healthcare context, peer support describes the work of healthcare staff who provide emotional and social support for colleagues who share a common work experience. Peer support can be provided in both group and one-to-one relationships, and can take place in community groups, clinical settings, and workplaces. Regardless of its setting, peer support is considered to have value, either on its own or as a complement to clinical care.

An important corollary is the necessity for practitioners who offer and receive peer support to recognise the limitations of this approach, and to understand what it is not. For example, it is not a form of counselling or psychotherapy, and, quite properly, there are limitations to the confidentiality that one member of staff should offer another. The specifics of a peer support relationship are unique to each person.

Peer support is rooted in the knowledge that hope is the starting point from which a journey of recovery must begin [1]. Peer supporters can inspire hope and demonstrate the possibility of recovery. They are valued for their authenticity because they are aware of and can relate to the challenges that colleagues face.

Recovery focuses on people regaining quality of life while striving to achieve their full relationship potential [1]. Recovery goes beyond reducing symptoms, and considers each person's wellness from a holistic point of view that includes their relationships, their involvement within the communities of work and family, their general wellbeing, and their sense of empowerment. Peer support focuses on health and recovery rather than on illness and disability.

The Value of Peer Support

If they are to be effective, peer supporters need to be able to relate to the experiences of the people whom they are supporting and have the ability to create relationships that promote empathy and connectedness as well as the possibility of recovery. As we point out here, various authors have identified the power of peer support. Creating a relationship with people with comparable experience can result in the formation of a real bond for a person who is facing particular issues [2,3]. Peer support can be preventative, enabling the moderation of disruptive and distressing life events [4], and it can provide a sense of empowerment [5–7]. Peer support can provide a social setting that enables symptoms and quality of life to improve [8]. The assistance that comes from someone who can see through one's eyes what one is experiencing can help to provide practical and emotional help as part of the process of recovery [9]. In Chapter 28, the SIRE study is reported as identifying that peer support offered by people who have shared experiences provides mutual support and can be a catalyst for social validation, information exchange, and social processes such as local identification [10].

The social connectedness and associated networks that enable support from colleagues are cited as being an important means of mitigating adverse events in the workplace [11]. A project undertaken at Johns Hopkins Hospital, called Resilience in Stressful

Events (RISE), concerns a peer support programme that was designed to assist healthcare professionals who had experienced mildly stressful events [12]. It has been reported that this and similar programmes have the potential to reduce nurse turnover and to underpin consequential budget savings.

In 2017 the Faculty of Pre-Hospital Care of the Royal College of Surgeons of Edinburgh commissioned work to develop guidance on psychosocial and mental health topics that would support the work of pre-hospital care practitioners and first responders. That programme published an introduction to peer support [13]. The emergence of the COVID-19 pandemic punctuated the work of the project but did allow components of the psychosocial care that was being considered to be evaluated, and this brought peer support to the fore. Training for peer supporters proceeded with an online programme. Later in this chapter we describe an example of peer support in practice from a critical care unit that was one of the pioneers in the online training.

In a literature review of peer support and how it facilitated post-traumatic growth in first responders, the findings were that the type of support a first responder receives after an incident can influence their response [14]. The review notes that different organisations use different types of peer-led support, which range from more universally recognised systems, such as the Critical Incident Stress Management (CISM) programme, to local stand-alone systems. The review focused on discovering and describing the benefits of these programmes in facilitating post-traumatic growth (PTG) among participants. PTG has been defined in various ways, one example being a 'coping process of positive reinterpretation, positive reframing, interpretive control, or reconstrual of events' [15]. In describing peer support, the review draws a distinction between the more informal support given by friends, and the more formal crisis interventions, such as CISM and stand-alone peer support. Stand-alone peer support has a broader focus. It can encompass workplace and personal issues, be available at any time, and people who are trained as peer supporters have training in mental health matters, including being able to access more formal mental health interventions, and receive supervision. Peer support, unlike professional mental health interventions, creates no difference in status between the people who participate.

Table 48.1 lists five themes that Nicola Donovan identified as resulting from peer support interfaces.

Table 48.1 Five main themes emerging from studies relating to interactions between peer support and first responders that support growth (Donovan N. Peer support facilitates post-traumatic growth in first responders: a literature review. *Trauma* 2022; 14604086221079441 [14]. Reproduced with the permission of Sage under Creative Commons Licence CCBY.)

1. Peer support assists with processing of traumatic events

2. Peers provide support with organisational stressors

3. Social support increases the use of coping strategies

4. Active engagement with peers encourages growth

5. Relational safety encourages disclosure

The Guiding Values and Principles for Peer Supporters

The most effective peer support schemes aim to ensure that the people who are recruited to the role are able to demonstrate a range of competencies considered to be important. We have described the necessity for peer supporters to have similar working backgrounds and current work experiences in common with their peers who request support. These similarities enable connection and understanding.

Building on this, peer supporters should be able to think critically, to connect with the issues that are presented, and to fit their responses to the needs of the people who consult them. This may include signposting people to outside help, if appropriate. Peer supporters should therefore be able to sift and scrutinise what they hear. At the heart of peer support is the requirement to practise effective and appropriate communication skills. This includes working in the context of a team, being able to build trust, and being able to end peer support relationships well. All encounters between supporters and people who are supported should be informed by an ethical approach with regard, for example, to information sharing.

Good working models of peer support are able to demonstrate other essential values, including the ability to create environments that offer physical and emotional safety, and supervision. Systems that are set up to deliver peer support should ensure that colleagues who are seeking this have choice, and that they are able to exercise control over how they engage in the process. These features emphasise human connection and freedom to be oneself.

Providing support for peer supporters requires clear definitions of what the process provides and, crucially, of what it does not provide. The support offered to peer supporters should also be capable of offering advice about methods that are appropriate for handling difficult situations.

Peer support can come in many guises. It may be offered in the context of a formal system established within an organisation or part of an organisation. The more formal schemes are usually characterised by creating a pool of people who are prepared to make themselves available for this work. They should have undergone (and continue to undergo) training, and receive supervision.

Formal peer support programmes aim to ensure that there is not a power imbalance in the relationship between the peer supporter and the peer. The approach should be based on equality and self-determination within the relationship.

Engaging managers is a crucial element in establishing a peer support service, which ideally should be one part of, and integral to, a strategy for delivering the wellbeing and psychosocial agendas for the organisation or service described in Chapters 28 and 44, by building on skills and services that are already available. A peer support programme developed within such a strategic approach has the aim of sustaining staff who are thriving, and responding to the needs of staff who are struggling. Later, in Chapter 50, we see team leaders being encouraged to ask teams to engage in peer support as one means of dealing with complex situations and stressful experiences.

As we have seen in earlier chapters, particularly Chapters 12, 27, and 28, the Stevenson/Farmer review proposes a stepped approach that employers can use to help employees to thrive [16]. It suggests that there are three groups of employees – those who are thriving, those who are struggling and may require targeted support, and those who are possibly ill and may require targeted assessment and treatment.

A key role for leaders in enabling peer support to occur is developing a governance structure for their departments' peer support programmes. Research has shown that successful peer support programmes have well-developed governance structures. Important components of a successful governance structure include creating clear statements about what the programme is intended to achieve, what outcomes are expected, and what features and approaches characterise those outcomes. One of the key roles for senior managers, including those at Board level, is to support programmes of this nature in the context of the wider strategy for wellbeing and psychosocial care. It is not

the role of managers to participate themselves as peer supporters, as their presence might lead to misunderstanding and discomfort among those people who are seeking peer support.

Training Peer Supporters

Training for peer supporters is essential, as is the requirement for peer supporters to be able to practise their methods in a safe manner. The objective of training for peer supporters is to harness their life skills and enhance their professional experiences by contributing to their learning and developing skills. We propose that the key themes that need to be addressed in training are an understanding of:

- what peer support is
- why peer support is needed
- the principles of psychosocial care and peer support, including those relating to values and ethics
- the background knowledge
- the competencies required by peer supporters
- the principles of practice and its governance, and having opportunities to practise methods and techniques.

The Skills of Peer Supporters

There is a range of skills for peer supporters, which include their ability to demonstrate the relevant competencies that are outlined in this chapter. In addition, peer supporters should be able to encourage their peers to co-create solutions to problems, and show clarity about the importance of boundaries to confidentiality. They must be willing to participate in continuing professional development and personal development.

It is important that organisers of peer support schemes focus on maintaining the wellbeing of peer supporters, and that they support peer supporters in maintaining high ethical standards.

Peer Support in Practice

We offer observations and thoughts from a senior nurse about the experience of introducing and implementing a peer support programme in the CCU at a hospital in south-west England.

The Critical Care Unit (CCU)

A great deal of groundwork surrounding staff wellbeing had been laid at the CCU prior to introducing peer support. A spectrum of support had already been put in place, from staff simply offloading to one another over coffee and cake in a wellbeing café, to more formal Trauma Risk Management (TRiM) assessments that occurred after one-off traumatic events. We had the support of our managers and, crucially, their trust to develop and implement a peer support programme from the bottom up, rather than it being imposed as a 'good idea' from the top down.

It became apparent during the planning phase in response to COVID-19 that what we were witnessing in February 2020 across Europe, and subsequently in the UK, was going to be traumatic for healthcare staff. However, unlike any other traumatic event, we could see that this was going to continue for a prolonged period and with an unknown end point. It begged the question of how we were going to support staff immediately.

We were fortunate to gain an introduction to peer support in the spring of 2020, and a subsequent invitation to be a pilot site for the training programme seemed too good to be true. Much of the wellbeing work that had been carried out in the CCU in the preceding 4 years had focused on staff resolving issues as a team, using a bottom-up approach, empowering individual people to help themselves and their colleagues. The concept of peer support felt familiar.

Lessons Learned

We learned from initially setting up the programme that it was crucial to ensure that the staff who were being trained were able to demonstrate the competencies required of a peer supporter. Members of the nursing and allied health professional (AHP) teams were asked to submit a statement of interest, allowing us to select the people we felt would best fit the criteria for a peer supporter as described in this chapter.

Following on from training, careful thought and consideration were given to providing peer support and the governance supporting it. How would it be accessed? When and where would support sessions take place? Would records be kept? What was the process of disclosure? When would one refer on? Who was responsible for the supervision of the peer supporters? Together the wellbeing lead and the unit psychologist wrote a standard operating procedure (SOP) that addressed these questions and would serve as a guide for staff involved in delivering peer support.

A key part of the peer support programme has been to ensure that those staff who act as peer supporters have access to professional supervision.

Overall, we learned that establishing peer support as a wellbeing strategy is not a quick process, especially during a pandemic. On reflection, the groundwork that was carried out in the CCU stood us in good stead, and the team members were already open to the idea of supporting one another. Without this buy-in, we are confident that other units are likely to struggle to get a project such as this off the ground.

Peer support does not replace previously established support systems for staff, but acts as another rung on the ladder. However, we also know that having a wellbeing strategy in place, including peer support, has improved our staff turnover and retention.

Time (or more specifically the lack of it) was and remains the greatest obstacle. During the early waves of the pandemic, the CCU was working at high intensity, with little or no prospect of reprieve, which made it incredibly challenging to meet the needs of the team.

We had been told on numerous occasions that, as a profession, nurses are notoriously bad at self-care. Perhaps that is because it is in our nature and that of our role to put the needs of others first. However, we believe that the challenges of the initial waves of the pandemic led to a shift in attitude. We feel that we are more in tune with our own mental health, and no longer reluctant or fearful to ask for help. There has been a steady stream of nurses accessing peer support, the feedback is incredibly positive, and they are not afraid to tell colleagues how beneficial they find it.

The true test of peer support came shortly after it was implemented, with the tragic and untimely death of a colleague. Instinct suggested that external support was required, yet very few members of the team accessed it. Instead they turned to each other for support, to someone who understood what they were experiencing, without the need for explanation. This was truly peer support in practice.

Conclusion

Peer support is a proven method of helping both staff who are thriving and staff who are struggling. It gives staff another means of managing their own wellbeing and responding to colleagues who are struggling. A crucial element of peer support is that staff share their experiences with a person who understands their working environment. It also provides a way of ensuring that staff do not have to risk becoming isolated. Peer supporters should have an intrinsic understanding because of their lived experience. Peer support also has the flexibility to provide support either after a one-off stressful event or following a day-to-day accumulation of events.

Research also shows that peer support in the context of a wider wellbeing strategy has the power to improve the experience of staff at work, as well as reducing absenteeism and staff turnover [1,2,6,8,9,14].

The best schemes are characterised by having been developed using a bottom-up approach. There is management support, but peer support has not been imposed on any service or department.

References

1. Sunderland K, Mishkin W. *Peer Leadership Group, Mental Health Commission of Canada Guidelines for the Practice and Training of Peer Support*. Mental Health Commission of Canada, 2013.

2. Creamer M, Varker T, Bisson J, Darte K, Greenberg N, Lau W, et al. Guidelines for peer support in high-risk organizations: an international consensus study using the Delphi method. *J Trauma Stress* 2012; 25: 134–41.

3. Varker T, Creamer M. *Development of Guidelines on Peer Support Using the Delphi Methodology*. Australian Centre for Posttraumatic Mental Health, University of Melbourne, 2011.

4. Figley CR, Nash WP. Introduction: for those who bear the battle. In *Combat Stress Injury: Theory, Research, and Management* (eds CR Figley, WP Nash): 1–10. Routledge, 2007.

5. Corrigan PW. Impact of consumer-operated services on empowerment and recovery of people with psychiatric disabilities. *Psychiatr Serv* 2006; 57: 1493–6.

6. Dumont JM, Jones K. Findings from a consumer/survivor defined alternative to psychiatric hospitalization. *Outlook* 2002: spring issue: 4–6.

7. Resnick SG, Rosenheck RA. Integrating peer-provided services: a quasi-experimental study of recovery orientation, confidence, and empowerment. *Psychiatr Serv* 2008; 59: 1307–14.

8. Ochocka J, Nelson G, Janzen R, Trainor J. A longitudinal study of mental health consumer/survivor initiatives: Part III – a qualitative study of impacts on new members. *J Community Psychol* 2006; 34: 273–83.

9. Watkins J. The value of peer support groups following terrorism: reflections following the September 11 and Paris attacks. *Aust J Emerg Manag* 2017; 32: 35–9.

10. Stancombe J, Williams R, Drury J, Collins H, Lagan L, Barrett A, et al. People's experiences of distress and psychosocial care following a terrorist attack: interviews with survivors of the Manchester Arena bombing in 2017. *BJPsych Open* 2022; 8: e41.

11. McDonald G, Jackson D, Vickers MH, Wilkes L. Surviving workplace adversity: a qualitative study of nurses and midwives and their strategies to increase personal resilience. *J Nurs Manag* 2016; 24: 123–31.

12. Edrees H, Connors C, Paine L, Norvell M, Taylor H, Wu A. Implementing the RISE second victim support programme at the Johns Hopkins Hospital: a case study. *BMJ Open* 2016; 6: e011708.

13. Williams R, Kemp V, Stokes S, Lockey D. *Peer Support: An Introductory or Briefing Document*. Faculty of Pre-Hospital Care, The Royal College of Surgeons of Edinburgh, 2020 (https://fphc.rcsed.ac.uk/media/2841/peer-support.pdf).

14. Donovan N. Peer support facilitates post-traumatic growth in first responders: a literature review. *Trauma* 2022; 24: 1–9.

15. Tedeschi RG, Calhoun LG. The Posttraumatic Growth Inventory: measuring the positive legacy of trauma. *J Trauma Stress* 1996; 9: 455–71.

16. Stevenson D, Farmer P. *Thriving at Work: The Stevenson/Farmer Review of Mental Health and Employers*. Department for Work and Pensions and Department of Health and Social Care, 2017.

Chapter

49

Preparing Effectively for Emergencies, Incidents, Disasters, and Disease Outbreaks

David E Alexander, Tim Healing, Verity Kemp, and Richard Williams

Introduction

This chapter considers the 'architecture' – the components and organisation – of civil protection. It endeavours to answer the question 'What is needed in order to keep us safe?' These are important issues as the world is going through a period of intense change and instability. Considerable improvements are required in the way we view, understand, and respond to major emergencies. Chapter 50 develops several of the themes in this chapter, particularly the role of leaders in responses to emergencies, incidents, terrorist events, disasters, disease outbreaks and conflicts (EITDDC).

The first part of the chapter includes key definitions of terms. Then we define civil protection as a discipline, a service, and a form of organisation of emergency responses to EITDDC and resources, and ask what is needed in order to create and maintain a civil protection system that is capable of an effective response to impacts and contingencies. The third part of this chapter provides a critical review of the basis of emergency planning, an indispensable part of crisis response. In the fourth part we look at various aspects of emergency preparedness.

Good, robust, and detailed emergency planning usually involves developing likely future scenarios based on 'reference events', usually past EITDDC [1,2]. Problems are likely to arise if future EITDDC differ from those of the documented past, and, in the fifth part, we ask the key question about whether the past really is still an adequate guide to the future. If it is not, then ingenuity is required in order to exercise the required degree of foresight in emergency planning. Following on from this debate, the sixth part looks at the growing field of risk and disaster science and why this is needed in order to endow emergency planning and management with an adequate profile, and give it legitimacy as a discipline of synthesis and a set of rigorous techniques for promoting human safety.

As in other countries, so in the UK, the response to the COVID-19 pandemic was and remains the greatest test of the world's emergency management for the past 75 years [3, p. 432]. Failure and inefficiencies in this response underline the need for disaster science.

The key concluding message of this chapter is that, given the changing landscape of hazards and threats, civil protection needs to be at least an order of magnitude more potent in the future.

Some Important Definitions

Emergency Preparedness

In England, emergency preparedness concerns the extent to which emergency planning enables the effective and efficient prevention, reduction, control, and mitigation of risks, and responses to incidents and emergencies. The United Nations Office for Disaster Risk Reduction (UNDRR) defines emergency preparedness as 'the knowledge and capacities developed by governments, response and recovery organisationss, communities and individuals to effectively anticipate, respond to and recover from the impacts of likely, imminent or current disasters'[4]. In annotations to its definition, UNDRR notes that 'Preparedness action is carried out within the context of disaster risk management and aims to build the capacities needed to efficiently manage all types of emergencies and achieve orderly transitions from response to sustained recovery'. It also notes that:

> Preparedness is based on a sound analysis of disaster risks and good linkages with early warning systems, and includes such activities as contingency planning, the stockpiling of equipment and supplies, the development of arrangements for coordination, evacuation and public information, and associated training and field exercises. These must be supported by formal institutional, legal and budgetary capacities. The related term 'readiness' describes the ability to quickly and appropriately respond when required.

The UNDRR online glossary [5] also defines a preparedness plan as 'a plan that establishes arrangements in advance to enable timely, effective and appropriate responses to specific potential hazardous events or emerging disaster situations that might threaten society or the environment'.

Emergencies

Emergencies are the point at which damage, destruction, casualties, losses of goods and money, and interruptions of human activities occur. The term emergency is also difficult to define [6]. The UNDRR online glossary [5] notes that it is 'sometimes used interchangeably with the term disaster, as, for example, in the context of biological and technological hazards or health emergencies, which, however, can also relate to hazardous events that do not result in the serious disruption of the functioning of a community or society'.

Responses

In the UK, responses are decisions and actions taken in accordance with the strategic, tactical, and operational objectives defined by emergency responders, including those associated with recovery. In the UNDRR online glossary, responses are defined as 'Actions taken directly before, during or immediately after a disaster in order to save lives, reduce health impacts, ensure public safety and meet the basic subsistence needs of the people affected' [5].

Crises

A crisis is a fast-evolving situation with a high level of uncertainty and a high likelihood of negative effects. It may imply an emergency, but it does not necessarily become a disaster [7].

Incidents

With regard to healthcare services in the UK, the various types of incident are defined as follows.

Business Continuity Incident

This is an event or occurrence that disrupts, or might disrupt, an organisation's normal service delivery to below acceptable pre-defined levels. This would require special arrangements to be put in place until services can return to an acceptable level. Examples include a surge in demand requiring temporary re-deployment of resources within the organisation, breakdown of utilities, significant equipment failure, or hospital-acquired infections. There may also be impacts from wider issues, such as supply chain disruption or provider failure.

Critical Incident

This is any localised incident in which the level of disruption results in an organisation temporarily or permanently losing its ability to deliver critical services, or where patients and staff may be at risk of harm. It could also be due to the environment potentially being unsafe, requiring special measures and support from other agencies to restore normal operating functions. A critical incident is principally an internal escalation response to increased system pressures/disruption to services.

Major Incidents

In the UK, the Joint Emergency Services Interoperability Programme (JESIP) defines a major incident as 'An event or situation with a range of serious consequences that require special arrangements to be implemented by one or more emergency responders'. It adds that 'The severity of the consequences associated with a major incident are likely to constrain or complicate the ability of responders to resource and manage the incident, although a major incident is unlikely to affect all responders equally. The decision to declare a major incident will always be a judgement'.

Disasters

Several of the definitions given earlier include the term disaster, which the UNDRR defines as 'A serious disruption of the functioning of a community or a society at any scale due to hazardous events interacting with conditions of exposure, vulnerability and capacity, leading to one or more of the following: human, material, economic and environmental losses and impacts' [5]. In annotations to this definition the UNDRR notes that 'The effects of the disaster can be immediate and localized but are often widespread and could last for a long period of time. The effects may test or exceed the capacity of a community or society to cope using its own resources, and therefore may require assistance from external sources, which could include neighbouring jurisdictions, or those at the national or international levels'.

Table 49.1 Classification of hazards (Adapted from IFRC [8,9])

Natural hazards		Human-made/technological hazards
Naturally occurring physical phenomena		Events caused by humans that occur in or close to human settlements
· **Geophysical:**	Earthquakes, landslides, and volcanic activity	• Industrial accidents • Transport accidents • Environmental degradation and pollution
· **Hydrological:**	Floods and avalanches	
· **Climatological:**	Droughts and wildfires	Non-technological and human-made
· **Meteorological:**	Cyclones and storms	• Wildfires
· **Biological:**	Caused by exposure to living organisms and their toxic substances or diseases; they may carry disease epidemics/animal plagues	Armed conflicts and other situations of social instability or tension that are subject to international humanitarian law and national legislation: • Complex emergencies • Conflicts • Terrorism

Disasters can be precipitated by natural, human-made, and technological hazards, as well as by factors that influence the exposure and vulnerability of a community [8]. Hazards, and the types of disaster that they cause, are sometimes divided into natural hazards (i.e., those incidents caused by environmental events) and human-made hazards (i.e., those incidents caused by the failure of a human structure or activity), but these definitions overlap because any disaster implies human involvement (see Table 49.1) [9].

Every year, approximately 400 disasters resulting from natural hazards are reported worldwide [10]. Added to these are 40–50 armed conflicts, and numerous disasters resulting directly from human activities [11].

As readers can see, emergencies, incidents, crises, and disasters represent a definitional minefield despite attempts to standardise these definitions, but whatever these events are called, they require a form of response that differs from routine approaches [12,13]. This puts responders into unfamiliar situations, and may require organisations to work together that do not normally do so, or at least not in the mode required to bring an emergency under control. This is a theme that is developed in Chapter 50.

There are thresholds in particular impacts, and organisational and operational effects, and the gravity of social and political issues. Any of these can turn a dynamic situation into an emergency, but it is not easy to establish rules for specific levels at which a normal exigency becomes an emergency. Many emergencies are unexpected events, but are not necessarily so if hazard and threat monitoring and warning systems are well developed. Most emergencies are likely to require people to use local resources to reduce their effect on human welfare. Some are likely to require a much broader intake of resources.

It is evident that these terms overlap because they are based on different criteria. Thus in the UK some emergencies are major incidents. All major incidents and disasters are emergencies, but not all emergencies are large enough or sufficiently serious to be termed a disaster. Table 49.2 endeavours to quantify the distinction between incidents, major incidents, disasters, and catastrophes in semantic terms with reference to processes and the effects of different sizes of event, but it is by no means an infallible guide.

Complex Emergencies

The type of disaster that generally has the greatest impact is the complex emergency. This is defined by the Inter-Agency Standing Committee (IASC) (a forum of UN and non-UN humanitarian partners founded to strengthen humanitarian assistance) as 'A humanitarian crisis in a country, region or society where there is total or considerable breakdown of authority resulting from internal or external conflict and which requires an international response that

Table 49.2 Differentiation of size of event by process and impact (Reproduced by permission of Dunedin Academic Press, Edinburgh. Source: Alexander, 2016 [14 p. 15].)

Partly after Tierney [see 14]	Incidents	Major incidents	Disasters	Catastrophes
Impact	Very localised	Generally localised	Widespread and severe	Extremely large
Response	Local efforts	Some mutual assistance	Inter-governmental response	Major international response
Plans and procedures	Standard operating procedures	Emergency plans activated	Emergency plans fully activated	Plans potentially overwhelmed
Resources	Local resources	Some outside assistance	Inter-regional transfer of resources	Local resources overwhelmed
Public involvement	Very little involvement	Mainly not involved	Public very involved	Extensively involved
Recovery	Very few challenges	Few challenges	Major challenges	Massive challenges

goes beyond the mandate or capacity of any single agency and/or the ongoing United Nations country program' [15].

At the time of publication of this book, a major complex emergency is in progress in the Ukraine, caused by the Russo-Ukrainian War. This involves all the features of a true complex emergency, being characterised by:

- extensive violence, injury, and loss of life
- widespread damage to societies and economies
- massive population displacement
- mass food shortages and risk of famine
- the need for large-scale humanitarian assistance of many types
- political and military activities hindering or preventing the humanitarian assistance programme
- significant security risks for aid workers.

Civil Protection

Civil protection is the care and defence of the civilian population against a wide range of threats, hazards, and civil contingencies [16]. They include so-called white emergencies, unthreatening events that require at least some of the same techniques to manage them and ensure the safety of large numbers of people as are required during disasters. The funeral of Her Majesty Queen Elizabeth II in September 2022 is an example of a white emergency, because attendees at her Lying-in-State and lining the route of her funeral

processions required a major operation to be mounted to ensure security and the safety of the crowds. Other forms of emergency vary widely in duration and geographical scope. Most are localised (e.g., transportation crashes, structural collapses, landslides, minor flooding), but some are of a far larger scale, extending from the regional dimensions of major storms and floods and some complex emergencies to the global reach of pandemics. Regardless of the area covered by the event, in all disasters and major incidents, local areas are the theatres of operations. This emphasises the importance of both national and local organisation and preparedness, coordination at regional levels, and harmonisation at the national level to ensure that local responses follow nationally established operating procedures.

Civil defence is, *sensu stricto*, the protection of a non-combatant population against armed aggression, including warfare, insurrection, and terrorism [16]. It now includes cyber-attacks, whether of the presence-based or event-based kind, and other online influences designed to destabilise society in the target country [17]. Civil defence is essentially a national concern with a top-down structure. As it depends upon gathering and interpreting military and civilian intelligence, much of it involves actions that are not devolved to the public, but are in the domain of national secrets that are governed by laws on reserved information.

Despite these distinctions, many countries use the terms civil protection and civil defence loosely or interchangeably and may not have separate systems for each. Nevertheless, they are two different sets of processes. In the broadest terms, civil defence is concerned with threats and security, and civil protection is concerned with hazards and safety. This part of this chapter concentrates largely on civil protection, with some references to civil defence. Paradoxically, despite the emphasis on local organisation, the global reach, persistence, and dynamism of a pandemic such as COVID-19 underlines the need for an integral and integrated civil protection system [18,19].

What Constitutes a Good Civil Protection System?

In response to the question 'What is civil protection?', the simplest answer is that we all are part of it. The challenge of the twenty-first century is to encourage people to assume greater responsibility for the risks that they run, whether deliberately, inadvertently, or unavoidably. Major risks are now too great and too many to be managed only by specialists and government. What is required is participatory democracy. The guarantee and exercise of human rights, which must be codified, enshrined in law, and respected, are central to this endeavour. They ensure that people can access information in order to make decisions about risks and have the liberty to act in favour of risk management and reduction. The right to knowledge and education is fundamental because these matters are vital resources for creating a culture of prudence and readiness [20].

A good civil protection system must have local, regional, and national components. Each country needs legislation that defines the system and specifies how it is expected to function. For example, the USA has the Robert T. Stafford Disaster Relief and Assistance Act 1988 (as amended) at the federal level, India has the All-India Disaster Management Act 2005, and the UK has the Civil Contingencies Act 2004 (as amended). In this type of legislation, organs of government are created to make national decisions and give support and resources to efforts on the ground to prepare for, respond to, and, at least in the early stages, recover from disasters. The legislation predisposes the system to responses to EITDDC at lower levels of government and in the regions and municipalities of the country [21].

A fully functional system should have several essential characteristics [2]. It should:

- maintain a strong presence at local level, particularly in places subject to frequent or potentially serious hazard impacts
- emphasise planning and preparedness to ensure that resources are used effectively during an emergency
- incorporate organised voluntarism
- ensure that planning for business continuity, managing hazardous materials, and plans for critical facilities (e.g., hospitals, airports, major infrastructure) are compatible and mutually reinforcing
- emphasise local autonomy and coordination managed by the intermediate, or regional, tiers of government.

The role of national government is to create and maintain the system, harmonise arrangements at lower levels of public administration, and ensure that the system is equitable and adequately resourced. The role of all higher levels of government should be to support, not supplant, local efforts, and to augment them if local resources are overwhelmed [22].

There is usually tension between centralisation and devolution of powers in creating a system of readiness for major emergencies. Local autonomy is vital. Local authorities know indigenous conditions and respond more directly to the local population than do more remote powers. The degree of control that central government would like to exercise over the system varies with the prevailing political culture. Generally, highly centralised forms of civil protection work badly because they deprive local forces of autonomy and the ability to take the initiative [16].

An interesting question concerns what should be the role of military forces. In emergencies in well-organised, rich or relatively rich countries, they are domestic forces. In internationally declared disasters in low-income countries, or those with unstable governments, they may be foreign forces, which may operate under the banner of the UN. In both cases it is important to separate the military and humanitarian roles of armed forces. There are two key UN documents governing the use of military assets in disaster relief. The MCDA Guidelines cover the use of military and civil defence assets to support UN humanitarian activities in complex emergencies [23], and the Oslo Guidelines cover the use of foreign military and civil defence assets in disaster relief [24]. The latter specify that military forces should be under civilian command when so used. NATO has guidelines for this type of activity [25], and many nations have their own doctrines (e.g., the UK [26]). In recent years, foreign military units have been deployed to public health emergencies with an emphasis on their role in public health or healthcare rather than on broadly humanitarian activities (e.g., the Ebola outbreak in West Africa; see Chapters 17 and 18). In some countries, there are concerns that existing guidelines governing deploying forces for humanitarian purposes are inadequate or inappropriate for the health role [27]. Military forces have autonomy, skills, and equipment, but often lack detailed knowledge of local conditions, nor may they have long continuity of operations in disaster areas [28]. However, this may not apply to UN units that may have been in an area for years.

Economists sometimes regard disasters as a form of accelerated consumption of goods and services [29]. There is a risk of major emergencies turning into a form of barter market. Central government must necessarily ration scarce emergency resources. Local government will argue for more support. Regional governments will exercise both functions. Thus the success of emergency operations depends rather critically on the ability to make good, rational decisions about how available resources are deployed, used, and consumed.

Emergency Planning

The main purpose of emergency planning is to anticipate needs arising during a crisis and devise how to satisfy them. This appears to be codified common sense, but in fact is a complex and delicate process requiring considerable expertise so that vital needs are not overlooked [30].

An emergency plan should match urgent needs with available resources, and must be realistic and concrete. Each task should be assigned to emergency responders and coordinators, and all participants in the emergency response must have a role. The plan must cover situational awareness, and constructing, maintaining, and sharing the common operating picture [31]. It should ensure interoperability between services and organisations, including ensuring that they can communicate with a common language and interchangeable technology. They should share information and tasks, have conflict resolution procedures, and follow the same operational rules. An example is the need, when confronted by a serious impact, to declare a major incident or emergency

across all responding agencies so that they move into emergency mode simultaneously and rapidly [14].

In structural terms, emergency planning is akin to urban and regional planning. Both have a strong basis of geographical science and should be connected endeavours [32]. The connections relate particularly to control of land use in order to reduce the effect of hazards and maintain lifelines that enable relief to be brought to where it is needed, or people to be evacuated to safety and medical care.

Standards for Emergency Planning and Preparedness

Standards, or at least common procedures and benchmarks, are required in order to make plans compatible, to ensure that all relevant contingencies are covered, and to guarantee quality in the planning process [33]. Plans can be evaluated according to a number of criteria, including the following:

- Structure: does the plan have a clear, complete, and consistent structure?
- Functionality: are its provisions realistic and workable?
- Compatibility: is it compatible with legislation, other plans, including those of neighbouring jurisdictions, higher public administration levels, and critical installations such as hospitals and airports and the procedures that it governs?
- Dissemination: is it known to all participants and accepted by them?
- Maintenance: does the plan include provisions for updating and exercising it regularly?

It is important that emergency planning is taken seriously by all civil authorities. It should be a proper profession with stability of employment and career progression, and it should be well placed in the structure of public administration. Ideally at its head, it is a centralised dependency – for example, the UK's Civil Contingencies Secretariat in the Cabinet Office. As emergency preparedness and responses require the participation of many different competencies, it is not necessarily a good idea to make emergency planning a department of a single ministry, often a Home Office or Ministry of the Interior. Instead it needs to be able to reconcile the contributions of a wide variety of government departments or ministries [21].

A third question is whether the emergency planners should be the crisis managers. Against this is that there may be an agency (e.g., the police or fire service) that is accustomed to taking the lead in emergencies, and with accumulated expertise to do so. However, emergency planners could be expected to be natural emergency managers, as they would put their plans into action. Modern emergency management does not necessarily require much command authority. It is about coordinating resources and task forces while providing them with a constantly updated common operating picture in order to promote situational awareness. The planners are likely to be most familiar with the provisions of their plans, the environment in which the planning takes place, including legislation, public administration, social and economic factors, and the nature of available local resources. Combining planning and management is facilitated where there are dedicated emergency operations centres (see Chapter 50) [34,35].

Mass Gatherings

A useful microcosm of emergency planning is that required for mass gatherings, including the white emergencies mentioned earlier in this chapter. This is a part of public health science that has been developed and codified extensively during the last two decades [36]. Mass gatherings can vary in size from a few hundred people to millions, and can involve purely local actors or involve services at national level. Like all emergency planning, planning for mass gatherings must take into account a wide range of potential outcomes and possible events, including natural disasters, technological disasters, and health and social related matters, as well as logistics, transportation, and security.

One example is the extensive planning that went into preparing for the Olympic Games in the UK in 2012 [37], but there are many others (e.g., planning for the Football World Cup, the Hajj pilgrimage). If the event involves participants and/or attendees from many nations, extensive cooperative international planning, often within the framework of the International Health Regulations [38], may be involved.

In addition to its vital role in ensuring that the range of needs generated by a defined activity is met, planning for mass gatherings does allow planning methods and concepts to be tested in a real situation although, hopefully, planning for major incidents associated with the event remains in the realm of theory! In addition, a well-planned mass gathering can result in valuable legacies – including, for example, developing emergency services, changes to healthcare services, improvements in diagnostic and public health laboratory services, and improvements in disease surveillance – that benefit the host nation long after the event. It can also help to develop international links, as it is often based on activities that are not particularly politically controversial.

Emergency Preparedness and Logistic Preparedness

Degrees of organisation for protecting civilian populations have existed at least since the formation of the Vigiles Urbani in ancient Rome in AD 6. Commonly, they had a military or paramilitary origin. Into the late twentieth century the principal source of disaster relief was commonly the national armed forces, or even foreign equivalents [16]. Industrial and financial organisations have been involved in civil protection in the past, and still are. For example, in the UK, private fire services (e.g., airport fire services) operate with local authority fire services in some circumstances.

Generally, in any country, emergency preparedness and response systems tend to be mosaics of different degrees of initiative and development. This is because they depend on the acumen and initiative of individuals, who can be either enlightened and capable or uninterested and incapable [39].

Healthcare

All disasters carry with them the risk of health problems. Damage to infrastructures such as water and sewage systems, damage to buildings with loss of shelter, crowding, interruptions to fuel and food supply, and breakdowns of healthcare provision and disease control measures can combine to produce increases in the prevalence of diseases, leading to possible outbreaks. The risk factors for outbreaks of communicable disease after disasters are associated primarily with population displacement [40,41]. Certain groups – children (especially those under 5 years old and unaccompanied), women (especially pregnant women and nursing mothers), older people, and disabled people – are at especially high risk, and planning must take this into account.

Logistic Preparedness

A vital part of emergency preparedness is providing stocks of the materials and equipment necessary for effective responses to different types of disaster. These stores should be located and stocked on the basis of the likely types of disaster that might occur in a particular area.

Providing emergency stocks of this sort can pose both logistical and political problems. The process is not cheap. Items have to be purchased and stored safely and securely in appropriate conditions. Staff are required to maintain the stores and equipment, and stocks need to be rotated to ensure that items remain in date. Transport may be needed as part of the maintenance programme. Arrangements for purchasing perishable or short shelf-life items at short notice must be arranged.

Emergency preparedness of this sort requires firm political support. Preparing for incidents and disasters that may happen at long time intervals is potentially expensive and may seem wasteful (e.g., items may exceed use-by dates, vehicles require maintenance even if they are not regularly used). Stocks may be run down or not replenished if the preparative action appears unnecessary and maintaining stocks is no longer seen as an urgent matter. A classic example is the situation in the UK with regard to personal protective equipment (PPE) for disease outbreaks at the beginning of the COVID-19 pandemic. When the disease broke out in the UK, it rapidly became clear that the stocks of PPE for health workers had been allowed to run down or deteriorate, leaving many healthcare personnel without adequate protection [3].

Is the Past a Reliable Guide to the Future?

Good, robust, and detailed emergency planning is usually based on scenarios about what is likely to happen in the future based on 'reference events', which are usually disasters from the past [1,2]. This section seeks to answer the key question about whether, in a time of rapid change and upheaval, the past is still an adequate guide to the future.

Accelerating climate change is likely to intensify the impacts of meteorological disasters [42]. It is expected that in the future the following events are likely to increase:

- general effects: interruption of services, supplies, and basic infrastructure; escalation of costs associated with damage and interruption of activities; loss of natural and anthropogenic assets; more casualties

- wildfires: loss of forest, woodland, and natural environments; damage to agriculture; damage to local communities, increased risk of casualties; impact on tourism
- droughts: water shortages for agricultural, domestic, and industrial uses; environmental change and impoverishment of ecosystems; reduced crop yields; potential conflicts over access to water
- floods: damage to and destruction of infrastructure; destruction of houses and businesses; drownings; environmental damage
- flash floods: urban damage and casualties
- storms: damage to infrastructure, houses, and businesses; damage to forests and the natural environment; casualties
- storm surges: coastal and estuarine flooding; increased coastal erosion and damage to defences, plus the effects of sea-level rise
- tornadoes: urban damage and casualties
- snowfalls: increased levels of paralysation, isolation, and risk of casualties; isolation of and danger to livestock; increased risk of destructive avalanches
- cold waves: increased energy demand and strain on supply; more fatal cases of exposure
- heatwaves: heat-related casualties and associated health emergencies; increased energy demand and strain on supply; damage to transport systems.

Other major challenges include the following:

- proliferating failure of critical infrastructure, including interruption of vital transport, and 'space weather' (coronal mass ejections from the sun) which can affect power distribution and communications systems
- cyber warfare and online contamination of democratic processes with false information
- unplanned mass migrations
- collapse of economic confidence and the banking system
- generalised unrest among disadvantaged and disaffected populations.

As we live in increasingly networked societies, cascading impacts are likely to become common [43]. They will have to be modelled in the light of concurrent and coincident events [44]. One of the defining characteristics of cascading disasters is the presence of escalation points, at which interactions of different kinds of situations that cause vulnerability (physical, social, economic, psychological, etc.) worsen the impact. Many future disasters are likely to have secondary impacts that are more serious and profound than their primary triggers.

Detailed emergency planning is dependent on scenario building to reveal what needs to be done during a crisis. The scenarios are usually based on a 'reference event', usually taken from past experience of the hazard or threat in question, often the worst impact in the past for which clear descriptions and adequate data are available regarding its causes and consequences [14]. The question is whether future disasters will be so different in magnitude, impacts, and consequences from past events that this methodology is no longer sufficient. Much depends on how we exercise foresight in preparing for emergencies [45].

A special case is represented by so-called 'existential events'. There is little that emergency preparedness services can do to cope with an asteroid impact. Severe challenges would be posed by a non-seasonal influenza pandemic with a mortality rate of, say, 80%. A VEI-7 (volcanic explosivity index) eruption might cause 'multiple bread-basket failure', with severe worldwide consequences for the production and availability of food [46].

Risk and Disaster Science

Risk and disaster science is needed in order to endow emergency planning and management with an adequate profile, give it legitimacy as a discipline of synthesis, and give it a set of rigorous techniques for promoting human safety.

Investigation of disasters from a social science point of view began in the late 1910s and continued with applying principles of human ecology, or adaptation to environmental extremes [47,48]. Since the Second World War there has been an accumulation of studies and information on how to plan for, manage, and respond to emergencies [49]. As society has become more complex, the population of the world has grown, and disasters have proliferated. There has been an accompanying need to train professionals to deal with extreme events and to turn responding to disasters into a fully fledged profession. Disaster science is not the same as hazards sciences such as volcanology, hydrology, and seismology, and engineering risk management. Disaster science deals with logistics, stockpiling and warehousing, emergency

and mass communication, scheduling, coordinating resources, and so on. Its students learn how to assess, quantify, and reduce risks and manage emergencies. They gain a broad knowledge that embraces elements of more than 40 disciplines and professions.

Disaster science, as currently defined, mainly concentrates on so-called natural disasters and catastrophic events caused by nature or natural processes. It involves characterisation of risk based on understanding natural hazards, an appreciation of causes of vulnerability and exposure, and ways to reduce disaster risks. The severity of a disaster is measured in lives lost, economic loss, and the ability of the affected population to rebuild. Disaster science aims to increase the capacity of people and societies to prepare for, respond to, and recover from disasters at all levels, from individual people to communities.

The interdisciplinary nature of disaster science spans the natural, social, and applied sciences; it incorporates engineering (e.g., civil, mechanical, nuclear) and many other disciplines, including planning, medicine, healthcare and public health, and public administration. Training in disaster science involves:

- examining the influence of disasters on the environmental, social, cultural, political, and economic aspects of human life
- developing skills and knowledge in topics including disaster preparedness, responses to disasters, post-disaster reconstruction and recovery, and methods of disaster mitigation in the public, private, and non-profit sectors
- developing decision-making skills in the fields of policies, plans, and regulations
- developing skills in communication and cooperation at local, national, and global levels
- modelling and using statistical methods to quantify aspects of disasters such as risk and exposure.

Several MSc and Diploma courses in this topic now exist, and there are increasing numbers of journals that deal with this subject. Human-made disasters, particularly complex emergencies, are just as demanding of expertise, and numerous courses exist to help to prepare people to work effectively in these situations.

In order to improve disaster responses we need to bring disparate services together by developing a shared culture and a common approach to training

[50]. Developing courses such as those in disaster science can contribute to this process.

Conclusions

It is common to treat the past as a guide to the future, and to assume continuity over time. In the field of major incidents and disasters, this means using past impacts as reference events for the scenarios upon which emergency plans are based. The problem we face is that the pace of change is so fast that the past is no longer a reliable guide to the future.

Climate change, emerging risks, mass migration, strategic threats, and proliferating technological failure all demand a new, more flexible approach based on foresight rather than hindsight. Emergency preparedness systems need to be an order of magnitude larger and more effective than they are at present. Despite the fully justified emphasis on mitigation and prevention, one cannot underfund responses to emergencies. In the future, responding to emergencies will not be solely about rescuing and caring for people – it will have an increasing role in damage limitation. The question is whether this will be learned the hard way by implementing change during an escalating crisis, or whether foresight will prevail, and the system will be transformed in advance of what is to come.

References

1. Harrald JR, Mazzuchi T. Planning for success: a scenario-based approach to contingency planning using expert judgment. *J Contingencies Crisis Manag* 1993; 1: 189–98.

2. Alexander DE. Principles of emergency planning. In *Building Safer Communities: Risk Governance, Spatial Planning and Responses to Natural Hazards* (ed. U Fra Paleo): 162–74. IOS Press, 2009.

3. Calvert JG, Arbuthnott G. *Failures of State: The Inside Story of Britain's Battle with Coronavirus*. Mudlark, 2021.

4. UN Office for Disaster Risk Reduction (UNDRR). *UNISDR Terminology on Disaster Risk Reduction*. UNDRR, 2009 (www.undrr.org/publication/2009-unisdr-terminology-disaster-risk-reduction).

5. UN Office for Disaster Risk Reduction (UNDRR). *Online Glossary* (www.undrr.org/terminology).

6. CIPedia. *Emergency (Definitions)*. Fraunhofer, 2020 (https://websites.fraunhofer.de/CIPedia/index.php/Emergency).

7. Shaluf I, Ahmadun F, Said AM. A review of disaster and crisis. *Disaster Prev Manag* 2003; 12: 24–32.

8. IFRC. *What Is A Disaster?* (www.ifrc.org/what-disaster).

9. IFRC. *Hazards*. IFRC, 2021 (www.ifrc.org/sites/default/files/2021-06/04-HAZARD-DEFINITIONS-HR.pdf).

10. Emergency Event Database (EM-DAT). *Disasters in Numbers*. Emergency Event Database, 2021 (https://reliefweb.int/report/world/2021-disasters-numbers).

11. Wikipedia. *List of Armed Conflicts*. Wikipedia, 2022 (https://en.wikipedia.org/wiki/List_of_ongoing_armed_conflicts).

12. Kelman I. Lost for words amongst disaster risk science vocabulary? *Int J Disaster Risk Sci* 2018; 9: 281–91.

13. ReliefWeb. *Glossary of Humanitarian Terms*. ReliefWeb, 2008 (https://reliefweb.int/report/world/reliefweb-glossary-humanitarian-terms-enko).

14. Alexander DE. *How to Write an Emergency Plan*. Dunedin Academic Press, 2016.

15. UN Office for the Coordination of Humanitarian Affairs and the Inter-Agency Standing Committee. *Civil-Military Guidelines and Reference for Complex Emergencies*. UN Office for the Coordination of Humanitarian Affairs, 2008.

16. Alexander DE. From civil defence to civil protection – and back again. *Disaster Prev Manag* 2002; 11: 209–13.

17. Moore D. *Offensive Cyber Operations: Understanding Intangible Warfare*. Hurst & Company, 2022.

18. Mykhalovskiy E, Kazatchkine C, Foreman-Mackey A, McClelland A, Peck R, Hastings C, et al. Human rights, public health and COVID-19 in Canada. *Can J Public Health* 2020; 111: 975–9.

19. Hararia S, Vitacca M. COVID-19 spread: the Italian case. *Respir Med Res* 2020; 78: 100771.

20. Lauta KC. Human rights and natural disasters. In *Research Handbook on Disasters and International Law* (eds SC Breau, KLH Samuel): 91–110. Edward Elgar, 2016.

21. Handmer J, Dovers S. *Handbook of Disaster Policies and Institutions*. Earthscan, 2007.

22. Kapucu N, Arslan T, Demiroz F. Collaborative emergency management and national emergency management network. *Disaster Prev Manag* 2010; 19: 452–68.

23. UN Office for the Coordination of Humanitarian Affairs (UNOCHA). *Guidelines on the Use of Military and Civil Defence Assets to Support United Nations*

Humanitarian Activities in Complex Emergencies. MCDA Guidelines. UNOCHA, 2006.

24. UN Office for the Coordination of Humanitarian Affairs (UNOCHA). *Guidelines on the Use of Foreign Military and Civil Defence Assets in Disaster Relief – Oslo Guidelines (Revision 1.1)*. UNOCHA, 2007.

25. NATO. *NATO Standard AJP-3.4.3 Allied Joint Doctrine for the Military Contribution to Humanitarian Assistance*. NATO Standardization Office, 2016.

26. Ministry of Defence. *Disaster Relief Operations Overseas: The Military Contribution* 3rd ed. Ministry of Defence, 2016.

27. Boland ST, McInnes C, Gordon S, Lillywhite L. Civil–military relations: a review of major guidelines and their relevance during public health emergencies. *BMJ Mil Health* 2021; 167: 99–106.

28. Simm G. Disaster militarism? Military humanitarian assistance and disaster relief. In *Max Planck Yearbook of United Nations Law* (eds E de Wet, KM Scherr, R Wolfrum): 347–75. Brill, 2019.

29. Hallegatte S, Przyluski V. The economics of natural disasters. *SSRN* 2010; 11: 14–24.

30. Pullium JK, Roble GS, Raymond MA. Emergency planning: be prepared. *Nature* 2014; 514: 430.

31. O'Brien A, Read GJM, Salmon PM. Situation awareness in multi-agency emergency response: models, methods and applications. *Int J Disaster Risk Reduct* 2020; 47: 101634.

32. Wang J. Integrated model combined land-use planning and disaster management: the

structure, context and contents. *Disaster Prev Manag* 2012; 21: 110–23.

33. Alexander DE. Towards the development of a standard for emergency planning. *Disaster Prev Manag* 2005; 14: 158–75.

34. Haddow GD, Bullock JA, Coppola DP. *Introduction to Emergency Management* 6th ed. Butterworth-Heinemann, 2017.

35. Canton LG. *Emergency Management: Concepts and Strategies for Effective Programs* 2nd ed. Wiley, 2020.

36. World Health Organization. *Public Health for Mass Gatherings: Key Considerations*. World Health Organization, 2015 (www.who.int/publications/i/item/public-health-for-mass-gatherings-key-considerations).

37. McCloskey B, Endericks T. *Learning from London 2012: A Practical Guide to Public Health and Mass Gatherings*. Health Protection Agency UK, 2013.

38. World Health Organization. *International Health Regulations*, 3rd ed. World Health Organization, 2005 (www.who.int/publications/i/item/9789241580496).

39. Berke P, Smith G. Hazard mitigation, planning, and disaster resiliency: challenges and strategic choices for the 21st century. In *Building Safer Communities: Risk Governance, Spatial Planning and Responses to Natural Hazards* (ed. UF Paleo): 1–20. IOS Press, 2009.

40. Noji EK, ed. *The Public Health Consequences of Disasters*. Oxford University Press, 1997.

41. Watson JT, Gayer M, Conolly MA. Epidemics after natural

disasters. *Emerg Infect Dis* 2007; 13: 1–5.

42. O'Brien G, O'Keefe P, Rose J, Wisner B. Climate change and disaster management. *Disasters* 2006; 30: 64–80.

43. Pescaroli G, Alexander D. A definition of cascading disasters and cascading effects: going beyond the 'toppling dominos' metaphor. *Planet@Risk* 2015; 3: 58–67.

44. Pescaroli G, Alexander D. Understanding compound, interconnected, interacting and cascading risks: a holistic framework. *Risk Anal* 2018; 38: 2245–57.

45. Jahangiri K, Eivazi M-R, Mofazali AS. The role of foresight in avoiding systematic failure of natural disaster risk management. *Int J Disaster Risk Reduct* 2017; 21: 303–11.

46. Denkenberger DC, Pearce JM. Feeding everyone: solving the food crisis in event of global catastrophes that kill crops or obscure the sun. *Futures* 2015; 72: 57–68.

47. Prince S. *Catastrophe and Social Change: Based Upon a Sociological Study of the Halifax Disaster*. Colombia University Press, 1920.

48. Barrows HH. Geography as human ecology. *Ann Am Assoc Geogr* 1923; 13: 1–14.

49. Drabek TE. *Human System Response to Disaster: An Inventory of Sociological Findings*. Springer-Verlag, 1986.

50. Laakso K, Palomäki J. The importance of a common understanding in emergency management. *Technol Forecast Soc Change* 2013; 80: 1703–13.

Chapter

50

Leadership, Organisation, and Implementation of Emergency Preparedness

Stefan Schilling, Richard Williams, Verity Kemp, Tim Healing, and David E Alexander

Introduction

Emergencies, incidents, terrorist events, disasters, disease outbreaks and conflicts (EITDDC) may be large, such as the COVID-19 pandemic, Hurricane Irma, or the terrorist attacks of 9/11, or more localised, such as the Manchester Arena bombing in 2017 or the Miami Surfside condominium collapse in 2021. They have in common that they are sudden, unexpected, urgent, and often cause loss of life and significant damage to many people's livelihoods and the local infrastructure.

Organisations responsible for responding to the difficulties and consequences for human life of EITDDC share many strategic, logistic, and administrative similarities. These similarities are exemplified by the UK's response in 2017 to Hurricane Irma's destruction of the British Overseas Territories in the Caribbean (OPERATION RUMAN). The response to the disaster was characterised by a myriad of complex multi-sectoral tasks that required interprofessional/interdisciplinary cooperation and a distribution of responsibility to lower levels in the hierarchy. Simultaneously, it challenged pre-existing communication, command, control, and information (C3I) structures. Many of these problems have also been visible during the COVID-19 pandemic.

EITDDC are expected to increase in the future, posing unique challenges to leaders of responses to EITDDC and preparedness at the strategic and tactical levels [1–3]. Despite these known risks and requirements, research in this area is far from unified. Academic articles on disaster management are published in more than 900 journals, with most articles on specific disasters being anecdotal and descriptive single case studies. Articles on professional competencies in managing EITDDC are dominated by research on mostly Western healthcare staff [4,5]. Corresponding regulatory frameworks show vast differences between Western countries and low- to middle-income nations, as well as between regulations for domestic

management of EITDDC and expeditionary disaster responses [6,7]. The situation is similarly Western dominated in countries' responses to pandemics (e.g., COVID-19, Ebola), with few or no public health or clinical management guidelines for high-consequence infectious viral diseases being published in low- and middle-income countries, making rapid pandemic responses extremely difficult [8–10].

Whereas Chapter 49 addresses the components and organisation of civil protection at the strategic level, this chapter moves towards the operational and tactical levels, by collecting lessons from the literature to outline concrete steps necessary for organising and leading responses to EITDDC. First, this chapter summarises common problems experienced in responding to EITDDC. Second, it describes what steps should be taken at the policy level to prepare organisations for the challenges. Third, it outlines ways in which teams could be better organised to respond. Finally, it addresses the specific role of people who lead and manage EITDDC in preparing their teams, developing capacity, and ensuring a collaborative emergency network.

Although often separated into the different phases of preparedness, response, recovery, and rehabilitation, this chapter focuses on organisation and leadership in preparing for and responding to EITDDC. In the military, operational leadership sits above the tactical; in UK civilian services, including healthcare, the term operational is used to describe the hands-on work at the frontline of emergencies. This chapter adopts the terms strategic and tactical to delineate the top- and higher-level multi-agency coordination efforts from the frontline or operational work at the site of the incident or disaster. Similarly, the term strategic is used to describe the work of senior leaders in incident command centres who coordinate responses. The term organisation is used throughout to acknowledge that, in most cases, non-governmental organisations (NGOs) are involved in responding to EITDDC.

Common Problems Experienced When Responding to EITDDC

The key barriers to successful responses to EITDDC range from situational and environmental demands to organisational and personal problems. Effective responses to EITDDC are often hindered by degrees of uncertainty and constraints to developing situational awareness. In total, 55% of the world's population live in cities, with the number expected to grow in the next decades (see Chapter 7). In such an environment, acute and already complex tasks are likely to be made more difficult by the expected inaccessibility of the location affecting delivery of critical resources and dealing with displaced populations [11]. At the same time, low-income countries tend to be at higher risk for natural disasters, due in many instances to their location in low-elevation coastal zones or in seismic hazard zones – areas which, due to their accessibility and trade opportunities, are regularly inhabited by higher numbers of migrant workers and urban poor people [11–13].

Often mitigation, early warning, and disaster responses are also hampered by political and organisational hierarchies, decentralised command structures, and ineffective emergency medical systems [14]. For example, although Western countries have national response frameworks (e.g., the US National Response Framework [NRF], established in 2008, and the UK's Joint Emergency Services Interoperability Programme [JESIP], established in 2012 and renamed with the same acronym in 2015), situational awareness may still be affected by systems that differ by country, province, state, or county. This creates situations whereby similar and adjacent counties can have dissimilar emergency response networks in place, making large-scale disaster management and leadership across the smallest local setting difficult [15]. The COVID-19 pandemic highlighted the difficulty of establishing concrete health and safety guidelines and standardised clinical treatment plans, due to the complexity of the multi-system effects of the disease due to SARS-CoV-2 that was characterised by its multi-organ symptoms as well changing variants. The spread and impacts of the disease required a surge of multidisciplinary healthcare personnel, engagement of many agencies, and a rapid focus on and investment in research.

Responses to EITDDC are often obstructed by a lack of communication and information exchange, which undermines interoperability. Each phase in successful responses to EITDDC requires a complicated set of national and local structures that facilitate integration and coordination of the organisations involved into existing emergency plans, early warning systems, and C3I systems. Given this complexity, communication and information exchange often arise as an issue in responses to EITDDC. A recent systematic review of 302 academic articles and after-action reports on disasters found that although communication, connectivity, and capacity for data analysis were ranked as the biggest issues by members of disaster response agencies, the academic literature pays little attention to these issues [13]. In the UK, for example, inadequate communication and coordination, as well as confusion over command and control between professional responders, hindered responses during the Hillsborough Stadium disaster in 1989, the London bombings in 2005, the Manchester Arena bombing in 2017, and the Grenfell Tower fire in 2017 [16–18]. The poor responses to the last two of these disasters occurred despite the prior introduction of the JESIP joint doctrine, which is aimed at ensuring that responders have the ability to respond to major or complex incidents [19].

Due to the multi-sectoral complexity of many disasters and emergencies, multidisciplinary and multi-agency collaboration, at both the strategic and the tactical levels, has become the norm. In this environment, team members from other professions are often unaware of specific experiences, regulations, responsibilities, or resources of partnered organisations, resulting in misconceptions about occupational roles that routinely lead to goal confusion, interpersonal conflict, and retreat into occupational identities and formal hierarchies. Similarly, organisational and operational differences often hinder teamwork in multidisciplinary healthcare teams and multi-agency response teams through asynchronous shift patterns, spatial–temporal separation of team members, debriefs within a single occupation rather than the wider team, or failure to share risk assessments [16,20]. These issues are exacerbated by the hierarchical nature of some of the main organisations involved in responding to EITDDC, with entrenched organisational conditioning leading to misalignment of roles, and unclear boundaries [20].

The increasing complexity of disasters means that single leaders cannot handle the entirety of decision making that is required, especially if the response occurs over long periods of time and demands rapid changes, well-established procedures regulating information exchange, and existing social connections between organisations' managers [11]. The challenges to responding successfully to EITDDC include addressing difficulties in establishing situational awareness in complex, chaotic, and often impoverished environments, as well as barriers to effective communication and information exchange that can impede successful collaboration and interoperability between different organisations. Importantly, there are leadership challenges and inadequate training. The next section of this chapter outlines steps that can mitigate some of these issues.

Policy Level Preparation for Preventing, Mitigating, and Responding to EITDDC

Any response to EITDDC is characterised by the existing emergency and disaster response systems in place, the social, political, and cultural environment, and the network structure and organisational culture of the agencies involved [11,14]. Consequently, mitigation of and preparation for EITDDC contains three elements: developing emergency plans and surveillance; establishing systems, procedures, guidelines, and protocols; and providing resources and education. We overview these elements and provide organisational examples to identify the functions required.

The purpose of emergency plans is to anticipate the needs that are likely to arise during a crisis, and those plans should consider not only the direct consequences of disasters for the population, but also the long-term and indirect impacts. For example, after disasters, respiratory, gastrointestinal, and ophthalmic diseases are likely to occur; they are not immediately related to the disaster itself, but need to be anticipated in the response [21,22]. Similarly, during the COVID-19 pandemic the long duration of the lockdowns in the UK and elsewhere reduced people's access to primary care services and specialty consultants, contributing to backlogs in elective care, with long-term negative health impacts [23,24]. Therefore emergency planning must consider secondary effects of EITDDC, anticipate unusual developments, and monitor changing risks and organisational readiness, so that organisations are optimally prepared to cope with them. However, it is important to note that the development of plans and the identification of risks can be affected by the lack of surveillance systems, national prioritisation of risks, bureaucratic politics,

and the absence of international involvement. For example, despite regular outbreaks, Indonesia lacks both surveillance systems and diagnostic resources for the Chikungunya virus, so the true incidence rates are unknown, resulting in both a low prioritisation of the virus and the absence of clinical management guidelines and dedicated authorities. In particular, viral outbreaks and cross-border natural disasters show that plans cannot be purely national or regional, but must anticipate and integrate legal and statutory structures beyond regional and national borders.

Once potential risks have been identified and emergency plans developed, response systems for EITDDC, procedures, and protocols must be developed to create a unified system of preparedness and response. These procedures call for integration of different authorities and levels of public administration, facilities, and functions. For example, developing a robust C3I system requires the responsible authorities to identify potential risks, actors, tasks, responsibilities, resources, laws, and policies to act as an early warning system prior to events as well as a command-and-control centre during the emergency. These protocols and systems must be developed with consideration for local EITDDC requirements, and available agencies and resources, and should be consistently reviewed and adapted. This means that while, in many western countries, hierarchical systems have been found to under-perform in complex emergency situations, low- and middle income countries, which may not have the capacity to develop or maintain complex systems, would be ill-advised to develop decentralised systems for responding to EITDDC. For example, guidelines for managing pandemic patients that were developed in wealthy Western countries cannot easily be adopted in low- and middle-income countries, but need to be adapted to each local setting by considering locally available facilities, equipment, therapeutics, and healthcare staff to tackle viral outbreaks. An example of a localised adaptation of a C3I system is highlighted in Organisational Example 1 in Box 50.1.

Establishing a system for the command and control of an incident requires that there are detailed guidelines and procedures developed for how relevant personnel are activated and post-event lessons are integrated and disseminated across the network of people who are potentially involved [11,25]. Severe droughts and floods are forecast to occur more frequently, requiring accurate atmospheric forecasting

Box 50.1 Organisational Example 1: the Incident Command System

One example of a localised command and control system is the Incident Command System (ICS), most widely used in the USA, which is organised around one leader overseeing different functional teams the mix of which can be adapted based on the incident (e.g., operations, health and safety, planning, logistics, administration). In larger incidents, the teams may be supported by safety officers and public information staff.

During COVID-19, the respondent interviewed described the work in an Incident Control Centre in the UK as follows:

> Anything that happened was managed by gold, silver, and bronze level commands. Operational teams were at the bronze level, managing their resources, working out where things are. If they get a problem and they can't manage something, they flag it up to three operational directorates and a corporate one, with each one of those having a silver team. If they'd got emerging issues they couldn't manage, they would flag that up to the gold commander. We'd be managing issues that were coming up, like making sure PPE [personal protective equipment] is in the right place, responding to levels of staff sickness, closing certain services, and moving them online, responding to NHS England requests, [or] liaising with the police. ... We suspended our [normal] strategies and changed our focus to preserving life. Everything we were doing every day was focused on 'Are we doing the best we can to preserve life?'
>
> Interview with an NHS Hospital Trust Senior Leader, NHS COVID Teams Study

and early warning systems that must integrate not only emergency responders, but also the responsible authorities to minimise loss of lives, damage to roads, and destruction of property, while increasing positive effects such as replenishing water reservoirs [26,27]. Nevertheless, recognising that in many EITDDCs, a lack of clearly identified lead agencies can result in unpredictable capacity and response gaps, it is important to have protocols in place to ensure that appropriate aid is provided in suitable quantities, that responders can operate safely, and that the needs of residents and displaced populations can be met. This task is huge and difficult, as is illustrated by Organisational Example 2 in Box 50.2.

Box 50.2 Organisational Example 2: the UN Cluster approach

One example of the coordination between organisations is the United Nations (UN) Cluster approach, which may involve international and local civilian agencies, military personnel, the UN, and foreign NGOs on the ground. In complex emergencies (see Chapter 49), access to beneficiaries may be seriously compromised due to combat and destruction of dwellings and infrastructures. In the Cluster system, coordination of aid activities is based on 11 field-level clusters, each led by a UN agency functioning as 'provider of last resort' and accountable to the UN Humanitarian Coordinator (see Table 50.1).

Although the cluster approach has been developed for humanitarian interventions, it provides a useful example for national or regional emergency response systems, as it aids in coordinating between different functions and offers a well-tested system for leadership and accountability, strengthening partnerships, and prioritising roles.

Table 50.1 The UN Cluster approach

Cluster	Lead agency
Nutrition	UNICEF
Health	WHO
Water/sanitation/hygiene (WASH)	UNICEF
Emergency shelter	IFRC/UNHCR
Camp coordination/management	IOM/UNHCR
Protection	UNHCR
Early recovery	UNDP
Logistics	WFP
Emergency telecommunications	WFP
Education	UNISEF and Save the Children
Food security	WFP/FAO

UNICEF, United Nations Children's Fund; WHO, World Health Organization; IFRC, International Federation of Red Cross and Red Crescent Societies; UNHCR, United Nations High Commissioner for Refugees; IOM, International Organization for Migration; UNDP, United Nations Development Programme; WFP, World Food Programme; FAO, Food and Agriculture Organization.

Box 50.3 Organisational Example 3: local resilience forums

A good example of a system for planning and preparing for local incidents and emergencies is the 38 local resilience forums (LRF) in the UK. These multi-agency partnerships between Category 1 responders (i.e., emergency services, NHS hospitals, and local authorities) and Category 2 responders (e.g., utilities or transport companies) have a collective responsibility to plan, prepare, and communicate in a multi-agency environment. During an emergency, strategic coordinating groups (SCGs), formed by and from the LRFs, take overall responsibility for the multi-sectorial management of an emergency and develop the strategic framework in which tactical command and control centres operate. However, it is important to note that SCGs do not have authority over Category 1 or 2 organisations, as they retain their own command authority.

Protocols should address interoperability guidelines across different disaster categories (see also Chapter 49), and develop plans for restoring critical infrastructure, emergency medical care and healthcare preparedness, casualty and fatality management, health and safety protocols, community preparedness, and distress [28,29]. These plans should incorporate both legal and public ethical considerations (see Chapter 52), because limited resources as well as uncertainty during an incident may require unforeseen moral decisions, or legal ramifications may reduce the timely release of crucial information to the public. Box 50.3 provides an example of a system for planning and preparing for local emergencies and incidents.

The last component of successful mitigation of and preparedness for EITDDC is adequate resourcing and training of people and organisations. Careful selection of staff is crucial for the immediate response and for relief efforts, as response teams are often required to be self-sufficient for a period, as they cannot expect to rely on local infrastructure. In the long term this requires stockpiling materials and establishing robust supply chain systems that may potentially include private companies.

Simultaneously, communication systems and information infrastructure must deliver early warnings to communities, ensure shared situational awareness, and coordinate and ensure interoperability and information exchange between national, regional, and local organisations and response teams. Real-time exchange of information between decision-makers, experts, and the public is especially crucial in geographically widespread and rapidly changing incidents or emergencies. For example, the novelty, complexity, and mutability of the SARS-CoV-2 virus and of the disease that it causes – COVID-19 – necessitated rapidly changing medical advice and safety guidelines to be communicated across all actors from governmental public health agencies to local public health departments and hospitals and on to frontline staff and the public.

In many instances, technological tools can be useful for supporting situational awareness and communication, but fail-safe systems and alternative plans must be incorporated in case communications fail or staff lack experience or cannot access computer-based systems [13,30]. It is useful to establish a coordinated programme of standardised education, specialised training, and periodic simulations to allow familiarisation with procedures and communication systems, build inter-agency collaboration, establish shared mental models, and stress-test organisations.

At the policy and strategic levels, periodic exercises are required based on scenarios established during contingency planning in the form of walkthroughs, tabletop exercise, drills, functional exercises, and full-scale exercises. For this reason, countries periodically conduct national and regional exercises to stress-test and optimise the strategic response of federal and state agencies as well as that of critical infrastructure providers and emergency and healthcare organisations. At the tactical level, preparedness and multidisciplinary teamwork have been found to benefit from educational programmes that use active learning, simulation training, and reviews [31,32]. All levels of educational programmes, be they for personal skills development, operational simulations, or strategic exercises, require adequate funding.

Figure 50.1 provides a diagrammatic summary of the policy levels that we have described here.

Organising Teams to Respond to EITDDC

Interprofessional/interdisciplinary teamwork, defined as the combined, collaborative action of a group of people from different occupational backgrounds [20], has a range of beneficial outcomes, as such a group can be more efficient and innovative by bringing a variety of skills and expertise. In clinical settings this is associated with improvement in patients' satisfaction, and a

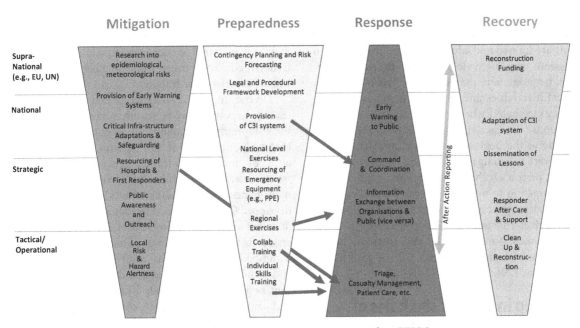

Figure 50.1 Policy levels for mitigating, preparing for, responding to, and recovering from EITDDC.

reduction in mortality, readmission, adverse drug events, length of inpatient stays, and clinical error rates [20]. Feeling connected and socially supported by other colleagues within teams has repeatedly been found to improve job satisfaction, enhance wellbeing and resilience, and protect against depression and post-traumatic stress disorder (PTSD) [33,34]. However, as such effects rely on stable and well-trained teams with functioning communication processes and shared mental models in place, we must caution against the notion that 'ad-hoc', 'task-orged', or 'flash' teams lacking prior training and familiarisation will achieve similarly positive effects. Our research on interprofessional/interdisciplinary COVID-19 teams highlighted that personnel from different occupational backgrounds who were not prepared for working on a COVID-19 ward, and did not know their colleagues prior to deployment, reported not only lower levels of teamwork, social support, and identification with the team, but also more negative mental health outcomes and career intentions.

As the immediate response to EITDDCs is usually coordinated at the tactical level, success is often impaired by a lack of preparedness and adequate training by the people involved in the response. Most people who are called upon in EITDDCs are primarily trained for a multitude of roles, which are not related to disasters or pandemics. Lack of preparedness has a considerable impact on job performance and potential patient care, and also on the wellbeing of responders [20]. Several systematic reviews found that healthcare staff are frequently ill-prepared for disaster responses, which in turn has been associated with higher levels of mental health problems and detrimental effects on people's ability to do their jobs [7,33,35,36].

Effective teamwork and a socially supportive work climate require an emphasis on the contributions of each team member, and the development of a shared identity and shared mental models. This has been supported by recent work on cross-organisational leadership, in which leaders who utilised prior organisational identities as a basis for subsequently developing a superordinate identity were able to increase support of the wider organisation's shared strategies [16]. Structural factors, such as co-location and alignment of work schedules, have been found to be beneficial to developing teamwork in multidisciplinary healthcare and military teams.

Although prior professional collaboration as well as friendships have been found to be useful in increasing collaboration, communication, and team cohesion, these links beforehand may not always be possible [15,17]. In addition to personality and professional differences, interprofessional team members also come with pre-existing concepts and procedures, and a general lack of detailed knowledge about colleagues' professional competence and experience. For example, as people from different occupational groups are trained and educated by and for their own profession, they often do not share the same operational language, and may revert to their own organisational hierarchies and identities in times of crisis. This is exacerbated when volunteers are involved in the response. In cases such as these, team members – especially at the beginning of their amalgamation – often revert to occupational stereotypes in order to discern a person's technical abilities and the benefit of their occupation to the team. Research has repeatedly shown that misperceptions of roles and responsibilities as well as role ambiguity increase conflict, negative outcomes for patients, and mental health problems in both mono-professional and multidisciplinary teams [20].

Leadership in EITDDC: The Roles of Emergency Leaders and Managers

Strategic leaders are the linchpins between governmental policies and their consequences on the ground. Their roles change based on the phase of the emergency response. During the mitigation and preparedness phases their role is mostly political and conceptual, coordinating between different agencies to establish the necessary structures, social networks, and processes. During the response, leaders are prone to micromanaging, but should try to refrain from coordinating every aspect of the response by themselves. Instead, they should ensure the smooth functioning of the response by delegating, resolving difficult problems that often have ethical ramifications, and supporting subordinate commanders. The environment also plays a part because leaders must often lead under substantially different circumstances. Research on leadership *in extremis* has shown that, at the frontline of an emergency, transactional leadership is more predictive of team members' performance, whereas transformational leadership may be more important in staff environments or when preparing for incidents [37–40].

Strategic leadership and management of EITDDC are often defined by a complex intergroup environment, which not only demands that leaders address perpetually shifting, competing goals, but also requires management and coordination of a network of different agencies and organisations, each of which has its own bureaucratic procedures, goals, and identities [41].

In such an environment, leaders seldom have professional expertise in every occupation of their team, and may be ill prepared to address occupational and organisational conflict between team members due to their lack of experience or training.

Diverse models of leadership and approaches to leading responses may be required in order to address the complexity of demands, the requirement for 24/7 leadership, the length of the response, and the importance of making efforts to prevent the response from deteriorating through burnout and micromanagement. Many traditional models of leadership – developed for permanent, stable organisations – may be ill-suited to disaster environments, which require leadership to be rotational and/or shared between several commanders of operations' centres. In these contexts, and without specific training, leadership is often emergent or transitory, especially when designated leaders and defined group goals are lacking [42]. Thus leaders emerge within the context of the tasks assigned to groups. This is often the case in more tactical or operational leadership scenarios and in interprofessional/ interdisciplinary teams. Thus, for example, NHS England created the Strategic Leadership in a Crisis course to better enable senior NHS managers to play their parts in managing incidents and major incidents. Its development is summarised in Box 50.4.

Additionally, health and safety guidelines, may limit senior leaders ability to be present on wards where patients who had COVID-19 were treated. In these instances, personnel without formal leadership training often took on leadership roles, based on having a particular clinical skill set relevant to their duties for patients who had COVID-19. Emergent leaders may be more prone to burnout due to higher workloads as a consequence of filling particular demands that others may not see or anticipate [43].

Research has shown that formalised leaders who empowered team members to take on peer-leadership roles were perceived as better leaders and were found to create a stronger sense of team cohesion and organisational identity [44]. This suggests that senior staff who invest in peer leadership among their contributing organisations are likely to generate a higher commitment to the common task. Similarly, use of inclusive language by leaders that utilises more invitations and appreciations has been found to be more beneficial to increasing the involvement and voices of healthcare professionals from different occupational backgrounds [45].

Box 50.4 Designing the NHS England Strategic
Leadership in a Crisis course

Box 50.4 **Designing the NHS England Strategic Leadership in a Crisis course**

Inquiries into major incidents, as defined in Chapter 49, often make recommendations and observations relating to the competency of incident commanders. In busy environments, such as acute hospitals, there are many, often conflicting, priorities for senior leaders that can result in training on the skills of command not being given sufficient priority.

In 2009 the Department of Health decided that it was important to train and exercise its most senior managers in the NHS locally in the roles and responsibilities required of them for emergency preparedness, resilience, and response (EPRR). Designing the training programme clearly identified who were the people in the roles that required command skills. The training became the Strategic Leadership in a Crisis course. Since then, the competencies required have been set out by NHS England.

The people to be trained were directors who were on-call and senior managers of the many NHS organisations. The objectives were to ensure that participants would understand EPRR planning and response arrangements in the NHS in the context of the Civil Contingencies Act 2004 and associated guidance, be able to evaluate the roles and responsibilities of partner organisations, review planning and response arrangements in their own organisation, and understand the defensible decision-making process and be able to assess the performance of their own response team.

In many parts of England, local NHS organisations created networks to share the training with neighbouring organisations; this enhanced collaboration and encouraged sharing knowledge, experience, and ideas.

At a personal level, leaders may be affected by long working hours, high levels of stress and uncertainty, and the inevitable shortages of resources. Emergency leaders and managers must be able to recognise their own limitations and those of their teams. The remainder of this section considers these personal, structural, and environmental difficulties in order to identify some of the key tasks and responsibilities that leaders should address.

Developing Collaborative Networks and Shared Spaces

Leaders should invest in developing a collaborative network between all possible actors involved in the response if they are to run a smooth response during an incident. Although many of the command structures are regulated and designated by the emergency plans and the C3I system adopted, the ability of strategic leaders to coordinate a response and facilitate interoperability hinges on relationships between actors that have been established prior to the incident.

Developing collaborative networks does not come easily to most leaders, because few professional development programmes provide the psychosocial skills for coordinating and communicating between people from different occupational backgrounds. In addition to psychosocial interventions, leaders also benefit from implementing spatial–temporal improvements, standardised work schedules across the responding agencies, and shared briefings and handovers. Many of these efforts are aimed at functional collaboration, but they also aid people to develop the necessary social relations and trust between members, which have been found to increase information exchange, speed of decision making, and stability of networks [11,17,25]. Increased social support in teams has been found to be beneficial for reducing distress and negative mental health outcomes [33,34].

Investing in Professional Skills and Psychosocial Staff Development

During the preparedness phase, managers should focus on developing staff by emphasising continuing professional development and multidisciplinary collaborative training, and ensuring widespread dissemination of lessons learned from responding to EITDDC. Managers and leaders must ensure that responders receive both specialised training in their own occupation and collaborative training with members from other professional groups. Exposure to personnel from other organisations during exercises and simulation training can aid in identifying weaknesses in the plan, but, more importantly, increases the understanding of each person's skills, roles, and responsibilities, which can reduce role ambiguity and help staff to develop shared goals [14,35,46].

Empowering Team Members and Shared Leadership

Leadership may also be emergent or of transitory character at the tactical level, with teams in dangerous situations often relying on shared leadership that allows knowledge, skills, and abilities from across the team to be pooled, and mutual influence between team members to improve performance [47]. Interprofessional/interdisciplinary teams have been found to benefit from shared leadership, which suggests that multiple team members sharing leadership contributed to team functioning by fulfilling a wider range of leadership functions than a single leader could do [48]. Shared leadership has also been found to increase work satisfaction, commitment, and goal attainment, while reducing stress, burnout, and interpersonal conflict within teams [20].

Building Capacity for Responses to EITDDC by Engaging Communities in the Planning Phase

Managers and leaders, particularly at the strategic level, are required to build public capacity through early engagement with local communities in the preparation phase. A recent review of responses to COVID-19 argued that communication with the public in a pandemic, or in any other type of disaster, should occur early, be decisive and open, and must not ignore any segments of society [49]. In many cases, this requires a dedicated public information team that can communicate using a range of different tools. However, community outreach and capacity building cannot merely consist of providing information from authorities, but should also integrate the population into the process of relieving EITDDCs. Examples of community outreach are provided in Box 50.5.

Strategic leaders, therefore, do not just make the decisions that need to be disseminated to the public, but also have much influence on which systems are employed and how they are implemented by responders and the public. They are also responsible for stress-testing these systems periodically, and for educating and involving communities.

Supporting the Health, Wellbeing, and Morale of Staff

Leaders have a substantial impact on the long-term health, morale, and efficiency of team members in responses to EITDDCs. Many of the stressors that commonly affect aid workers and responders to EITDDC are related directly and indirectly to workload, managers, and colleagues and other secondary

> **Box 50.5 Community engagement and capacity building before and during a disaster**
>
> **Prior to a disaster**
> The UK's Humanitarian Assistance and Disaster Relief (HADR) Troop, a unit of Royal Engineers and Royal Marines that is deployed in the Caribbean during the hurricane season, is a good example of early integration with the community, as it both allows familiarisation with the community and meets particular needs, but also provides an early warning system.
>
> **During a disaster**
> The Israeli approach to Search and Rescue places population intelligence at the centre of the rescue mission by utilising dedicated Population Intelligence Officers who not only provide information for the population but also integrate people into the search efforts and thus increase the effectiveness and success of locating survivors in a shorter amount of time, with substantial reduction of resources. This not only obtains critical information by questioning family members, but also – by pulling the population into the search and rescue process – allows continued psychosocial support for relatives' grief and bereavement.

stressors (see Chapter 9). Leaders have important roles in ensuring that team members can collaborate and function well. They have a substantial impact on the psychological safety of team members. Reducing incivility and conflict increases team performance and positive team climates (see www.civilitysaveslives.com/). As such, at every level, team leaders should have training in maintaining team members' wellbeing and in basic techniques of psychosocial care – for example, psychological first aid (PFA) and Trauma Risk Management (TRiM) [33,34,50] (see also Chapters 47 and 48 for operational information about caring for staff). However, positive outcomes have been shown to depend on leadership style, with dominant, passive, or authoritarian leadership styles decreasing teamwork and communication.

Leaders have a crucial role in informal chats with team members, which – especially in particularly difficult incidents – can provide a useful tool to help team members to make sense of complex situations and to reappraise and regulate stressful experiences (see Chapters 44, 47 and 48) [42,51,52]. Therefore team leaders should consider offering support for their teams to engage in peer support programmes (see Chapter 48). As mental health outcomes among responders to EITDDCs are linked to lack of preparedness, role ambiguity, and lack of confidence in one's professional competence, leaders can contribute positively to teams' level of preparedness by ensuring that they receive appropriate training.

Conclusion

Although preparedness for and responses to EITDDC are seldom discussed together, this chapter identifies some of the common challenges that organisations, leaders, and responders face across these endeavours. It provides key tasks and structures for developing people and organisations. It summarises some of the most pertinent problems for preparedness and responses, with a view to supporting readers to develop adequate preparedness and planning systems, procedures, and protocols. It also discusses some of the main difficulties that strategic leaders face in these environments, and it emphasises key tasks for leaders, in developing capacity, ensuring a collaborative emergency network, and supporting their staff.

References

1. Akter R, Hu W, Gatton M, Bambrick H, Cheng J, Tong S. Climate variability, socio-ecological factors and dengue transmission in tropical Queensland, Australia: a Bayesian spatial analysis. *Environ Res* 2021; **195**: 110285.

2. Coronese M, Lamperti F, Keller K, Chiaromonte F, Roventini A. Evidence for sharp increase in the economic damages of extreme natural disasters. *Proc Natl Acad Sci USA* 2019; **116**: 21450–55.

3. Otto FEL, Philip S, Kew S, Li S, King A, Cullen H. Attributing high-impact extreme events across timescales—a case study of four different types of events. *Climatic Change* 2018; **149**: 399–412.

4. Gallardo AR, Djalali A, Foletti M, Ragazzoni L, Corte FD, Lupescu O, et al. Core competencies in disaster management and humanitarian assistance: a systematic review. *Disaster Med Public* 2015; **9**: 430–39.

5. Smith EC, Burkle FM, Aitken P, Leggatt P. Seven decades of disasters: a systematic review of the literature. *Prehosp Disaster Med* 2018; **33**: 418–23.

6. Wolbers J, Kuipers S, Boin A. A systematic review of 20 years of crisis and disaster research: trends and progress. *Risk Hazards Crisis Public Policy* 2021; **12**: 374–92.

7. Shahrestanaki YA, Khankeh H, Masoumi G, Hosseini M. What structural factors influencing emergency and disaster medical response teams? A comparative review study. *J Educ Health Promot* 2019; **8**: 110.

8. Pilbeam C, Malden D, Newell K, Dagens A, Kennon K, Michelen M, et al. Accessibility, inclusivity, and implementation of COVID-19 clinical management guidelines early in the pandemic: a global survey. *Wellcome Open Res* 2021; **6**: 247.

9. Lipworth S, Rigby I, Cheng V, Bannister P, Harriss E, Cook K, et al. From severe acute respiratory syndrome (SARS) and Middle East respiratory syndrome (MERS) to coronavirus disease 2019 (COVID-19): a systematic review of the quality and responsiveness of clinical management guidelines in outbreak settings. *Wellcome Open Res* 2021; **6**: 170.

10. Dagens A, Sigfrid L, Cai E, Lipworth S, Cheung V, Harris E, et al. Scope, quality, and inclusivity of clinical guidelines produced early in the covid-19 pandemic: rapid review. *BMJ* 2020; **369**: m1936.

11. Kapucu N, Arslan T, Demiroz F. Collaborative emergency management and national emergency management network. *Disaster Prev Manag* 2010; **19**: 452–68.

12. Balk D, Montgomery MR, McGranahan G, Kim D, Mara V, et al. Mapping urban settlements and the risks of climate change in Africa, Asia and South America. In *Population Dynamics and Climate Change* (eds Guzman JM, Martine G, McGranahan G, Schensul D, Tacoli C): 80–103. UNFPA, IIED, 2009.

13. Kedia T, Ratcliff J, O'Connor M, Oluic S, Rose M, Freeman J, et al. Technologies enabling situational awareness during disaster response: a systematic review. *Disaster Med Public Health Prep* 2022; **16**: 341–59.

14. Jha A, Lin L, Short SM, Argentini G, Gamhewage G, Savoia E. Integrating emergency risk communication (ERC) into the public health system response: systematic review of literature to aid formulation of the 2017 WHO Guideline for ERC policy and practice. *PLoS One* 2018; **13**: e0205555.

15. Kapucu N, Hu Q. Understanding multiplexity of collaborative emergency management networks. *Am Rev Public Admin* 2016; **46**: 399–417.

16. Davidson L, Carter H, Drury J, Amlot R, Haslam SA. Advancing a social identity perspective on interoperability in the emergency services: evidence from the Pandemic Multi-Agency Response Teams during the UK COVID-19 response. *Int*

J Disaster Risk Reduct 2022: 77: 103101.

17. Manninham-Buller E, Smith L, Hunter P, Duffy B, Greenberg N, Rubin J, et al. *EPR Health Protection Research Unit Annual Review*. Health Protection Research Unit in Emergency Preparedness and Response at King's College London, 2022.

18. Saunders J. *Manchester Arena Inquiry Volume 2: Emergency Response*. Home Office, 2022.

19. JESIP. *JOINT DOCTRINE: The Interoperability Framework. Edition 3*. JESIP, 2021.

20. Schilling S, Armaou M, Morrison Z, Carding P, Bricknell M, Connelly V. Understanding teamwork in rapidly deployed interprofessional teams in intensive and acute care: a systematic review of reviews. *PLoS One* 2022; **17**: e0272942.

21. Banwell N, Rutherford S, Mackey B, Street R, Chu C. Commonalities between disaster and climate change risks for health: a theoretical framework. *Int J Environ Res Public Health* 2018; **15**: 538.

22. van Berlaer G, Staes T, Danschutter D, Ackermans R, Zannini S, Rossi G, et al. Disaster preparedness and response improvement. *Eur J Emerg Med* 2017; **24**: 382–8.

23. Mansfield KE, Mathur R, Tazare J, Henderson AD, Mulick AR, Carreira H, et al. Indirect acute effects of the COVID-19 pandemic on physical and mental health in the UK: a population-based study. *Lancet Digit Health* 2021; **3**: e217–30.

24. Moynihan R, Sanders S, Michaleff ZA, Scott AM, Clark J, To EJ, et al. Impact of COVID-19 pandemic on utilisation of healthcare services: a systematic review. *BMJ Open* 2021; **11**: e045343.

25. Du L, Feng Y, Tang LY, Kang W, Lu W. Networks in disaster emergency management: a systematic review. *Nat Hazards* 2020; **103**: 1–27.

26. NOAA Science Advisory Board. *A Report on Priorities for Weather Research*. NOAA Science Advisory Board, 2021.

27. Szönyi M, Roezer V, Deubelli T, Ulrich J, MacClune K, Laurien F, et al. *PERC Floods Following 'Bernd'*. Zurich Insurance Company, 2022.

28. Stikova ER. 2.8 Disaster Preparedness. *South East Eur J Public Health* 2016; Special Volume (A Global Public Health Curriculum).

29. Subbarao I, Lyznicki JM, Hsu EB, Gebbie KM, Markenson D, Barzansky B, et al. A consensus-based educational framework and competency set for the discipline of disaster medicine and public health preparedness. *Disaster Med Public Health Prep* 2008; **2**: 57–68.

30. Seppänen H, Virrantaus K. Shared situational awareness and information quality in disaster management. *Safety Sci* 2015; **77**: 112–22.

31. Floren LC, Donesky D, Whitaker E, Irby DM, Ten Cate O, O'Brien BC. Are we on the same page? Shared mental models to support clinical teamwork among health professions learners: a scoping review. *Acad Med* 2018; **93**: 498–509.

32. McEwan D, Ruissen GR, Eys MA, Zumbo BD, Beauchamp MR. The effectiveness of teamwork training on teamwork behaviors and team performance: a systematic review and meta-analysis of controlled interventions. *PLoS One* 2017; **12**: e0169604.

33. Brooks SK, Dunn R, Amlôt R, Greenberg N, Rubin GJ. Social and occupational factors associated with psychological distress and disorder among disaster responders: a systematic review. *BMC Psychol* 2016; **4**: 18.

34. Brooks SK, Dunn R, Amlôt R, Greenberg N, Rubin GJ. Training and post-disaster interventions for the psychological impacts on disaster-exposed employees: a systematic review. *J Ment Health* 2018; **0**: 1–25.

35. Labrague LJ, Hammad K, Gloe DS, McEnroe-Pettite DM, Fronda DC, Obeidat AA, et al. Disaster preparedness among nurses: a systematic review of literature. *Int Nurs Rev* 2018; **65**: 41–53.

36. Nafar H, Aghdam ET, Derakhshani N, Sani'ee N, Sharifian S, Goharinezhad S. A systematic mapping review of factors associated with willingness to work under emergency conditions. *Hum Resour Health* 2021; **19**: 76.

37. Geier MT. Leadership in extreme contexts: transformational leadership, performance beyond expectations? *J Leader Organ Stud* 2016; **23**: 1–14.

38. Sweeney P, Matthews M, Lester P. *Leadership in Dangerous Situations: A Handbook for the Armed Forces, Emergency Services, and First Responders*. Naval Institute Press, 2011.

39. Kolditz TA. Research in *in extremis* settings. *Armed Forces Soc* 2016; **32**: 655–8.

40. Yammarino FJ, Mumford MD, Connelly MS, Dionne SD. Leadership and team dynamics for dangerous military contexts. *Mil Psychol* 2010; **22**: S15–41.

41. Mühlemann NS, Steffens NK, Ullrich J, Haslam SA, Jonas K. Understanding responses to an organizational takeover: introducing the social identity model of organizational change. *J Pers Soc Psychol* 2022; **123**: 1004–23.

42. Schilling S. Visualizing the ties that bind us: a cross-sectional thematic and visual analysis of cohesion across three British military formations. *Armed Forces Soc* 2022: 38: 1–28.

43. Guastello SJ, Correro AN, Marra DE. Do emergent leaders experience greater workload? The swallowtail catastrophe model and changes in leadership in an emergency response simulation. *Group Dyn Theory Res Pract* 2018; **22**: 200–22.

44. Edelmann CM, Boen F, Fransen K. The power of empowerment: predictors and benefits of shared leadership in organizations. *Front Psychol* 2020; **11**: 582894.

45. Weiss M, Kolbe M, Grote G, Spahn DR, Grande B. We can do it! Inclusive leader language promotes voice behavior in multi-professional teams. *Leader Q* 2018; **29**: 389–402.

46. Farahani RZ, Lotfi MM, Baghaian A, Ruiz R, Rezapour S. Mass casualty management in disaster scene: a systematic review of OR&MS research in humanitarian operations. *Eur J Oper Res* 2020; **287**: 787–819.

47. Ramthun AJ, Matkin GS. Leading dangerously: a case study of military teams and shared leadership in dangerous environments. *J Leader Organ Stud* 2014; **21**: 244–56.

48. Bergman JZ, Rentsch JR, Small EE, Davenport SW, Bergman SM. The shared leadership process in decision-making teams. *J Soc Psychol* 2012; **152**: 17–42.

49. Nicola M, Sohrabi C, Mathew G, Kerwan A, Al-Jabir A, Griffin M, et al. Health policy and leadership models during the COVID-19 pandemic: review article. *Int J Surg* 2020; **81**: 122–9.

50. Milligan-Saville JS, Tan L, Gayed A, Barnes C, Madan I, Dobson M, et al. Workplace mental health training for managers and its effect on sick leave in employees: a cluster randomised controlled trial. *Lancet Psychiatry* 2017; **4**: 850–58.

51. Brown AD, Colville I, Pye A. Making sense of sensemaking in organization studies. *Organ Stud* 2015; **36**: 265–77.

52. Gilbar O, Ben-Zur H, Lubin G. Coping, mastery, stress appraisals, mental preparation, and unit cohesion predicting distress and performance: a longitudinal study of soldiers undertaking evacuation tasks. *Anxiety Stress Coping* 2010; **23**: 547–62.

Chapter

51

Caring for People who Have Disabilities and Are Affected by Emergencies, Incidents, Disasters, and Disease Outbreaks

David E Alexander, Verity Kemp, and Tim Healing

Introduction

This chapter focuses on caring for people who have disabilities who are affected by emergencies, incidents, terrorist events, disasters, disease outbreaks and conflicts (EITDDC). The World Health Organization (WHO) estimates that there are about 1.3 billion people (one in six of the world population) with some degree of disability [1]. People in this population display a wide spectrum of seriousness of disability, but the way data are collected and the lack of a clear definition of the term disability make it hard to be precise about the numbers and proportions of people with serious intellectual or developmental disability compared with those with a range of physical disabilities, or with both. We use the definition of disability given in the Council of Europe Working Paper on COVID-19 (published in 2021), as 'a state that may make it difficult for a person to carry out certain activities or to interact with their immediate environment. It may involve dependency in carrying out activities of daily living' [2].

With wide recognition of the need to support this highly disadvantaged group, the UN Convention on the Rights of Persons with Disabilities was adopted in 2006 [3]. This Convention introduced a new paradigm for people with disabilities. It moved policy and policy implementation from a charitable and medical approach to one based on rights. Article 1 of the convention states that 'The purpose of the present Convention is to promote, protect and ensure the full and equal enjoyment of all human rights and fundamental freedoms by all persons with disabilities, and to promote respect for their inherent dignity'. Article 25 requires that healthcare provision does not discriminate against people who have disabilities.

Equality, Equity, and People Who Have a Disability

Whereas the application of principles of equality would ensure that all would get the same resources, application of the principle of equity allows for people to have resources tailored to their needs. The concept of equity is an essential part of support for people who have a disability, but can be hard to apply in practice. This is especially so in EITDDC.

People with Disabilities in the Humanitarian Context

The *Sphere Handbook* notes that 'in the humanitarian context, persons with disabilities are more likely to face barriers and obstacles to the physical environment, transportation, information and communications and humanitarian facilities or services' [4]. Sarah Polack and Phillip Sheppard note that people who have disabilities are 'among the most marginalised and socially excluded in humanitarian disasters and displacement' [5]. For example, Maria Kett and colleagues studied the impact of the West African Ebola crisis in 2014–2015 on people who have disabilities. They found that disabled people were excluded from planning and response processes, and that in emergencies their needs were not met and care workers had little or no awareness or training in how to address those needs; all this was on top of existing inequalities and discrimination [6]. They reported that 'knowledge, preparation, and responses to the EVD [Ebola virus disease] epidemic was often markedly different among people who have disabilities due to limited resources, lack of inclusion by many mainstream public health and medical interventions and pre-existing discrimination, marginalisation and exclusion' [6]. They also noted that 'interviews with other key stakeholder revealed a lack of awareness of disability issues or sufficient training to include this population systematically in both Ebola response activities and general health services' [6].

Article 11 of the UN Convention of 2006 [3] focuses on situations of risk and humanitarian emergencies, and requires States to take 'all necessary measures to ensure that persons with disabilities are protected under international law in situations at risk, which include armed conflict, complex humanitarian emergencies and natural disasters'. The Article sets out what its intentions mean in practice, including keeping all people with disabilities at the centre of planning, interventions, and responses, as well as ensuring that all appropriate agencies are engaged in these processes.

A subsequent document, the Charter on Inclusion of Persons with Disabilities in Humanitarian Action, aims to significantly improve the living conditions of people with disabilities during emergencies [7]. It was developed by over 70 stakeholders from nation states, the United Nations (UN), agencies, humanitarian aid organisations, and organisations of people who have disabilities. It has been endorsed by more than 100 stakeholders who have committed themselves to implement practical measures to ensure that people who have disabilities can benefit fully from humanitarian aid. Its goal is to include people who have disabilities in humanitarian action by lifting the barriers they face in accessing relief, protection, and recovery support, and ensuring their participation in the development, planning, and implementation of humanitarian programmes.

More recently, the Inter-Agency Standing Committee (IASC) published guidelines in its document *Inclusion of Persons with Disabilities in Humanitarian Action* [8]. It set out 'essential actions that humanitarian actors must take in order to effectively identify and respond to the needs and rights of persons with disabilities who are most at risk of being left behind in humanitarian settings'. The document is a key contribution of the humanitarian sector to the United Nations Disability Inclusion Strategy (UNDIS), which was launched by the United Nations Secretary General in June 2019 [9].

An important agency supporting and advocating for people with disabilities is the International Disability and Development Consortium (IDDC), made up of more than 20 non-governmental organisations (NGOs) working across the world on disability and development [10]. It has the objective of 'promoting inclusive international development and humanitarian action with a special focus on the full and effective enjoyment of human rights by all people who have disabilities' [10]. It works through task groups, one of which, the Task Group on Conflict and Emergencies, worked to raise awareness of the needs of people who have a disability among people who work in emergency relief [11]. This task group published a paper designed to 'inform and raise awareness about the UN Convention of the Rights of Persons with Disabilities and explain the significance of the UN Convention to the work of emergency and humanitarian assistance'. It is intended for use by NGOs active in humanitarian aid, including emergency aid, rehabilitation, disaster preparedness, and conflict prevention. It is also designed to assist policymakers and donors in the fields of emergencies and humanitarian assistance to include disability issues in planning, and includes recommendations on how the needs of people who have disabilities and their families can best be addressed in emergency and humanitarian crisis situations.

A key feature of the changed approach to people who have disabilities in disasters has been the concept that they should be at the centre of humanitarian action, both as actors and as members of affected populations. The international system has become more inclusive with the adoption of the 2030 Agenda for Sustainable Development, which affirms that no one should be left behind, and that people who are furthest behind should be supported first [12]. The Sendai Framework for Disaster Risk Reduction affirms the same principles [13].

Risks of EITDDC to people who have a disability

Many emergencies and disasters (especially complex emergencies; see Chapter 49 of this book) lead to extensive population displacement. There are several groups of people among displaced populations who are especially at risk from the many hazards associated with displacement. One of those groups includes people who have a disability and who encounter challenges, including those of physical access, separation from families or other carers and other social support, discrimination, lack of recognition or identification of their particular needs, and a lack of access to the specialist services that they may need [3,14]. Camps for displaced people are often constructed rapidly in available spaces and without planning for people who have a disability and who may find it difficult or impossible to access the services that they need [5]. The International Disability Alliance (IDA) also points to the increased discrimination and risk faced by people with intellectual and psychosocial disabilities, and the difficulties of providing the specialist care that they may need in a situation where meeting the needs of able people is already posing severe problems [15].

People Who Have a Disability and the War in Ukraine

In April 2022 the UN Office of the High Commissioner for Human Rights reported that it was estimated that there were 2.7 million people who have disabilities in Ukraine who were being put at risk by the war [16]. Many agencies – for example, the IDA [15], the European Disability Forum, and UN agencies – have pointed to the obstacles that people who have a disability are facing in Ukraine in attempting evacuation, accessing humanitarian assistance, and maintaining their safety. One frequently cited example of this is that people with disabilities are unable to access shelters in Kyiv and elsewhere, and therefore have to stay at home.

Meeting the needs of people with intellectual and psychosocial disabilities, neurological problems, and substance abuse has proved a serious challenge in this situation. The WHO is working with the Ukrainian Health Ministry to scale up Mental Health Gap Action Programme (mhGAP) activities throughout the country. Primary care workers and others are being trained using the WHO's *mhGAP Humanitarian Intervention Guide*, which provides techniques for the 'clinical management of mental, neurological and substance use conditions in humanitarian emergencies' [17]. The WHO aims to train over 10% of Ukraine's primary health care staff by the end of 2023.

People Who Have a Disability and COVID-19

In June 2021 the Council of Europe published a Working Paper, *Disabled Persons in Viral Pandemics: The Example of Covid-19* [2]. It opens by stating that pandemics tend to heighten the impact of inequality

because their effects are not just medical but have an impact on all aspects of human life and activity. People who are already disadvantaged by reason of, for example, disability, illness, lack of immunity, or poverty may find themselves disproportionately affected by the impacts of a pandemic. The Working Paper emphasises that 'ethics, fairness and equity demand that efforts be made to counter the discriminatory effects of the [COVID-19] pandemic' [2].

Nicholas Evans and co-authors describe the story of equity in COVID-19 as one of failure [18]. Glaring examples of this include the global inequities in availability of vaccine, variations in supporting employment, and the disproportionate impact on marginalised communities. In its evidence brief, the WHO reports how the inequalities in the social determinants of health have been emphasised by COVID-19 giving rise to stark inequities in health outcomes [19]. This is a matter that is raised by Chapters 9 and 52. Furthermore, it is reported that the effects of the pandemic have had an unequal impact on the social determinants of health, something that Richard Williams and his colleagues have characterised as the inverse socioeconomic gradient of the impact of COVID-19 [20]. (See also Chapters 42 and 52; the latter covers the public ethical aspects of this matter.)

The Council of Europe Working Paper, *Disabled Persons in Viral Pandemics: the Example of Covid-19*, notes that many people who have disabilities show an increased susceptibility to viral infection, and may also experience more serious illness if they become infected [2]. There may be reliance on others to do what is needed, and attendant worries that carers may succumb to the disease and be unable to provide care. People may be isolated, may not want to go out, and may not receive visitors such as carers. In addition, the day-to-day requirements of physical care for people who have a disability may make it harder to nurse them during an acute illness such as COVID-19.

The WHO working paper considers some specific aspects of the COVID-19 pandemic as they apply to people who have disabilities [2]. These are considered in turn here.

Care homes

Many people who have disabilities live in residential care. Several specific examples in Italy and the UK are cited in which people were discharged from hospitals into care homes to create capacity for COVID-19 patients without requisite testing, without supplying personal protective equipment (PPE), and without training staff in the use of PPE [2]. This led to the deaths of many residents, and some care workers carried the virus from one home to another.

Healthcare rationing

Frequently, at the height of the pandemic, overburdened hospitals were faced with the problem of how to allocate scarce resources, especially ventilators. Some hospitals used disability as one of the criteria for withholding potentially life-saving care – a solution that was illegal in many instances, and certainly was against the spirit and the letter of the major international agreements on disability mentioned earlier in this chapter [21].

In the UK in March 2021 the National Institute for Health and Care Excellence (NICE) published guidelines for critical care [22]. A triage device suggested was a frailty score that assesses a person's ability to withstand invasive treatment. Other nations adopted similar methods of assessing people for treatment. The guideline was withdrawn later in March 2021, because frailty is often associated with comorbidity, and frailty scales were found to deny treatment to people who have a disability based on predicted outcomes of treatment.

Ageism and ableism

COVID-19 has had a disproportionately severe impact on elderly people, who include people who have disabilities. In part this was due to the issue of ageism, in which younger lives seemed to carry more value than older lives. It also involved ableism, in which a person whose body is deemed to match some concept of normality has a higher value than one whose body does not achieve this norm and who might not, for example, be offered a ventilator because of this perception.

Workers who are people with a disability

Rates of employment of people who have a disability declined during the pandemic. Even with the increase in remote working, people who have disabilities formed a smaller proportion of the working population than before the pandemic.

Other forms of discrimination

These include:

- the negative impacts that restrictions on transborder commerce during the COVID-19 pandemic had on procurement of materials, including medicines
- discrimination due to some countries restricting pandemic-related payments to people who were already in receipt of disability payments.

The Need for Data

Information is often collected and used during a viral pandemic without considering the needs of people who have disabilities [23]. Data are needed to ensure that the whole population has access to appropriate health protection, to improve measures, and to ensure equity in access to and quality of care [24].

The WHO working paper considers and describes how people with particular disabilities are affected and might be helped during a viral pandemic [2]. The particular disabilities described are:

- cognitive impairment – intellectual disabilities and mental health conditions
- young people who have disabilities
- spinal cord injury
- osteoarthritis
- visual and hearing impairment
- other issues.

COVID-19 as a Source of Impairment

The WHO working paper acknowledges the potential long-term effects of infection with the SARS-CoV-2 virus, and the negative impacts that these are likely to have for many people who have disabilities. It notes the need for specialist support to assist their recovery from rare but serious effects of the infection, including damage to the central and peripheral nervous systems and to the respiratory system.

Solutions to Problems

The pandemic highlighted the need to develop changes in the long term to enable people who have disabilities to gain equitable access to services. These changes include legislation, regulation, and technology, as well as a focus on more customised solutions. The WHO has made a series of recommendations for actions that should be taken by people who have a disability, by governments, by carers, and by healthcare workers [25].

The Working Paper concludes by identifying three problems that particularly affect people who have disabilities during a pandemic:

1. triage that may negatively affect the priority for care afforded to people who have disabilities, in contravention of basic medical ethics
2. restriction or withdrawal of routine support
3. application of measures intended for the general population that do not take account of the needs of people who have disabilities.

Conclusions

Thomas Abrams and David Abbott state that 'disability is a way of life and it should not prevent people from living through a pandemic to the best of their potential and abilities' [26]. The principal of equity demands that people who have disabilities must have individual plans for their care. This is resource intensive, and requires multi-organisational cooperation across civil protection services. Therefore emergency planning must take account of the needs of vulnerable people, and people who have a disability must have a role in planning, preparing, and also delivering responses.

People who have disabilities endure negative experiences during emergencies. The Ebola outbreak in West Africa, the war in Ukraine, and the COVID-19 pandemic have all highlighted not just the needs of people who have a disability but also, sadly, the difficulties faced in meeting their needs, and the extent to which people who have a disability are still seriously disadvantaged in pandemics and disasters.

To quote the WHO working paper, 'Disability is not a problem: it is a challenge. Facing up to that challenge can help to build a better, fairer society for all' [2].

References

1. World Health Organization. *Disability*. World Health Organization, 2022 (www.who .int/news-room/fact-sheets/detail/ disability-and-health).

2. Alexander D. *Disabled Persons in Viral Pandemics: The Example of COVID-19*. Council of Europe, 2021 (https://rm.coe.int/ publication-disabled-persons-in-viral-pandemics-the-example-of-covid-1/1680a44c46).

3. United Nations. *Convention on the Rights of Persons with Disabilities*. Treaty Series 2515. United Nations, 2006.

4. Sphere Association. *The Sphere Handbook: Humanitarian Charter and Minimum Standards in Humanitarian Response* 4th ed. Sphere Association, 2018 (www .spherestandards.org/handbook).

5. Polack S, Sheppard P. Disability. In *Handbook of Refugee Health for Healthcare Professionals and Humanitarians Providing Care to Forced Migrants* (ed. Orcutt M): 134–7. CRC Press, 2021.

6. Kett M, Cole E, Beato L, Carew M, Ngafuan R, Konneh S, et al. The Ebola crisis and people with disabilities' access to healthcare and government services in Liberia. *Int J Equity Health* 2021; **20**: 247.

7. World Humanitarian Summit. *Charter on Inclusion of Persons with Disabilities in Humanitarian Action*. World Humanitarian Summit, Istanbul, 23–24 May 2016.

8. Inter-Agency Standing Committee (IASC). *Guidelines on Inclusion of Persons with Disabilities in Humanitarian Action*. IASC Task Team on Inclusion of Persons with Disabilities in Humanitarian Action. Inter-Agency Standing Committee, 2019 (https:// interagencystandingcommittee .org/system/files/2020-11/IASC% 20Guidelines%20on%20the% 20Inclusion%20of%20Persons% 20with%20Disabilities%20in% 20Humanitarian%20Action%2C% 202019_0.pdf).

9. United Nations. *Disability Inclusion Strategy*. United Nations, 2019 (www.un.org/en/ content/disabilitystrategy/).

10. International Disability and Development Consortium (www .iddcconsortium.net/).

11. International Disability and Development Consortium Task Group on Conflict and Emergencies. *Emergency & Humanitarian Assistance and the UN Convention on the Protection and Promotion of the Rights and Dignity of Persons with Disabilities*. International Disability and Development Consortium, 2007 (www.alnap .org/system/files/content/ resource/files/main/iddc-conflict-and-emergencies-taskgroup.pdf).

12. United Nations Department of Economic and Social Affairs. *Transforming Our World: The 2030 Agenda for Sustainable Development*. United Nations Department of Economic and Social Affairs, 2015 (https://sdgs .un.org/publications/ transforming-our-world-2030-agenda-sustainable-development-17981).

13. United Nations Office for Disaster Risk Reduction. *Sendai Framework for Disaster Risk Reduction 2015–2030*. United Nations Office for Disaster Risk Reduction, 2015.

14. Shivji A. Disability in displacement. *Forced Migr Rev* 2010; **35**: 4.

15. International Disability Alliance. *Through This Conflict in Ukraine,*

What Happens to Persons with Disabilities? International Disability Alliance, 2022 (www.internationaldisabilityalliance.org/content/through-conflict-ukraine-what-happens-persons-disabilities).

16. UN Office of the High Commissioner for Human Rights. Ukraine: 2.7 million people with disabilities at risk, UN committee warns. 14 April 2022 (www.ohchr.org/en/statements/2022/04/ukraine-27-million-people-disabilities-risk-un-committee-warns).

17. World Health Organization. *mhGAP Humanitarian Intervention Guide (mhGAP-HIG).* World Health Organization, 2015.

18. Evans NG, Berger ZD, Phelan AL, Silverman RD. COVID-19, equity, and inclusiveness. *BMJ* 2021; 29; n1631.

19. World Health Organization. *COVID-19 and the Social Determinants of Health and Health Equity: Evidence Brief.* World Health Organization, 2021 (www.who.int/publications/i/item/9789240038387).

20. Williams R, Kaufman KR. Narrative review of the COVID-19, healthcare and healthcarers thematic series. *BJPsych Open* 2022; 8: e34.

21. Bagenstos SR. May hospitals withhold ventilators from COVID-19 patients with pre-existing disabilities? Notes on the law and ethics of disability-based medical rationing. *130 Yale Law Journal Forum*, 24 March 2020 (http://dx.doi.org/10.2139/ssrn.3559926).

22. National Institute for Health and Care Excellence. *COVID-19 Rapid Guideline: Managing COVID-19. NICE Guideline [NG191].* National Institute for Health and Care Excellence, 2021 (www.nice.org.uk/guidance/ng191).

23. Kuper H, et al. Disability-inclusive COVID-19 response: what it is, why it is important and what we can learn from the United Kingdom's response. *Wellcome Open Res* 2020; 5: 79.

24. Boyle CA, et al. The public health response to the COVID-19 pandemic for people with disabilities. *Disabil Health J* 2020; 13: 100943.

25. World Health Organization, Regional Office for the Eastern Mediterranean. *Protecting People with Disability during the COVID-19 Pandemic.* World Health Organization, Regional Office for the Eastern Mediterranean, 2020 (https://apps.who.int/iris/handle/10665/332329).

26. Abrams T, Abbott D. Disability, deadly discourse, and collectivity amid coronavirus (COVID-19). *Scand J Disabil Res* 2020; 22: 168–74.

Chapter 52

Public Ethics in Emergencies: Learning from the COVID-19 Pandemic

Jonathan Montgomery

Introduction

This chapter explores the lessons that can be drawn from the ways in which bioethical governance operated during the COVID-19 pandemic. First, it examines the way in which our thinking is framed because this may substantially determine the policy choices that we make. We need to align the ways in which we think in order to respond collectively to challenges. Second, it explores the contemporary context of public reasoning. Assumptions about public information and communications from previous pandemic planning frameworks proved unreliable during COVID-19. The ways in which we talk about issues are crucial to successful public engagement as we coordinate responses. Third, this chapter examines the governance of ethical concerns. During COVID-19 the institutions that public health experts anticipated would protect against the risks of pandemics dissolved at the very moment when they were expected to come into their own. Lessons can be drawn to help us to prepare better for the governance of bioethical deliberations in future emergencies. If we can think more consistently, talk more effectively, and act more coherently, then we can hope to respond better.

Thinking in Emergencies: The Importance of Ethical Frameworks

Ethical frameworks can be used to increase ethical awareness, provide guidance for action, and improve deliberation [1]. They can also provide a benchmark against which to assess plans, including when holding individual people, organisations, and governments to account for their actions [2]. COVID-19 has proved particularly challenging because there has been no consensus on the best way to frame the ethical and political problems that we have faced. This section outlines four dimensions in which frameworks need to operate when societies face all-consuming emergencies.

Clinical Ethics

Typically, discussions about resource scarcity assume that responsibility sits with frontline clinicians to determine what care should be offered to which patients, perhaps with institutional or clinical ethics support [3,4]. Their actions are judged against ethical principles such as those proposed by Ezekiel Emanuel and colleagues of maximising benefits, treating people equally, promoting and rewarding instrumental value (although avoiding the risk that people's wealth should determine whether they live or die), and giving priority to those people who are worst off [5]. From a similar starting point, and building on significant previous conceptual and public engagement work, Douglas White and colleagues express concern about categorical exclusions and point out the need to avoid 'morally irrelevant considerations, such as sex, race, religion, intellectual disability, insurance status, wealth, citizenship, social status, or social connections' [3]. Their solution is a points system based on capacity to benefit. They propose adapting it to prioritise those people who are vital to the public health response, although the definition of this category and the rationale are unclear. Where scores are equal, life cycle considerations would justify the prioritisation of young patients so that they get an opportunity to pass through life stages.

However, the key ethical questions that COVID-19 makes us confront go beyond individual clinician–patient transactions.

Public Health Ethics

Public health ethics does not sit in opposition to the focus on specific patients, but it supplements it with additional consideration of the social and system contexts in which it rapidly becomes apparent that trade-offs may be necessary [6]. It emphasises rights to health and security, recognises interdependencies, and is concerned with exacerbation of vulnerabilities that are associated with public health emergencies [7–9].

These emergencies may include matters within the scope of health systems. Thus guidance from the Intensive Care Society in the UK sets out a capacity management matrix that identifies the responsibilities of leaders within the health system to provide mutual aid in order to avoid the need to consider the prospects of a patient surviving and receiving 'sustained benefit' if admitted to critical care [10]. More broadly, it is necessary to consider whether to limit some services in order to increase the resources of another (e.g., intensive care for patients who have COVID-19), or whether to prioritise one aspect of wellbeing over another (e.g., survival over mental health for people who are advised to self-isolate). There may be pressures to adapt regulatory systems, such as emergency authorisations for medicines with reduced efficacy and safety data [11].

Processes are important. Vaccination ethics recognises that the need for collective action requires oversight by a politically legitimate authority [12]. Usually authorisation is additional to consent. However, if the urgency of the situation is thought to justify mandatory immunisation, the decision of the legitimate authority may be alternative to patient's consent [13,14]. Similar principles apply to other interventions, including non-pharmaceutical ones such as quarantine and contact tracing. Good governance requires evaluation to see whether interventions can reasonably be expected to achieve their objectives [15], and that options are submitted for decision to an appropriate authority [16]. This body should be accountable for the reasonableness of its decisions by reference to criteria that are acceptable to the public who are affected, and ideally tested through some form of deliberative democratic process [17–19].

Public health ethics recognises that this involves deploying state power [20]. Health is not the only legitimate goal, and citizens retain rights against interference [21]. Governments should seek to use the least restrictive or coercive means to achieve public health gains [22–24]. Therefore public health ethics is underpinned by political theory [25].

Justice Approaches

The UK Pandemic Influenza Planning Ethical Framework, on which the response to COVID-19 has drawn, sets out the fundamental principle that 'everyone matters equally'. This egalitarian commitment does not require each person to be treated identically, but it does mean that their interests are the concern of us all, and of society, and that they must be treated fairly and with respect [26].

Generic social distancing requirements (including lockdown, stay-at-home, and shelter-in-place) may seem to treat everyone in the same way, but the practical and psychosocial impacts can be widely different. Some jobs enabled people to work effectively at home with reduced outgoings but stable income. Those people will have experienced net economic benefits. Other people have seen dramatic reductions in income, or lost their jobs, but they must continue to eat and pay rent.

Health and social impacts are also not uniform. Staying at home may not be particularly isolating for people with strong social networks that are maintained remotely through social media and video links. For lonely people and for some who have mental health conditions, the cost of social distancing may be much greater [27]. Equal treatment may not be fair or equitable if it has harsher impacts on some than on others.

Fairness may require that people who are adversely affected are compensated so that impacts are equalised. Some have argued that those most vulnerable to the adverse effects of the virus should get greater protection in order to equalise their chances of surviving [7,8]. Governments in rich nations have responded with expensive support packages, sometimes subsidising employers to keep people in work, and sometimes providing direct payments.

Justice considerations are particularly important when trade-offs are required, choosing who will gain and who will lose as well as assessing net impacts. An aggregate benefit may obscure very different impacts on individual people. COVID-19-related deaths occur mainly in older age groups, but it is younger people who suffer most directly from economic recession, and this raises questions of intergenerational justice.

The impact of the virus has been more severe in communities that have suffered historical injustices and to whom we may have an obligation to put right those structural disadvantages and restore an equality of respect and dignity. In the UK, people in Black communities have been more likely to become ill, and less likely to survive [28]. Death rates in the most deprived areas of England are more than double those in the least deprived areas [29]. The principles at stake can be articulated in terms of the proper response to vulnerability [30], health justice in realising capabilities [31], or the 'right to health' [32,33].

The Good Society

Finally, we should frame our thinking about public ethics in an emergency by considering our vision of the sort of society in which we aspire to live. The European Group on Ethics in Science and New Technologies argued that 'Good leadership in times of crisis is dependent upon protecting and promoting democracy, and human rights and the rule of law' [34]. It stressed the value of social solidarity, which it described as a 'social vaccine', and it noted how the pandemic had elicited acts of kindness that must be encouraged. The emphasis on solidarity and state responsibility can be contrasted with the focus on liberty and the limits of governmental power in the debates across the USA. In the UK, tensions have been apparent between libertarian approaches that shy away from state diktat, and support for collective and mutual responsibility.

We need to align these domains of thinking if we are to frame our collective response effectively. Clinical and public health ethical frameworks and decision-support tools should be consistent with a common understanding of the justice issues that is in turn compatible with our shared sense of the idea of a well-functioning society. This is very difficult to achieve in the current context of democratic deliberation.

Challenges of Public Reason

Effective public reason was particularly challenging during the COVID-19 pandemic. It operated in a political context in which trust in experts had been undermined, and a social context in which there had been an explosion of channels for public debate. Lack of transparency undermined confidence further, and the need to address societal taboos over discussing death and dying exacerbated the challenges.

Dwindling Faith in Expertise and Lack of Transparency?

The established practice of the UK when presented with a major threat is to convene the Scientific Advisory Group for Emergencies (SAGE). This brings together relevant expertise, tailored to the circumstances, under the leadership of the Government Chief Scientific Adviser. SAGE had been activated eight times since 2009, including in relation to threats from the Zika, Ebola, and swine flu viruses. COVID-19 required a much more extensive and intensive coordination of expertise. SAGE met 74 times during 2020 alone, whereas for Zika it met only five times in total, and for Ebola there were three meetings. Even during the H1N1 swine flu pandemic there were only 22 meetings between May 2009 and January 2010.

The complexity of COVID-19 can be seen in the additional expert groups that fed into SAGE, namely the New and Emerging Respiratory Virus Threats Advisory Group (NERVTAG), the Independent Scientific Pandemic Insights Group on Behaviours (SPI-B), the Scientific Pandemic Infections Group on Modelling (SPI-M), the PHE Serology Working Group, the COVID-19 Clinical Information Network (CO-CIN), the Environmental Modelling Group, COVID-19 Genomics UK (COG-UK), Health Data Research UK (HDR UK), the Children's Task and Finish Working Group, the Hospital Onset COVID-19 Working Group, the Ethnicity Subgroup, and the Social Care Working Group (SCWG).

Despite this mobilisation of expertise, and high public trust in science [35], the UK has struggled to maintain public trust in expert-driven decision making [36]. It was undermined by lack of transparency. Although SAGE first convened for COVID-19 in late January 2020, the membership, minutes, and papers remained obscure until May. Among the consequences of this early lack of transparency was establishment of a rival 'Independent SAGE' (Indie SAGE) in early May 2020. This group aims 'to provide independent scientific advice to the UK government and public on how to minimise deaths and support Britain's recovery from the COVID-19 crisis', and 'was founded with the intention of putting scientific facts and debate into the public domain'. The implications of this way of explaining the mission of 'Independent Sage' are, of course, that government advisers lack independence and therefore should not be trusted, and that there is a conspiracy against the public to keep them in the dark about the science.

Anti-Societal Media?

As COVID-19 hit, contemporary politics had become aggressively divisive, and public health measures such as mask wearing became treated as indicative of ideological allegiances. This trend might decrease as we reflect on the experience, but other factors are likely to present enduring challenges.

First, social media has dissolved, or at least diluted, trusted sources of truth in public discourse. During COVID-19, governments, scientists, and clinicians have struggled to be heard above the clamour of competing claims to be the voice of truth. Conspiracy theories abound, ranging from denial of the existence of the virus through its deliberate introduction (including from China into the USA or vice versa, by Bill Gates or by Big Pharma) to dissemination via 5G [37]. False news travels further and faster than scientific truth [38]. People who rely on social media for information are more likely to hold conspiracy beliefs about COVID-19, and those who hold such beliefs are less likely to exhibit health-protective behaviours [39], or to comply with government guidelines [40].

Second, demand for soundbites and slogans makes measured, timely responses hard to communicate. Simplicity is valued at the expense of accuracy on complex and uncertain issues. In the UK, public health messages were distilled into slogans such as 'Stay Home, Protect the NHS, Save Lives'. These are unhelpful to those people whose circumstances depart from the assumed norm, such as essential workers who must leave home to support the NHS, or those for whom economic or social circumstances make compliance unrealistic. However, debate about these issues is suppressed in the public sphere for fear of undermining the impact of the 'nudges' that are being applied. They are behavioural interventions rather than vehicles for conveying information, and their use gives credence to people who are concerned that they are coercive impositions rather than health advice.

Third, the desire of media outlets constantly to report success and failure and to hold people to account led to perverse incentives and premature certainty. From the early stages of the pandemic, governments felt compelled to promote numbers of tests without regard either to the reliability of the tests (some of which had to be withdrawn from the market) or to whether the results would prompt any action [41–43]. Testing became an end in itself. In the UK, high numbers of tests were not matched with efficient contact tracing or with effective encouragement of people to self-isolate. This departed even further from the scientific rationales for testing when it played into the need of the media to find people to blame for not achieving the promised number. The context of scrutiny therefore served to incentivise poor public health practice.

'Tragic Choices'

The third contextual element that hampered public reason during COVID-19 concerned the difficulties that officials face when exploring 'tragic choices', in which all of the available options present uncomfortable ethical problems. In private ethics, it is acceptable to privilege your own values or the needs of people close to you. In academic ethics, it is permissible to explore the taboo and unpalatable. However, in public ethics, the first is regarded as selfish and the second rapidly exposes officials to attack rather than debate. Academics and clinicians can readily debate matters such as prioritising scarce critical care resources without attracting criticism – it is the essence of their role [5,44,45]. Things are trickier for official bodies.

In late March 2020, the UK's Moral and Ethical Advisory Group (MEAG) discussed a draft document on critical care prioritisation that built on an evidence review of the significance of age in predicting prognosis. In the event this was not progressed, as it became apparent that there was sufficient critical care unit (CCU) capacity to avoid the need for rationing. At much the same time, the National Institute for Health and Care Excellence (NICE) was preparing a rapid guideline but did not include any data on the extent to which age was an independent predictor of outcomes. These events are linked by the understandable fear among public bodies of being accused of discrimination, as indeed they were [46,47].

We should be worried about discrimination, but the effect of these pressures was to prevent a public discussion, and to drive the work into an obscure section of a professional society website [10]. Given the evidence of poor survival of older people with COVID-19 admitted to intensive care, it is plausible to argue that, where resources are scarce, it is unethical to discriminate against young people by ignoring evidence of their better chances of successful treatment. However, such nuances are obliterated by the weaponisation of media slogans such as those typifying attempts to apply ethical guidelines as being 'death panels' [48]. There are important ethical issues to be explored, and survey work by academics suggests that there would have been broad support for maximising survival [49]. However, the media and political climate mitigated against public reasoning on this issue.

The dynamics of power and accountability link only very loosely and unstably with the concerns of public ethics as we have presented them. This presents formidable challenges in ensuring that politics and the wellbeing of the people come together. Therefore we turn to consider how governance has worked during the pandemic.

Governance and Coordination Problems

During COVID-19, anticipatory governance was exposed as inadequate [50]. The structures in place for bioethics governance [51] have largely given way to broader politics. Failures of government responses have led to ethical matters becoming subsumed into partisan politics and market forces, and subjected to the threat of judicial determinations. The weaknesses of our processes for coordination of society for the common good were exposed.

How It Was Supposed to Work

Viral pandemics have been on national risk registers for decades. The International Health Regulations of 2005 specifically provide for 'public health emergencies of international concern' (PHEIC). Although under protracted discussion since 1995, it was the challenges of severe acute respiratory syndrome (SARS) in 2003 that prompted the agreement of the new Regulations [52]. Further learning from the H1N1 flu pandemic and from Ebola prompted the World Health Organization (WHO) to assert the idea of a shared global sovereignty to better protect the world from threats of pandemic diseases [53]. Scholars identified the opportunities for 'adaptive governance' in which reflexive learning could enhance the ability of health policy to deliver outcomes that respond to the values, interests, and concerns of stakeholders [54]. Problems were modelled in late 2019 during a simulation exercise convened by the Johns Hopkins Bloomberg School of Public Health, the World Economic Forum, and the Gates Foundation.

The international experience shows that the bioethics governance could operate as anticipated. The WHO declared that COVID-19 met the criteria for a PHEIC on 30 January 2020, when 98 cases had been identified outside China across 18 countries, of which four had seen local human-to-human transmission (Germany, Japan, Viet Nam, and the USA). Since that

period, it has issued regular briefings and developed materials to support states in responding. By February 2020 the WHO had established a Working Group on Ethics and COVID-19, which published on resource allocation, various aspects of research ethics, and digital contact tracing [55–57]. In April 2020 an ethical statement from the UNESCO Bioethics Committee, a body charged with advancing a shared understanding of global bioethics that transcends cultural differences, stressed the vulnerabilities that COVID-19 was exposing [58]. In a number of countries the mechanisms for bioethics governance worked as anticipated. The French standing advisory Comite Consultatif National d'Ethique produced an opinion on ethical issues by 13 March 2020 [59]. An opinion on solidarity and responsibility in COVID-19 was published by the German ethics committee towards the end of March, and another on immunity certification was published in September 2020 [60,61]. In Italy the national bioethics committee published opinions on triage criteria in early April [62], and on matters of public health, freedom, and solidarity in June 2020 [63].

How It Happened

However, this pattern was not seen in the UK. According to the Global Health Security Index, the two best prepared countries in the world were the USA and the UK. Both have long traditions of public health and bioethical leadership, and both have extensive resources. The UK had undertaken a careful review of learning from the H1N1 flu pandemic [64]. It had publicly reaffirmed its commitment to the Ethical Framework that had been drawn up in 2007. It convened the MEAG, although its existence was not announced for many months after its first meeting, as a successor to the Committee on the Ethical Aspects of Pandemic Influenza. The Nuffield Council on Bioethics, the nearest the UK has to a national bioethics committee, published a very timely report, *Research in Global Health Emergencies* [65]. However, despite the resources of the UK, the expected mechanisms for bioethics governance failed to inform the government response effectively [66,67].

MEAG met frequently to discuss issues and provide informal advice to officials, but its minutes reveal little of the substance of that advice, raising concerns about transparency. Although COVID-specific statements of principle were issued for Scotland and Wales

[68,69], MEAG published no specific opinion. In part this reflects a divergence of views and approaches within the group that made it hard to reach a consensus in the time available. However, it may be connected with a concern about expert advice being used to criticise the government.

There was also a tendency of the governments in the UK and the USA to resist using existing expert bodies. Rather than building on the experience of PHE, a new Joint Biosecurity Centre was established and, in the midst of the pandemic, it was announced that PHE would be dissolved and a new National Institute for Health Protection established (subsequently set up with the title UK Health Security Agency). Despite the UK's long-established public health services, the government was quick to seek private sector involvement in personal protective equipment (PPE) procurement, data analysis, testing, and contact tracing.

This interplay between science and politics was manifested in the context of vaccine delivery, illustrated by the prioritisation of first doses for many people over the twin doses recommended by the manufacturers. In the UK a detailed scientific review led to an independent recommendation by the Joint Committee on Vaccination and Immunisation to take this step, in order to increase the short-term impact of vaccination in the face of a rapidly escalating wave of infections. However, this decision was quickly politicised. It was raised in an intervention by former Prime Minister Tony Blair prior to the data being clear, and attacked by French President Emmanuel Macron, who in turn was attacked in an outbreak of vaccine nationalism [70]. An apocalyptic post on Twitter suggested that the UK was doing exactly what the virus needed to create resistance to vaccines [71]. Vaccine diplomacy has become as much a political tool as a public health measure [72].

Conclusion

COVID-19 has shown us that we lack an accepted conceptual approach to balance and mediate the competing demands that the pandemic has made on states. The UK government has been unable to articulate the rationales for its responses, and has lurched, consequentially, between health and economic perspectives. The problems that we have discussed about suspicion of expertise and the degradation of public discourse are global. COVID-19 may have rekindled our faith in science, but it is also possible that rising mortality is blamed on failure of science. Some social media

platforms are beginning to recognise the damage that they have done to the common good by failing to address misinformation and allowing the algorithms that drive targeted dissemination to stoke conspiracy theories. The pandemic has exposed the weaknesses of our collective thinking, our readiness to discuss the issues rationally and effectively, and our ability to act effectively in the public good. Rebuilding effective public ethics in its wake will present a monumental challenge. We must attempt it, but it is imperative that we do not underestimate the task if we are to respond better to future pandemics than we have to COVID-19.

In the wake of the COVID-19 pandemic, there is an increasing awareness that health security will depend on improved recognition of the interdependence of human and animal health, universal access to healthcare, and reduction in inequality. Global health governance needs to develop accordingly [73]. In public ethics, trust in the integrity and ethical orientation of decision-makers is of fundamental importance. Unless people believe that decisions are driven by values that they recognise as appropriate, they will not take the advice given to them. Two principles follow from this. The first is that there must be openness and transparency about the ethical issues and approaches that are being applied. Without this, people cannot trust that decisions are ethically informed. The second principle concerns the democratic legitimacy of those values in pluralist societies. People do not necessarily need to agree with government decisions, but they do need to accept that they are reasonable and responsible. This requires deliberative processes that generate commonly accepted ethical guidance. These principles can be brought together by using the techniques of deliberative democracy to review the ethical frameworks that have been developed during the pandemic for revision as necessary. Government should then reaffirm its commitment to using them.

In the short term, this offers a mechanism for addressing the fragmentation of values that is currently seen in many Western societies. Whether it has an impact in future pandemics will depend largely on whether governments stick to their plans or abandon them. No amount of ethical preparedness can prevent leaders believing that the situation is unique and that the plan has to be ignored. Improved planning does not guarantee that the lessons will be learned, but this should not prevent us from trying. The success of our future responses to emergencies is probably more dependent on the renewal of democratic government than on any specific steps taken within public ethics. Thus the integration of clinical and public health ethics with wider concerns about social justice is crucial.

Acknowledgment

This chapter has been informed by collaboration with Professor Kenneth Kaufman and Professor Richard Williams in the production of our research paper: Montgomery J, Kaufman K, and Williams R. *Thinking, Talking and Acting about Public Health Ethics in the COVID-19 Pandemic* (9 April 2021). Faculty of Laws University College London Law Research Paper No. 4/2022 (available at https://ssrn.com/abstract=4144692 or http://dx.doi.org/10.2139/ssrn.4144692).

References

1. Coggon J, Syrett K, Viens AM. *Public Health Law: Ethics, Governance and Regulation.* Routledge, 2017.

2. Montgomery J, Williams R. Public health values and evidence-based practice. In *Social Scaffolding: Applying the Lessons of Contemporary Social Science to Health and Healthcare* (eds R Williams, V Kemp, A Haslam, C Haslam, K Bhui, S Bailey): 227–43. Cambridge University Press, 2019.

3. White DB, Lo B. A framework for rationing ventilators and critical care beds during the COVID-19 pandemic. *JAMA* 2020; **323**: 1773–4.

4. Arie S. COVID-19: can France's ethical support units help doctors make challenging decisions? *BMJ* 2020; **369**: m1291.

5. Emanuel E, Persad G, Upshur R, Thome B, Parker M, Glickman A, et al. Fair location of scarce medical resources in the time of COVID-19. *N Engl J Med* 2020; **382**: 2049–55.

6. UK Faculty of Public Health. *Tackling the Social, Professional, and Political Challenges of COVID-19: The Crucial Role of Public Health Ethics.* UK Faculty of Public Health, 2020 (www.fph.org.uk/media/2922/fph-statement-of-public-health-ethics-and-covid-19.pdf).

7. Buccieri K, Gaetz S. Ethical vaccine distribution planning for pandemic influenza: prioritizing homeless and hard-to-reach populations. *Public Health Ethics* 2013; **6**: 185–96.

8. Kaposy C, Bandrauk N. Prioritizing vaccine access for vulnerable but stigmatized groups. *Public Health Ethics* 2012; **5**: 283–95.

9. Lee C, Rogers WA, Braunack-Mayer A. Social justice and pandemic influenza planning: the role of communication strategies. *Public Health Ethics* 2008; **1**: 223–4.

10. Montgomery J, Stokes-Lampard H, Griffiths M, Gardiner D, Harvey D, Suntharalingam G. Assessing whether COVID-19 patients will benefit from critical care, and an objective approach to capacity challenges during a pandemic: an Intensive Care Society clinical guideline. *J Intensive Care Soc* 2021; **22**: 204–10.

11. Ortolani C, Pastorello EA. Hydroxychloroquine and dexamethasone in COVID-19: who won and who lost? *Clin Mol Allergy* 2020; **18**: 17.

12. Schwartz JL, Caplan AL. *Vaccination Ethics and Policy.* The MIT Press, 2017.

13. Harmon SHE, Faour DE, MacDonald NE, Graham JE, Steffen C, Henaff L, et al. Immunization governance: mandatory immunization in 28 Global NITAG Network countries. *Vaccine* 2020; **38**: 7258–67.

14. Cassimos DC, Effraimidou E, Medic S, Konstantinidis T, Theodoridou M, Maltezou HC. Vaccination programs for adults in Europe, 2019. *Vaccines (Basel)* 2020; **8**: 34.

15. Grill K, Dawson A. Ethical frameworks in public health decision-making: defending a value-based and pluralist approach. *Health Care Anal* 2017; **25**: 291–307.

16. Thompson AK, Faith K, Gibson JL, Upshar REG. Pandemic preparedness: an ethical framework to guide decision-making. *BMC Med Ethics* 2006; **7**: 12.

17. Daniels N. Accountability for reasonableness. *BMJ* 2000; **321**: 1300–301.

18. Daniels N. *Just Health: Meeting Health Needs Fairly.* Cambridge University Press, 2008.

19. Faust HS, Upshur R. Public health ethics. In *The Cambridge Textbook of Bioethics* (eds P Singer, AM Viens): 274–80. Cambridge University Press, 2009.

20. Gostin L. *Public Health Law: Power, Duty, Restraint* 2nd ed. University of California Press, 2008.

21. Kass N. An ethics framework for public health. *Am J Public Health* 2001; **91**: 1776–82.

22. Childres J, Faden R, Gaare R, Gostin L, Kahn J, Richard B, et al. Public health ethics: mapping the terrain. *J Law Med Ethics* 2002; **30**: 169–77.

23. Nuffield Council on Bioethics. *Public Health Ethics.* Nuffield Council on Bioethics, 2007.

24. Upshur R. Principles for the justification of public health interventions. *Can J Public Health* 2002; **93**: 101–3.

25. Coggon J. *What Makes Health Public?* Cambridge University Press, 2012.

26. Department of Health and Cabinet Office. *Responding to Pandemic Influenza: The Ethical Framework for Policy and Planning.* Department of Health, 2007.

27. Kaufman KR, Petkova E, Bhui KS, Schulze TG. A global needs assessment in times of a global crisis: world psychiatry response to the COVID-19 pandemic. *BJPsych Open* 2020; **6**: e48.

28. Public Health England. *COVID-19: Review of Disparities in Risks and Outcomes.* Public Health England, 2020 (www.gov.uk/government/publications/covid-19-review-of-disparities-in-risks-and-outcomes).

29. Office for National Statistics. *Deaths Involving COVID-19 by Local Area and Socioeconomic Deprivation: Deaths Occurring between 1 March and 17 April 2020.* Office for National Statistics, 2020 (www.ons.gov.uk/peoplepopulationandcommunity/birthsdeathsandmarriages/deaths/bulletins/deathsinvolvingcovid19bylocalareasanddeprivation/latest).

30. Bennet B, Carney T. Vulnerability: an issue for law and policy in pandemic planning? In *Law and Global Health* (eds M Freeman, S Hawkes, B Bennett): 121–32. Oxford University Press, 2014.

31. Venkatapuram S. *Health Justice: An Argument from the Capabilities Approach.* Polity Press, 2011.

32. Wolff J. *The Human Right to Health.* WW Norton & Company, 2012.

33. Tasioualas J. *Minimum Core Obligations: Human Rights in the Here and Now.* World Bank, 2017 (https://openknowledge.worldbank.org/handle/10986/29144).

34. European Group on Ethics in Science and New Technologies. *Statement on European Solidarity and the Protection of Fundamental Rights in the COVID-19 Pandemic.* European Group on Ethics in Science and New Technologies, 2020 (https://ec.europa.eu/info/sites/info/files/research_and_innovation/ege/ec_rtd_ege-statement-covid-19.pdf).

35. Wellcome Trust. *Wellcome Global Monitor: How Does the World Feel About Science and Health?* Wellcome Trust, 2019.

36. Newton K. Government communications, political trust and compliant social behaviour: the politics of COVID-19 in Britain. *Polit Q* 2020; **91**: 502–13.

37. Lynas M. *COVID: Top 10 Current Conspiracy Theories.* Alliance for Science, 2020 (https://allianceforscience.cornell.edu/blog/2020/04/covid-top-10-current-conspiracy-theories/).

38. Vosoughi S, Roy D, Aral S. The spread of true and false news online. *Science* 2018; **359**: 1146–51.

39. Allington D, Duffy B, Wessely S, Dhavan N, Rubin J. Health-protective behaviour, social media usage and conspiracy belief during the COVID-19 public health emergency. *Psychol Med* 2021; **51**: 1763–9.

40. Freeman D, Waite F, Rosebrock L, Petit A, Causier C, East A, et al. Coronavirus conspiracy beliefs, mistrust, and compliance with government guidelines in England. *Psychol Med* 2022; **52**: 251–63.

41. Service RF. Coronavirus antigen tests: quick and cheap, but too often wrong? *Science* 2020. Available at: https://doi.org/10.1126/science.abc9586.

42. US Food and Drug Administration. *Coronavirus (COVID-19) Update: FDA Revokes Emergency Use Authorization for Chembio Antibody Test.* US Food and Drug Administration, 2020 (www.fda.gov/news-events/press-announcements/coronavirus-covid-19-update-fda-revokes-emergency-use-authorization-chembio-antibody-test.).

43. Deeks JJ, Brookes AJ, Pollock AM. Operation Moonshot proposals are scientifically unsound. *BMJ* 2020; **370**: m3699.

44. Liddell K, Skopek J, Palmer S, Martin S, Anderson J, Sagar A. Who gets the ventilator? Important legal rights in a pandemic. *J Med Ethics* 2020; **46**: 421–6.

45. Newdick C, Sheehan M, Dunn M. Tragic choices in intensive care during the COVID-19 pandemic: on fairness, consistency and community. *J Med Ethics* 2020; **46**: 646–51.

46. Age UK. *Joint Statement on the Rights of Older People in the UK to Treatment During This Pandemic.* Age UK, 2020 (www.ageuk.org.uk/latest-press/articles/2020/03/rights-of-older-people-during-pandemic/).

47. Popescu D, Marcoci A. Coronavirus: allocating ICU beds and ventilators based on age is discriminatory. *The Conversation*, 22 April 2020 (https://theconversation.com/coronavirus-allocating-icu-beds-and-ventilators-based-on-age-is-discriminatory-136459).

48. Luthi S. Trump administration steps in as advocacy groups warn of Covid 'death panels'. *POLITICO*, 10 August 2020 (www.politico.com/news/2020/08/10/coronavirus-treatment-death-panels-392463).

49. Wilkinson D, Zohny H, Kappes A, Sinnot-Armstrong W, Savalescu J. Which factors should be included in triage? An online survey of the attitudes of the UK general public to pandemic triage dilemmas. *BMJ Open* 2020; **10**: e045593.

50. Lincoln M. A special self-image is no defence against COVID-19. *Nature* 2020; **585**: 325.

51. Montgomery J. Bioethics as a governance practice. *Health Care Anal* 2016; **24**: 3–23.

52. Fidler D. *SARS, Governance and the Globalisation of Disease.* Palgrave Macmillan, 2004.

53. World Health Organization. *Report of the Ebola Interim Assessment Panel.* World Health Organization, 2015 (www.who .int/csr/resources/publications/ ebola/report-by-panel.pdf).

54. Onzivu W. Reinforcing global health normative frameworks and legal obligations: can adaptive governance help? In *Global Health and International Community: Ethical, Political and Regulatory Challenges* (eds J Coggon, S Gola): 233–48. Bloomsbury, 2013.

55. World Health Organization. *Ethics and COVID-19: Resource Allocation and Priority-Setting.* World Health Organization, 2020 (www.who.int/ ethics/publications/ethics-and-covid-19-resource-allocation-and-priority-setting/en/).

56. World Health Organization. *Ethical Standards for Research During Public Health Emergencies: Distilling Existing Guidance to Support COVID-19 R&D.* World Health Organization, 2020 (www .who.int/publications/i/item/ WHO-RFH-20.1).

57. World Health Organization. *Ethical Considerations to Guide the Use of Digital Proximity Tracking Technologies for COVID-19 Contact Tracing.* World Health Organization, 2020 (www.who .int/publications/i/item/WHO-2019-nCoV-Ethics_Contact_tracing_apps-2020.1).

58. International Bioethics Committee and World Commission on the Ethics of Scientific Knowledge and Technology. *Statement on COVID-19: Ethical Considerations from a Global Perspective.* UNESCO, 2020 (https://unesdoc .unesco.org/ark:/48223/ pf0000373115).

59. Comite Consultatif National d'Ethique. *Ethical Issues in the Face of a Pandemic.* Comite Consultatif National d'Ethique, 2020 (www.ccne-ethique.fr/en/ publications/contribution-french-national-consultative-ethics-committee-covid-19-crisis-ethical).

60. Deutsher Ethikrat. *Solidarity and Responsibility During the Coronavirus Crisis.* Deutsher Ethikrat, 2020 (www.ethikrat.org/ en/publications/publication-details/?tx_wwt3shop_detail% 5Bproduct%5D=135&tx_ wwt3shop_detail%5Baction%5D= index&tx_wwt3shop_detail% 5Bcontroller%5D=Products& cHash=a37377aedcc6b8b1 31fce9a9146f9095).

61. Deutsher Ethikrat. *Immunity Certificates During the COVID-19 Pandemic.* Deutsher Ethikrat, 2020 (www.ethikrat.org/fileadmin/ Publikationen/Stellungnahmen/ englisch/opinion-immunity-certificates.pdf).

62. Comitato Nazionale per la Bioética. *COVID-19: Clinical Decision-Making in Conditions of Resource Shortage and the 'Pandemic Emergency Triage' Criterion.* Comitato Nazionale per la Bioética, 2020 (http://bioetica .governo.it/en/opinions/opinions-responses/covid-19-clinical-decision-making-in-conditions-of-resource-shortage-and-the-pandemic-emergency-triage-criterion/).

63. Comitato Nazionale per la Bioética. *COVID-19: Public Health, Individual Freedom, Social Solidarity.* Comitato Nazionale per la Bioética, 2020 (http:// bioetica.governo.it/en/opinions/ opinions-responses/covid-19-public-health-individual-freedom-social-solidarity/).

64. Hine D. *The 2009 Influenza Pandemic: An Independent Review of the UK Response to the 2009 Influenza Pandemic.* Cabinet Office, 2010.

65. Nuffield Council on Bioethics. *Research in Global Health Emergencies.* Nuffield Council on Bioethics, 2020.

66. Whittall H. *COVID, Transparency and Trust.* Nuffield Council on Bioethics, 2020 (www .nuffieldbioethics.org/blog/covid-transparency-and-trust).

67. Gadd E. *Is the Government Using its Own Ethical Framework?* Nuffield Council on Bioethics, 2020 (www.nuffieldbioethics.org/ blog/is-the-government-using-its-own-ethical-framework).

68. Rutter A, Bell D, Cole S. *COVID-19 Guidance: Ethical Advice and Support Framework.* Scottish Government, 2020 (www.gov .scot/publications/coronavirus-covid-19-ethical-advice-and-support-framework/).

69. Welsh Government. *Coronavirus: Ethical Values and Principles for Healthcare Delivery Framework: Guidance for Healthcare Services When Making Decisions During the Coronavirus Outbreak.* Welsh Government, 2020 (https://gov .wales/coronavirus-ethical-values-and-principles-healthcare-delivery-framework-html).

70. Hawker L. Take that, Macron! French President's 'ludicrous' Oxford vaccine claims brutally backfire. *Daily Express*, 3 February 2021 (www.express.co.uk/news/ world/1392542/Emmanuel-macron-news-covid-Vaccine-oxford-AstraZeneca-jab-coronavirus-uk).

71. Bieniasz P. Musings of an anonymous, pissed off virologist. *Virology Blog*, 5 January 2021 (https://twitter.com/PaulBieniasz/ status/1345195420033691648).

72. Safi M. Vaccine diplomacy: west falling behind in race for influence. *The Guardian*, 19 February 2021 (www .theguardian.com/world/2021/ feb/19/coronavirus-vaccine-diplomacy-west-falling-behind-russia-china-race-influence).

73. Gostin L. *Global Health Security: A Blueprint for the Future.* Harvard University Press, 2022.

53

Compliance with UK Government Measures During the COVID-19 Pandemic: Patterns, Predictors, and Consequences

Liam Wright, Elise Paul, and Daisy Fancourt

Introduction

In the absence of effective treatment or vaccines, the primary strategy for managing viral pandemics is reducing interpersonal transmission by changing citizens' behaviour. During the COVID-19 pandemic, governments implemented public health measures ranging from campaigns promoting regular hand washing, wearing face masks, and practising social distancing, to closing businesses, placing restrictions on travel, prohibiting household mixing, and implementing shelter-in-place lockdown orders. Although many of these measures were backed with the threat of fines or imprisonment, ultimately compliance requires active cooperation on the part of citizens, and some of these measures, notably closing businesses and implementing lockdown orders, entailed significant disruption to citizens' lives, with potentially large material, financial, and psychosocial costs.

This chapter summarises the early literature on the patterns, determinants, and consequences of citizen's preventive behaviours during COVID-19, paying particular attention to the role of socioeconomic factors in determining compliance. It also offers some general lessons that may be applied to future pandemics.

Patterns of Compliance

The COVID-19 pandemic generated and is generating an explosion of research on compliance using a variety of disciplinary approaches and a multitude of data sources, including online surveys and experiments, aggregate GPS data, direct observation (e.g., via CCTV), and other novel datasets.

One of the main sources of data on compliance during the pandemic came from the polling company YouGov, which carried out surveys on self-reported preventive behaviours in over 25 mostly East Asian and Western countries [1]. Although there was considerable variation between and within countries, self-reported compliance with behavioural measures such as social distancing was generally high. For instance, in Italy, one of the countries hardest hit by COVID-19, throughout 2020 approximately 80% of people reported avoiding crowded places, whereas in the USA, where compliance was relatively low, the figure was closer to 65%, with the number declining as the vaccine was rolled out. In the UK, shortly after measures were put in place for the first lockdown, around four in five YouGov respondents reported avoiding crowded places and practising improved personal hygiene (Figure 53.1A).

Masks were increasingly adopted in countries without established cultures of mask wearing, particularly when recommended or mandated by governments and health authorities [3]. Levels of compliance in previous epidemics appear to have been much more variable [4].

Although there is evidence that survey responses are correlated with real-world behaviour [5], self-reports are likely to be subject to social desirability bias, recall errors, and limitations in knowledge. For example, in one study from Japan, a country with a strong mask-wearing culture, 80.9% of people reported wearing a face mask, but only 23.1% were found to wear, take off, and dispose of the mask according to guidelines [6]. Nevertheless, the high compliance reported during the COVID-19 pandemic does not appear to have been driven by inaccurate self-reporting. More objective data collected from smartphones also showed steep drops in routing requests and visits to retail locations, transit stations, and workplaces during the COVID-19 pandemic, compared with before it [2]. Importantly, large drops in mobility occurred prior to the introduction of stay-at-home lockdown orders and in areas where no lockdown orders were ultimately put in place,

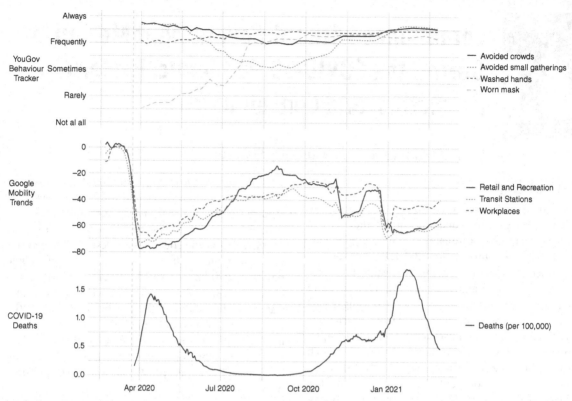

Figure 53.1 (A) Average self-reported frequency of practising preventive behaviours [1]. (B) Seven-day rolling average trends in visits to locations in the UK [2]. (C) Seven-day rolling average new deaths from COVID-19. Broken line represents the imposition of national lockdown in the UK on 23 March 2020.

highlighting the fact that behaviours were to a certain extent self-initiated (see Figure 53.1B).

Although compliance has remained high across the COVID-19 pandemic, levels did change over time [1,2]. Whether citizens would be able to maintain high compliance was an issue of considerable importance to policymakers. In early March 2020, as infection rates were rising across the UK, England's Chief Medical Officer cited the possibility of behavioural fatigue as a reason to delay lockdown in the UK. This was widely criticised by groups of behavioural scientists as being poorly elucidated and relatively untested at the time [7,8]. Published studies testing for behavioural fatigue during the COVID-19 pandemic generally found small and gradual declines in adherence with preventive measures over extended periods of the pandemic [9–11]. For example, one study using international data found progressively increased mobility and lower compliance with behaviour measures, controlling for differences in the stringency in lockdown measures and trends in deaths

across time [10]. Using data from the COVID-19 Social Study, a large non-representative panel survey of UK adults over the pandemic, we also identified a group (15%) of participants who show sustained declines in self-reported compliance – a figure that is likely to underestimate prevalence in the wider population, given the sample's bias towards individuals with high compliance [11]. However, a major issue in interpreting these results is that several potentially important factors changed across the pandemic, including knowledge about the virus and efficacy in following the rules. Furthermore, decreasing compliance may be attributable to other factors, such as economic necessity [8]. Sustained compliance was also found to be related to non-economic factors, such as age and personality traits [11].

Another important question for policymakers was the extent to which compliant behaviours co-occur within individual people – that is, whether people perform, or intend to perform, some behaviours and not others, or all behaviours or none [9,12–15]. In general, studies found that although compliance levels depended on the specific behaviour in question, behaviours were positively correlated within individual people, although some studies also identified idiosyncratic patterns, such as differences in compliance according to distancing and hygiene behaviours [9,12,13,15].

These results highlight concerns that individual people would offset one preventive behaviour with lower compliance with other behaviours – a phenomenon known as risk compensation. The potential for risk compensation was central to debates over mandating face masks in public places [16]. There is, however, little evidence that face masks had a negative impact on other behaviour. Although one study found that mobility increased after the introduction of mask mandates in the USA [17], this result was not replicated in similar studies [18]. Furthermore, a review of experimental studies from before the COVID-19 pandemic on mask usage found no negative impact on hygiene behaviour [16]. Two reasons why wearing masks may not have reduced compliance with other behaviours are that masks may act as a visual cue for people to remain vigilant, and that they may be a 'hassle factor', making activity outside the home less appealing [18]. Moreover, there is evidence from direct observation studies that people give mask wearers more space when passing them [19], which suggests that they can have positive externalities.

Concerns about risk compensation have also arisen with the rollout of the COVID-19 vaccine. An issue is that vaccines are much more effective than masks, and so the incentives to comply may be much lower among vaccinated people. Evidence from an influenza vaccination programme showed reduced compliance with some protective behaviours [20], but evidence from the COVID-19 pandemic is more equivocal. Although there is survey evidence that people's anticipated intention to comply following COVID-19 vaccination was low [21], using COVID-19 Social Study data we found no robust evidence of changes in compliance in vaccinated people compared with a matched non-vaccinated group [22]. However, an unresolved issue is that the existence of a vaccine programme could decrease compliance among unvaccinated people, if their motive for complying was to protect others.

Predictors of Compliance

A wide range of theoretical models have been used to understand the causes of high and low compliance

[23]. One often cited model among health psychologists and medical researchers is the Health Belief Model (HBM) [24]. The HBM posits that differences in people's health behaviours are determined by them weighing the (perceived) costs and benefits (perceived effectiveness, importance of health to themselves) of different courses of action against beliefs about one's ability to carry out these actions (e.g., through differences in skills and beliefs about self-efficacy). The main prediction of the HBM is that people are more likely to comply when (i) the risk of illness is high or (ii) susceptibility is larger.

During COVID-19, the empirical evidence in support of the HBM model's predictions was relatively strong, although most of this literature relied on cross-sectional data and used convenience samples, which may generate biases in associations due to selection effects [23]. In relation to risk of illness, fear of COVID-19 was shown to be related to greater behaviour change [25], and reducing personal risk was the most endorsed motivation for compliance [26]. This finding was supported by evidence from previous epidemics that perceived risk and susceptibility are related to more preventive behaviours [27]. In relation to susceptibility, several studies also looked at the role of age, given that this is a strong predictor of mortality risk from COVID-19. In general, studies showed greater compliance among older people, although this is not uniform [28]. However, despite men being on average more at risk from COVID-19, females on average complied more [28]. This association with gender has also been observed during previous respiratory pandemics [29]. One explanation for this could be that women *perceived* the risk to be higher than men did during COVID-19 [27].

The HBM also predicts that features of the environment or characteristics of individual people (e.g., social pressure, low self-efficacy, financial constraints, poor knowledge) can make it more difficult to perform a given behaviour, leading to lower compliance. Regarding external impediments, during COVID-19, complying with lockdown orders entailed significant loss of income for some people [8]. Although some governments sought to recompense employees for temporary loss of work (e.g., through furlough schemes), these measures were not in place in all countries, and typically did not fully replace all lost income, often involved bureaucratic obstacles, and had eligibility criteria that did not cover everyone (e.g., self-employed people). These financial challenges appeared to affect compliance – for example, reductions in mobility were greater in areas of the USA that received more pandemic-related federal income support, and an Israeli study showed that hypothetical compensation for isolation increased intentions to comply from 71% to 96% [30]. Lack of compensation was also suggested by members of the UK Government's Committee on Behavioural Science, SPI-B, as a reason for low adherence to the test, trace, and isolate system in the UK [8].

Another external impediment to compliance can be the actions of other people. In recent work analysing free-text data from the COVID-19 Social Study, the main reported barrier to compliance was other people violating social distancing rules [31]. Also important were social pressures from families and friends to violate rules, and the consequences of isolation for mental health and feelings of loneliness. Low knowledge was also a substantial hurdle to compliance, but this appears to be partly a result of failures in public health communication. Quantitative work has identified considerable misunderstanding about some government rules [32], and in our work a sizeable proportion of participants discussed difficulties in keeping abreast of changing rules and tracking differences in rules across localities.

Two features of viral pandemics are, arguably, not well incorporated into the HBM framework. First, prosocial incentives are important, given that for many sections of the populace their personal health risks can be low. Second, preventive behaviours are not solely self-generated or voluntary, but are mandated or recommended by authorities. Thus several studies have focused on the role of prosocial motivations, obedience to authority, legitimacy, and cooperation with the law in explaining compliant behaviour [33,34]. In one study, over 80% of respondents reported being motivated to socially distance in order to protect others or out of a sense of responsibility to the wider community [26,31]. Another study showed that geographical mobility decreased faster in regions with more interpersonal trust [35,36].

Regarding political motivations to comply, a number of studies, including some using longitudinal approaches, have looked at the role of confidence in government. They have found that people who had higher trust or confidence were more likely to comply [37], and this includes the studies that used longitudinal approaches [38]. These studies are troubling given the decline in confidence that has been observed in several countries. Although mask mandates and shelter-at-home rules appeared to increase compliance [39], there is not much evidence that fear of getting caught was what motivated behaviour changes [33]. Government mandates can act as signals as well as creating social norms that citizens feel compelled to follow. Lockdowns may also have created what is known as a 'strong situation', in which the range of people's behaviours is restricted and their expected behaviour is clear, which is argued to support compliance and thus reduce interpersonal differences in compliance levels [34].

Another widely studied part of the literature has been motivated by the increased political polarisation in Western democracies. Several studies suggest a role of partisan news sources (e.g., Fox News) [40], COVID-19-sceptical pronouncements by politicians [41], and belief or trust in science [42] in predicting compliance levels. Studies on the role of partisan media are bolstered by the ability to use quasi-experimental designs. However, it should be noted that even in areas with high viewership of partisan news, mobility still declined by a sizeable amount.

Consequences of Compliance

Although compliance with rules during pandemics is essential from a public health perspective, a key question is what impact such compliance can have on people and society. There is evidence from COVID-19 that behavioural mitigation measures can cause significant psychosocial consequences in the short and long term. Most of this literature focuses on the impact of lockdowns and stay-at-home orders, and emphasises increases in secondary stressors (e.g., financial loss, domestic abuse, loneliness, boredom, prolonged uncertainty, infection fears) as correlates and risk factors for psychological distress. A review of the psychological impact of quarantine in pandemics prior to COVID-19 found that people who had been quarantined reported more symptoms of acute stress disorder, anxiety, anger, post-traumatic stress, and exhaustion compared with those who had not been quarantined [43] (see Chapter 32 in this book). Among people who were quarantined, specific stressors included longer quarantine duration, infection fears, frustration, boredom, inadequate supplies, inadequate information, financial loss, and stigma.

There was also some evidence that psychosocial effects did not fully abate with the end of quarantine. Echoing these findings, a review of longitudinal, repeated cross-sectional, and nationally representative studies published from the start of the COVID-19 pandemic to December 2020 found that although loneliness, life satisfaction, and self-harm were relatively stable over the first year of the pandemic, symptoms of depression, anxiety, and psychosocial distress increased in the early months and then declined [44].

Certain subgroups within the wider population were more adversely affected than others. Some studies found that keyworkers (e.g., people working in the health and social care sectors, teachers, delivery workers) broadly suffered greater psychosocial distress [45], anxiety, and depression than the rest of the population during the COVID-19 pandemic [46], but other studies did not replicate this finding [47–49]. However, keyworkers were a heterogeneous group. Most research on the mental health of different keyworker subgroups focused on healthcare workers [50,51], who were assumed to be at greater risk for poor mental health and distress than the general population, due to their increased likelihood of infection. However, an analysis using data from the UCL COVID-19 Social Study found that of four groups of keyworkers, only those in essential services (e.g., utility, food chain, public safety) had consistently higher anxiety and depression symptom levels than non-keyworkers across the first 12 months of the COVID-19 pandemic [52].

In addition to the direct psychosocial costs of lockdown rules, there may have been long-term indirect consequences from COVID-19 through sharp rises in unemployment across the globe as countries entered economic recessions. Although some of these consequences were unavoidable costs of personal behaviour change during the pandemic, government policies mandating the closure of businesses are likely to have played a part. Some of the economic declines may prove to have been relatively short term, but they could nevertheless have long-term effects on individual people, known as scarring effects, particularly among young people (e.g., through worsening their trajectories of career earnings) [53]. Besides economic costs, there is also evidence that graduating during a recession can have long-term effects on health outcomes, notably mental health [53]. In the UK, the reduction in pay, working hours, and employment during COVID-19 was greater among young people and those initially in low-paid work [54].

Conclusion and Lessons for Future Pandemics

Common pandemic strategies such as quarantine, social distancing, and lockdowns are associated with people developing emotional and psychosocial distress [4], and the economic costs can be substantial and potentially persistent. We learned from COVID-19 that groups who were at particularly high risk and who might therefore require additional levels of support during future pandemic lockdowns were young adults, people with pre-existing mental health problems, people living with children, and people with lower household incomes. Many of these psychosocial and mental health consequences of the COVID-19 pandemic have to be addressed by mental health professionals in the long term.

The experience of the COVID-19 pandemic offers several lessons for planning future pandemic situations. Foremost of these is that, although there has been variation across countries and over time, it appears possible to achieve high compliance with preventive behaviours over extended periods of the pandemic. There is some evidence of behavioural fatigue, but it appears less widespread or immediate than was perhaps feared by policymakers, and less significant than other barriers to compliance, such as difficulty understanding complex, frequently changing rules, and the cost that compliance can have for people who are struggling financially. Furthermore, people are generally consistent in their stated compliance with preventive behaviours; individuals comply with all measures to similar extents, rather than complying with some measures but not others. This suggests that changing general motivation is important to influencing behaviour. To the extent that it has to be tested, there is little evidence for risk compensation, particularly as applied to masks. However, more research is required on the consequences of vaccination for other behaviours. Overall, large-scale behaviour changes can be achieved through voluntary action on the part of citizens, often with widespread support despite the huge toll for some individual people [55]. In times of emergency, people are willing to act as 'we' above 'me'.

References

1. YouGov. *Personal Measures Taken to Avoid COVID-19.* YouGov, 2021 (https://yougov.co.uk/topics/international/articles-reports/2020/03/17/personal-measures-taken-avoid-covid-19).

2. Google LLC. *COVID-19 Community Mobility Reports.* Google LLC, 2021 (www.google.com/covid19/mobility/).

3. Haischer MH, Beilfuss R, Hart MR, Opielinski L, Wrucke D, Zirgaitis G, et al. Who is wearing a mask? Gender-, age-, and location-related differences during the COVID-19 pandemic. *PLoS One* 2020; 15: e0240785.

4. Usher K, Jackson D, Durkin J, Gyamfi N, Bhullar N. Pandemic-related behaviours and psychological outcomes; a rapid literature review to explain COVID-19 behaviours. *Int J Ment Health Nurs* 2020; 29: 1018–34.

5. Gollwitzer A, Martel C, Marshall J, Höhs JM, Bargh JA. Connecting self-reported social distancing to real-world behavior at the individual and U.S. state level. *Soc Psychol Pers Sci* 2021; 13: 1–13.

6. Machida M, Nakamura I, Saito R, Nakaya T, Hanibuchi T, Takamiya T, et al. Incorrect use of face masks during the current COVID-19 pandemic among the general public in Japan. *Int J Environ Res Public Health* 2020; 17: 6484.

7. Hahn U, Chater N, Lagnado D, Osman M, Raihani N. Why a group of behavioural scientists penned an open letter to the U.K. government questioning its coronavirus response. *Behavioral Scientist*, 16 March 2020 (https://behavioralscientist.org/why-a-group-of-behavioural-scientists-penned-an-open-letter-to-the-uk-government-questioning-its-coronavirus-response-covid-19-social-distancing/).

8. Reicher S, Drury J. Pandemic fatigue? How adherence to COVID-19 regulations has been misrepresented and why it matters. *BMJ* 2021; 372: n137.

9. Ayre J, Cvejic E, McCaffery K, Copp T, Cornell S, Dodd RH, et al. Contextualising COVID-19 prevention behaviour over time in Australia: patterns and long-term predictors from April to July 2020 in an online social media sample. *PLos One* 2021; 16: e0253930.

10. Petherick A, Goldszmidt R, Andrade EB, Furst R, Hale T, Pott A, et al. A worldwide assessment of changes in adherence to COVID-19 protective behaviours and hypothesized pandemic fatigue. *Nat Hum Behav* 2021; 5: 1145–60.

11. Wright L, Steptoe A, Fancourt D. Trajectories of compliance with COVID-19 related guidelines: longitudinal analyses of 50,000 UK adults. *Ann Behav Med* 2022; 56: 781–90.

12. Breakwell GM, Fino E, Jaspal R. The COVID-19 Preventive Behaviors Index: development and validation in two samples from the United Kingdom. *Eval Health Prof* 2021; 44: 77–86.

13. Brouard S, Vasilopoulos P, Becher M. Sociodemographic and psychological correlates of compliance with the COVID-19 public health measures in France. *Can J Polit Sci* 2020; 53: 1–6.

14. Tomczyk S, Rahn M, Schmidt S. Social distancing and stigma: association between compliance with behavioral recommendations, risk perception, and stigmatizing attitudes during the COVID-19 outbreak. *Front Psychol* 2020; 11: 1821.

15. Wright L, Steptoe A, Fancourt D. Patterns of compliance with COVID-19 preventive behaviours: a latent class analysis of 20,000 UK adults. *J Epidemiol Community Health* 2022; 76: 247–53.

16. Mantzari E, Rubin GJ, Marteau TM. Is risk compensation threatening public health in the COVID-19 pandemic? *BMJ* 2020; 370: m2913.

17. Yan Y, Bayham J, Richter A, Fenichel EP. Risk compensation and face mask mandates during the COVID-19 pandemic. *Sci Rep* 2021; 11: 3174.

18. Kovacs R, Dunaiski M, Tukiainen J. *Compulsory Face Mask Policies Do Not Affect Community Mobility in Germany.* Aboa Centre for Economics, 2020.

19. Marchiori M. *COVID-19 and the social distancing paradox: dangers and solutions.* University of Padova, 2020 (http://arxiv.org/abs/2005.12446).

20. Reiber C, Shattuck EC, Fiore S, Alperin P, Davis V, Moore J. Change in human social behavior in response to a common vaccine. *Ann Epidemiol* 2010; 20: 729–33.

21. YouGov. *YouGov/Sky Survey Results.* YouGov, 2020.

22. Wright L, Steptoe A, Mak HW, Fancourt D. Do people reduce compliance with COVID-19 guidelines following vaccination? A longitudinal analysis of matched UK adults. *J Epidemiol Community Health* 2022; 76: 109–15.

23. Noone C, Warner NZ, Byrne M, Durand H, Lavoie KL, McGuire BE, et al. A scoping review of research on the determinants of adherence to social distancing measures during the COVID-19 pandemic. *Health Psychol Rev* 2021; 15: 350–70.

24. Rosenstock IM, Strecher VJ, Becker MH. Social learning theory and the health belief model. *Health Educ Q* 1988; 15: 175–83.

25. Harper CA, Satchell LP, Fido D, Latzman RD. Functional fear predicts public health compliance in the COVID-19 pandemic. *Int J Ment Health Addict* 2021; 19: 1875–88.

26. Coroiu A, Moran C, Campbell T, Geller AC. Barriers and

facilitators of adherence to social distancing recommendations during COVID-19 among a large international sample of adults. *PLoS One* 2020; **15**: e0239795.

27. Bish A, Michie S. Demographic and attitudinal determinants of protective behaviours during a pandemic: a review. *Br J Health Psychol* 2010; **15**: 797–824.

28. Perra N. Non-pharmaceutical interventions during the COVID-19 pandemic: a review. *Phys Rep* 2021; **913**: 1–52.

29. Moran KR, Valle SYD. A meta-analysis of the association between gender and protective behaviors in response to respiratory epidemics and pandemics. *PLoS One* 2016; **11**: e0164541.

30. Bodas M, Peleg K. Income assurances are a crucial factor in determining public compliance with self-isolation regulations during the COVID-19 outbreak – cohort study in Israel. *Isr J Health Policy Res* 2020; **9**: 54.

31. Wright L, Paul E, Steptoe A, Fancourt D. Facilitators and barriers to compliance with COVID-19 guidelines: a structural topic modelling analysis of free-text data from 17,500 UK adults. *BMC Public Health* 2022; **22**: 34.

32. Smith LE, Potts HWW, Amlôt R, Fear NT, Michie S, Rubin GJ. Adherence to the test, trace, and isolate system in the UK: results from 37 nationally representative surveys. *BMJ* 2021; **372**: n608.

33. Murphy K, Williamson H, Sargeant E, McCarthy M. Why people comply with COVID-19 social distancing restrictions: self-interest or duty? *Aust N Z J Criminol* 2020; **53**. Available at https://doi.org/10.1177/0004865820954484.

34. Wright L, Fancourt D. Do predictors of adherence to pandemic guidelines change over time? A panel study of 22,000 UK adults during the COVID-19 pandemic. *Prev Med* 2021; **153**: 106713.

35. Barrios JM, Benmelech E, Hochberg YV, Sapienza P, Zingales L. Civic capital and social distancing during the Covid-19 pandemic. *J Public Econ* 2021; **193**: 104310.

36. Jørgensen F, Bor A, Petersen MB. Compliance without fear: individual-level protective behaviour during the first wave of the COVID-19 pandemic. *Br J Health Psychol* 2021; **26**: 679–96.

37. Bargain O, Aminjonov U. Trust and compliance to public health policies in times of COVID-19. *J Public Econ* 2020; **192**: 104316.

38. Wright L, Steptoe A, Fancourt D. Predictors of self-reported adherence to COVID-19 guidelines. A longitudinal observational study of 51,600 UK adults. *Lancet Reg Health Eur* 2021; **4**: 100061.

39. Askitas N, Tatsiramos K, Verheyden B. Estimating worldwide effects of non-pharmaceutical interventions on COVID-19 incidence and population mobility patterns using a multiple-event study. *Sci Rep* 2021; **11**: 1972.

40. Ananyev M, Poyker M, Tian Y. The safest time to fly: pandemic response in the era of Fox News. *J Popul Econ* 2021; **34**: 775–802.

41. Ajzenman N, Cavalcanti T, Da Mata D. More than words: leaders' speech and risky behavior during a pandemic. *Am Econ J* 2020. Available at: https://doi.org/10.2139/ssrn.3582908.

42. Plohl N, Musil B. Modeling compliance with COVID-19 prevention guidelines: the critical role of trust in science. *Psychol Health Med* 2021; **26**: 1–12.

43. Brooks SK, Webster RK, Smith LE, Woodland L, Wessely S, Greenberg N, et al. The psychological impact of quarantine and how to reduce it: rapid review of the evidence. *Lancet* 2020; **395**: 912–20.

44. Aknin L, De Neve J-E, Dunn E, Fancourt D, Goldberg E, Helliwell J, et al. Mental health during the first year of the COVID-19 pandemic: a review and recommendations for moving forward. *Perspect Psychol Sci* 2022; **17**: 915–36.

45. Pierce M, Hope H, Ford T, Hatch S, Hotopf M, John A, et al. Mental health before and during the COVID-19 pandemic: a longitudinal probability sample survey of the UK population. *Lancet Psychiatry* 2020; **7**: 883–92.

46. Murphy J, Spikol E, McBride O, Shevlin M, Hartman TK, Hyland P, et al. The psychological wellbeing of frontline workers in the United Kingdom during the COVID-19 pandemic: first and second wave findings from the COVID-19 Psychological Research Consortium (C19PRC) Study (www.researchgate.net/publication/342251558_The_psychological_wellbeing_of_frontline_workers_in_the_United_Kingdom_during_the_COVID-19_pandemic_First_and_second_wave_findings_from_the_COVID-19_Psychological_Research_Consortium_C19PRC_Study).

47. Ayling K, Jia R, Chalder T, Massey A, Broadbent E, Coupland C, et al. Mental health of keyworkers in the UK during the COVID-19 pandemic: a cross-sectional analysis of a community cohort. *BMJ Open* 2020; **10**: e040620.

48. Iob E, Frank P, Steptoe A, Fancourt D. Levels of severity of depressive symptoms among at-risk groups in the UK during the COVID-19 pandemic. *JAMA Netw Open* 2020; **3**: e2026064.

49. Kwong AS, Pearson RM, Adams MJ, Northstone K, Tilling K, Smith D, et al. Mental health before and during the COVID-19 pandemic in two longitudinal UK

population cohorts. *Br J Psychiatry* 2021; **218**: 334–43.

50. Cai Q, Feng H, Huang J, Wang M, Wang Q, Lu X, et al. The mental health of frontline and non-frontline medical workers during the coronavirus disease 2019 (COVID-19) outbreak in China: a case-control study. *J Affect Disord* 2020; **275**: 210–15.

51. Rossi R, Socci V, Pacitti F, Di Lorenzo G, Di Marco A, Siracusano A, et al. Mental health outcomes among frontline and second-line health care workers during the coronavirus disease 2019 (COVID-19) pandemic in Italy. *JAMA Netw Open* 2020; **3**: e2010185.

52. Paul E, Mak HW, Fancourt D, Bu F. Comparing the mental health trajectories of four different types of keyworkers with non-keyworkers: a 12-month follow-up observational study of 21,874 adults in England during the COVID-19 pandemic. *Br J Psychiatry* 2022; **220**: 1–8.

53. Cutler DM, Huang W, Lleras-Muney A. *Economic Conditions and Mortality: Evidence from 200 Years of Data*. National Bureau of Economic Research, 2016.

54. Brewer M, Cominetti N, Henehan K, McCurdy C, Sehmi R, Slaughter H. *Jobs, Jobs, Jobs: Evaluating the Effects of the Current Economic Crisis on the UK Labour Market*. Resolution Foundation, 2020.

55. Ipsos. Most Britons continue to say they are following coronavirus rules; almost half believe lockdown measures are not strict enough. *Ipsos*, 17 January 2021 (www.ipsos.com/ipsos-mori/en-uk/most-britons-continue-say-they-are-following-coronavirus-rules-almost-half-believe-lockdown).

54

The Threat of Pandemics to Interwoven Material, Social, Health, and Political Resources: Conservation of Resources as a Strategy for Avoiding Repeating Past Failure

Stevan E Hobfoll

Resilience in the Face of Terrorism: Linking Resource Investment with Engagement

Since the attacks on the World Trade Center on 11 September 2001 there has been an emerging awareness of the nature of mass casualty threats and society's need to respond politically, medically, with potential police and military efforts, and socially. One might think that pandemics and disasters do not have a police or military component, and academics and public health officials have pretended to be apolitical in their approach to health crises and disasters. However, it is my thesis that this is not only a naive approach, but also one that led to what has mostly been a failure to respond effectively to the COVID-19 pandemic. Major health crises and disasters differentially affect people of different regions, social classes, races, and ethnic groups, because the distribution of resources is vastly unequal due to historical sociopolitical distribution of resources. Furthermore, because the allocation of resources after the threat or actuality of a major health crisis or disaster is the response of a sociopolitical process, nearly every part of the mental health, medical, and logistical response is orchestrated and implemented through power structures. Finally, major health crises and disasters have always been fodder for manipulating sociopolitical forces, sadly usually exploited, and often exploited for hate. To be clear, I believe the failure to recognise this was the determining failure in the global and country-by-country response to the COVID-19 pandemic, and the near complete failure of both the medical and mental health community to anticipate and response to the socio-political-

economic-medical interwoven ramifications of the pandemic.

We can better understand a complex social problem or condition by looking at past ones. The Black Death in the fourteenth century was the most devastating health crisis in human history, killing a sizeable percentage of the population of Europe and Asia (see Chapter 16). Historical records allow estimates that as much as half the population of Europe died of the plague [1]. As today with the response to COVID-19, religious influences were marked, and fanaticism bloomed in the USA. Renewed religious fervour and fanaticism bloomed in the wake of the Black Death. As occurred during the COVID-19 pandemic, the politics of political exclusion and blame emerged in the targeting of Jews, foreigners, homeless people, and Romani. Jews were actually blamed for the plague, both due to historical anti-Semitism that was deeply ingrained in Catholic theology and its millennium-long social manifestations, and due to the fact that Jews were less susceptible to the plague as a result of their cleanliness practices and quick and less invasive burial practices. Riots and murders of Jews were pervasive. In 1349 the Jewish communities in Cologne and Mainz were virtually annihilated, and hundreds of other communities were attacked and Jews slaughtered [2]. Since the Catholic Church was itself under assault for a failure to protect against God's wrath, blaming Jews diverted anger with the Church.

Using the worst world crisis exposes magnified social processes, and one might argue that our modern world is more educated and advanced. Therefore let us consider a modern smaller health crisis, namely the polio epidemic of the 1950s [3]. Poliomyelitis has existed since ancient times, but its presence in Europe and the USA increased in the early part of the twentieth century, and it became a significant health threat in the 1950s. Parents avoided sending their children to public spaces and swimming pools, and sizeable segments of the population were affected by this often devastating disease. Again, as with COVID-19, issues surrounding the vaccine became deeply politicised. In the early 1950s, US scientist Jonas Salk developed an injectable vaccine. By 1955, over 4 million school children had been inoculated, but this number was small given the level of threat and the difficulty in distributing an injection-requiring vaccine. Albert Sabin, an immune scientist who worked at the University of Michigan and then the University of Pittsburgh, developed an oral vaccine which could be easily distributed by non-medical personnel, enabling its distribution in school and other public settings. It was blocked for nearly 5 years, and in some areas of the country it was resisted thereafter as a 'communist vaccine', because it did not require physician administration. The Eisenhower administration resisted requiring vaccination or making government-sponsored programmes, due to it being an act of state socialism. Oveta Culp Hobby, the first Secretary of Health, Education and Welfare, aggressively fought any federal involvement or leadership in the polio response, associating it with communism. This impeded the saving of lives and reduction of the impact of this crippling disease for years, until a wiser and less dogmatic President Eisenhower acted to intervene, but the battle was hard won.

A Theory of Resource Loss: Setting a Guiding Strategy

This chapter maps out a theoretical framework that has been employed in multiple areas of stress research, and applied in particular to loss related to mass casualties. It applies it, in this instance, to the threat and loss that follow global pandemics, and it focuses on the COVID-19 pandemic in 2020–2021. Conservation of resources (COR) theory has been used across the continuum of levels of stress [4–7]. COR theory has been particularly applied to traumatic stress, and has been used as a framework for understanding disasters [8–10] and terrorism [11,12].

Conservation of Resources Theory

COR theory is based on several principles and corollaries that should be delineated in order to understand

the theory and move forward in applying it to mass casualties and to our more informed understanding of responding to pandemics. In contrast to other stress theories, COR theory emphasises the centrality of both loss and gain cycles, and an understanding of both is critical to understanding how populations are likely to respond to the multiple levels of a pandemic crisis.

COR theory begins with the tenet that people strive to obtain, retain, foster, and protect those things that they value centrally. People employ key resources in order to conduct this self-, social, and societal regulation in everyday life, and it becomes energised and particularly focused upon when they either are threatened with loss or experience salient loss.

This tenet places COR theory as a motivational theory that extends beyond times of stress and challenge, but one that becomes particularly powerful in times of threat and loss. It should be underscored that what is centrally valued is universal and includes health, wellbeing, peace, family, self-preservation, and a positive sense of self, even if these elements do vary in their expression within different cultures. Importantly, this also means that humans exist in, build, foster, and protect social and societal systems that enable these same valued ends, and, when either a threat or the response to that threat in turn threatens sociopolitical force, they are likely to be resisted, as has clearly occurred with the COVID-19 pandemic.

COR Theory States Several Key Principles

These principles have been supported in hundreds of studies of people who have been affected by stress and trauma. The principles and their corollaries have been delineated in detail in many earlier publications.

Principle 1: The primacy of resource loss

The first principle of COR theory is that resource loss is disproportionately more salient than resource gain. Resources include object resources (e.g., car, house), condition resources (e.g., employment, long-term relationship), personal resources (e.g., key skills and personal traits such as self-efficacy and self-esteem), and energy resources (e.g., credit, knowledge, money). The disproportionate impact of resource loss on psychological, emotional, and behavioural intermediaries and outcomes is seen in both the degree and speed of impact, as losses have a large impact and typically also have a rapid impact. The issue of speed of response does not exist generally in theories of psychology, but is common in biological theories and physics, where not only degree of impact but also speed of impact is often relevant. By stating the primacy of loss, we are paradoxically emphasising the central challenge of resilient responding, which is to offset the powerful, rapid, and often long-term impact of resource loss as it affects psychological wellbeing, behavioural responsiveness, social processes, and material resources.

Resource loss is primary across all stress levels, from everyday hassles to threats of death. That said, there are both quantitative and qualitative differences when stress threat and loss are more traumatic. Furthermore, when traumatic threat and loss occur communally in situations of mass trauma, it can result in dynamics that might not otherwise have the opportunity to affect individual people and at less traumatic levels. First, the process of resource loss following traumatic stress occurs with marked rapidity, as people's worlds can literally be altered fundamentally and at core levels of life, family, and society, as we have seen with COVID-19. Furthermore, as a pandemic, by definition, operates at the level of community, the extent of resource breakdown affects the full continuum of society, resulting in fundamental resource losses in people's and families' reserves, and across community and organisational structures. Indeed, if great enough or chronic, as has occurred with COVID-19, they are likely to quickly challenge and deplete the reserves established for treatments and interventions, as well as the structural guard-rails of a society, which can become rapidly overwhelmed.

Principle 2: Resource investment

The second principle of COR theory is that people, including how they are nested in organisations and societal structures (e.g., government, political parties), must invest resources in order to protect against resource loss, recover from losses, and gain resources. This resource investment acts to limit both immediate and anticipated loss cycles that occur on the psychological, behavioural, social, sociopolitical, and organisational and structural levels in response to stressful challenge.

Principle 3: Gain's increased impact under high loss conditions

The third principle of COR theory is paradoxical. Although resource loss is disproportionately more powerful than resource gain, when resource loss increases markedly, resource gain increases the impact of loss substantively. In other words, in normal stress periods, resource gain has few psychological, emotional, or behavioural impacts on people or groups. However, when resource loss accumulates, resource gain increases the impact substantively.

Related corollaries of COR theory include the following.

1. Those people who have greater resources are less vulnerable to resource loss and more capable of orchestrating resource gain, thus limiting negative outcomes and resource loss spirals. Conversely, those people with fewer resources are more vulnerable to resource loss and less capable of resource gain.

2. Initial loss begets further loss, as fewer resources are available for defence and coping, and this accelerates loss cycles.

3. Those people who possess greater resources can offset initial loss, and are more likely to hold reserve resources that can counter ongoing losses, at least up to a point, and that point is often significant, but may be overwhelmed.

4. When resources become markedly depleted, people enter a defensive posture that may include extreme and irrational acts, in order to conserve their few resource reserves.

The principle and corollary related to resource investment and gain are central to any understanding of our stress responses, as well as our ability to respond resiliently. There has been widespread failure of both scientists and governments to fully understand this. Each tends to divide the world into health versus the economy, when they are in fact entirely intertwined and essential to sociopolitical processes and the fabric of people's lives, and they posit that effective responses to the severe threat of a global pandemic involve an active process and one that demands personal, social, and societal resources that reverberate throughout other fundamental sociopolitical processes.

As a life- and economy-threatening pandemic results in profound resource loss, the means of protection of resources or their reinstatement in the aid of our responses places fundamental pressures on the self, families, and society. Indeed an effective response strategy is beyond individual people's capacity, and requires major influx of social and material support, as well as therapeutic and resource interventions from government and non-governmental organisations

(NGOs) that were never structured to respond to this level of crisis. We are not structured into competent communities on any level to respond to any 'worst ever' or 'among the worst ever' levels of communal crisis.

Fran Norris and colleagues [10] provided evidence illustrating clearly that following a brief period of altruistic sharing of resources, people and social systems become more neutral and potentially antagonistic about sharing resources, and move from a possible salutogenic honeymoon period into a potentially pathogenic and socially destructive competitive period. As the COVID-19 pandemic was inherently also economically devastating, and quickly became a bizarre but predictable factor in ongoing politics of populism and nationalism movements, the competitive components were rapidly made more salient than the health and safety of the public. Moreover, for those people who are most disenfranchised in a society, the altruistic period of resource sharing was never allowed to occur, and in Europe and the USA they were merely offered as sacrificial lambs, and even now have no priority for receiving a vaccine as they risk their lives daily (see Chapter 40 for more information from the UK). Families and care agencies attempted to take care of their communities, but having been offered limited political leadership and resources, their efforts have been minimally effective. The psychological, economic, material, and sociocultural consequences have been enormous, and continue to cascade at the time of publication of this book.

The processes of resource gain to aid resilience are also challenged by the nature of resource conservation. Specifically, COR theory states that individual people, families, and organisations have a strong motivation to withhold resource reserves, and consequently tend to be conservative in their resource investment. With a pandemic the course of which even experts could not accurately predict, resource conservation was a safer strategy, especially given that economic loss and, for some, political loss were seen as more easily definable. Even in instances of massive loss, there is motivation and logic in withholding resources for the unknown challenges that are yet to come. Even as depression, anxiety, belief in government, and a sense of personal and community agency wane, it is rational to withhold limited resources if people do not know what challenges and losses are yet to come. The threat to the reserves of people who are resource rich may have been theoretically challenged

by COVID-19, and the steep early stock-market plunges did spell possible economic depression. However, for people who lacked basic resource reserves on social, economic, or emotional levels, COVID-19 posed immediate threats that the strategy of shelter in place did not answer. Furthermore, to be very clear, societies demanded that staff of healthcare services, transportation services, public services, food processing, and delivery services should sacrifice themselves without being offered more than minimal protection (e.g., resource investment). Even when vaccines became available, only healthcare workers, and not these other working-class populations, were prioritised.

Defensive Responding Under Conditions of Lack of Resources

The fourth corollary of COR theory posits that those people who lack resources are likely to adopt a defensive posture to conserve their resources. It is this corollary that was most seriously ignored by government and health experts. Indeed, President Trump may have been the most visible person to understand this, even if he exploited it for his own political ends. That is, he seemed to recognise that the massive threat of resource loss would lead to a defensive posture that was open to being organised as a powerful political force. By adding the warning that health efforts constituted part of an ongoing threat to loss of freedom and his 'Making America Great Again' themes, he was able to garner powerful political forces to help to propel his presidency and his authoritarian tactics.

The fourth corollary of COR theory is fundamental to an understanding of mass casualty trauma, and became fundamental in the (mostly failed) efforts in places like the USA and Brazil, where fodder was added to the pandemic's fire. Following periods of personal and communal onslaught of resource loss, individuals, families, and organisations shift to a defensive posture. Although these postures often look magical or illogical, they do fit the imposed logic that can occur through grass-roots interpretations of events, or can be harnessed by political explanations offered by authoritarian leadership in particular. Under such circumstances a new logic occurs – the logic of defence – and it was this defensive posture, which quickly becomes irrational, competitive, and even violent, that characterised much of the public's response to the pandemic.

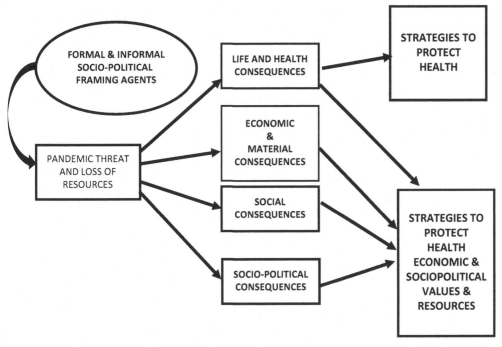

Figure 54.1 The impact of pandemic resource threats and loss on interwoven resource outcomes and the strategies that they engender. (Reproduced with the permission of the author.)

Conclusions

In conclusion, COR theory demands that we examine the full spectrum of potential resource loss and resources at risk in any given situation in order to predict and respond to psychological, social, material, financial, and sociopolitical outcomes (see Figure 54.1).

In the case of the COVID-19 global pandemic, health experts and academics had few of their own resources threatened, other than of course their health and even their lives due to COVID-19. Many of the population at risk faced more significant threats to their lives, and in addition their employment, ability to feed themselves and their families, and housing and shelter were threatened. Furthermore, authoritarian political processes spread the belief that health efforts were part of an ongoing process of taking away their freedom, with catchwords such as 'deep state' and 'socialism' added to the script. Given a death rate of about 167 per 100,000 in the USA, 200 per 100,000 in Belgium, 189 per 100,000 in the UK, and 180 per 100,000 in Italy, as Western exemplars [13], the risk of death was quite low for those people who were at high risk of losing their homes and their families becoming food insecure, leading to an obvious strategy of semi-cautiousness, at best.

When a threat to fundamental freedoms becomes the frame, however false that frame is, the choice of ignoring those threats to freedom becomes obvious. Thus as soon as grass-roots, right-wing forces and authoritarian leadership both framed the pandemic as blown out of proportion in terms of its threat, and framed the countermeasures that were offered by health experts as being efforts to impose socialism and rob the population of fundamental freedoms, the stage was set for what has occurred. That health experts and academics failed to see this as the likely outcome of unfolding events was both because they exist in siloed medical, psychological, economic, and political ivory towers, and because they logically saw themselves as immune from the dire economic consequences that were surely going to occur, and indeed have occurred.

References

1. Cohen SK. *The Black Death Transformed: Disease and Culture in Early Renaissance Europe.* Oxford University Press, 2002.

2. Foa A. *The Jews of Europe after the Black Death* (trans. A Grover). University of California Press, 2000.

3. Oshinsky DM. *Polio: An American History.* Oxford University Press, 2005.

4. Hobfoll SE. Conservation of resources: a new attempt at conceptualizing stress. *Am Psychol* 1989; **44**: 513–24.

5. Hobfoll SE. Traumatic stress: a theory based on rapid loss of resources. *Anxiety Res* 1991; **4**: 187–97.

6. Hobfoll SE. *Stress, Culture, and Community: The Psychology and Philosophy of Stress.* Plenum, 1998.

7. Hobfoll SE. Social and psychological resources and adaptation. *Rev Gen Psychol* 2002; **6**; 307–24.

8. Benight CC, Ironson G, Klebe K, Carver CS, Wynings C, Burnett K, et al. Conservation of resources and coping self-efficacy predicting distress following a natural disaster: a causal model analysis where the environment meets the mind. *Anxiety Stress Coping* 1999; **12**: 107–26.

9. Freedy JR, Shaw DL, Jarrell MP, Masters CR. Towards an understanding of the psychological impact of natural disasters: an application of the conservation resources stress model. *J Trauma Stress* 1992; **5**: 441–54.

10. Norris FH, Perilla JL, Riad JK, Kaniasty K, Lavizzo EA. Stability and change in stress, resources, and psychological distress following natural disaster: findings from Hurricane Andrew. *Anxiety Stress Coping* 1999; **12**: 363–96.

11. Hobfoll SE, Canetti-Nisim D, Johnson RJ. Exposure to terrorism, stress-related mental health symptoms, and defensive coping among Jews and Arabs in Israel. *J Consult Clin Psychol* 2006; **74**: 207-18.

12. Hobfoll SE, Canetti-Nisim D, Johnson RJ., Palmieri PA, Varley JD, Galea S. The association of exposure, risk, and resiliency factors with PTSD among Jews and Arabs exposed to repeated acts of terrorism in Israel. *J Trauma Stress* 2008; **21**: 9–21.

13. Wikipedia. *COVID-19 Pandemic by Country and Territory.* Wikipedia, 2021 (https://en.wikipedia.org/wiki/COVID-19_pandemic_by_country_and_territoryopened4-5-21).

Chapter

55

Using Social Media to Reduce the Risks of Community-Wide Emergencies, Incidents, Disasters, and Disease Outbreaks

Neil Dufty

Introduction

Social media consist of tools that enable open exchange of information through conversation and interaction. Unlike the traditional internet sites, social media manage the content of the conversation or interaction in the online environment. 'Social media rely on peer-to-peer (P2P) networks that are collaborative, decentralised and community driven. They transform people from content consumers into content producers' [1].

Over half of the global population are active social media users [2]. However, a limitation of using social media in community-wide emergencies, incidents, terrorist events, disasters, disease outbreaks and conflicts (EITDDC) is that many of the most vulnerable developing countries in the world have relatively low social media usage rates [2]. Apart from the low internet connection rates, a contributing factor is the level of total or partial censorship of social media in several countries [3]. On the other hand, an important factor in the recent increase in the use of social media, particularly in emerging and developing countries such as the Philippines and Indonesia, is the upsurge in smartphone ownership [4]. Additionally, there is evidence showing that the COVID-19 pandemic has significantly stimulated social media usage globally, due mainly to the limitations on people's mobility and to home lockdowns [5].

Another limitation in comparison with other means of emergency communication (e.g., newspapers, radio, television) is that social media usage tends to be skewed towards younger age groups [6]. These age differences generally extend to use of specific platforms – for example, people aged 18 to 24 years tend to use Instagram, Snapchat, and TikTok more than do older age groups [6].

Social media have been used extensively before, during, and after community-wide EITDDC, with

Facebook (launched in 2004) and Twitter (2006) platforms particularly utilised. David Alexander identified seven broad ways in which social media can be used in disaster risk reduction and crisis responses [7]:

1. as a listening function – social media enable disaster managers to listen to people affected by disasters
2. to monitor a situation – in order to improve reactions to events and to better help affected people by learning what they are thinking and doing
3. to integrate social media into emergency planning and crisis management – social media are used with traditional media (e.g., to issue warnings)
4. for crowdsourcing and collaborative development – information provided from social media by people affected can be very valuable to disaster managers (e.g., through crisis mapping)
5. to create social cohesion and promote therapeutic initiatives – social media can help people to feel part of certain initiatives and promote volunteerism
6. for the furtherance of causes – social media can be used to launch fundraising appeals for disasters
7. for research – understanding of social reactions to stress, risk, and disaster can be enhanced by using social media.

A large proportion of the research into using social media in managing EITDDC has focused on Twitter, even though the global uptake of Facebook is substantially higher [2], and despite the fact that Facebook has been used more extensively in disasters to date [8]. This is largely because Twitter has some unique characteristics that are, at this stage, more useful in disaster management and research [9].

A literature exploration of Twitter in disaster management, including that for pandemics, found several uses [9]. Apart from public communication and education, uses of Twitter in disaster management include providing psychosocial support, conducting risk assessment, threat detection, promoting situational awareness, damage assessment, and post-disaster evaluation.

Of concern to emergency managers and health service providers is that social media can attract fake news and false information, given the number of people who are creating information at the same time, often with different interests and viewpoints. Outdated, inaccurate, or false information can complicate situational awareness of an incident and consequently hinder or slow response efforts [10]. Authentication of information from credible sources is therefore crucial to effective responses and recovery, and to allaying possible high levels of public distrust of social media [11].

Within this context, the next section of this chapter examines the uses of social media for managing three serious diseases – influenza, Ebola virus disease (Ebola), and COVID-19. These three illnesses were chosen due to their variation in spatial coverage, seasonality, and challenges for affected communities and healthcare providers.

Social Media and Community-Wide Diseases

The use of social media for managing the three diseases is largely in concert with that identified for other hazards. Much of the social media use by authorities has been for risk communication and crisis communication related to these diseases [12]. However, for the Ebola outbreaks in 2013–2016 in west African countries there was limited use of social media for communications, due to the low uptake rate. Moreover, according to some research, community engagement for 'rapid assessment, contact tracing, isolation of infected individuals, safe cremation/burial of the deceased and access to laboratory services which were hampered initially' could have been improved if there were higher rates of social media use [13].

In contrast, worldwide between 30 September and 29 October 2014 there were approximately 26 million tweets that contained the word 'Ebola', many of which originated from news outlets [14].

As is the case for other public safety hazards, social media offer more uses than health risk and crisis communications. For example, an analysis of 81 studies

found five overarching public health themes concerning the role of online social media platforms and COVID-19 [15]. These themes focused on:

1. surveying public attitudes
2. identifying infodemics
3. assessing mental health, and detecting or predicting COVID-19 cases
4. analysing government responses to the pandemic
5. evaluating the quality of health information in prevention education videos.

There are numerous examples of research that gauged the attitudes and emotions that were expressed by social media users regarding the three diseases. For example, a study was conducted in order to better understand blame related to the 2014-16 Ebola outbreaks. The study concluded that 'In the early stage of the epidemic, blame directed at the affected populations was more prominent. However, during the peak of the outbreak, the increasingly perceived threat of inter-continental spread was accompanied by a progressively proximal blame tendency, directed at figures with whom the social media users had pre-existing biopolitical frustrations' [16].

A total of 167,073 unique English tweets were analysed in order to learn about public sentiment towards the overall COVID-19 pandemic and its interventions. The findings were divided into four categories – origin, source, regional and global effects on people and society, and methods of reducing transmission. Tweets regarding economic loss had the highest mean number of likes, whereas travel bans and warnings had the lowest number of likes [17].

Sentiments about vaccination can strongly affect vaccination decisions made by individual people. Online social media provide unprecedented access to data, allowing inexpensive and efficient tools to identify target areas for intervention efforts and to evaluate their effectiveness.

The analysis of attitudes and emotions enables public health authorities to explore social media users' understanding of epidemics in order to better grasp their concerns, preoccupations, and sentiments and adjust the online communication strategies targeting the public.

The term infodemic – a combination of information and epidemic – refers to rapid and widespread dissemination of both accurate and inaccurate information about an epidemic. Several studies have investigated infodemics stimulated by social media for illnesses, including COVID-19 [15]. This research can 'help to design more efficient epidemic models accounting for social behaviour and to design more effective and tailored communication strategies in time of crisis' [18].

Social media are increasingly becoming a tool for predicting and detecting outbreaks, and providing resultant early warnings for the public. For influenza, social media analysis 'represents an advancement in accuracy of assessments, prediction of future flu activity accurately and an ability to combine big social data and observed health data to build predictive models' [19].

Data collected via social media sites have typically been used as a complementary source of surveillance data for existing outpatient, hospital, and laboratory-based systems. This can be extremely useful because traditional surveillance systems rely on tracking individual people who are seeking care, and they tend to underestimate the total disease burden due to lack of representativeness. However, digital surveillance systems need to be developed in ways that avoid the numerous potential pitfalls associated with biases, and to meet ethical standards.

Social media data can be used to detect the spread of epidemics or pandemics, such as influenza, Ebola, or COVID-19, which can assist in providing early warnings. New techniques for analysis of search engine logs and social media data can be used to obtain real-time analysis, creating better services [20].

There is increasing evidence to show that social media can elicit positive behaviour changes from the public, and therefore help to reduce the risk of infection in the population. For example, one study examined the relationships between social media use, social media as a source of health information, and influenza vaccination status [21]. The results indicated that people who used Twitter and Facebook as sources of health information were more likely to be vaccinated than users who did not use Twitter or Facebook as sources of such information.

Social media are an excellent means of evaluating uptake of health messages and the effectiveness of education programmes. An example of the potency of social media in this respect is described in a study from the USA [22]:

African Americans and Hispanics have significantly lower vaccination rates, and large-scale education campaigns have had difficulty increasing vaccination among these two groups. This study assessed the feasibility of delivering a flu vaccination promotion campaign using influencers, and

examined shifts in social norms regarding flu vaccine acceptability after a social media micro influencer campaign. Influencers were asked to choose from vetted messages and create their own original content promoting flu vaccination, which was posted to their social media pages. Content was intentionally unbranded to ensure that it aligned with the look and feel of their pages. Cross-sectional pre- and post-campaign surveys were conducted within regions that received the campaign and control regions to examine potential campaign impact. Digital metrics assessed campaign exposure. Overall, 117 influencers generated 69,495 engagements. Results from the region that received the campaign showed significant increases in positive beliefs about the flu vaccine, and significant decreases in negative community attitudes toward the vaccine. This study suggests that flu campaigns using a ground-up rather than top-down approach can feasibly reach at-risk groups with lower vaccination rates, and shows the potentials of using an influencer-based model to communicate information about flu vaccination on a large scale.

Building Community Resilience

There is emerging evidence that social media can help to build community resilience to all EITDDCs. The main way that this is achieved is through the role of social capital formation via the development of the social networks encased in social media [23].

Social capital has been defined as the 'networks, norms, and social trust that facilitate coordination and cooperation for mutual benefit' [24]. It consists of those bonds created by belonging to a group that instils trust, solidarity, and cooperation among members.

Disaster scholars have consistently demonstrated that communities with strong levels of social capital are better at recovering after a disaster. Daniel Aldrich identified three mechanisms by which social capital contributes to resilience before, during, and after disasters [25].

1. Deep levels of social capital serve as informal insurance and promote mutual assistance after a disaster.

2. Dense and numerous social ties help survivors to solve collective action problems that stymie rehabilitation.

3. Strong social ties strengthen the voices of survivors and decrease the probability of leaving.

Online social networks can support and enhance face-to-face networks, and have been found to be critical before, during, and after a disaster. For example, in a study of the impacts of Hurricane Harvey on

Houston, USA, it was found that 'hyperlocal social media activity was a statistically significant predictor of the rate of rebuilding in these geographically based online communities' [26]. 'These findings suggest that policy and decision-makers should invest into online and offline hyperlocal social networks well before a disaster strikes, and leverage resources and legislation to maintain and strengthen the telecommunications and energy infrastructure that supports access to social media and telecommunications infrastructure during a time of crisis' [26].

With the health requirement to physically isolate in pandemics, such as the COVID-19 pandemic, the ability of social media to enable online social networks to help people to respond to and recover from the crises becomes critical. Studies have shown the role of social capital in reducing mortality from COVID-19 and obtaining other positive health outcomes, such as high vaccination rates [27]. Although the effects of social media-based social capital are less well understood, 'digital and other mediated forms of communication must be utilised as a means of creating and nurturing social connections' [28]. Furthermore [29], 'considerations of social capital – including virtual community building, fostering solidarity between high-risk and low-risk groups, and trust building between decision-makers, healthcare workers, and the public – offer a powerful frame of reference for understanding how response and recovery programs can be best implemented to effectively ensure the inclusive provision of COVID-19 health services'.

Discussion

There are five general principles that emerge from the science.

1. Social media are important risk communication and crisis communication tools for community-wide EITDDC that should be used in conjunction with traditional means such as media releases, websites, and fact sheets.
2. Emergency management authorities and health service professionals need to manage social media misinformation infodemics and fake news by providing consistent, credible, and clear messaging before, during, and after a crisis.
3. Social media can provide authorities with insights that assist with predicting crises, and with providing early warnings and responses, and also promote recovery related to crises.

4. Social media are a useful conduit for promoting risk reduction interventions, including vaccinations.
5. Social media provide a means of forming social capital, which has been shown to build community resilience to disasters and illnesses.

The short-term impacts of using social media in community-wide EITDDC are well summarised by the following quote [20]:

> Social media is an omnipresent part of today's world. We suggest that moving forward, it should be considered as a part of the larger body of preventative social tools that can be used to spread awareness and mitigate the disease, and be synergistically used with other measures and policies to be most effective. Although misinformation, amongst other factors, are large drawbacks in the usage of social media during endemics and pandemics, it is vital to understand how we can use this tool to benefit public health, especially during an infectious disease outbreak.

Although there is extensive evidence to show that social media help to amplify health messages, their direct impact on appropriate behaviours is more problematic, and more research is required. 'Understanding the complexities between social media and subsequent changes in behaviour in the context of infectious disease can aid the advancement of public policy regarding social media utilisation in healthcare communication' [20].

In the longer term, social media are highly likely to be extended to many of those countries and communities that currently have low uptake rates [2]. Hopefully this will include developing countries, particularly in Africa and Asia, many of which are vulnerable in a complex hazardscape. Even in developed countries such as the USA, there are poorer people who should be able to access social media in the future as smartphones and mobile connections become more affordable [6].

Social media platforms are constantly evolving and have provided support in EITDDC (e.g., Facebook Local Alerts). 'Social media companies may wish to have empirical information to better understand how their platforms do and could aid in other emergency situations' [20]. Furthermore, in the future, new social media platforms are likely to become available, and they should be reviewed by emergency managers and health service providers to assess their potential for use in crises.

In terms of the implications for interventions, there have been multiple studies examining aspects of social media use in EITDDCs, yet few that synthesise the research into meaningful and digestible advice for emergency managers and health service providers [15]. There are few books or meta-analyses on the research. This is mainly due to the disparate nature of investigations and the rapidly evolving social media platforms and analytical technologies, which mean that a research book could quickly become dated.

A major practical aspect of implementing the principles identified in this chapter is to provide training and guidance on the use of social media for emergency managers and health service providers. This training is widespread around the world, although it tends to be confined to the use of social media in risk and crisis communication, mainly due to the apparent disconnect between research and practice. However, there are some examples of guidance that encapsulates some of the opportunities that social media provide [30].

Conclusion

This chapter explores the use of social media in community-wide EITDDCs. It shows that the global reach of social media is rapidly increasing, ironically spurred on by the COVID-19 pandemic. Due to poverty and social media censorship in some countries, some vulnerable communities are excluded from social media uptake.

Social media have numerous uses that can support authorities in communicating and better understanding risk prevention and emergency responses. However, this value is tempered by the misinformation and fake news that are spread via social media, leading to distrust in them as credible news sources.

Social media also have benefits in forming social capital, which has been found to build resilience to crises. Further research is required in order to understand these relationships in specific communities and situations.

Research into applying social media in EITDDC is growing and rapidly evolving with new social platforms and analytical technologies. However, there appears to be a disconnect between the research and practical training of emergency managers and health service providers in the full gamut of social media use.

References

1. Keim ME, Noji E. Emergent use of social media: a new age of opportunity for disaster resilience. *Am J Disaster Med* 2011; **6**: 47–54.

2. We Are Social. *Digital 2022*. We Are Social, 2022 (https://wearesocial.com/uk/blog/2022/01/digital-2022/).

3. Shahbaz A, Funk A. *Freedom on the Net 2019: The Crisis of Social Media*. Freedom House, 2019 (https://freedomhouse.org/report/freedom-net/2019/crisis-social-media).

4. Pew Research Center. *Smartphone Ownership and Internet Usage Continues to Climb in Emerging Economies*. Pew Research Center, 2016 (www.pewglobal.org/2016/02/22/smartphone-ownership-and-internet-usage-continues-to-climb-in-emerging-economies/).

5. We Are Social. *Digital 2021: April Global Snapshot Report*. We Are Social, 2021 (https://wearesocial.com/blog/2021/04/60-percent-of-the-worlds-population-is-now-online).

6. Pew Research Center. *Social Media Use in 2021*. Pew Research Center, 2021 (www.pewresearch.org/internet/2021/04/07/social-media-use-in-2021/).

7. Alexander DE. Social media in disaster risk reduction and crisis management. *Sci Eng Ethics* 2014; **20**: 717–33.

8. Irons D, Paton D, Lester L, Scott J, Martin A. Social media, crisis communication and community-led response and recovery: an Australian case study. In Proceedings of the Research Forum of the Bushfire and Natural Hazards CRC and AFAC Conference, Wellington, New Zealand, 2 September 2014.

9. Dufty N. Twitter turns ten: its use to date in disaster management. *Aust J Emerg Manag* 2016; **31**: 50–54.

10. Lindsay BR. *Social Media and Disasters: Current Uses, Future Options, and Policy Considerations*. Congressional Research Service, 2011 (https://digital.library.unt.edu/ark:/67531/metadc93902/).

11. Pew Research Center. *News Use Across Social Media Platforms in 2020*. Pew Research Center, 2020 (www.journalism.org/2021/01/12/news-use-across-social-media-platforms-in-2020/).

12. Benis A, Khodos A, Ran S, Levner E, Ashkenazi S. Social media engagement and influenza vaccination during the COVID-19 pandemic: cross-sectional survey study. *J Med Internet Res* 2021; **23**: e25977.

13. Hossain L, Kam D, Kong F, Wigand R, Bossomaier T. Social media in Ebola outbreak. *Epidemiol Infect* 2016; **144**: 2136–43.

14. Househ M. Communicating Ebola through social media and electronic news media outlets: a cross-sectional study. *Health Inform J* 2016; **22**: 470–78.

15. Tsao S-F, Chen H, Tisseverasinghe T, Yang Y, Li L, Butt ZA. What social media told us in the time of COVID-19: a scoping review. *Lancet Digit Health* 2021; **3**: e175–94.

16. Roy M, Moreau N, Rousseau C, Mercier A, Wilson A, Atlani-Duault L. Ebola and localized blame on social media: analysis of Twitter and Facebook conversations during the 2014–2015 Ebola epidemic. *Cult Med Psychiatry* 2019; **44**: 56–79.

17. Abd-Alrazaq A, Alhuwail D, Househ M, Hamdi M, Shah Z. Top concerns of tweeters during the COVID-19 pandemic: infoveillance study. *J Med Internet Res* 2020; **22**: e19016.

18. Cinelli M, Quattrociocchi W, Galeazzi A, Valensise CM, Brugnoli E, Schmidt AL, et al. The COVID-19 social media infodemic. *Sci Rep* 2020; **10**: 16598.

19. Lee K, Agrawal A, Choudhary A. Forecasting influenza levels using real-time social media streams. IEEE International Conference on Healthcare Informatics (ICHI), Park City, UT, USA, 23–26 August 2017.

20. Kumar S, Xu C, Ghildayal N, Chandra C, Yang M. Social media effectiveness as a humanitarian response to mitigate influenza epidemic and COVID-19 pandemic. *Ann Oper Res* 2022; **319**: 823–51.

21. Ahmed N, Quinn SC, Hancock GR, Freimuth VS, Jamison A. Social media use and influenza vaccine uptake among White and African American adults. *Vaccine* 2018; **36**: 7556–61.

22. Bonnevie E, Rosenberg SD, Kummeth C, Goldbarg J, Wartella E, Smyser J. Using social media influencers to increase knowledge and positive attitudes toward the flu vaccine. *PLoS One* 2020; **15**: e0240828.

23. Dufty N. Using social media to build community disaster resilience. *Aust J Emerg Manag* 2012; **27**: 40–45.

24. Putnam R. Bowling alone: the collapse and revival of American community. *J Democr* 1995; **6**: 65–78.

25. Aldrich DP. *Building Resilience: Social Capital in Post-Disaster Recovery.* University of Chicago Press, 2012.

26. Page-Tan C. The role of social media in disaster recovery following Hurricane Harvey. *J Homel Secur Emerg Manag* 2021; **18**: 93–123.

27. Fraser T, Aldrich DP, Page-Tan C. Bowling alone or distancing together? The role of social capital in excess death rates from COVID-19. *Soc Sci Med* 2021; **284**: e114241.

28. Pitas N, Ehmer C. Social capital in the response to COVID-19. *Am J Health Promot* 2020; **34**: 942–4.

29. Wong AS, Kohler JC. Social capital and public health: responding to the COVID-19 pandemic. *Global Health* 2020; **16**: 88.

30. Newberry C. *How to Use Social Media in Healthcare: A Guide for Health Professionals.* Hootsuite, 2021 (https://blog.hootsuite.com/social-media-health-care/).

56

'Plans Are Worthless, but Planning is Everything': Lessons from Science and Experience

Richard Williams, Keith Porter, Tim Healing, Verity Kemp, and John Drury

Major Incidents, Pandemics, and Mental Health

The Scope of This Book

Despite its length, this book is but a snapshot of a very broad thread of related experiences, societal and personal endeavours, health and social care practices, and research. Although its contents cover a substantial number of topics, the chapters reflect the editors' choices. Although we narrowed the field substantially by focusing most on the psychosocial experiences and needs of people affected by emergencies, incidents, terrorist events, disasters, disease outbreaks and conflicts (EITDDC), there remain many topics that we could have developed more. The need for us to make choices reflects just how diverse is awareness of EITDDC and how rapidly science has moved forwards in the last century. All of these matters are affected by people's wide-ranging perspectives. The Lord Alderdice reflects on this matter in Chapter 3, where he states:

As I trained in psychiatry, I learned how biological, psychological, and sociological perspectives competed for allegiance in the profession. Later the diversity of views within our scientific communities was brought home to me when I was invited by the World Federation of Scientists to help them with a major division that had opened up as they tried to apply their expertise in the aftermath of the 9/11 terrorist attacks. Western scientists wanted to assist in the fight against Al Qaeda, whereas those from Eastern countries insisted that we must understand why the attacks were taking place. These conflicting perspectives among scientists showed how, even within the rational scientific community, we develop different narratives to explain and explore traumatic events and major incidents.

We see similar divergence with ... COVID-19 ... Epidemiologists give a response based on their developing understanding of the community transmission of the virus. Clinicians focus on treating the disease resulting from the over-reaction of the immune system that occurs in a minority of individual patients, and which may lead to serious illness and death. The impact on the healthcare system as a whole is the concern for people on lengthening waiting lists, and government officials are constantly balancing these pressures and the economic and societal consequences.

We intend this book to offer readers a broad and comprehensive picture that should help them to understand the nature of people's experiences before, during, and after disastrous and other untoward events. As Chapter 1 says, we set out to find common themes across different natures of EITDDC, to reflect our belief that there are features shared in common in the ways that people react to events. We also believe that there are general approaches to meeting their needs. That is not to say that we think that the impacts of terrorist attacks and disease outbreaks are the same as people's reactions to, say, road traffic collisions, which are much more common, but there are similarities in their experiences and the care that they need. We conclude this work believing that we were correct in our presumptions of a decade ago [1].

In this book, we emphasise social and psychological perspectives, and the diversity of narratives becomes evident. Yet there are also common themes even if they are expressed in different ways by different authors. The mental health field is broad. We focus most on the challenges to people's wellbeing and their psychosocial needs, whether they be members of the public or staff of organisations that endeavour to assist the public. We adopt these foci because we think that the social and psychological aspects of the matters that trouble people before, during, and after EITDDCs are, or should be, malleable – that is, open to modification.

We consider in detail people's experiences and their psychosocial needs with a view to developing a contemporary approach to understanding and responding to people's suffering consequent on their exposures to EITDDC. There are substantial commonalities. We outline four here.

First, it is clear that our authors endorse sustaining people's wellbeing before, during, and after the adversities they face, with the intention of aiding them to prepare for, struggle with the challenges of, and recover as rapidly as possible after their exposures to EITDDC. Preparing and supporting people should also aid them to respond rapidly when they do develop psychosocial needs or diagnosable disorders.

Second, we include several chapters and case studies in the mental health domain of caring for people who develop mental health disorders consequent on their experiences and on the epidemiology of mental health disorders relating to EITDDC. We are aware that there are many books, papers, and leaflets that cover aspects of the psychiatric topics within the mental health canon [2–4].

Third, we recognise that most people who are involved in or affected by EITDDC do not develop a mental health disorder, but, nonetheless, their experiences affect their mental health. Despite not attracting diagnoses, those experiences may be extremely upsetting, and those upsets may persist for a sizeable minority of people exposed to EITDDC. The people affected may experience perplexing and anxiety-inducing distress during and after EITDDC that may make them feel as if they are unwell. Indeed, research involving people affected by the Manchester Arena bombing of 2017 shows the importance of hearing and 'validating' people's distress and the misunderstandings that may arise from alternative terminology, termed 'normalising' people's experiences, which has similar intentions. But, the latter approach can leave some people feeling worse rather than better (see Chapters 5 and 28). Furthermore, being affected by an EITDDC affects the quality of people's lives and heightens awareness of the impacts of the social causes of mental ill health. These impacts spread out to affect relatives and friends of the people who are directly involved. The topic of psychosocial care has received less attention in responses to EITDDC than do the risks of people developing mental health disorders, but everyone affected by persisting effects deserves our care. These situations do not, alone, mean that sufferers have a diagnosable disorder. However, we fear that the duration and impacts of these psychosocial experiences have been underestimated; some people

who are distressed do require psychosocial care, and, as Chapter 42 portrays, kindness and social support lie at the centre of meeting their needs.

Fourth, the impacts of COVID-19 on societies have accentuated our awareness of what we term the inverse gradient of socioeconomic disadvantage, in which people who have fewer resources to rely on tend to fare much less well in the face of EITDDC than do people in more advantageous and affluent circumstances. This gradient is one of the social determinants of mental health upon which a companion book focuses [5].

In this closing chapter, we look back into the book to identify some broad lessons that stand out for us. We also look forward by endeavouring to identify what are the challenges that countries, jurisdictions, regions, and researchers must face if we are to stay ahead of the rapid progression of history into the future. What is plainly evident from this book is that nothing stands still. Aiming to bring our services to the level of the best that current science, practice, and humanity can justify is insufficient for the future, because the goalposts will continue to move in front of us; this work is a constant effort of preparedness. Is this not a key lesson from the UK's management of and responses to the COVID-19 pandemic, which found parts of our planning and preparation wanting when the SARS-CoV-2 virus hit?

The topics that we cover are heterogenous, but they have a commonality in wanting to bring equitable care of increasing quality to people who are affected by EITDDCs; that common theme is caring sensitively for everyone involved. As Montgomery comments in Chapter 52, a core public ethical value in designing and delivering responses is that 'everyone matters equally'. He continues, 'This egalitarian commitment does not require each person to be treated identically, but it does mean that their interests are the concern of us all, and of society, and that they must be treated fairly and with respect'.

Historical Developments in Pre-Hospital Emergency Medicine

Medical and social responses to emergencies have developed over many centuries. Chapters 13, 14, and 16 serve to remind us of the importance of studying history. The quote 'Those who cannot remember the past are condemned to repeat it', attributed to Santayana, sums up a key message about this matter [6].

The parable of the Good Samaritan describes the importance of immediate care. It recognises the care that a member of the public was sufficiently kind (see Chapter 42), generous and brave to offer that clearly integrated the physical care required by the survivor with responding to his psychosocial needs.

That parable begins to identify why it is important to use well and safely the willingness of a proportion of the public in attendance at an emergency to contribute to rescue and recovery. This theme emerges strongly in Chapter 22. We see the term first responder as applying to anyone who intervenes at the scene of an incident or is first to come to the aid of someone in need. Of course, we also recognise the special expertise and responsibilities of certain professional groups across several sectors of response by referring to them as professional first responders. Thus we have the citizenAID initiative in the UK, which aims to familiarise members of the public with the basic techniques of first aid and resuscitation. It is important, we think, that these approaches integrate the contributions of public first responders and professional first responders and psychosocial and physical healthcare at the scenes of incidents large and small, as Chapters 4 and 5 identify.

Older approaches and assertions that emergencies are the sole province of highly trained professional practitioners are not maximally effective, and the Manchester Arena bombing highlighted the challenges imposed by delays in availability of professional first responders. Time and again, we have heard the argument for cordoning and asking apparently extraneous people to leave incident sites because those sites are crime scenes, for health and safety reasons, or because of the risk of an incident escalating. We respect that reasoning, but it also runs the risk of denying the help and expertise of many bystanders. We argue for a fresh look at managing well the sites of incidents.

Furthermore, the maxim of 'no health without mental health' applies fully to EITDDC, and it is clear that patients and responders concur. Integration of the physical and mental health aspects of trauma care should be emphasised whatever the circumstances. It should begin at the point of injury and continue through successive steps in care. However, few local emergency plans outline steps to achieve this, and all too often mental healthcare, broadly defined, has been an afterthought. The patient in Chapter 4 calls for a designated hand-holder in the team of responders –

that is, a member of the team charged with focusing on the psychosocial needs of conscious casualties. The trainee in pre-hospital emergency medicine (PHEM), a hugely experienced doctor although still junior, describes just how important is his continuing psychosocial support in doing such a challenging job. The interesting finding from our work with practitioners of pre-hospital care is that the enormity of patients' injuries and illnesses, although challenging, is not necessarily the most stressful feature of an incident, and environmental, contextual, and interpersonal features may cause as much or more stress.

Our aspiration for integrated care does not require mental health practitioners to attend the frontline, although that is a model used in some countries, as Chapter 35 shows. However, we think that prior training should sensitise professional first responders to messages about simple ways of recognising and responding to people's emotional needs early on. Similarly, there are many approaches to caring for staff that do not rely on mental health practitioners for direct care, but rather for their input into training and supervising practitioners who offer informal peer support as a first step (see Chapters 44 and 48).

The Rhythm of Advances in Clinical Practice and Service Developments

The chapters in Section 2 provide important information about the nature of traumatic injuries, which are very common, and describe the huge leaps forward in the twentieth century in techniques that enable us to keep seriously injured people alive during and after even the most dangerous and serious events. Chapters 13, 14, and 15 point out that there is in the UK an almost rhythmical exchange of technique, practice, and service organisation that runs between healthcare practitioners who work in the military and go to war or attend conflicts and staff of the facilities that are offered by civilian healthcare systems. Hippocrates was recorded as saying that 'war is the only proper school of the surgeon', and this resonates with the Hertford Consensus of 2015, which stated that 'he who wishes to be a surgeon should go to war' [7].

The creation of the Red Cross in 1863 led to the introduction of standardised care of injured people and adoption of the first Geneva Convention for the Amelioration of the Condition of the Wounded in

Armies in the Field in 1864. Modern PHEM is based on standardised protocols of care. The First World War is credited with creating the concept of modern ambulances, and with advancing antiseptic and anaesthetic practice, and the Second World War saw the introduction of penicillin and great advances in blood transfusion. Innovation and treatments devised during warfare in Afghanistan, which have now been adopted as standard practice in civilian healthcare in the UK and elsewhere, include integrated trauma systems and networks, trauma centres with consultants available 24/7 as trauma team leaders, and resuscitative endovascular balloon occlusion of the aorta (REBOA).

This rhythm of mutual learning between the civilian and military health services is set to continue in the UK, because they are joined together through clinical personnel in the Defence Medical Services being embedded in civilian NHS services in order for them to practise and maintain their skills and conduct research in peacetime.

Definitions

In other texts, two of us (RW and VK) have called for definitions to be agreed at all levels, including between agencies that contribute to responses to EITDDC, across the departments of contributing agencies, and within teams [8]. This is because it is common to find in practice that the same and similar terms are used to describe different matters, and for different terms to be used to refer to the same thing. This contributes powerfully to misunderstandings, and also impedes service design and practice. Matters such as these should be worked on, and a language agreed within and between organisations long before events occur. We illustrate the importance of definitions by looking at terminology for the mental health impacts of EITDDC.

The Nature of the Impacts of EITDDC on People Who Survive and on Staff of the Rescue and Responding Services

The Lord Alderdice points to a clinical perspective on this matter when he says in Chapter 3:

A further problem of expectation, specifically with regard to mental wellbeing, has been created by widening the meaning of 'mental health problem'. In the past, disturbed mental functioning was regarded as being caused by moral weakness or the influence of evil spirits. More recently, mental illnesses, which might have physical, psychological, or social contributors, have been viewed through a medical lens that sees definable categories of mental illness whose diagnoses have pathological and therapeutic implications. Such an approach regarded low spirits and anxiety as symptoms of mental illness only when they were experienced in an inappropriate context or to an excessive degree.

Thus The Lord Alderdice identifies an important matter of definition that affects service design and the expectations of the public. It relates to how we use terms such as health and wellbeing, mental health problem, and mental health, as well as other related terms. Sometimes these terms are all used to refer to the same broad construct, but their meaning is not always clear. We suggest that terminology should be used more specifically with a view to promoting service development. Thus, in this book, we have adapted the report by Dennis Stevenson and Paul Farmer to create a more explicit but practical approach [9]. We suggest adopting a nomenclature that identifies the following three agendas for mental healthcare, in its broadest meaning [10].

- The wellbeing agenda assists people to thrive at home, in work, or at school. Wellbeing is about feeling good and functioning well, and is influenced by each person's experience of life.
- The psychosocial agenda supports people who are struggling. Psychosocial care describes interventions for people who are distressed or struggling, or who have symptoms of mental health problems that do not meet the criteria for a diagnosis, whether or not they also suffer social or work dysfunction.
- The mental health agenda enables people whose needs appear to go beyond struggling to access mental healthcare for timely assessment and, if necessary, treatment and recovery, and support with returning to work or school [10].

It is worth pausing for a moment to consider in a little more detail what we mean by wellbeing. Recovery of healthcare staff to wellbeing at the current stage of the COVID-19 pandemic is a matter for concern in many countries. It is clear that, at the time of publication of this book, in 2024, many staff feel that they are not thriving at work or at home and that their lives are not as fulfilling as they would wish. Financial difficulties driven by inflation and people's incomplete recovery from the burnout that they experienced during the pandemic are components. However, other important concerns can be traced back to well before the pandemic. Malcolm Gladwell, an author, considers fulfilment at work, and in his explorations the importance emerges of people being given opportunities for personal development and to find work meaningful. In his book, Gladwell illustrates three criteria for work being meaningful [11]:

- complexity – having a job that engages and challenges us
- autonomy – having a sense of self-directedness in our work
- there being a clear relationship between the effort we put into our work and its impact.

These are all matters to which we could return with benefit in creating jobs in the future that may protect people when they face the challenges of EITDDC.

Services for Survivors of EITDDC

We are keen that this book appraises people's needs consequent on their exposure to EITDDCs from broad perspectives that enable a strategic approach to be taken to meeting those needs whether they represent distress or disorder. Chapter 12 offers a framework, based on the three agendas identified earlier, for a general approach to how policy, planning, and service development might be developed to create a new and better balanced public approach to recognising and responding to people's wellbeing needs, meeting their psychosocial needs, and preventing and responding to their possible development of mental health disorders. We reproduce that framework here, in Figure 56.1, but refer readers to Chapters 12, 27, and 28 for more detail. Section 4 of this book adds depth to these endeavours to better define the assistance that survivors require.

However, before we proceed, it is important to consider a fallacy. This is that survivors of disasters who have been affected by EITDDC previously are likely to cope better than do people who are experiencing an emergency for the first time. Chapter 11 covers aspects of this topic. We conclude from that chapter and the work of Hanna Zagefka that this fallacy is inaccurate because 'repeated exposure to severe adversity makes it harder, not easier, for disaster ... [survivors] to cope with a new negative event' [12]. This is an important consideration because adherence to the fallacy could result in less support being offered to police officers, paramedics, and PHEM practitioners, for example.

Preparing and Caring for the Workforce of Responding Agencies

A vital matter is the necessity for fully including in emergency planning and delivery the mental wellbeing, psychosocial, and mental health needs not only of people affected, but also of responders to EITDDC. We now know a great deal about the risks that people face because of their exposure to many events. The single most important matter that is often not recognised, or is omitted, is the length of the timescale over which the impacts may affect people, as Chapters 35, 36, and 42 show [13]. The result is that wellbeing, psychosocial, and mental health interventions tend to be offered late and for insufficient periods after EITDDC [14]. However, there are hopeful signs emerging from COVID-19. Figure 56.2 is reproduced from Chapter 44. It shows how the general framework in Figure 56.1 might be adapted by the responsible authorities and turned into strategy to ensure comprehensive responses to the needs of staff of responding agencies.

Chapter 46 offers a view of endeavours that were put in hand to support staff by NHS England and NHS Improvement early in the COVID-19 pandemic. It bears testament to how some of the learning covered by this book was used to inform managers and leaders and instigate support services early on. It gives hope that wellbeing, psychosocial care, and mental healthcare are now more openly on the agenda. What is required now is for these topics to become integral to emergency planning and preparedness and workforce development.

We believe that preparing and caring for the workforce from all sectors that respond to EITDDCs is an important matter. This includes preparing and informing not just professional first responders but also all staff of all services who might be engaged in responding later to an EITDDC. We have recognised the importance of creating an alliance with the public by recognising their contributions to managing EITDDCs, at least in the initial phase before professional first responders arrive. Thus we provide a case study in Chapter 45 that shows how Blue Light services might be prepared and cared for using the principles identified in this book. Chapter 47 provides a good example of actioning these principles during the COVID-19 pandemic. Of course, preparing the public and staff should be a matter of co-production, so that they receive the forms of advice that they wish

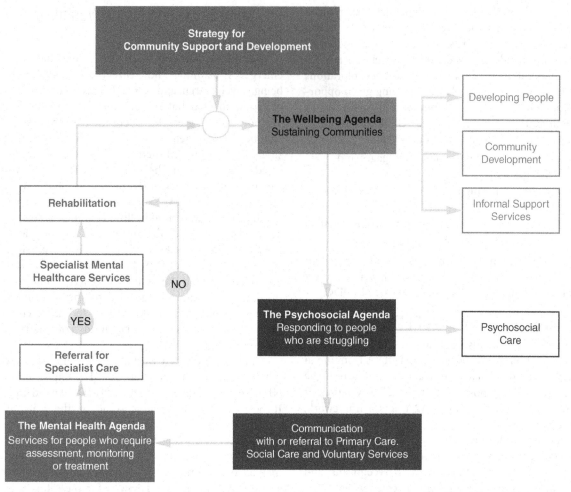

Figure 56.1 A strategic approach to meeting the needs of communities for support for their mental health, psychosocial care, and mental healthcare. (© R Williams and V Kemp, 2020. All rights reserved.)

to receive [15]. If that were the case, mitigation of the risks to people's mental health might be advanced by developments to emergency preparedness that incorporate people's psychosocial and mental health as prominent topics.

Environmental Changes

We should also be aware of the huge effects of societal changes and their impacts on the risks of people being exposed to EITDDCs. Many people now occupy habitats that we would regard as marginal, and one example of the consequences is that of people being more exposed to flooding because of climate change, and communities being more prepared to create housing on flood plains. Furthermore, Chapter 7 draws our attention to increasing urbanisation across the world. Although this may have many advantages, there are also disadvantages and impacts on the risks of EITDDCs. Both of these matters affect civilian and military practice in emergencies, as the earthquakes in Turkey and Syria in 2023 have shown.

However, we must also recognise and take into planning the imperatives posed by climate change and global warming. They contribute increasingly massively to the risks of EITDDC, and they also affect planning for responding effectively. As the impacts of climate change manifest, the nature and scale of emergencies may well change, and there is likely to be a greater number of complex emergencies in which there is the potential for shortages of water and food across the world.

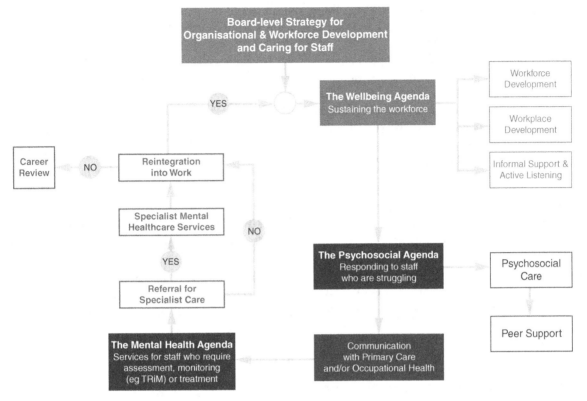

Figure 56.2 A model of care. (© R Williams and V Kemp, 2021 all rights reserved.)

As Chapter 49 shows, complex emergencies are disasters that generally have the greatest impacts. They are defined by the Inter-Agency Standing Committee (IASC), a forum of United Nations (UN) and non-UN humanitarian partners founded to strengthen humanitarian assistance, as follows: 'A humanitarian crisis in a country, region or society where there is total or considerable breakdown of authority resulting from internal or external conflict and which requires an international response that goes beyond the mandate or capacity of any single agency and/or the ongoing United Nations country program'.

It is clear that climate change and its impacts are a complex emergency. We do not deal with this matter directly in this book, but we think that the principles for intervention that we outline could be applied to planning for the psychosocial and mental health aspects of complex emergencies, including climate change.

The Social Cure Approach, Resilience, and Social Capital

Social Cure

Another vitally important avenue of development in recent years has come from the social sciences. Consequentially, we now understand a lot more about: how people's behaviours are affected by EITDDC and their backgrounds; about the nature of their responses; and about how we should use the learning gained to develop more sophisticated responses. Earlier, we spoke of integrating psychosocial care with physical healthcare, and this is one component of responses that has benefited from psychological research. We have found that much of this learning has yet to find its way into emergency planning, and so we devoted Section 3 to summarising the actual and potential contributions of social psychology to better understanding and responding to EITDDC. One theoretical approach that has been extensively tested in research on EITDDC is the social cure approach. It is important in:

1. taking forward the science of group psychology
2. showing the relevance and usefulness of the psychology of groups in an increasing number of health, mental health, and organisational contexts, where it suggests new and relatively cost-effective solutions to many old problems
3. enhancing our understanding of the precise mechanisms whereby social groups help, and sometimes hinder, the health and wellbeing of people affected by EITDDCs [5,16].

Specifically, work under the social cure banner has expanded from addressing the role of social identity in symptom appraisal and response, health-related norms and behaviour, social support, coping, and clinical outcomes [17], to a very broad range of topics, including stress and 'trauma', loneliness, depression, addiction, eating behaviour, ageing, and emergency response [18]. We have used this approach to better understand what we were told by people directly affected by the Manchester Arena bombing about their experiences, responses, and what helped them [19–21]. This work is influencing policy and practice in the UK and internationally.

Resilience

As Chapter 19 shows, the emergence of the resilience agenda as applied to EITDDC since the 9/11 terrorist attacks in the USA, and particularly the concept of community resilience, has opened the way for modern social psychological approaches to be acknowledged and included. On the one hand, the approaches that pathologise public responses, such as mass panic (see Chapters 8 and 19), are still influential, but are in retreat because they are inaccurate and counter-productive. On the other hand, the widely accepted sociologically based concept of social capital is seen as necessary but insufficient psychologically. It leaves open, for example, where social capital comes from, and does not explain the evidence of supportive behaviour among survivors in an emergency who have no prior connections.

Discussions about psychosocial resilience have developed in the last 15 years. First, Chapter 19 summarises the case against assumptions of inherent psychological frailty and vulnerability that have traditionally informed emergency planning and

treatment of the public. Second, more recent discussions have drawn attention to the different meanings, definitions, and usages of the term resilience, and suggested that they are not always useful and can sometimes be problematic [22], or even ideological [23]. We argued from early on that it was helpful to understand collective psychosocial resilience as a social process and not simply a disposition [24]. Now we caution against over-using the term resilience, especially when it implies some unidentified force for good that keeps people well when they meet adversity, or when it is used as a synonym for good outcomes.

Emergency Preparedness, Response, and Recovery (EPRR)

Emergency Preparedness

We tend to assume that planning how we might meet EITDDCs well ahead of their happening is self-evidently important to all services that might contribute to meeting people's extraordinary needs. We note that, time and again, communities and the responding services are insufficiently prepared for the challenges that they meet. Surely then, isn't the answer to develop all-enveloping plans? However, doing so would threaten to consume so much of our resources, which might otherwise be used to respond to people's existing needs. Plainly there is a balance to be achieved. In our opinion, the pendulum has swung too far away from emergency preparedness. However, experience shows that if we were to take the approach of creating rigid plans, we would inevitably prepare better for the last event, but not necessarily for the big event that is next to occur. We are aware of the old military maxim that no plan survives first contact with the enemy. It embodies the sentiment that we need to be able to plan well, but not for our response to EITDDC to be hampered by inflexibility, rigidity, and inability to adapt rapidly. That said, we have come across instances of key components being omitted from planning cycles, and we have already noted that matters concerning the wellbeing, psychosocial care, and mental healthcare of survivors and responders are routinely omitted from emergency planning. Yet they are crucial for sustaining effective responses.

The quote in the title of this chapter, which is attributed to Dwight D Eisenhower, summarises the risks of creating plans that are over-rigid and over-prescriptive. Churchill used a similar statement in the

Second World War. We opine that it is the *process* of planning that should be rehearsed and tested rigorously in exercises that rehearse the cross-disciplinary, interdepartmental, multi-agency elements that require coordination to the full. Resources should be allocated in the planning cycle for stockpiling and replenishing materiel that cannot be procured at short notice.

This is one of the reasons why the military in many countries now stresses training on the doctrine of mission command. That is, people are taught how to command, plan, and exercise together, and are offered tables to make easier managing readiness states, and the computational and logistic components of the process. As Chapter 50 shows, people should exercise together to build relationships with other people in key positions in their own and other organisations in order to learn: how to get things done; how to engage effectively with the organisations that should be partners; and how to reduce to manageable levels the different cultures of partners and their impacts on interoperability.

Policy Development

Achieving comprehensive wellbeing, psychosocial care, and mental health services for moderate and large-scale EITDDCs requires that lessons learned through research and experience are translated into integrated, ethical, evidence-based policies and plans at four levels [8]. They are:

- governance policies at national, regional, and local levels, which should set the overall aims and objectives for responses to EITDDC
- strategic policies for service design, which translate political requirements into the purpose and content of plans, and are based on research, past experience and knowledge of the population, geography, and services affected
- service delivery policies, which are evidence and values based, and are focused on particular services and knowledge of how specific services function and are likely to be used
- policies for good clinical practice, which are based on clinical practitioners taking account of the needs of individual patients and the contexts in which they are cared for (person-centred care).

In Chapter 52, Jonathan Montgomery examines the links between ethical planning and practice and science. He describes his observations of problems that emerged in the UK during the COVID-19 pandemic in which, in our words, the influences of social media and populism appeared to create complications in harnessing science into finding solutions to problems, and trusting experts. As a partial solution, Figure 56.3, reproduced from a recent paper, illustrates an approach that is based on aligning policy with science and practice [25]. It portrays two linked processes whereby emergency preparedness may be advanced, and also how rapid adjustments of policy and existing plans can be made that are based on lessons from science and practice to solve contemporary problems. This figure comes from a paper that appraises guidelines for evidence-based mental health and psychosocial support [25].

However, what is also required for the future is a sophisticated approach to communicating plans, and the reasoning that supports them, that takes into account the challenges of democratisation of science and expansion of what constitutes knowledge and use of social media.

Organisational Preparedness

Organisational preparedness calls for us to develop trust in what our own organisations and what others can be relied upon to contribute effectively. As we have implied, for example, the beginning of an incident is not the time to discover matters of definition and terminology, the need for cross-disciplinary training of team members, or lack of rehearsed multi-agency leadership and coordination. Similarly, certain matters such as supply chains for expendable items require negotiation and rehearsal, and stores of certain items need to be procured, held in reserve, and cycled through use and resupply. Many countries found themselves in very difficult positions regarding supply of personal protective equipment (PPE) as the COVID-19 pandemic got under way and spread rapidly.

Psychological Safety

Another lesson from the COVID-19 pandemic is that although many people might not recognise the term psychological safety, they do recognise the working environment that it creates, and they know that it is a hugely important aspect of organisational culture. Psychological safety in workplaces means that people feel assured that they can take appropriate interpersonal risks while working. As well as being good for the wellbeing of everyone, there is additional evidence that psychologically safe working environments are less

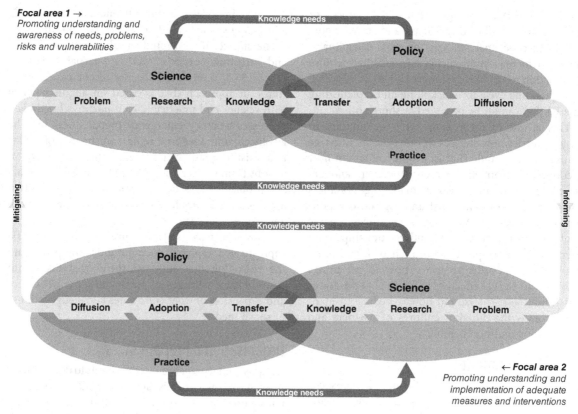

Figure 56.3 Promoting awareness, understanding, and implementation of EPRR. (Reproduced under licence CC BY.)

likely to result in errors of judgement or mistakes [26]. Edmondson has stated that 'in psychologically safe environments, people believe that if they make a mistake others will not penalize or think less of them for it ... [and] ... that others will not resent or penalize them for asking for help, information or feedback' [27].

Horizon Scanning, Assessment, and Surveillance

Certain matters can be better predicted than others sufficiently early to make detailed preparation of people and resources more effective. During the flu pandemic of 2009–2010, this was the case in the UK, but much less so before the the COVID-19 pandemic. All of this requires a sufficient capacity for horizon scanning, assessment, and surveillance as tools to support emergency planning and preparedness. Again these facilities should be planned, developed, and tested well before untoward events occur, but learning to trust them and use them well calls for mature organisations. Chapter 52 identifies that

organisations in the UK were not prepared for the changes in public culture that had arisen during the period between the flu and COVID-19 pandemics, including the accumulated impact of populist politics, and greater access to and use of social media. Reduced levels of trust in experts made handling information about SARS-CoV-2 relatively more difficult, and trust between scientists, surveillance agencies, the public, politicians, and experts very much more difficult to achieve. Managing inter-agency relationships in these circumstances is an important matter for the long term, and requires repeated exercises.

Mitigation of Risks, Partnerships, and Good Communications

We know from research that preparation for, response to, and recovery from EITDDCs are common problems (e.g., failures in communications, supply chains, policy, and values), as well as differences in the ability of organisations to respond according to available resources.

Partnerships are key matters in planning and preparing. Good communications are also vital, and very frequently the inadequacy of communications is remarked on by inquiries after major incidents. They involve having good public health services available that include the needs of people affected and responders for sufficient wellbeing, psychosocial care, and mental healthcare provision being legitimate concerns. Again, we have witnessed a trajectory of progress in this regard. More frequently in the last 10 years, we have been contacted for advice about these matters and necessary provisions as incidents, and especially major incidents, occur. However, that is still some way from public health services being fully confident about what they should do. Now we sense a consensus about the importance of public mental health in EITDDC that should enable development of greater confidence in which services should be involved in emergency planning with a view to their preparing to go live at short notice.

Coordinated and consistent communications between all responding organisations at local, regional, and national levels are fundamental to managing EITDDC. Using available information about the demographics of the populations involved should shape communications that should contain appropriate messages for the public to ensure physical and psychological safety using a variety of methods, appropriate to the target audience. This requires agencies to know about the composition of communities and to have forged good relationships with, and the confidence of community leaders. Messages are likely to include information about possible risks, their mitigation, and where to find further information and assistance.

Public-facing messages should:

1. involve people because communication is more effective in influencing people when they feel involved; this means:
   - acknowledging the gravity of events and the tragedy for people affected
   - recognising public concern and the efforts of the public to manage the risk
   - assuring the public that officials are doing all they can, provided that this is true
2. express a coherent, consistent approach
3. be open and transparent, particularly with reference to:
   - the likely course of the incident
   - how the incident is being handled
   - what people can do to protect themselves [28,29].

Contributions from Psychology to Developing EPRR and Its Role in Wellbeing, Psychosocial Care, and Mental Healthcare

Our opinion is that people who are responsible for and involved in emergency planning and practice need to understand that several branches of psychology can contribute to modern approaches to emergency planning and preparedness, adapting responses to novel circumstances and solving problems with behaviour by using lessons from the social sciences. As we expounded earlier in this chapter, this means that the psychosocial domain should no longer be regarded as an add-on but as an essential component of emergency responses and recovery. There should be continued further embedding of psychosocial principles and insights in training personnel of the emergency services (see Chapter 25) [30]. It also means mainstreaming psychosocial care for survivors and their families and for staff of responding services across all relevant sectors. Importantly, a debate is needed about the sources of and funding for psychosocial care, because much that is required lies outwith the present responsibilities, capabilities, and funding for mental healthcare, social care, and public health services.

We go further by calling for consistent and coherent approaches to including psychology and behavioural science in emergency responses. We note, for example, that the Scientific Advisory Group for Emergencies (SAGE) system of providing advice to government departments in the UK's response to COVID-19 did recognise the importance of psychology in that it involved the behavioural science subgroup, SPI-B, in advising SAGE. However, advice of this nature was not so available to practitioners on the ground locally. Also, some of the advice generated for SPI-B was undermined by advice from elsewhere that was not based on the same scientific appraisals [31]. An example is when senior advisers in other specialties rationalised policy decisions with unevidenced folk psychological concepts such as behavioural fatigue. We argue that the contributions of psychology might be advanced and better recognised if there were senior advisers in this field as there are in medicine and nursing.

In the future, practice could be improved if there was greater recognition of the value of advice from psychologists by formalising relationships between psychology advisers and local public health teams [32].

Similarly, we call for development of the science of emergency planning and for including planners and mental health specialists in advisory structures at all levels. Greater resources are required to train advisers and provide an infrastructure to support them [33].

Teams and Leadership

Very often, we take individual people as the unit of consideration. It is easy to understand how that might arise in healthcare from the focus of pathological processes on individual people as the primary substrate for history taking, examination, investigation, diagnosis, and treatment. However, we also know that this approach does not adequately recognise the importance of other people to how index people suffer, and their roles in people's recoveries and the degree to which they are impaired by residual problems. Section 3 of this book provides an overview of the most important matters from science that have stood out before and during the COVID-19 pandemic. In our view, the most important are social relationships, social support, and teams.

Social Scaffolding, a book in which RW, VK, TH, and JD were involved as authors and/or editors, includes several chapters about teams and how people work together [5]. We distinguish between teams and groups of people who work together, and, in our opinion, an important difference between teams and groups lies in whether the people involved have a shared social identity. Plainly, this is not the way in which the term teams is used by most organisations, and although some work groups are teams, many more groups that are designated as teams do not meet our definition. We point out the distinction because our experience is that there is so much more that teams are able to contribute to working collaboratively and achieving demanding objectives in challenging circumstances. Frequently, teams are more able to offer support to members than are ad-hoc groups of people who happen to be working together.

One of us (RW) has learned first-hand the problems that may emerge when moving people between teams. These observations should be borne in mind by managers and leaders who consider reorganising their workforce when they are faced with extreme challenges. That kind of reorganisation is not a simple matter, as relocating staff during the pandemic has shown (see Chapters 40 and 41 in this regard). This is not to say that reorganisation should not be contemplated, because that would limit organisations' flexibility, but it does call for substantial planning, preparation, training, and support to be put in place as people are asked to adopt changed roles and working relationships.

As Chapters 44, 47, and 50 show, feeling connected with and socially supported by other colleagues within teams has repeatedly been found to improve job satisfaction, enhance wellbeing, and protect against depression and post-traumatic stress disorder [34,35]. These effects rely on stable and well-trained teams with functioning communication processes and shared mental models in place.

Effective teamwork and socially supportive work climates require emphasis of the contributions of each team member and, importantly, development of a shared identity and shared mental models. This has been supported by recent work on cross-organisational leadership, in which leaders who utilised prior organisational identities as a basis for subsequently developing a superordinate identity were able to increase support of the wider organisations' shared strategies [36]. Structural factors, such as co-location and alignment of work schedules, have been found to be beneficial to developing teamwork in multidisciplinary healthcare teams. Again, Chapter 50 speaks to these challenges.

Achieving positive activity on all of the agendas that we identify in this chapter calls for effective leadership. It should be supported by policy and plans at all levels. That policy must reflect the moral architecture that is required (see Chapter 37). Leadership is important no matter what the circumstances, but particularly during and after EITDDC. Recent events (e.g., the COVID-19 pandemic, the terrorist attacks in Manchester and at Bataclan, severe weather events) have served to remind us that we live, and perhaps have always lived, in uncertain times.

This takes us to the notion of extreme teaming. As the research cited in Chapter 50 shows, responses to more substantial emergencies require groups of people from different teams and agencies to work collaboratively and effectively at strategic, tactical, and operational levels. There are enormous challenges in doing so. According to Amy Edmondson and Jean-François Harvey, 'complex technical and social problems nearly always require experts from different organisations and sectors to collaborate ... what we have called extreme teaming' [37]. They offer a model that is based on four leadership functions. Two of them target emotions and relationships and involve building an engaging vision and 'cultivating a psychologically safe environment for learning (displaying authentic care and framing cross-boundary work as a resource)' [37]. The other two leadership functions 'target the technical challenges of integrating knowledge and skills across expertise domains' [37]. Thus this model resonates with material about strategic leadership developed previously by Christopher Heginbotham and Richard Williams [38].

Policy for EPRR should recognise that, in the course of EITDDC, leaders are more than likely to be operating without complete, accurate information. This may mean that they have to change course and acknowledge that they have done so and why, even if that means accepting that initial actions might not have been the right ones. Again, this emphasises the importance of training leaders and managers in the *processes* of emergency planning and preparedness rather than reifying the plan itself. We must recognise that the capacity to work in these circumstances requires the ability to tolerate ambiguity while trying to create order and effective ways forward from uncertainty. This requires us to select and train leaders to prepare, respond, and recover from EITDDCs. Not everyone, no matter how senior or skilled, is able to lead well in emergency planning and preparation and during the response and recovery phases of EITDDC.

During EITDDC, many people may find themselves fulfilling a role as a leader in a crisis, and representing their service, organisation, function, or profession. However, this does not obviate the need to have a core of professional staff who are trained to plan, respond, and recover from EITDDCs, with some of them further trained to provide leadership at times of crisis. It is important to ensure that leaders who are not EPRR professionals are identified, receive training, and are able to practise responding to EITDDC scenarios. Priority should be given to planning and preparation for EITDDCs, and not just by emergency practitioners. This also requires widening understanding of the critical importance of the wellbeing, psychosocial, and mental health agendas driven by awareness of the needs of people who are involved in and affected by EITDDC, whether as members of the public or as professional practitioners, responders, leaders, and managers.

Research

As we hope this book illustrates, research and evaluation should be an integral part of planning for and responding to EITDDC. Research should be started at the earliest opportunity in emergencies, working on assessment and measurement of the psychosocial care and mental healthcare needs of the people affected. Another important topic for further research is the power of peer support for people's psychosocial care and their wellbeing as well as practice.

Two Recent Circumstances

The Manchester Arena Bombing in 2017

Chapter 36 is a brief case study of the Manchester Arena bombing in the UK in 2017, and Chapter 28 provides examples of research conducted over the 4 years that followed. These chapters focus on practical approaches to delivering psychosocial care and mental healthcare for the public and professional staff, and consider the generic lessons identified from the experience. They conclude that the impacts on people's wellbeing and their psychosocial and mental health needs, should form part of emergency preparedness plans. Training and exercising these arrangements should involve people who are likely to deliver these functions.

The SIRE project was established to enhance understanding of the experience of distress among people present at the Manchester Arena bombing, identify their experiences of psychosocial care after the incident, and learn how to better deliver and target effective psychosocial care after major incidents. The project extends our understanding of how people react to terrorist incidents. Aspects of its findings are reported in Chapters 5 and 28. There is a substantial agenda for developing awareness of people's needs for psychosocial interventions, and for training practitioners to deliver them. The findings have substantial implications for policy and service delivery [19–21].

The War in Ukraine

At the time of publication of this book, a major complex emergency is in progress in the Ukraine. Owen Matthews states that 'the Russo-Ukrainian War is the most serious geopolitical crisis in Europe since the Second World War, and one which will result in far greater global consequences than 9/11. The world's security architecture, food and energy supply, balance of power and alliances will be altered forever' [39]. This is the time to describe the impacts and responses to this war among the people, save to say that several of us have advised healthcarers in Ukraine. Our experiences remind us that that war shows all the features of a complex emergency. It also reminds us of our assertion earlier in this chapter of the rhythm of mutual learning between civilian and military services.

Conclusion

This chapter draws to a close *Major Incidents, Pandemics, and Mental Health: The Psychosocial Aspects of Emergencies, Incidents, Disasters, and Disease Outbreaks.*

The quote in the title of this chapter, which as mentioned earlier is attributed to Dwight D Eisenhower, summarises the importance of creating plans that are not over-rigid. Our opinion overall is that it is the *process* of planning that should be rehearsed again and again and tested in exercises with adequate resources being allocated for materiel that

cannot be procured at short notice. And the planning processes that are taught, experienced, and learned must recognise the importance of prompt and lasting attention to the wellbeing, psychosocial, and mental health needs of everyone who is affected. There is no health without mental health.

Creating this book has drawn on a huge amount of expertise from 91 contributors. We, the editors, take this opportunity to thank each of them for the years of care and enterprise that they have put into accruing the wisdom and experience that they have presented in their chapters.

The editors have been a tower of strength to the leading and managing editors of this book. Richard Williams and Verity Kemp wish to express their gratitude to Keith Porter, Tim Healing, and John Drury, who have done so much as editors, authors, advisers, and section editors. Without them, this book might well never have been completed.

References

1. Williams R, Bisson J, Kemp V. *OP94: Principles for Responding to the Psychosocial and Mental Health Needs of People Affected by Disasters or Major Incidents.* Royal College of Psychiatrists. 2014.

2. Scott HR, Stevelink SAM, Gafoor R, Lamb D, Carr E, Bakolis I, et al. Prevalence of post-traumatic stress disorder and common mental disorders in health-care workers in England during the COVID-19 pandemic: a two-phase cross-sectional study. *Lancet Psychiatry* 2023; 10: 40–49.

3. Ursano RJ, Fullerton CS, Weisaeth L, Raphael B, eds. *Textbook of Disaster Psychiatry* 2nd ed. Cambridge University Press, 2017.

4. Goenjian A, Steinberg A, Pynoos R. *Lessons Learned in Disaster Mental Health: The Earthquake in Armenia and Beyond.* Cambridge University Press, 2022.

5. Williams R, Kemp V, Haslam SA, Haslam C, Bhui KS, Bailey S. *Social Scaffolding: Applying the Lessons of Contemporary Social Science to Health and Healthcare.* Cambridge University Press, 2019.

6. Santayana G. *The Life of Reason.* From the series Great Ideas of Western Man. The MIT Press, 1905/2013.

7. Woodson J. *Hertford Consensus.* American College of Surgeons, 2015.

8. Williams R, Bisson JI, Kemp V. Health care planning for community disaster care. In *Textbook of Disaster Psychiatry* 2nd ed. (eds RJ Ursano, CS Fullerton, L Weisaeth, B Raphael): 244–60. Cambridge University Press, 2017.

9. Stevenson D, Farmer P. *Thriving at Work: The Stevenson/Farmer Review of Mental Health and Employers.* Department for Work and Pensions and Department of Health and Social Care, 2017.

10. Murray, E, Kaufman KR, Williams R. Let us do better: learning lessons for recovery of healthcare professionals during and after COVID-19. *BJPsych Open* 2021; 7: e151.

11. Gladwell M. *Outliers: The Story of Success.* Penguin Books, 2009.

12. Zagefka H. The habituation fallacy; disaster victims who are prepeatedly victimised are assumed to suffer less, and they are helped less. *Eur J Soc Psychol* 2022; 52. Available at https://doi.org/10.1002/ejsp.2843

13. Smith EC, Burkle FM. Paramedic and emergency medical technician reflections on the ongoing impact of the 9/11 terrorist attacks. *Prehosp Disaster Med* 2019; 34: 56–61.

14. Brewin CR, DePierro J, Pirard P, Vazquez C, Williams R. Why we need to integrate mental health into pandemic planning. *Perspect Public Health* 2020; 140: 309–10.

15. San Juan NV, Aceituno D, Djellouli N, Sumray K, Regenold N, Syversen A, et al. Mental health and well-being of healthcare workers during the COVID-19 pandemic in the UK: contrasting guidelines with experiences in practice. *BJPsych Open* 2021; 7: e15.

16. Jetten J, Haslam SA, Cruwys T, Greenaway KH, Haslam C, Steffens NK. Advancing the social identity approach to health and

well-being: progressing the social cure research agenda. *Eur J Soc Psychol* 2017; 47: 789–802.

17. Haslam SA, Jetten J, Postmes T, Haslam C. Social identity, health and well-being: an emerging agenda for applied psychology. *Appl Psychol* 2009; 58: 1–23.

18. Haslam C, Jetten J, Cruwys T, Dingle GA, Haslam SA. *The New Psychology of Health: Unlocking The Social Cure*. Routledge, 2018.

19. Stancombe J, Williams R, Drury J, Collins H, Lagan L, Barrett A, et al. People's experiences of distress and psychosocial care following a terrorist attack: interviews with survivors of the Manchester Arena bombing in 2017. *BJPsych Open* 2022; 8: e41.

20. Drury J, Stancombe J, Williams R, Collins H, Lagan L, Barrett A, et al. The role of informal social support in recovery among survivors of the 2017 Manchester Arena bombing. *BJPsych Open* 2022; 8: e124.

21. Stancombe J, Williams R, Drury J, Hussey L, Gittins M, Barrett A, et al. Trajectories of distress and recovery, secondary stressors and social cure processes in people who used the resilience hub after the Manchester Arena bombing. *BJPsych Open* 2023; 9: e143.

22. Ntontis E, Drury J, Amlôt R, Rubin GR, Williams R. Community resilience and flooding in UK guidance: a critical review of concepts, definitions, and their implications. *J Contingencies Crisis Manag* 2019; 27: 2–13.

23. Drury J, Novelli D, Stott C. Representing crowd behaviour in emergency planning guidance: 'mass panic' or collective resilience? *Resilience* 2013; 1: 18–37.

24. Williams R, Drury J. Psychosocial resilience and its influence on managing mass emergencies and disasters. *Psychiatry* 2009; 8: 293–6.

25. Duckers M, van Hoof W, Willems A, Te Brake H. Appraising evidence-based mental health and psychosocial support (MHPSS) guidelines–Part II: a content analysis with implications for disaster risk reduction. *Int J Environ Res Public Health* 2022; 19: 7798.

26. Bleetman A, Sanusi S, Dale T, Brace S. Human factors and error prevention in emergency medicine. *Emerg Med J* 2012; 29: 389–93.

27. Edmondson AC. Managing the risk of learning: psychological safety in work teams. In *International Handbook of Organizational Teamwork and Cooperative Working* (eds MA West, D Tjosvold, KG Smith): 255–75. Wiley, 2003.

28. Morgan MG, Fischhoff B, Bostrom A, Atman CJ. *Risk Communication: A Mental Models Approach*. Cambridge University Press, 2002.

29. Pandemic Influenza Preparedness Team. *Principles of Effective Communication: Scientific Evidence Base Review*. Department of Health, 2011 (assets.publishing.service.gov.uk/government/uploads/system/uploads/attachment_data/file/215678/dh_125431.pdf).

30. Drury J, Carter H, Cocking C, Ntontis E, Tekin Guven S, Amlôt R. Facilitating collective psychosocial resilience in the public in emergencies: twelve recommendations based on the social identity approach. *Front Public Health* 2019; 7: 141.

31. Drury J, Carter H, Ntontis E, Tekin Guven S. Public behaviour in response to the COVID-19 pandemic: understanding the role of group processes. *BJPsych Open* 2021; 7: e11.

32. Chater AM, Whittaker E, Lewis L, Arden MA, Byrne-Davis L, Chadwick P, et al. *Health Psychology, Behavioural Science,*

and Covid-19 Disease Prevention. British Psychological Society, 2021.

33. Byrne-Davis LM, Turner RR, Amatya S, Ashton C, Bull ER, Chater AM, et al. Using behavioural science in public health settings during the COVID-19 pandemic: the experience of public health practitioners and behavioural scientists. *Acta Psychol (Amst)* 2022; 224: 103527.

34. Brooks SK, Dunn R, Amlôt R, Greenberg N, Rubin GJ. Social and occupational factors associated with psychological distress and disorder among disaster responders: a systematic review. *BMC Psychol* 2016; 4: 18.

35. Brooks SK, Rebecca D, Richard A, Greenberg N, James RG. Training and post-disaster interventions for the psychological impacts on disaster-exposed employees: a systematic review. *J Ment Health* 2018; 2018: 1–25.

36. Davidson L, Carter H, Drury J, Amlot R, Haslam SA. Advancing a social identity perspective on interoperability in the emergency services: evidence from the Pandemic Multi-Agency Response Teams during the UK COVID-19 response. *Int J Disaster Risk Reduct* 2022; 77: 103101.

37. Edmondson AC, Harvey J-F. *Extreme Teaming: Lessons in Complex Cross-Sectoral Leadership*. Emerald Publishing, 2017, pp. 110–11.

38. Heginbotham C, Williams R. Achieving service development by implementing strategy. In *Child and Adolescent Mental Health Services* (eds R Williams, M Kerfoot): 63–80. Oxford University Press, 2005.

39. Matthews O. *Overreach: The Inside Story of Putin's War Against Ukraine*. Mudlark, 2022, p. 7.

A Glossary of Selected Key Terms Used in This Book

Burnout
A syndrome conceptualised as resulting from chronic workplace stress that has not been successfully managed. It is characterised by three dimensions: feelings of energy depletion or exhaustion; increased mental distance from one's job or feelings of negativism or cynicism related to one's job; and reduced professional efficacy.

Business continuity incident (NHS England definition)
An event or occurrence that disrupts, or might disrupt, an organisation's normal service delivery to below acceptable pre-defined levels. This would require special arrangements to be put in place until services can return to an acceptable level.

Critical incident
Any localised incident in which the level of disruption results in an organisation temporarily or permanently losing its ability to deliver critical services, or where patients and staff may be at risk of harm. It could also result from the environment potentially being unsafe, requiring special measures and support from other agencies to restore normal operating functions.

Disaster (United Nations Office for Disaster Risk Reduction [UNDRR] definition)
A serious disruption of the functioning of a community or a society at any scale due to hazardous events interacting with conditions of exposure, vulnerability, and capacity, leading to one or more of the following: human, material, economic, and environmental losses and impacts.

The effect of a disaster can be immediate and localised, but is often widespread and could last for a long period of time. The effect may test or exceed the capacity of a community or society to cope using its own resources, and therefore may require assistance from external sources, which could include neighbouring jurisdictions, or those [jurisdictions] at the national or international levels.

Disease outbreak
The sudden occurrence of cases of a disease that has not previously or recently been recorded in a population, or where the disease is usually present but the number of cases normally fluctuates little over time.

See also Epidemic and Pandemic.

Distress
People are likely to feel stressed during and after emergencies, incidents, disasters, and disease outbreaks. Their experiences are described as distress when they are accompanied by emotions, thoughts, and physical sensations that are upsetting or which affect their relationships. Distress is not a diagnosis, but may accompany a disorder.

Recent research shows that common experiences that people describe as distress include feeling very upset, fear, anxiety, fear of recurrence of the event, vigilance at social gatherings and in public places, avoiding uncomfortable feelings, and social withdrawal. The main differences between distress and the symptoms of common mental health disorders lie in the severity and duration of these experiences, and the trajectory of people's recovery. Until recently, the literature has tended to underestimate the number of people who take a longer time to recover from distress.

Emergencies, incidents, terrorist events, disasters, disease outbreaks and conflicts (EITDDC)
This term is used as a collective description of all the kinds of events that are the subject of this book.

See also Emergency, Incident, Disaster, and Disease outbreak.

Emergency
The point at which damage, destruction, casualties, losses of goods and money, and interruptions of human activities occur.

Emotional labour
The suppression of a person's own feelings, while their outward appearance produces in others a sense of being cared for in a safe place. It is a key element in ensuring compassionate care.

Epidemic
The occurrence in a defined region of cases of a disease in the human population in excess of normal expected numbers.

First professional responder
A person with specialised training who is among the first to arrive and provide aid at the scene of an incident or emergency.

First responder
A person with or without specialised training who is among the first to arrive and provide aid at the scene of an incident or emergency. Most first responders are friends, family members, or members of the public, and usually they render invaluable assistance.

Immunisation
The process of getting a vaccine and becoming immune to the disease following vaccination.

See also Vaccination.

Incident

An event that might or does lead to disruption. It is not an emergency of itself, but rather it is an event that might trigger an emergency.

See also Business continuity incident, Critical incident, Major incident.

International Health Regulations (IHR)

An international legal instrument binding on the vast majority of countries in the world, including all of the Member States of the World Health Organization (WHO). It is designed with the aim of 'preventing, protecting against, controlling and providing a public health response to the international spread of disease in ways that are commensurate with and restricted to public health risks and avoid unnecessary interference with international traffic and trade'.

See also World Health Organization (WHO).

International Strategy for Disaster Reduction (ISDR)

A global framework established within the United Nations for the promotion of action to reduce social vulnerability and risks of natural hazards and related technological and environmental disasters.

Isolation

The separation of a person or persons suffering from a communicable disease from people who are healthy.

Major incident

Any occurrence that presents a serious threat to the health of the community, or that causes such numbers or types of casualties as to require special arrangements to be implemented. For the NHS, this includes any event defined as an emergency under the Civil Contingencies Act 2004 as amended.

Mental healthcare

Formal biomedical and psychological treatments for mental health disorders, which are delivered by trained mental health practitioners. Psychosocial care is often required at the same time, as a platform for these specialised treatments.

Mental health disorder

Also termed mental illness. A disorder that is characterised by a clinically significant disturbance in a person's cognition, emotional regulation, or behaviour, or a combination of these. The symptoms and signs should meet the criteria of an international classification (e.g., ICD-11 or DSM-5). It is usually associated with distress or impairment in important areas of functioning in social, work, or family activities. There are many different types of mental health disorders, and examples include depression, anxiety disorders, schizophrenia, eating disorders, and addictions. The term mental health condition is broader and covers mental health disorders, psychosocial impairments, and other mental states associated with significant distress, impairment in functioning, or risk of self-harm.

Moral distress

The emotional state that occurs when staff are unable to deliver the level of care that they would like to provide, due to organisational constraints. For example, failures in leadership, and the types of injury or illness treated in pre-hospital settings, hospitals, and communities, are linked to psychosocial distress in healthcare practitioners. Moral distress arises because the aspirations of staff to deliver high-quality care are not realised due to limitations in the quality of care that services are able or willing to support.

Moral injury

The psychological consequences of bearing witness to violence and human carnage and their aftermath.

It encompasses witnessing human suffering or failing to prevent outcomes that transgress deeply held beliefs, such as the rights of children to be protected by their parents, or the belief that life can and should be preserved by appropriate and timely medical interventions. It also recognises failings in leadership, where staff are not appropriately resourced, whether in terms of people, space, or equipment.

Needs

People's requirements for assistance because of their exposure to an emergency or incident.

See also Responses.

Pandemic

An epidemic that occurs worldwide, or over a very wide area, crossing international boundaries and usually affecting many people.

Post-traumatic growth

Positive psychological change experienced because of a person's struggle with challenging life circumstances. This can lead to them revising and developing new psychological and philosophical beliefs. It can stimulate growth across three domains – self-perception, interpersonal relationships, and their philosophy of life.

Post-traumatic stress disorder (PTSD)

A disorder that can develop after a major incident or other stressful event or situation of an exceptionally threatening or catastrophic nature. It may affect up to 25% of people of any age who have experienced an event of this nature. Symptoms include:

- re-experiencing (including nightmares)
- avoidance
- hyperarousal (including hypervigilance, anger, and irritability)
- negative alterations in mood and thinking
- emotional numbing
- dissociation
- emotional dysregulation
- interpersonal difficulties or problems in relationships
- negative self-perception (including feeling diminished, defeated, or worthless).

Primary stressors

The sources of worry, anxiety, and stress that stem directly from the events and consequential tasks that people, including survivors and the staff of services, face during their work. Primary stressors are inherent in EITDDC.

Psychological safety

One component of organisational and team culture.

In psychologically safe environments, people believe that others will not resent or penalise them for asking for help, information, or feedback. Psychological safety avoids blame, belittling, and undermining, and emphasises constructive learning that has substantial effects on the wellbeing of staff.

Psychosocial

Relating to the emotional, cognitive, social, and physical experiences of people in the context of their environments. This adjective describes the interactions between psychological and social processes within and between people and across groups of people.

Psychosocial care

Interventions for people who are distressed or struggling, whether or not their distress is accompanied by thoughts and feelings that interfere with their day-to-day functioning, and if they have symptoms of a mental health problem that do not reach a diagnosis.

Public Health Emergency of International Concern (PHEIC)

Defined by the WHO as 'an extraordinary event which is determined to constitute a public health risk to other States through the international spread of disease and to potentially require a coordinated international response', formulated when a situation arises that is 'serious, sudden, unusual or unexpected', which 'carries implications for public health beyond the affected state's national border' and 'may require immediate international action'. Under the International Health Regulations 2005 (IHR), states have a legal duty to respond promptly to a PHEIC.

Quarantine

Restriction of the movement of well people who may have been exposed to a disease, in order to prevent the spread of the disease to healthy people.

Responses

The ways in which societies, communities, relatives, formal services, and practitioners act to meet the needs of people and communities during and after EITDDC.

See also Needs.

Secondary stressors

Circumstances, events, or policies that are not inherent in events. Secondary stressors are (1) social factors and people's life circumstances (including policies, practices, and social, organisational, and financial arrangements) that exist prior to and impact people during an emergency or major incident, and/or (2) societal and organisational responses to an incident or emergency. Often secondary stressors are as impactful as, and in some circumstances they are more stressful than, the primary stressors.

Stress

A term that is used widely and often inconsistently; sometimes it refers to a stimulus, which is more appropriately described as a stressor, and sometimes it refers to people's responses. In this book, the term stress describes a collection of common human psychological, physical, and behavioural responses to external and internal challenges. Stress can be positive when it motivates people, but is a problem when the level of stress that people experience is overwhelming and unpleasant. The experiences are then described as distress. Most people experience stress in EITDDC because these events may

undermine their positive perceptions of the environment, themselves, their sense of control, and their feelings of worth.

Stressor

An event, circumstance, other occurrence, attitude, response, or something else that stimulates people to experience a stress response, or which causes a state of strain or tension.

Triage

The process of sorting patients, especially battle and disaster survivors, and allocating treatment priorities to them according to a system designed to maximise the number of survivors.

United Nations High Commissioner for Refugees (UNHCR)

The UN Refugee Agency, which has a mandate to protect and aid refugees, forcibly displaced persons, and stateless people, and to assist in their voluntary repatriation, local integration, or resettlement to a third country.

United Nations Office for the Coordination of Humanitarian Affairs (UNOCHA)

A UN agency that contributes to principled and effective humanitarian responses through coordination, advocacy, policy, information management, and humanitarian financing tools and services. It coordinates humanitarian responses to expand the reach of humanitarian action, improve prioritisation, and reduce duplication, ensuring that assistance and protection reach the people who need them most.

United Nations Office for Disaster Risk Reduction (UNDRR)

The UN agency with the mandate to ensure the implementation of the International Strategy for Disaster Reduction.

Vaccination

The process of getting a vaccine – for example, either by getting the injection or by taking an oral vaccine dose.

See also Immunisation.

Validation

People who are affected by emergencies and incidents regard social and professional acknowledgement of their experiences as key to their psychological recovery.
It emphasises the importance of ensuring that opportunities are created for other people, whose opinions are respected, to recognise and acknowledge the experiences of, for example, Blue Light staff.

Wellbeing

The ability of people to continue to develop, to enjoy the stimulation of their relationships and work, and to flourish. The term is used in this book in relation to everyone's needs for certain sources of support to ensure their wellbeing.

World Health Organization (WHO)

The directing and coordinating authority for health within the UN system. It is responsible for providing leadership on global health matters, shaping the health research agenda, setting norms and standards, articulating evidence-based policy options, providing technical support to countries, and monitoring and assessing health trends.

Index

Printed in the United States
by Baker & Taylor Publisher Services